AF515773

Atlas of

Magnetic Resonance Imaging

Atlas of Magnetic Resonance Imaging

Editors

Hariqbal Singh MD DMRD
Professor and Head
Department of Radiology
Smt Kashibai Navale Medical College and General Hospital
Pune, Maharashtra, India

Vikash Ojha MD
Consultant
Department of Radiology
Apollo Jehangir Hospital
Pune, Maharashtra, India

Santosh Konde MD
Associate Professor
Department of Radiology
Smt Kashibai Navale Medical College and General Hospital
Pune, Maharashtra, India

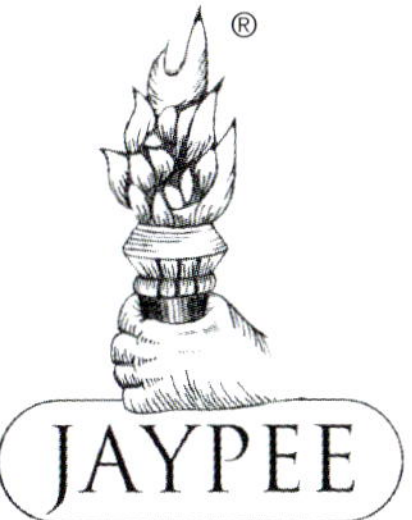

JAYPEE BROTHERS MEDICAL PUBLISHERS (P) LTD

New Delhi • London • Philadelphia • Panama

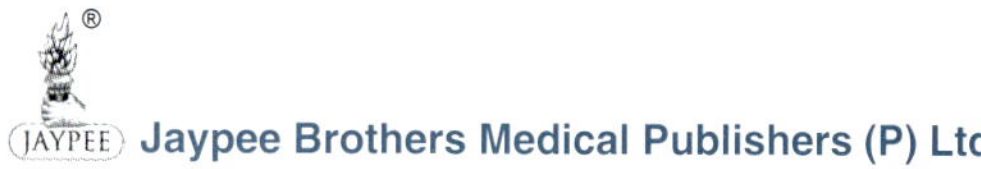

Jaypee Brothers Medical Publishers (P) Ltd.

Headquarters
Jaypee Brothers Medical Publishers (P) Ltd.
4838/24, Ansari Road, Daryaganj
New Delhi 110 002, India
Phone: +91-11-43574357
Fax: +91-11-43574314
Email: jaypee@jaypeebrothers.com

Overseas Offices

J.P. Medical Ltd.
83, Victoria Street, London
SW1H 0HW (UK)
Phone: +44-2031708910
Fax: +02-03-0086180
Email: info@jpmedpub.com

Jaypee-Highlights Medical Publishers Inc.
City of Knowledge, Bld. 237, Clayton
Panama City, Panama
Phone: +1 507-301-0496
Fax: +1 507-301-0499
Email: cservice@jphmedical.com

Jaypee Medical Inc.
The Bourse
111, South Independence Mall East
Suite 835, Philadelphia, PA 19106, USA
Phone: +1 267-519-9789
Email: jpmed.us@gmail.com

Jaypee Brothers Medical Publishers (P) Ltd.
17/1-B, Babar Road, Block-B, Shaymali
Mohammadpur, Dhaka-1207
Bangladesh
Mobile: +08801912003485
Email: jaypeedhaka@gmail.com

Jaypee Brothers Medical Publishers (P) Ltd.
Bhotahity, Kathmandu, Nepal
Phone: +977-9741283608
Email: kathmandu@jaypeebrothers.com

Website: www.jaypeebrothers.com
Website: www.jaypeedigital.com

Inquiries for bulk sales may be solicited at: jaypee@jaypeebrothers.com

Atlas of Magnetic Resonance Imaging

First Edition: 2014

ISBN 978-93-5152-176-1

Printed at Replika Press Pvt. Ltd.

Dedicated to

Our dear wives

Arvind Babbal Hariqbal

Hariqbal Singh

Samta Singhania Ojha

Vikash Ojha

Leena Santosh Konde

Santosh Konde

Radiology is a kindergarten
of logical rational coherent exploration and
balanced learning
and not
dexterous adroit smugness
or learning egotism
cultivated by fake self-centeredness and egoism.

Hariqbal Singh

Contributors

Abhijit Pawar DNB (Radiology)
Assistant Professor
Smt Kashibai Navale Medical
College and General Hospital
Pune, Maharashtra, India

Aditi Dongre MD (Radiology)
Assistant Professor
Smt Kashibai Navale Medical College
and General Hospital
Pune, Maharashtra, India

Amol Sasane MD (Radiology)
Assistant Professor
Smt Kashibai Navale Medical
College and General Hospital
Pune, Maharashtra, India

Hariqbal Singh MD DMRD
Professor and Head
Department of Radiology
Smt Kashibai Navale Medical
College and General Hospital
Pune, Maharashtra, India

Manisha Hadgaonkar DNB (Radiology)
Assistant Professor
Smt Kashibai Navale Medical
College and General Hospital
Pune, Maharashtra, India

Parvez Sheik MD DMRE
Consultant
Department of Radiology
Smt Kashibai Navale Medical
College and General Hospital
Pune, Maharashtra, India

Santosh Konde MD
Associate Professor
Department of Radiology
Smt Kashibai Navale Medical
College and General Hospital
Pune, Maharashtra, India

Sikandar Sheikh MD DMR
Consultant
Department of Radiology
and PET-CT
Apollo Health City
Hyderabad, Andhra Pradesh, India

Subodh Laul DNB
Consultant
Department of Radiology
Smt Kashibai Navale
Medical College and General Hospital
Pune, Maharashtra, India

Varsha Rangankar MD (Radiology)
Associate Professor
Smt Kashibai Navale Medical College
and General Hospital
Pune, Maharashtra, India

Vikash Ojha MD
Consultant
Department of Radiology
Apollo Jehangir Hospital
Pune, Maharashtra, India

Preface

The advent of MR has revolutionized the field of medicine. This book provides a large bank of MR images. The importance of having a good knowledge of anatomy cannot be undermined. It has led us to include normal anatomy and a good range of MR imaging solutions routinely required. With these images in mind, it will help the residents, radiologists and practitioners to interpret the possible diagnosis during their routine practice. The intent has been to provide in-depth useful information material accounting for most of what is seen in clinical practice. It will be an ideal reference for anyone involved with MR image interpretation. The book, *Atlas of Magnetic Resonance Imaging* also includes a chapter on Assessment to make it more interest generating and gives the reader self-assessment to certain extend.

This book is meant for radiology residents, radiologists, general practitioners, other specialists, MR technical staff and those who have a special interest in MR imaging. It is meant for medical college and institutional libraries, departmental and MR stand-alone unit libraries.

Hariqbal Singh
Vikash Ojha
Santosh Konde

Acknowledgments

We thank Prof MN Navale, Founder President, Sinhgad Technical Education Society, Pune, Maharashtra, India, and Dr Arvind V Bhore, Dean, Smt Kashibai Navale Medical College and General Hospital, Pune, Maharashtra, India, for their kind acquiescence in this endeavor.

We profusely extend our gratefulness to the consultants Amit Ghawate, Yasmeen Khan, Shrikant Nagare, Anjali Sawant, Poonam Tambare, Swati Shah, Vikram Shende and Jarvis Pereira for their genuine help in building up this educational entity.

Our gratitude to Anna Bansode and Sachin Babar for their clerical help.

We are thankful to Musmade Bala, More Rahul, Demello Thomas, Gangoor Raghvendra, Shankar Gopale and Manjusha Chikhale for the plenteous help in data retrieval.

We express our thanks to the entire staff of M/s Jaypee Brothers Medical Publishers (P) Ltd., New Delhi, India, for their commitment to create highest standard of quality and state-of-the-art presentation with their excellence in publishing.

We are grateful to God Almighty and mankind who have allowed us to have this wonderful experience.

Contents

Introduction

Magnetic resonance imaging (MRI) is the most important diagnostic imaging discovery in medicine since the discovery of X-ray in 1895 by Wilhelm Conrad Röntgen (also spelt as Roentgen). The first MRI was commercially available in 1980. Since then, its importance in the field of medicine continues to grow at a tremendous pace and is now established beyond doubt. Before beginning a study, it is important to know a brief history of MRI.

Sir Joseph Larmor (1857-1942) developed the equation that the angular frequency of precession of the nuclear spins being proportional to the strength of the magnetic field referred as Larmor relationship. In the 1930s, Isidor Isaac Rabi of Columbia University succeeded in detecting and measuring single states of rotation of atoms and molecules, and in determining the magnetic and mechanical moments of the nuclei.

Working independently, Felix Bloch of Stanford University and Edward Purcell of Harvard University made the first successful nuclear magnetic resonance experiment to study chemical compounds in 1946, thus magnetic resonance phenomenon was discovered. They developed instruments, which could measure the magnetic resonance in bulk material such as liquids and solids. In 1946, they came up with the idea to use magnets to take pictures of a living being and called it magnetic resonance. Both Felix Bloch and Edward Purcell were awarded the Nobel Prize in 1952.

In 1971, Raymond Damadian, a physician and scientist of State University of New York, demonstrated that there are different T1 relaxation times between normal and abnormal tissues of the same type, as well as between different types of normal tissues on Nuclear Magnetic Resonance (NMR) device. In the same year, he proved that magnetic resonance could be used to help detect diseases by the different nuclear magnetic relaxation times between tissues and tumors thus motivating scientists to consider magnetic resonance for the detection of disease.

In 1973, Paul Christian Lauterbur (6 May 1929 – 27 March 2007) of State University of New York described a new imaging technique that he termed Zeugmatography. By utilizing gradients in the magnetic field, this technique was able to produce a two-dimensional image. Magnetic resonance imaging was first demonstrated on small test tube samples. He used a back projection technique similar to that used in CT.

In 1975, Richard Ernst introduced two-dimensional NMR using phase and frequency encoding, and Fourier transformier instead of Paul Lauterbur's back-projection, he timely switched magnetic field gradients. This basic reconstruction method is the basis of current MRI techniques.

On 3 July 1977, the first MRI body examination was performed through a finger of a human being, this was a cross-sectional image. It took almost five hours to produce one image. This machine was named by Raymond Damadien as "Indomitable". This machine is now in the Smithsonian Institution. Indomitable represents a milestone in the history of medical imaging (Fig. 1). Its story is a timeless one of a driven inventor who perseveres through every obstacle only to find that others are racing along similar paths, which in this case led to today's ubiquitous MRI machines.

Peter Mansfield further developed the utilization of gradients in the magnetic field and the mathematical analysis of these signals for a more useful imaging technique. In 1977, the first images taken of a cross section through a finger were presented by Peter Mansfield and Andrew Maudsley. Peter Mansfield also could present the first image through the abdomen. In the same year, Peter Mansfield developed the echo planar imaging (EPI) technique. This technique developed in later years to produce images at video rates (30 ms/image). Paul Lauterbur and Peter Mansfield were awarded the Nobel Prize in Medicine in 2003.

Raymond Damadien in 1978 founded the FONAR Corporation, which manufactured the first commercial MRI scanner in 1980. As late as 1982, there were a handful of MRI scanners in the world. Today, there are a million or even more MR scanners world over, and images can be created in seconds what used to take hours. Current MRI scanners produce highly detailed two-dimensional and three-dimensional images. The technique was initially called nuclear magnetic resonance imaging (NMR or NMRI) but because of the negative connotations associated with the word nuclear it is called magnetic resonance imaging.

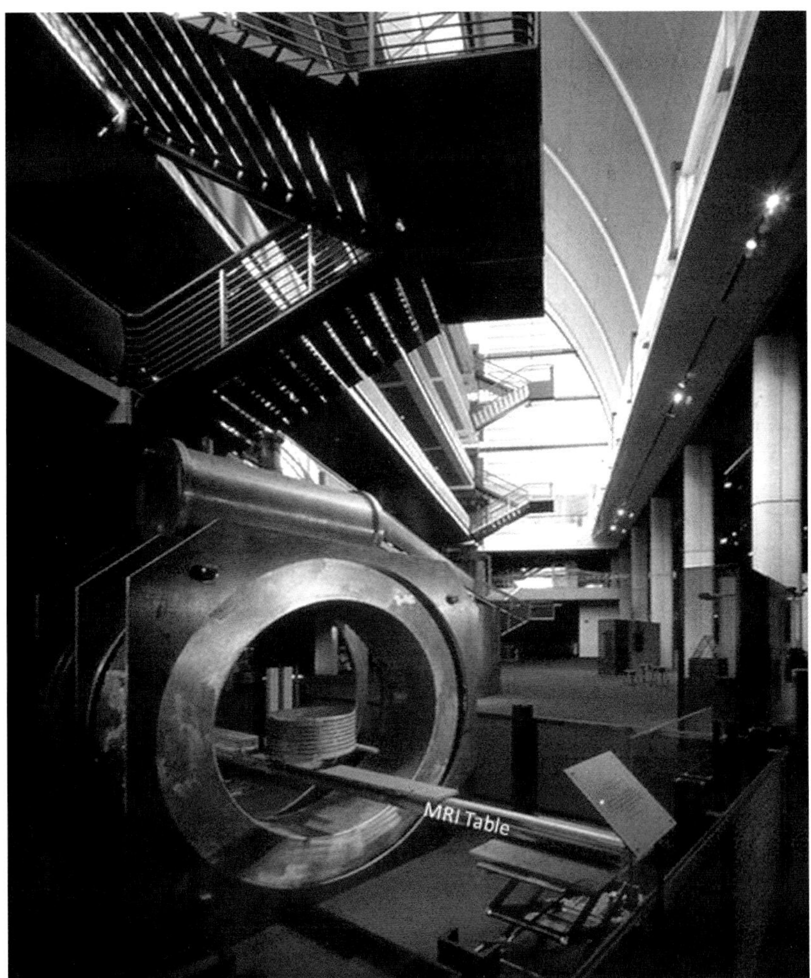

Fig. 1: "Indomitable" the first MRI machine invented by Raymond Damadian (*Source:* Jeff Goldberg/Esto)

PLATE 1

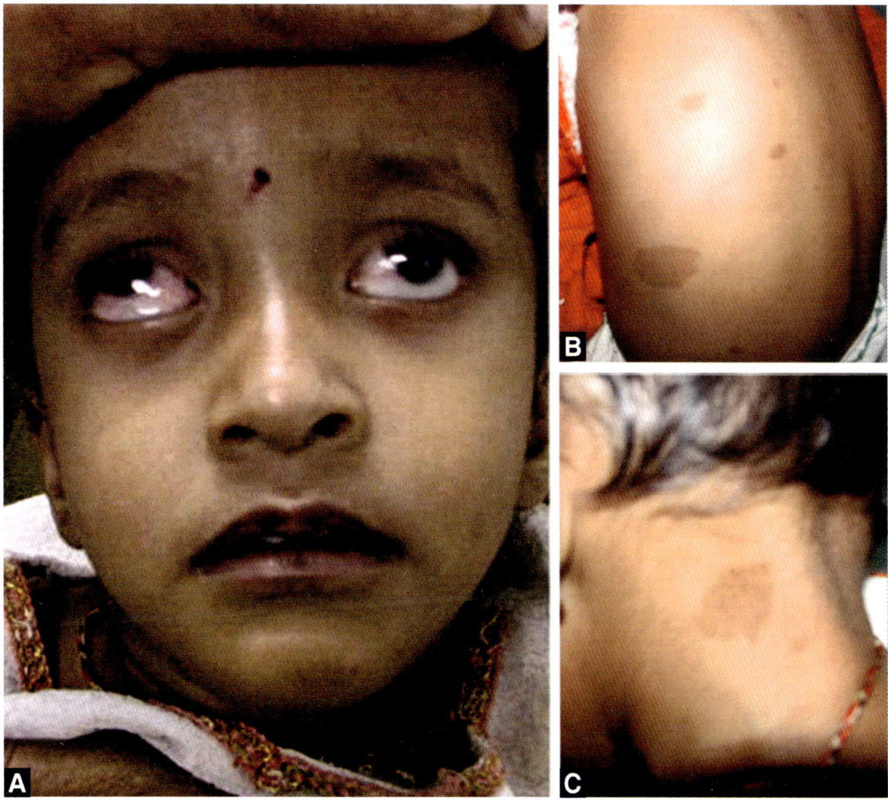

Figs 33A to C: Photographs of patient showing squint (A) and café-au-lait spots (B and C)

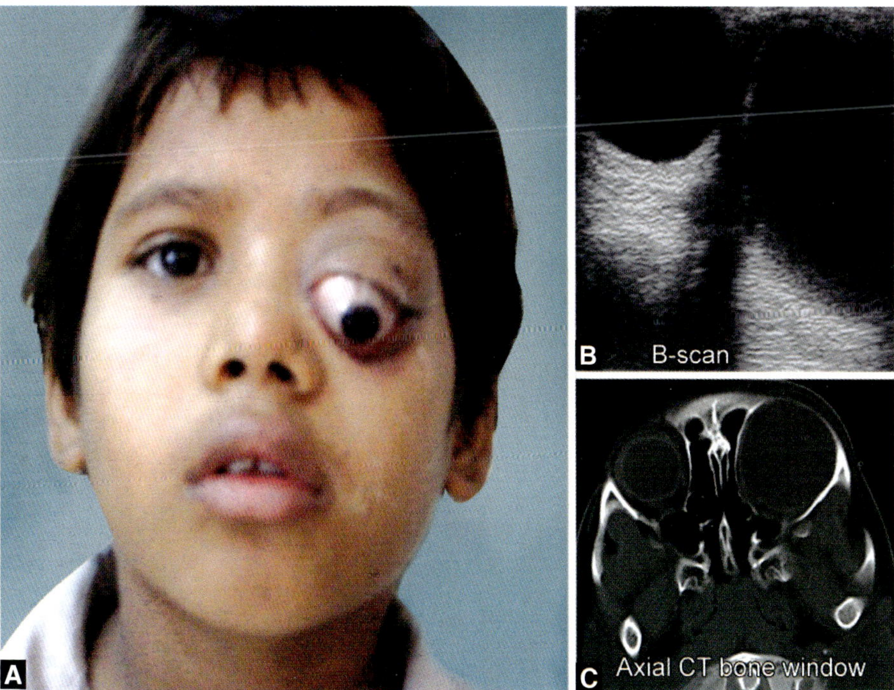

Figs 5A to C: (A) Photograph of the patient with proptosis of the eyeball downwards and medially; (B) B-scan image of left eyes show large cystic lesion in left orbit; (C) Orbital CT shows a large cystic lesion in left orbit causing expansion and scalloping of adjacent bones

PLATE 2

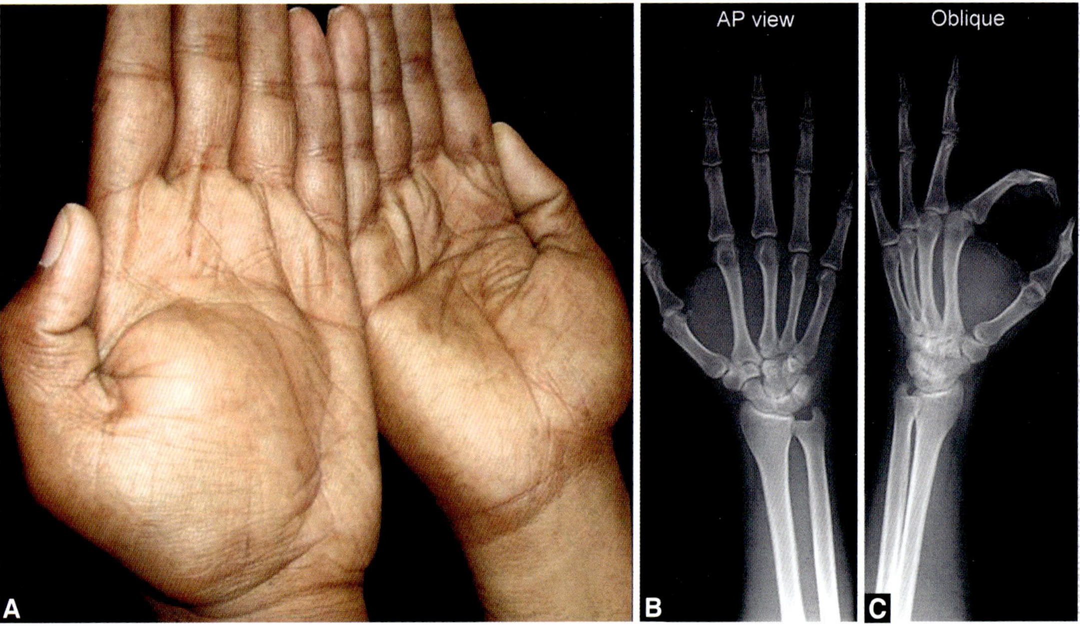

Figs 128A to C: 24-year-old male presented swelling of the left thenar eminence with pain on and off since 8 years, gradually increasing in size. Photograph of hands (A) X-ray AP and lateral views (B and C) of left hand shows soft tissue swelling in the region of thenar eminence

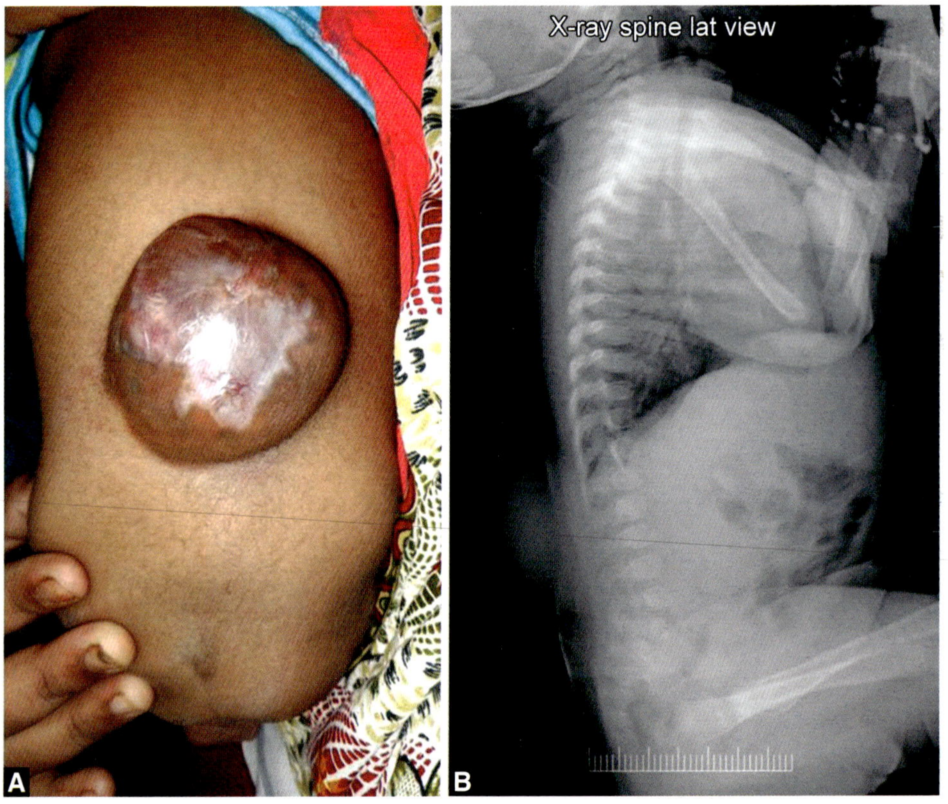

Figs 17A and B

Physical Principle of Magnetic Resonance Imaging

1

Parvez Sheik

Magnetic resonance imaging (MRI) is based on the principle of electromagnetic character of atomic nuclei which was first described by physicist Felix Bloch and Edward Purcell in 1946. They received a Nobel Prize for this in 1952. However, it was long after this that nuclear magnetic resonance was used for imaging. In 1973, Lauterbur showed that images of human body could be acquired by placing a magnetic field around it. First human images were published by Damadian et al in 1977. Since then use of MRI for medical imaging has seen an exponential growth and now it is a mainstay in the field of medical diagnostics.

Electromagnetism is at the core of MRI physics. When current is passed through a wire, a magnetic field is created around it. Similarly, in a nucleus with odd number of protons or neutrons, the electrons rotating around the nucleus produce a field around them. This gives a "charge" to the nucleus, also called as the spinning charge or "the spin". Thus these nuclei behave as tiny magnets. Hydrogen proton is the most favorable nucleus for MRI as it is widely available in the water molecules present in the body.

When these nuclei are placed in an external magnetic field (B_0), they either align along the magnetic field or against it. When the number of nuclei along the magnetic field is more as compared to those against the field, a net magnetization is created in the direction of the field.

In order to generate a signal from these spinning nuclei they have to be tipped out of alignment with B_0 (i.e. out of the longitudinal plane and towards the transverse plane). The signal generated by each rotating nucleus is much stronger if the nuclei precess in unison with each other at 90° to the main magnetic field. For this a second magnetic field is introduced and it is referred to as B_1. This B_1 should be applied perpendicular to B_0, and it has to be at the resonant frequency. Radiofrequency (RF) coils are used to transmit B_1. If sufficient RF pulse is applied the spins are flipped into the transverse plane. This is the 90° RF pulse and it generates the strongest signal. However, as this is a high energy state, the signal starts decaying quickly and is called free induction decay (FID). This decay or relaxation is of two types:

T1 relaxation is the relaxation in the longitudinal plane due to the spins returning to the normal equilibrium state and aligning with the main magnetic field. In T2 relaxation there is dephasing in the transverse plane (90° plane), each individual at slightly different speed. After a while, the signal from protons in transverse plane degenerates as protons start precessing out of phase with each other. This is T2 relaxation.

In human tissue T1 is usually 10 times longer than T2 which means that T2 decay occurs before T1 recovery. In actual practice the T2 dephasing time is much quicker than the 'natural' T2 due to inhomogenities in the magnetic field B_0. This reduced T2 is called T2*. T2* is decay of transverse magnetization because of spin-spin relaxation and inhomogeneity of the magnetic field. In GRE T2* sequence is the main determinants of image contrast and forms the basis of MR applications including perfusion imaging, and functional imaging and susceptibility-weighted imaging. A low flip angle, long echo time and long repetition time can make the GRE sequence T2*. Bleed, calcium and iron deposition in various tissues can be depicted on GRE with T2*.

Susceptibility-weighted imaging uses phase information in addition to T2* to develop the magnetic susceptibility differences of the blood, iron, and calcium in various tissues.

Perfusion MR imaging exploits the signal intensity decrease that occurs with the passage of high concentration of gadopentetate dimeglumine through the microvasculature. Change in oxygen saturation during specific tasks changes the local T2* which leads to the blood oxygen level dependent effect seen at functional MR imaging.

T1W and T2W images result by manipulating the manner and frequency in which RF pulses are applied (Repetition to Time), and by changing time to start signal acquisition after RF has been applied (Time to Echo), T1-weighted or T2-weighted images can be obtained (Tables 1 and 2).

Pulse sequences: (1) Partial saturation (PS)—It is also known as gradient echo or field echo and it uses a 90° RF pulse. (2) Spin echo (SE)—A 90° pulse is followed by 180° refocusing RF pulse. (3) Inversion recovery (IR)—180° pulse is followed by a 90° pulse.

In a typical image acquisition, the basic unit of each sequence (i.e. the 90°-180° signal detection) is repeated hundreds of times. By altering the time to echo (TE) or time to repetition (TR), i.e. the time between successive 90° pulses, the signal contrast can be altered or weighted. For example, if a long TE is used, inherent differences in T2 times of tissues will become apparent. Tissues with a long T2 (e.g. water) will take longer to decay and their signal will be greater (or appear brighter in the image) than the signal from tissue with a short T2 (e.g. fat). In a similar manner TR governs T1 contrast. Tissue, with a long TR (water) will take a long time to recover back to the equilibrium magnetization value, therefore, a short TR interval will make this tissue appear dark compared to tissue with a short T1 (fat). When TE and TR are chosen to minimize both these weightings, the signal contrast is only derived from the number or density of spins in a given tissue. This image is said to be proton density weighted (PDW).

Air is black in all sequences because of very few protons and cortical bone is always black due to no mobility of protons.

Each volume element in the body has a different resonant frequency which depends on the protons present within it. This produces a signal which is specific to the resonant frequency of that volume element. This signal is analyzed by the computers using a mathematical technique called as Fourier analysis.

Magnet forms the main component of the MRI, it is of two types: (1) Permanent or resistive magnets used in low field scanners and are usually referred to as open MRI, (2) Superconducting magnet are used in all scanners above 1.0 Tesla. It is wound from an alloy (usually Nb-Ti) that has zero electrical resistance below a critical temperature. To maintain this temperature the magnet is enclosed and cooled by a cryogen containing liquid helium which has to be topped-up on a regular basis.

RF coils are needed to transmit and/or receive the MR signal. The RF coil should cover only the volume of interest. This gives an optimal signal-to-noise ratio (SNR). To achieve this there are various types of RF coils with trade-offs in terms of coverage and sensitivity, e.g. head coil being smaller in size provides better SNR. Body coil is integrated into the scanner bore and is not seen by the patient. Both these coils act as transceivers, i.e. they transmit and receive. Surface coils are used for imaging anatomy near to the coil. They are simple loop designs and have excellent SNR close to the coil but the sensitivity drops off rapidly with distance from the coil. These are only used as receivers, the body coil acting as the transmitter. Quadrature or circularly-polarized coils comprise of two coils 90° apart to improve SNR by a factor of 2½.

Table 1: Time to echo and time to repetition for MR sequences

	Time to Echo (TE)	*Time to Repetition (TR)*
T1 weighted (T1W)	Short TE	Short TR
T2 weighted (T2W)	Long TE	Long TR
Proton density weighted (PDW)	Short TE	Long TR

Table 2: Signal intensity of various tissues at T1, T2 and proton density imaging

Tissue	*T1*	*T2*	*Proton density*
Fat	Bright	Bright (less than T1)	Bright
Water	Dark	Bright	Intermediate bright
Cerebral gray matter	Gray	Gray	Gray
Cerebral white matter	White	Dark	Dark
TR values	TR < 500	TR > 1500	TR > 1500
TE values	TE 50–100	TE > 80	TE < 50

Advanced applications include diffusion imaging, perfusion imaging, functional MRI, spectroscopy, interventional MRI.

Possible adverse effects of MRI can be due to static magnetic field, gradients, RF heating, noise and claustrophobia.

Caution needs to be exercised while selecting patients for MRI. Patients with pacemakers, metallic implants, aneurysm clips should be excluded. Metallic objects should not be taken near the magnet as they can be injurious to the patient, personnel and equipment.

SPECIAL SEQUENCES

Short Tau Inversion Recovery (STIR) Sequence

It is heavily T2 weighted imaging, as a result the fluid and edema return high signal intensity and it annuls out the signal from fat. The resultant images show the areas of pathology clearly. The sequence is useful in musculoskeletal imaging as it annuls the signal from normal fatty bone marrow.

Fluid Attenuated Inversion Recovery (FLAIR)

This is an inversion-recovery pulse sequence that suppresses or annuls out the signal from fluid/CSF. The sequence is useful to show subtle lesions in the brain and spinal cord as it annuls the signal from CSF. It is useful to bring out the periventricular hyperintense lesions, e.g. in multiple sclerosis.

Gradient Echo Sequence

This sequence reduces the scan times. This is achieved by giving a shorter RF pulse leading to a lesser amount of disruption to the magnetic vectors. The sequence is useful in identifying calcification and blood degradation products.

Diffusion-weighted Imaging

'Diffusion' portrays the movement of molecules due to random motion. It enables to distinguish between rapid diffusion of protons (unrestricted diffusion) and slow diffusion of protons (restricted diffusion). GRE pulse sequence has been devised to image the diffusion of water through tissues. It is a sensitive way of detecting acute brain infarcts, where diffusion is reduced or restricted.

MR Angiography

The most common MR angiographic techniques are time-of-flight imaging and phase contrast. In these sequences, multiple RF pulses are applied with short TRs which saturate the spins in stationary tissues. This results in suppression of the signal from stationary tissues in the imaging slab. In-flowing blood is unaffected by the repetitive RF pulses, as a result, as it enters the imaging slab, its signal is not suppressed and appears hyperintense compared with that of stationary tissue. Time-of-flight imaging may be 2D, with section-by-section acquisition, or 3D, with acquisition of a larger volume. Dynamic MRA can also be performed with intravenous gadolinium when in the vascular phase of enhancement.

Brain 2

Hariqbal Singh, Vikash Ojha

ANATOMY OF BRAIN

The human brain is most complex organ in the body. It develops from the neural tube, undergoes complex divisions (Flow chart 1) to form the forebrain (prosencephalon), midbrain (mesencephalon) and hindbrain (rhombencephalon) (Figs 1A to P).

The forebrain or prosencephalon consists of

- The telencephalon which comprises of the cerebral cortex, basal ganglion, corpus striatum and olfactory bulb
- The diencephalon, which is made up of the thalamus, subthalamus, hypothalamus epithalamus and metathalamus.

Cerebral hemispheres are on either side of the cranial cavity above the tentorium cerebelli. On MRI, the axial, coronal and sagittal sections provide excellent view of the various cerebral lobes and their pathology. The cerebral hemisphere is separated from each other in midline by the interhemispheric fissure. The interhemispheric fissure extends from the floor of anterior cranial fossa to the posterior cranial cavity. In the middle part of the interhemispheric fissure lies

Flow chart 1: Brain structure and their divisions

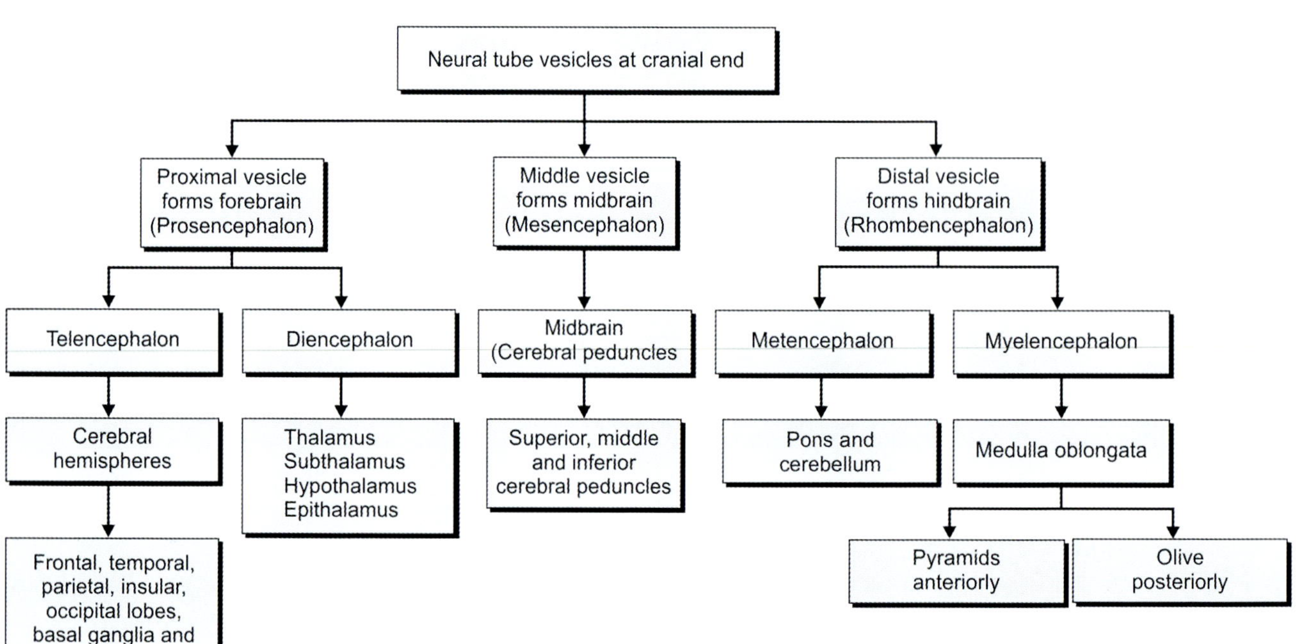

the corpus callosum which connects the two cerebral hemispheres in midline.

The gray matter and white matter are appreciated on axial, coronal and sagittal T1W images. The gray matter on cerebral hemispheres is located on the outer aspect while the white matter also called as centrum semiovale is located deep in cerebral hemispheres. Some white matter extends from centrum semiovale into the cortical gyri; these are called subcortical white matter. The cortical gyri are separated from each other by cleft like involutions known as cortical sulci.

The cortical sulci help in subdividing the cerebral hemispheres for descriptive purposes into:

- *Frontal lobe* (Figs 1L to O, 2C, and 3A and B) is the anterior part of cerebral hemisphere, it is limited posteriorly by the central sulcus (of Rolando) and inferiorly by the Sylvian fissure. The frontal lobe has prominent gyri like the superior frontal gyrus, medial frontal gyrus and lateral frontal gyrus appreciated on T1W sagittal and coronal sections.
- *Parietal lobe* (Figs 1L to P) lies posterior to the central sulcus (of Rolando) and extends up to the parieto-occipital sulcus beyond which the occipital lobe begins. The inferior border of parietal lobe is related to the Sylvian fissure.
- *Insular region* (central lobe) (Figs 1L, 2F and 3I) is a submerged area of cortical tissue in the posterior ramus of the Sylvian fissure (lateral sulcus). The insular region is appreciated on axial, coronal and sagittal sections on T1W and T2W images. The insular region receives contributions from the temporal, frontal, and parietal lobes. The insular region is surrounded by the circular sulcus (of Rolando). The insular region is supplied by branches from the middle cerebral artery. Middle cerebral artery infarcts characteristically reveal a hyperdense thrombus on axial T1W images in insular region (known as the "Insular ribbon sign").
- *Temporal lobe* (Figs 1E to I) is located below the sylvian fissure. It is visualized on T1W images in axial, coronal and sagittal sections. It has superior, middle and lower temporal gyri. The temporo-occipital gyrus is seen posterior aspect of temporal lobe. The hippocampal gyrus is seen on sagittal T1W sections. The upper part of the superior temporal gyrus contains the transverse temporal gyri of Heschl—the main auditory areas, Brodmann areas 41, 42. Lesions in the auditory areas usually do not lead to complete deafness because each auditory area receives auditory impulses from both the ears-each lateral lemniscus in the brainstem contains fibers derived from both the cochlear nuclei.
- *Occipital lobe* (Figs 1F, G, M and O) is located at the posterior aspect of cerebral hemisphere; it is limited anteriorly by the parieto-occipital sulcus. It is well visualized on T1W images in axial, coronal and sagittal sections. The tentorium cerebelli on its inferior aspect separates the occipital lobe from cerebellar hemispheres.

Basal ganglia are central gray matter nuclei in each cerebral hemisphere and consist of the caudate nucleus, lentiform nucleus, claustrum and amygdala. The basal ganglia are seen on T1W and T2W images in axial, sagittal and coronal sections. Corpus striatum is a collective term for the caudate nucleus and lentiform nucleus. The anterior and posterior limbs of internal capsule lie between the basal ganglia and thalamus.

The basal ganglia is subdivided for descriptive purposes into:

- *Caudate nucleus* (Figs 1K, 2F, G and 3G) has a head, body and tail. The head and body of caudate nucleus is seen on T1W axial, coronal and sagittal sections. The head of caudate nucleus abuts the frontal horn of lateral ventricle. The body of caudate nucleus lies along the periventricular region of lateral ventricles. The tail of caudate nucleus is seen on T1W sagittal and coronal images. The tail of caudate nucleus is narrow; it is superolateral to the thalamus.
- *Lentiform nucleus* (Figs 1K and 2G) appears as a wedge shaped nucleus. It is located lateral to the caudate nucleus and thalamus on T1W images in axial and coronal MRI sections. The lentiform nucleus is separated from the caudate nucleus by the anterior limb of internal capsule.

  The posterior limb of internal capsule separates the lentiform nucleus from thalamus. The lentiform nucleus has two components, an outer putamen and an inner globus pallidus. The sublentiform part of the internal capsule passes under the lentiform nucleus to the auditory cortex. The main afferent fibers come from the cortex, substantia nigra and thalamus. Fibers from the putamen mostly end in the globus pallidus. Efferent fibers from globus pallidus reach thalamus, subthalamic nuclei, hypothalamus, red nucleus, substantia nigra and reticular formation. The final outflow tracts reach the spinal cord via the rubrospinal and rubro-reticulospinal tracts. Lesions of the basal ganglia lead to extra-pyramidal effects such as dyskinesias, rigidity and tremor.

- *Claustrum* (Fig. 3I) is a thin strip of saucer-shaped nucleus which is located lateral to the putamen. It is easily seen on axial and coronal section in T1W images.
- *Amygdala* is located in the roof of the temporal horn of lateral ventricle. It contains nuclei which are connected to the tail of caudate nucleus and the limbic system. Stria terminalis is the efferent connection of amygdala connecting the amygdala to the anterior hypothalamus.
- *Internal capsule* (Figs 1L, 3G and H) is seen on axial and coronal sections on MRI. It is a compressed white band of projection fibers going to and from

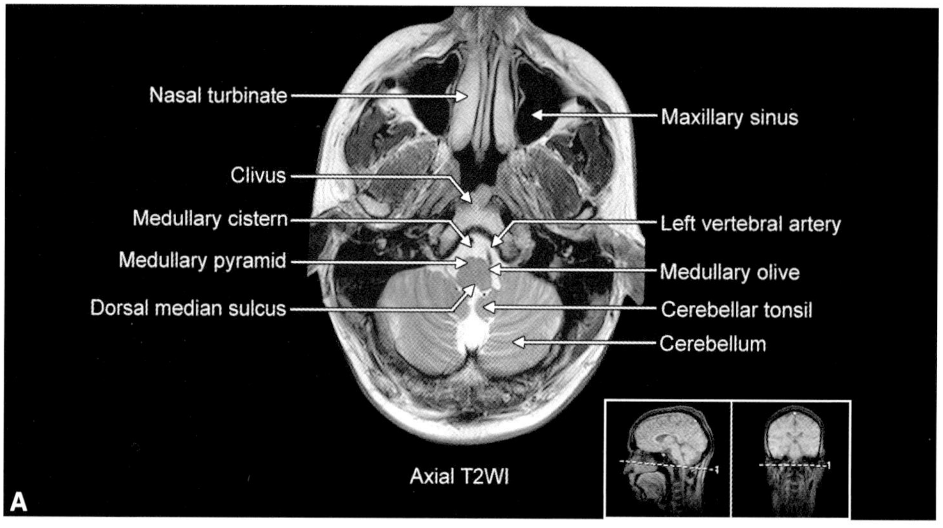

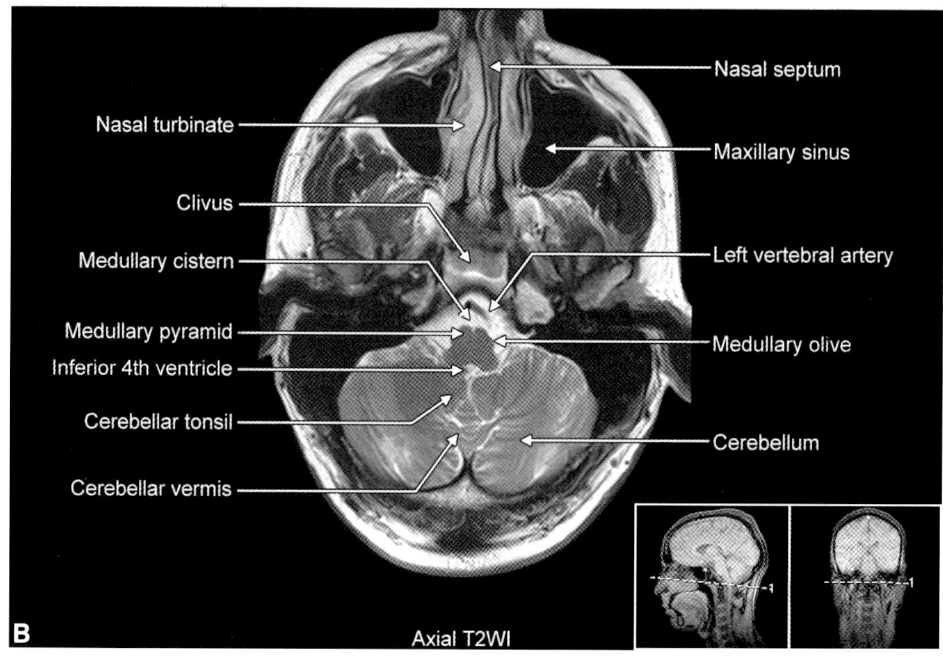

the brain. It lies medial to the lentiform nucleus and lateral to the caudate nucleus and thalamus. It has five parts: (1) Anterior limb; (2) Genu; (3) Posterior limb; (4) Retrolentiform part and (5) Sublentiform part.

The anterior limb, genu and posterior limb contain frontopontine fibers.

The retrolentiform part contains the occipitopontine fibers and a few parietopontine fibers.

The sublentiform part contains the parietopontine and the temporopontine fibers. The corticonuclear fibers are located in the genu of the internal capsule. The posterior limb contains corticospinal and corticorubral fibers. Vascular lesions of the internal capsule can cause extensive damage. Lesions of the genu can cause paralysis of face of the opposite side due to involvement of corticonuclear fibers for head and neck. Lesions of the posterior limb can cause extensive contralateral hemiplegia and loss of sensations on the opposite side of the body. Lesions of the retrolentiform and sublentiform parts can cause visual and auditory defects. By far the commonest cause of lesions is the rupture of one of the branches of the middle cerebral artery (Lenticulostriate arteries - Charcot's artery of cerebral hemorrhage).

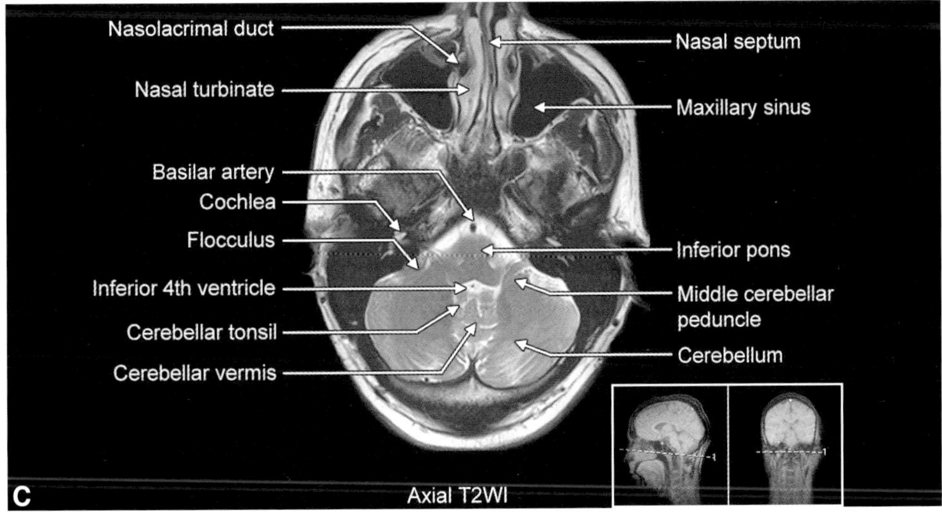

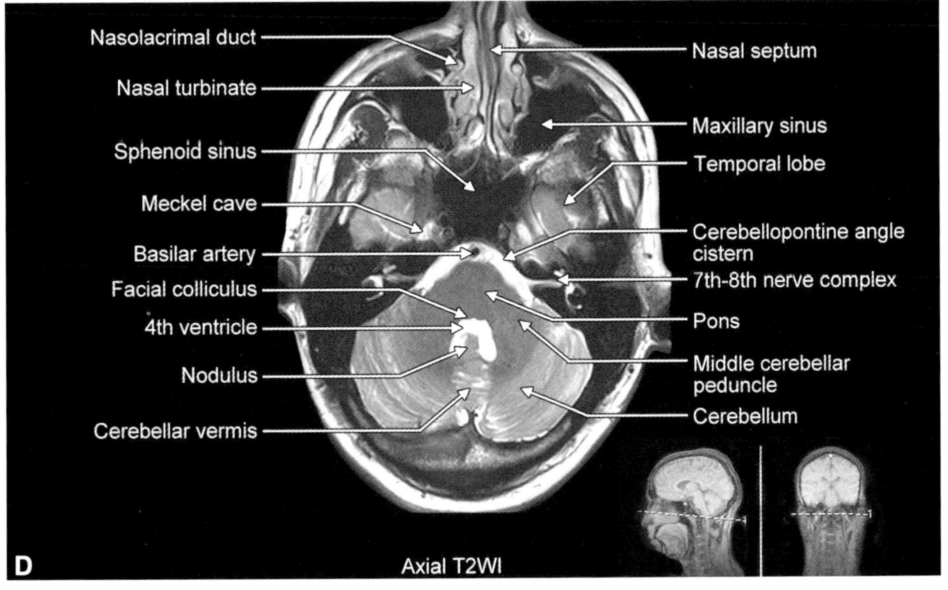

White matter tracts consist of corpus callosum, commissural fibers and corona radiata. The perivascular spaces (of Robin Virchow) surround the striatal vessels and appear as oval areas of bright signal intensity. The white matter tracts are subdivided for descriptive purposes into:

- *Corpus callosum* (Figs 1L to N, 2A and 3G) is the largest commissural white matter tract of the brain. It connects the two cerebral hemispheres. It consists of rostrum, genu, trunk and splenium. The large rounded splenium forms the posterior end of corpus callosum. The corpus callosum develops in an anterior to posterior end, the genu forms first followed by the body and splenium, the rostrum is the last to develop. On MRI images the genu and rostrum show slightly lower signal intensity as compared to the body and splenium. The rostrum of corpus callosum continues inferiorly to join the lamina terminalis. The body of corpus callosum lies over the roof of

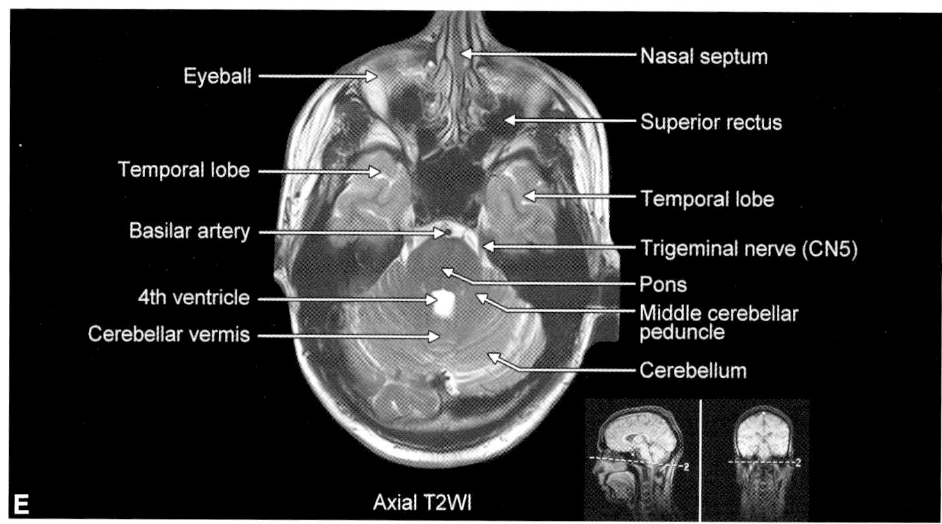

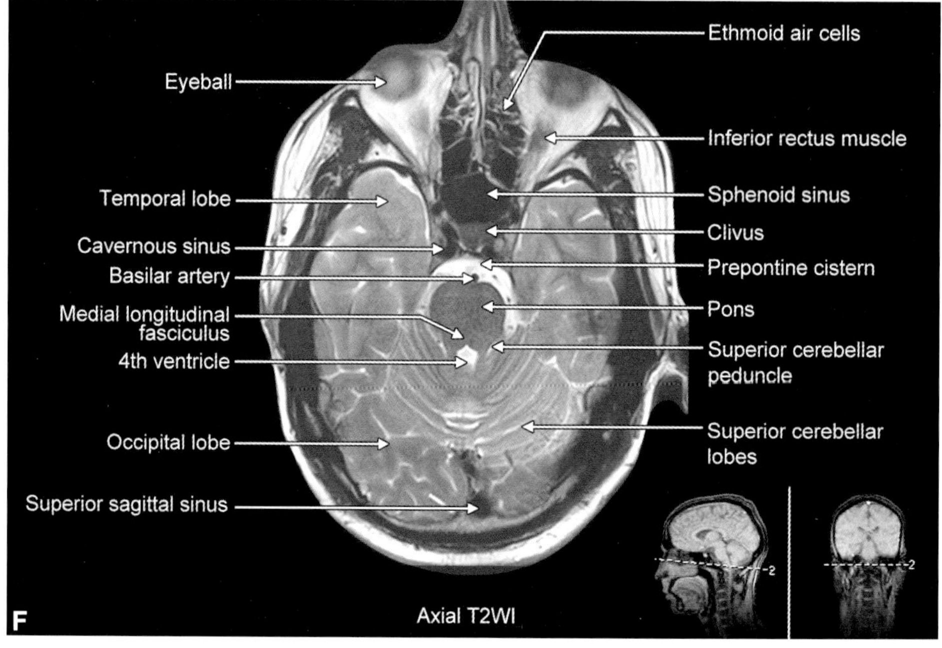

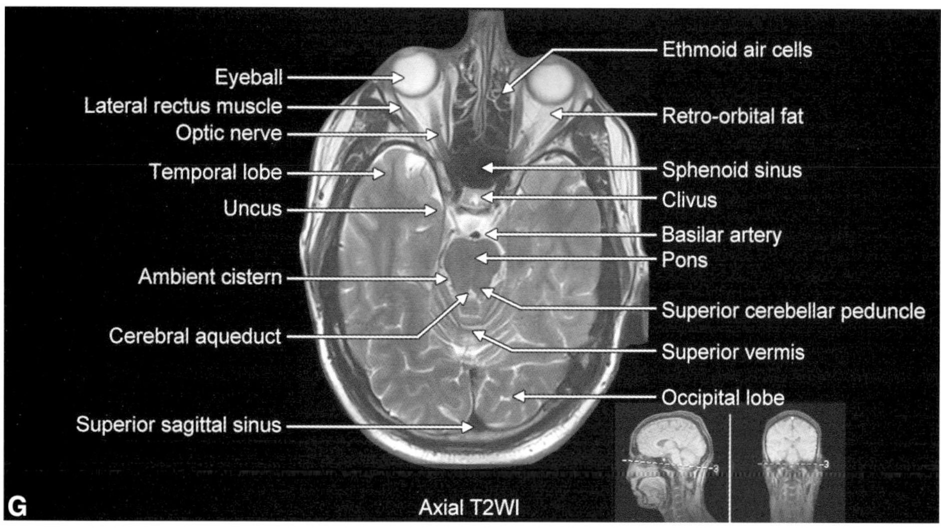
Eyeball
Lateral rectus muscle
Optic nerve
Temporal lobe
Uncus
Ambient cistern
Cerebral aqueduct
Superior sagittal sinus
Ethmoid air cells
Retro-orbital fat
Sphenoid sinus
Clivus
Basilar artery
Pons
Superior cerebellar peduncle
Superior vermis
Occipital lobe
G
Axial T2WI

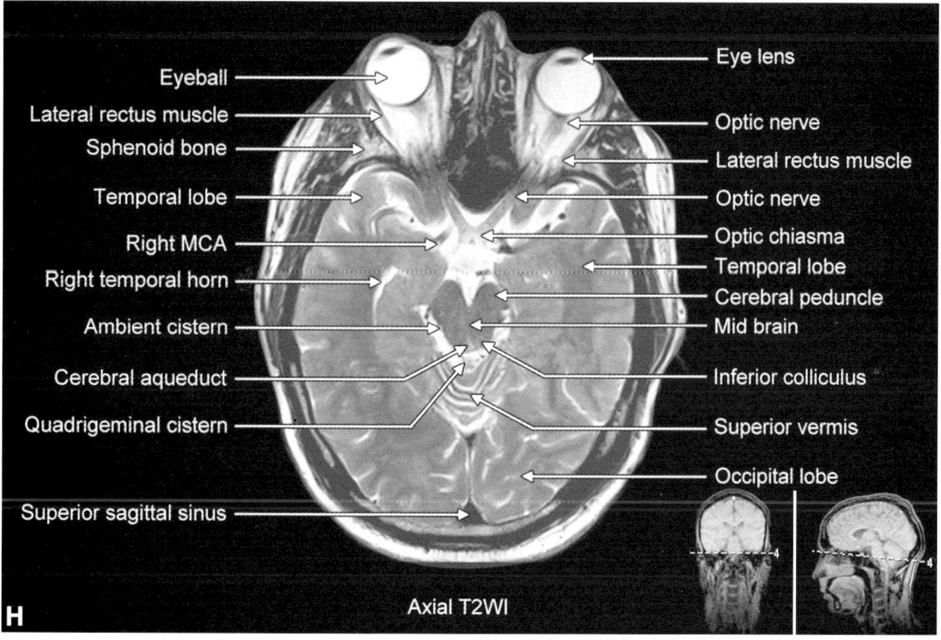
Eyeball
Lateral rectus muscle
Sphenoid bone
Temporal lobe
Right MCA
Right temporal horn
Ambient cistern
Cerebral aqueduct
Quadrigeminal cistern
Superior sagittal sinus
Eye lens
Optic nerve
Lateral rectus muscle
Optic nerve
Optic chiasma
Temporal lobe
Cerebral peduncle
Mid brain
Inferior colliculus
Superior vermis
Occipital lobe
H
Axial T2WI

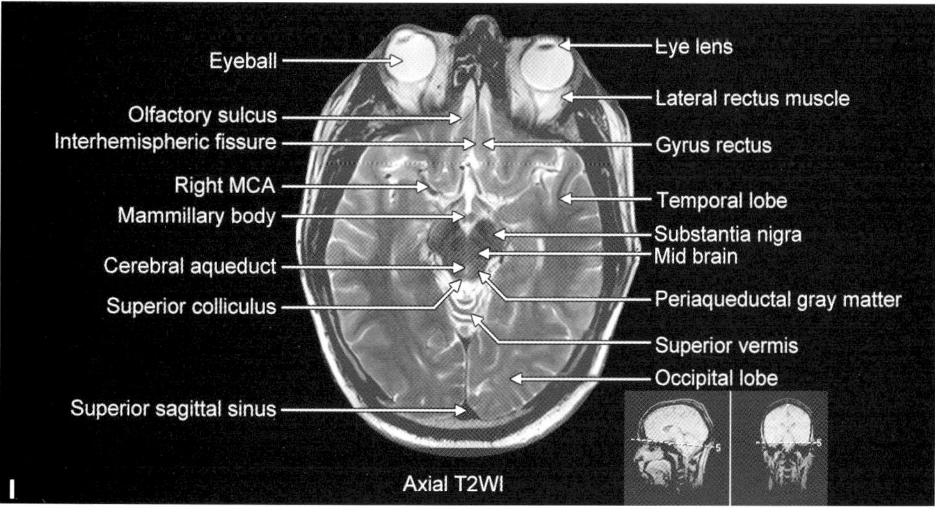
Eyeball
Olfactory sulcus
Interhemispheric fissure
Right MCA
Mammillary body
Cerebral aqueduct
Superior colliculus
Superior sagittal sinus
Eye lens
Lateral rectus muscle
Gyrus rectus
Temporal lobe
Substantia nigra
Mid brain
Periaqueductal gray matter
Superior vermis
Occipital lobe
I
Axial T2WI

lateral ventricle. The splenium of corpus callosum overlies the pineal body and colliculi. Fibers from the occipital lobes run forwards, cross to the opposite side in the splenium and reach the occipital lobe of the opposite side forming forceps major.

- *Forceps major* (Fig. 2F) are commissural fibers that run from the occipital lobe and loop through the splenium of corpus callosum to the opposite occipital lobe.
- *Forceps minor* (Fig. 2F) are commissural fibers that run from the frontal lobe and loop through the anterior part of corpus callosum to the opposite frontal lobe.

Diencephalon consists of the thalamus, hypothalamus, subthalamus, epithalamus and metathalamus.

- *Thalamus* (Figs 1L, 2B and D) is an ovoid structure of brain seen on axial, sagittal and coronal MRI sections. The thalamus lies lateral to the third ventricle and medial to the posterior limb of

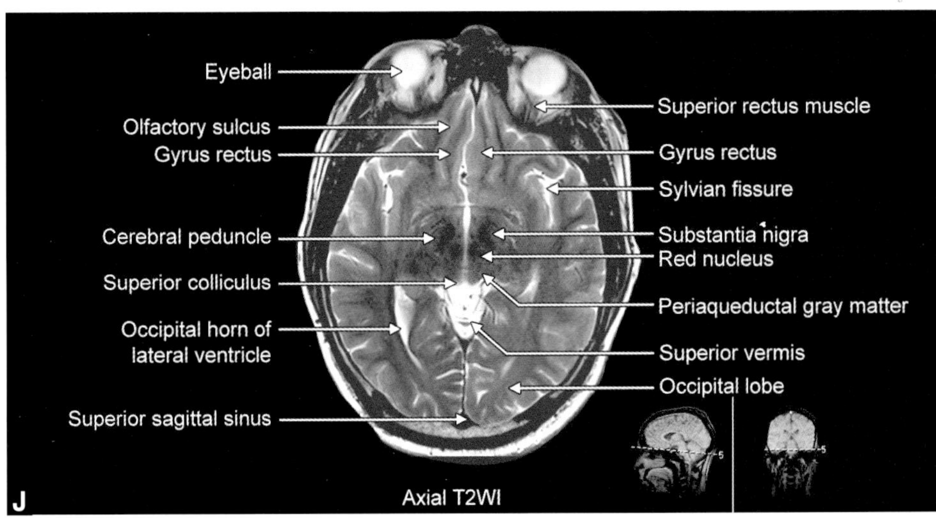

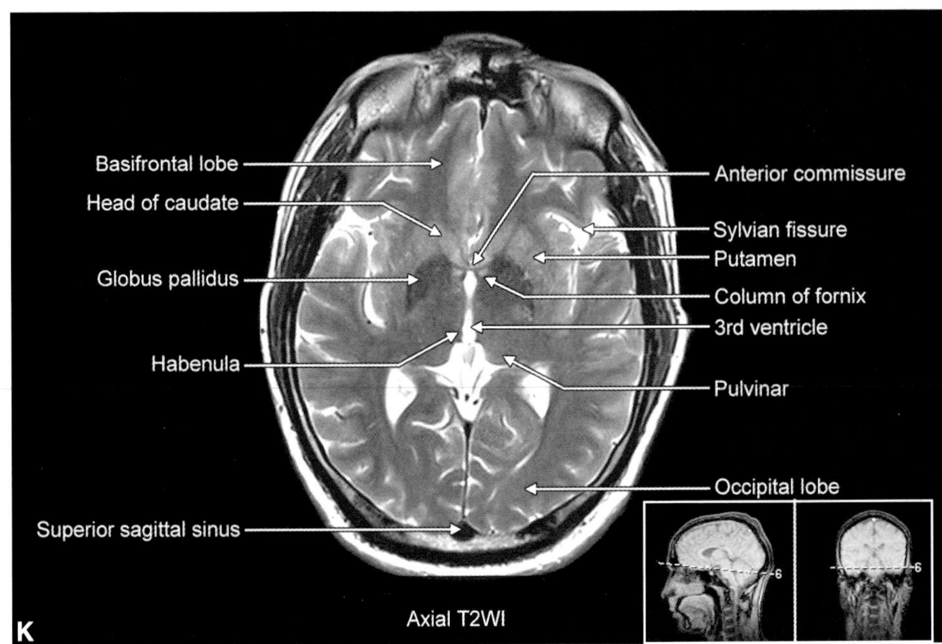

internal capsule. The thalamus contains a large number of nuclei. The important nuclear groups are lateral, medial and anterior nuclei. The ventral posterior nucleus is a part of the lateral nuclear group and receives inputs from medial, spinal and trigeminal lemniscus. Fibers from here pass to the sensory part of the cerebral cortex. Some parts of lateral nucleus receive fibers from the dentate nucleus of the cerebellum and globus pallidus. The fibers project to the motor areas of the cerebral cortex. The medial group of thalamic nuclei receives fibers from the hypothalamus, corpus striatum and frontal lobes. The medial group of nuclei appears to be concerned with emotions and memory. The anterior group of thalamic nuclei receives fibers mainly from the hypothalamus via

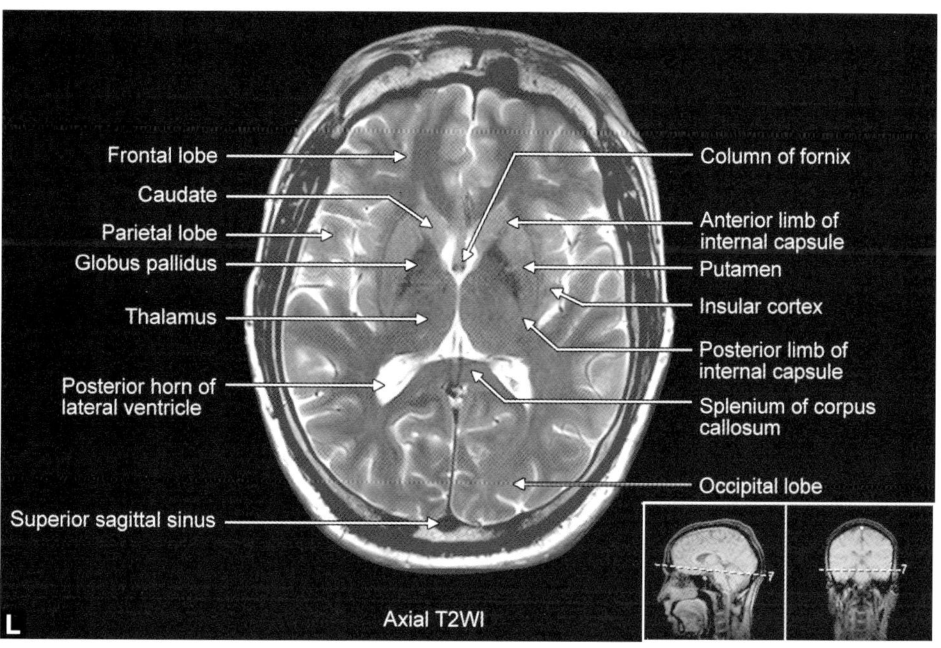

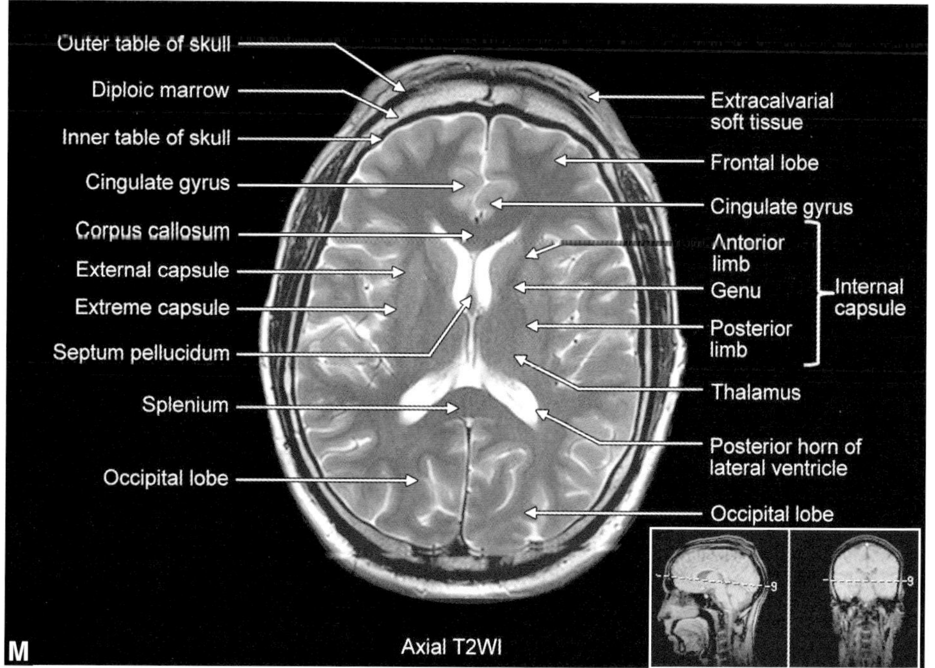

the mamillothalamic fasciculus. Most ascending tracts pass through and relay in the thalamus as they proceed towards the cortex of the cerebral hemispheres. Fibers from anterior nuclei project to cingulate gyrus—part of the limbic system. The geniculate bodies, medial and lateral are two rounded bodies forming the posterior aspect of the thalamus. The medial geniculate body is a relay station in the auditory pathway; the lateral geniculate body is a relay station in the visual pathway.

- *Metathalamus* is formed by the medial and lateral geniculate bodies. The geniculate bodies' main function is to serve as relay stations for the visual and auditory pathways. The medial geniculate body is a part of the auditory pathway; the inferior brachium connects the medial geniculate body to the inferior colliculus. The medial geniculate

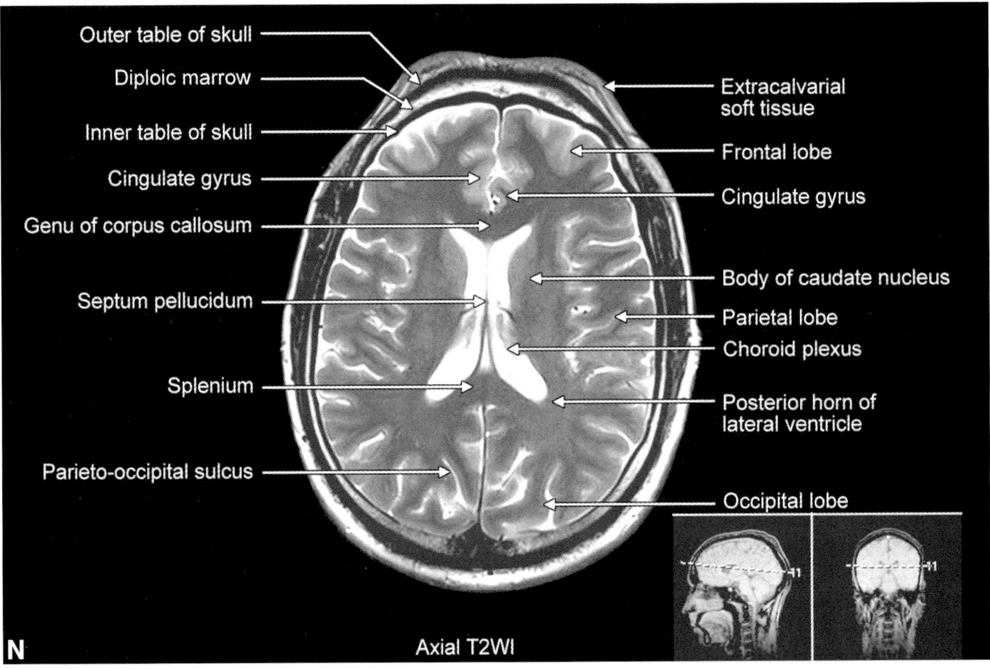

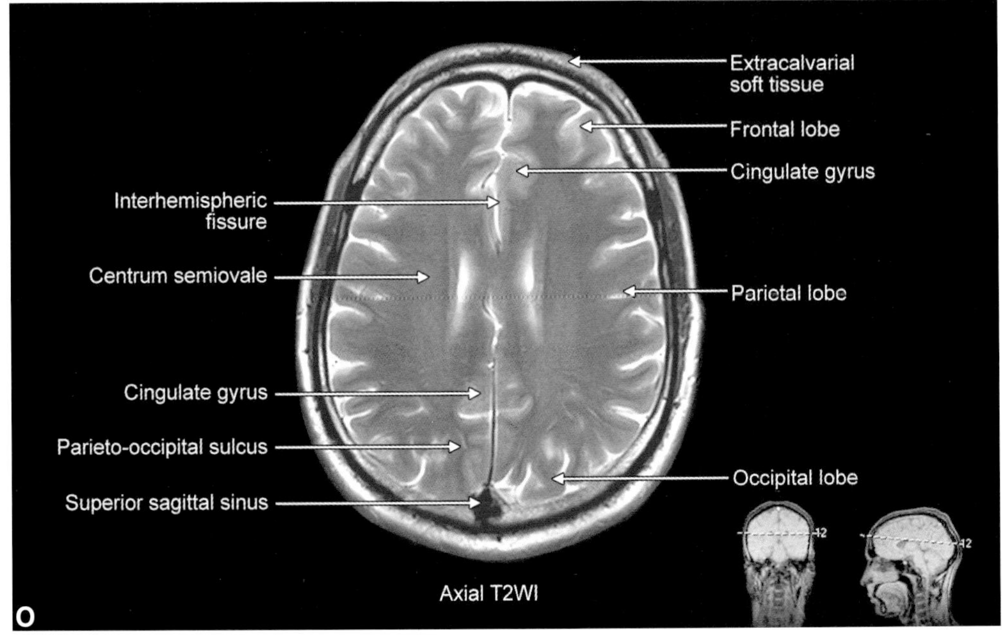

body relays the information to the auditory cortex located on the superior temporal gyrus. The lateral geniculate body is a part of the visual pathway; the superior brachium connects the lateral geniculate body to superior colliculus. The lateral geniculate body relays the information to the visual cortex located in occipital lobe.

- *Epithalamus* is formed by the habenula, pineal body and posterior commissure seen on T1W and T2W images in axial, coronal and sagittal sections. The pineal stalk has a superior and inferior lamina. The habenula forms the superior lamina. The posterior commissure forms the inferior lamina. The pineal recess is located between the superior and inferior lamina.

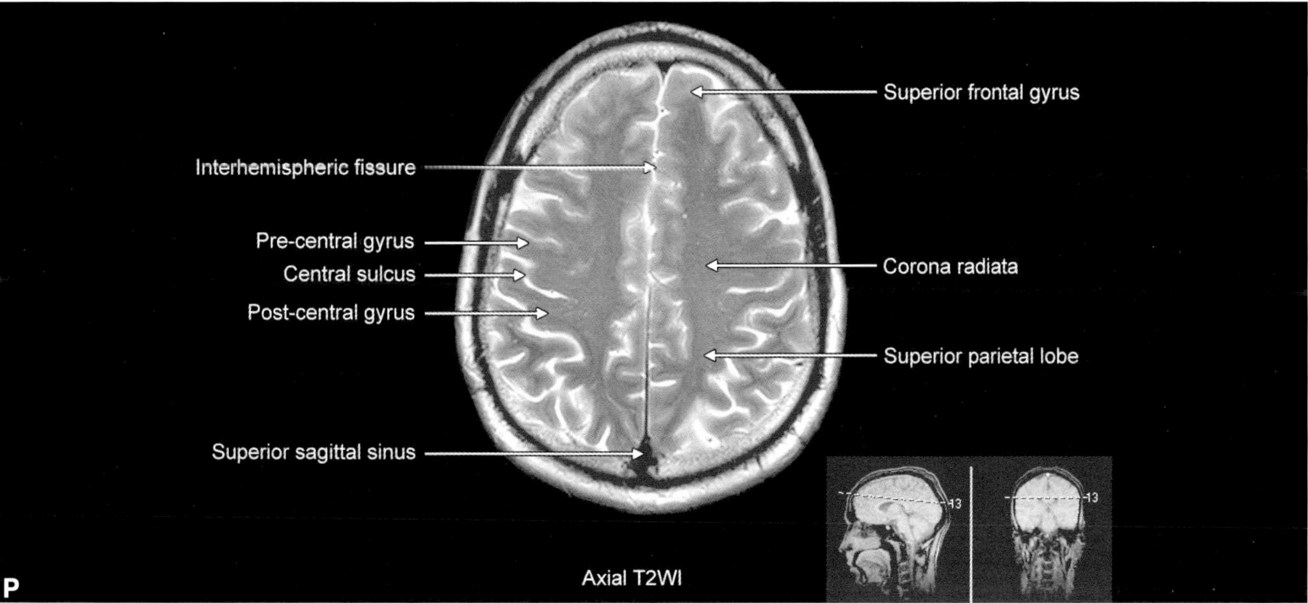

Figs 1A to P: MRI head axial section T2 weighted images

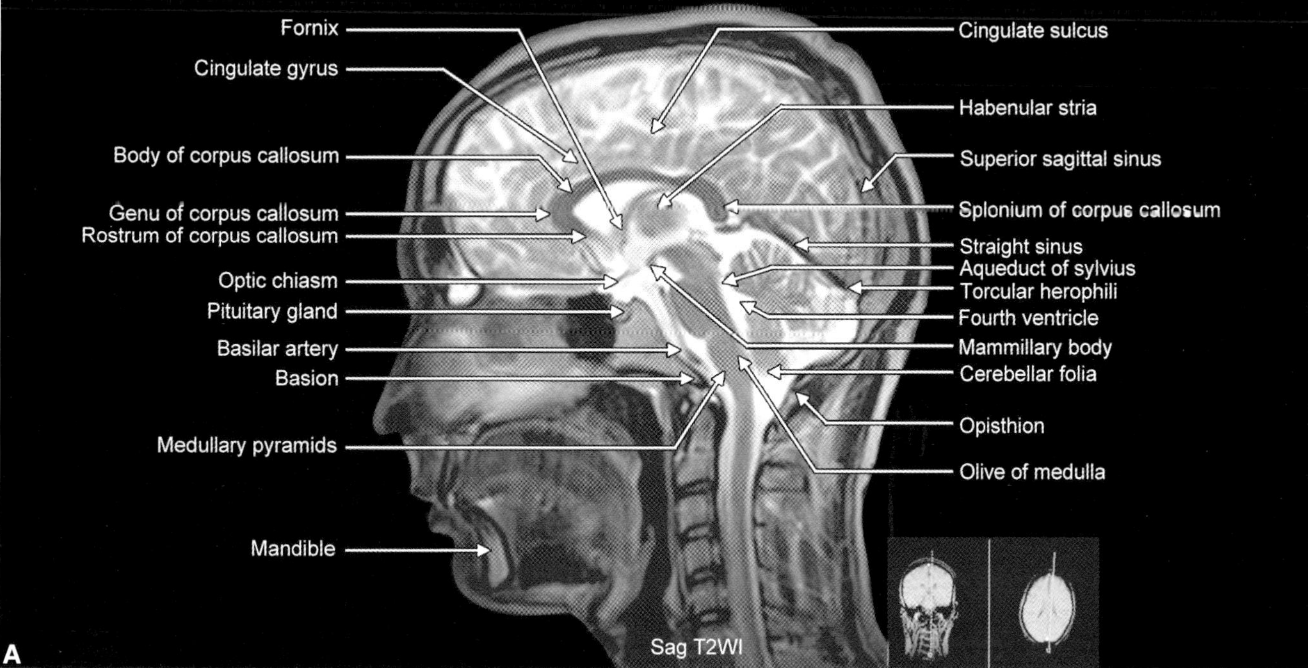

- *Hypothalamus* (Fig. 2D) is a triangular brain structure inferior to the anterior part of the thalamus is seen on sagittal and axial MRI sections. It consists of the mammillary bodies, tuber cinereum, infundibulum, hypophysis and optic chiasm. In a sagittal MRI section, the hypothalamus is separated from the thalamus by an oblique hypothalamic sulcus which extends from the aqueduct of Sylvius to the interventricular foramen of Monro. The anterior part of the hypothalamus is connected to the infundibular stalk of pituitary. The mammillary bodies form the most posterior part of the hypothalamus. The hypothalamic groove is seen on the lateral walls of the third ventricle and extends from the aqueduct of Sylvius to the interventricular foramen. The hypothalamus has important roles in autonomic functions (modulation of visceral activities like thermoregulation, appetite, thirst, sexual responses and emotions), endocrine

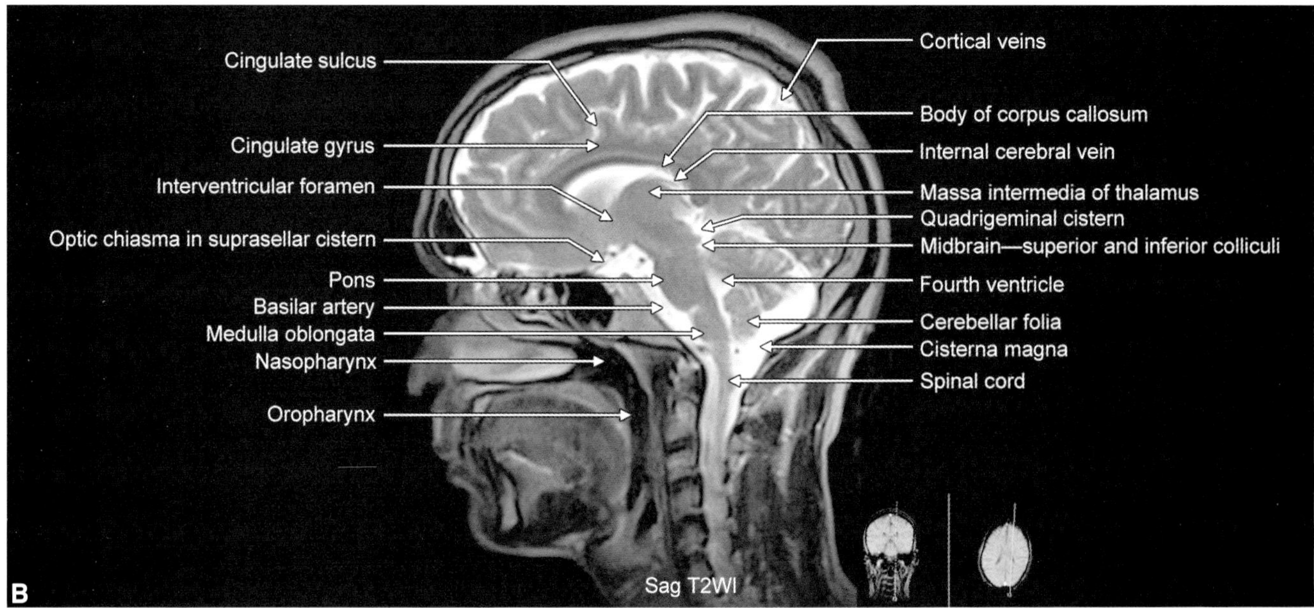

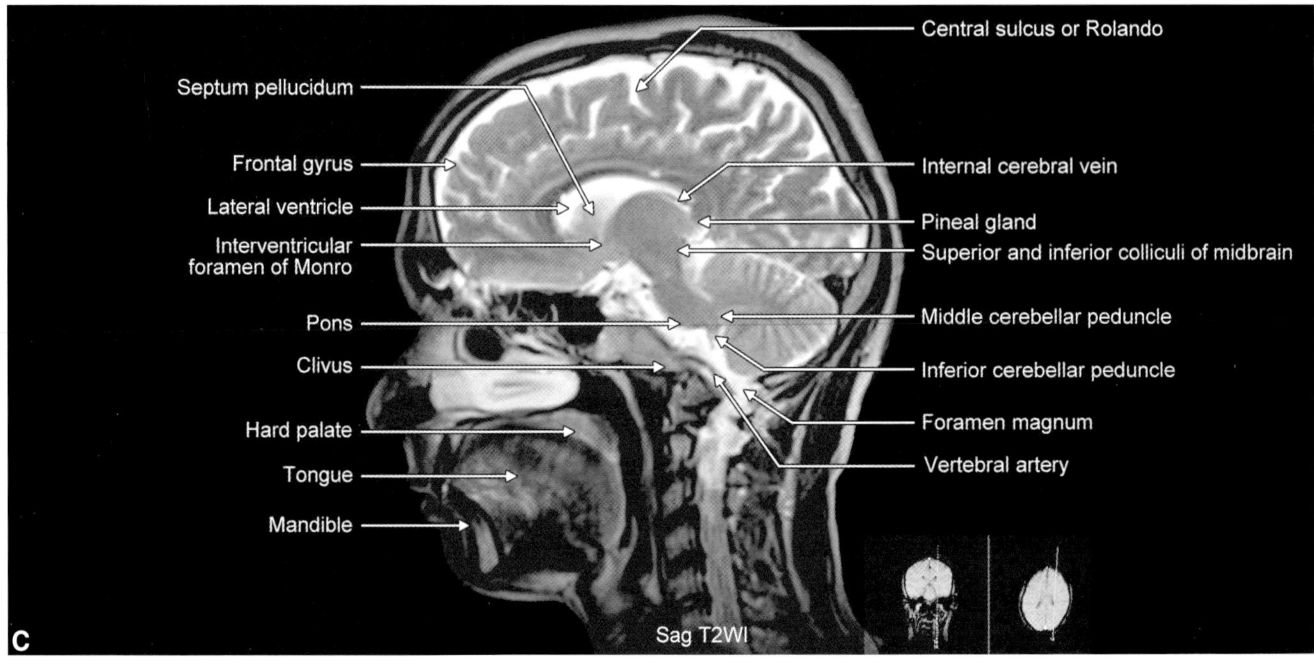

functions (regulates release of hormones from the pituitary gland) and pain response such as blunting of painful stimuli by releasing endorphins and encephalin.

- *Subthalamus* is seen on T1W and T2W images on sagittal and coronal sections as a thin zone of transition between the thalamus and tegmentum of the midbrain.

Limbic System

The limbic system is concerned with emotional and personality aspects of each individual. The limbic system is made up of various nuclei and interconnecting fibers. The olfactory nerves, olfactory bulb and tract, hippocampal gyrus, fornix, fimbriae, dentate gyrus, mammillary body, uncus, cingulate and parahippocampal gyri, amygdaloid body, septal

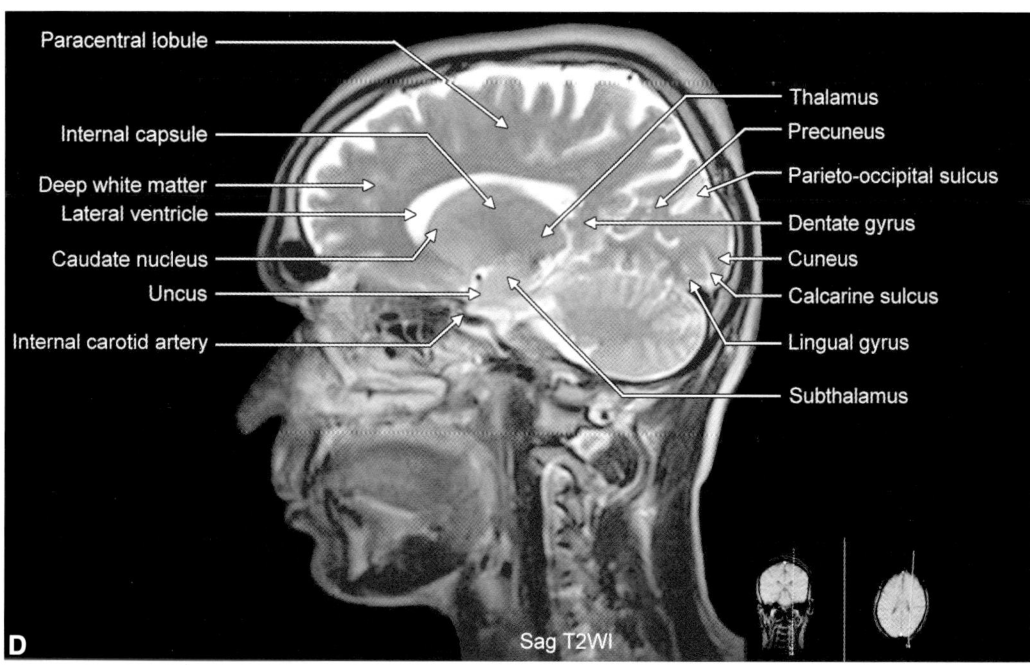

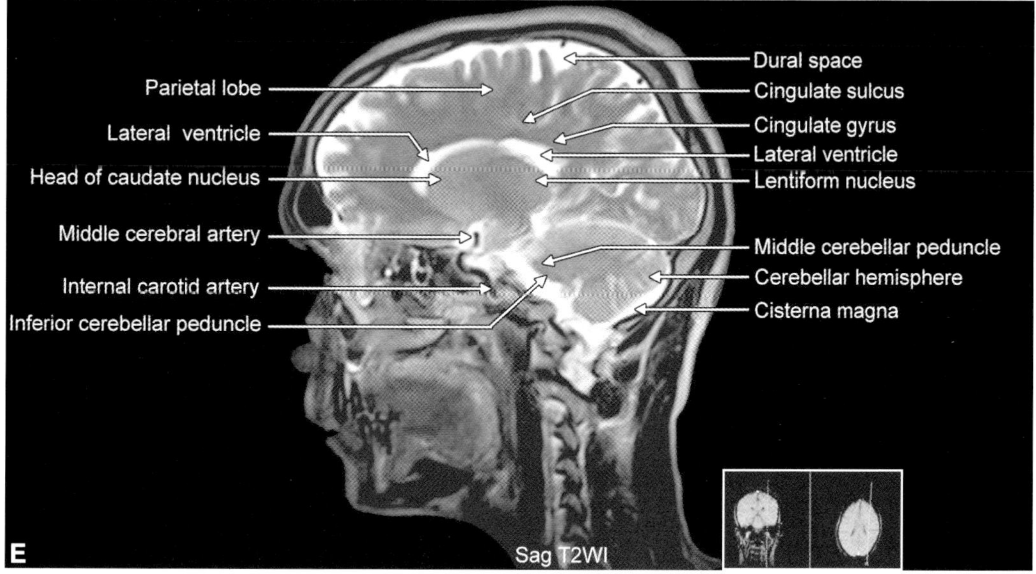

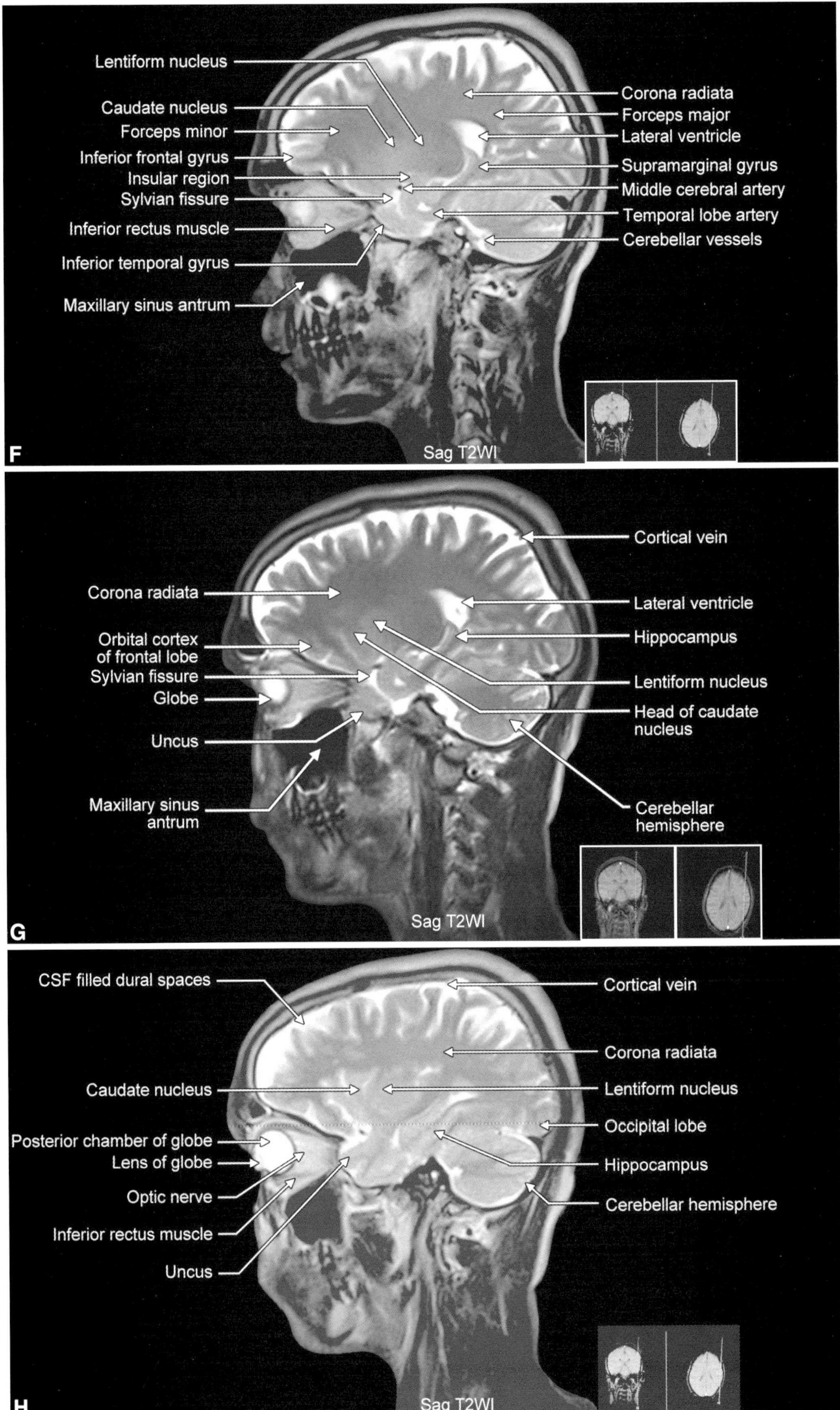

Figs 2A to H: MRI head sagittal T2 weighted images

and piriform areas of cortex near lamina terminalis and anterior thalamic nuclei.

- *Hippocampal gyrus* (Figs 2E and G, H, 3G and H) is seen on T1W images in sagittal and coronal MRI sections. The hippocampal gyrus is located in temporal lobe and receives input from the mammillary body, the septal region, amygdala, superior and middle frontal gyri, superior temporal and cingulate gyri, precuneus, lateral occipital cortex, occipitotemporal gyri and subcallosal cortical areas.
- *Mammillary body* (Figs 1I and 2A) is seen well on T1W images in sagittal MRI sections. It is located as a small nodular area in the anterior aspect of interpeduncular cistern. The mammillary body is connected with the dorsal and ventral tegmental nuclei, anterior thalamic nucleus (via the mamillothalamic tract), septal nuclei, tegmental pontine and reticulotegmental nuclei.
- *Amygdaloid complex* is seen well on T1W images in sagittal and coronal MRI sections at the roof of temporal horns of lateral ventricles. The amygdaloid nuclear complex receives input from and projects to the brainstem and forebrain centers via the stria terminalis and ventral amygdalofugal pathway. Corticoamygdaloid and

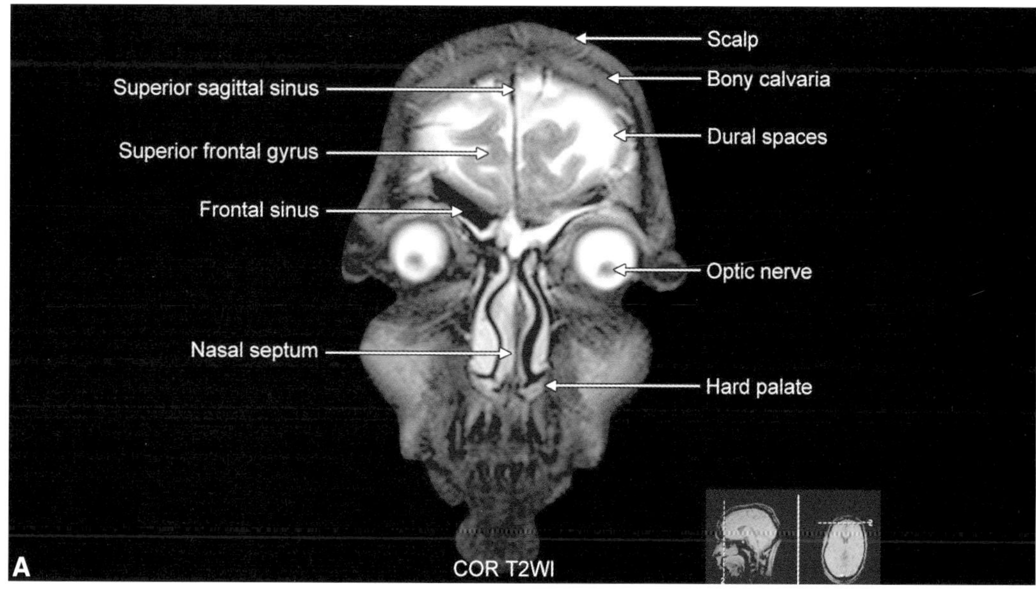

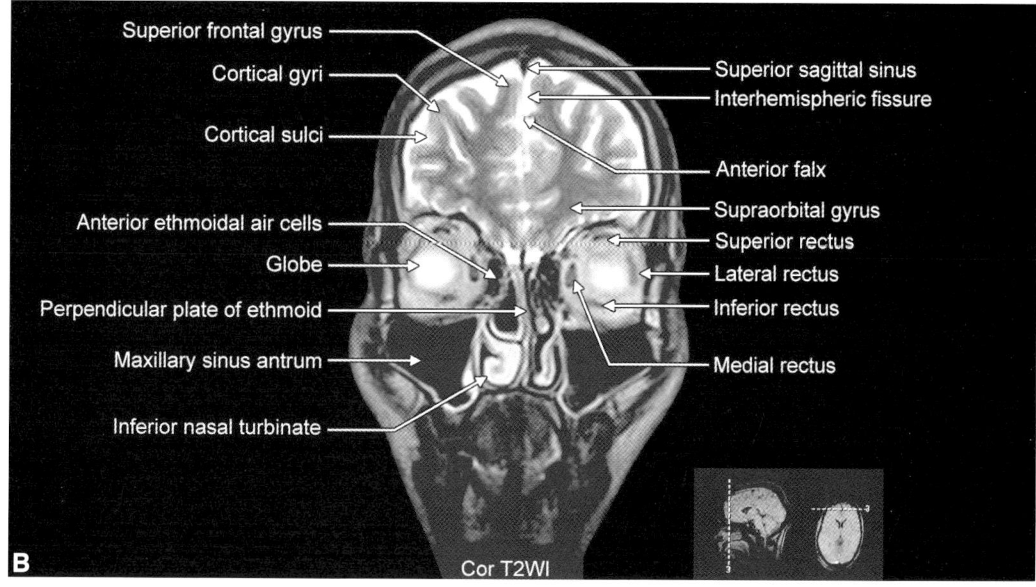

amygdalocortical fibers interconnect the basal and lateral amygdaloid nuclei to cerebral cortex.

- *Fornix* (Figs 1L and 2A) is an important part of the limbic system by providing efferent connections. The body of fornix is a bundle of white matter mass beneath the corpus callosum in midline and communicates with fibers from the other side of brain. The fornix has anterior and posterior fibers, the anterior fibers of fornix connect to the septal nuclei near lamina terminalis and the posterior fibers connect to anterior thalamic nuclei or to the mammillary bodies.

Mesencephalon and Rhombencephalon

For convenience of description and understanding mesencephalon and rhombencephalon are dealt with together.

- *Brainstem* is formed by midbrain, pons and medulla oblongata. It is seen on T1W and T2W images in axial, coronal and sagittal MRI sections.
  - *Midbrain* (Figs 1H, I and 3K) is also called as mesencephalon. It is seen on T1W images in axial, coronal and sagittal MRI sections as

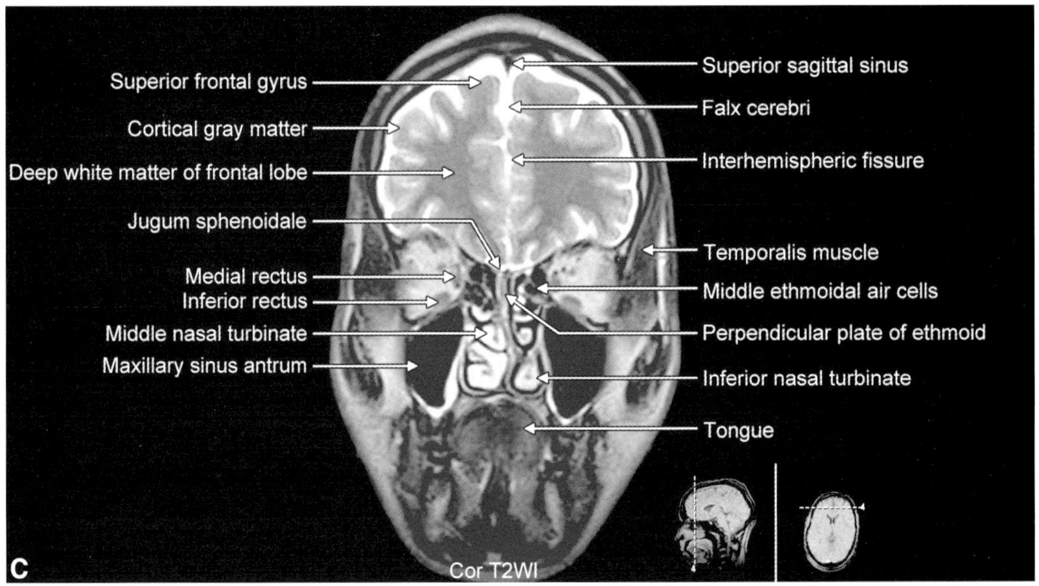

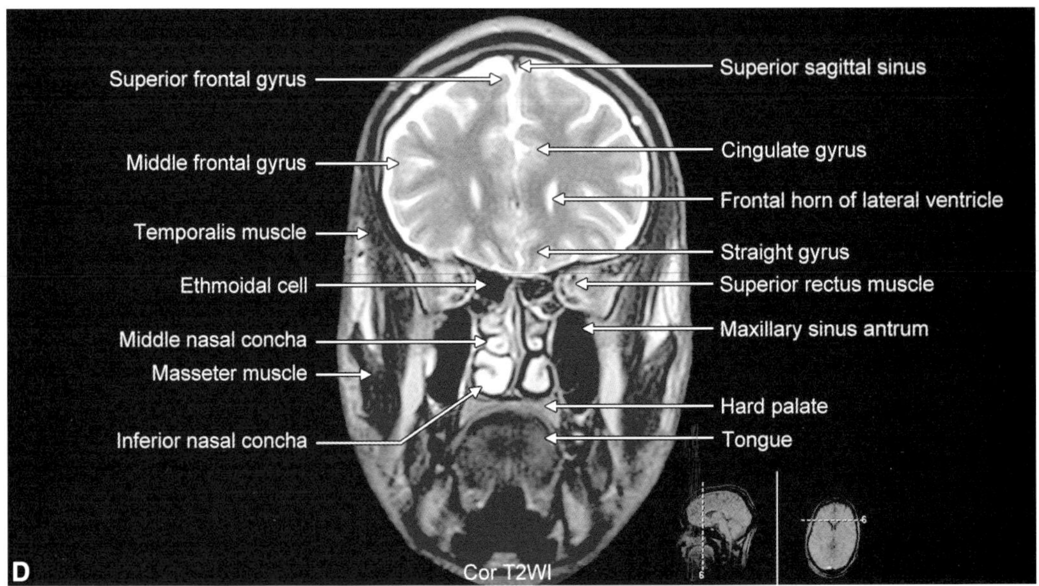

a short upper segment of the brainstem at the level of tentorial inscisura. The midbrain on T1W axial sections can be subdivided by an imaginary passing horizontally through the central canal into cerebral peduncles anteriorly and tectum posteriorly. Between the cerebral peduncles and tectum is a central gray matter which surrounds aqueduct of Sylvius passing through the substance of midbrain, this is seen on T1W midsagittal sections. The interpeduncular fossa containing the interpeduncular cistern is located anteriorly between the cerebral peduncles. The cerebral peduncles of midbrain has two parts, the ventral part is called the crus, the dorsal part is called the tegmentum.

- The tectum of midbrain has nodular prominences (corpora quadrigemina), they are four in number which are called as superior and inferior colliculi. Behind the corpora quadrigemina is the quadrigemina cistern. The fibers of the superior colliculi are connected to the lateral geniculate body in the visual pathway. The fibers of the inferior colliculi are connected to the medial geniculate body in the auditory pathway.

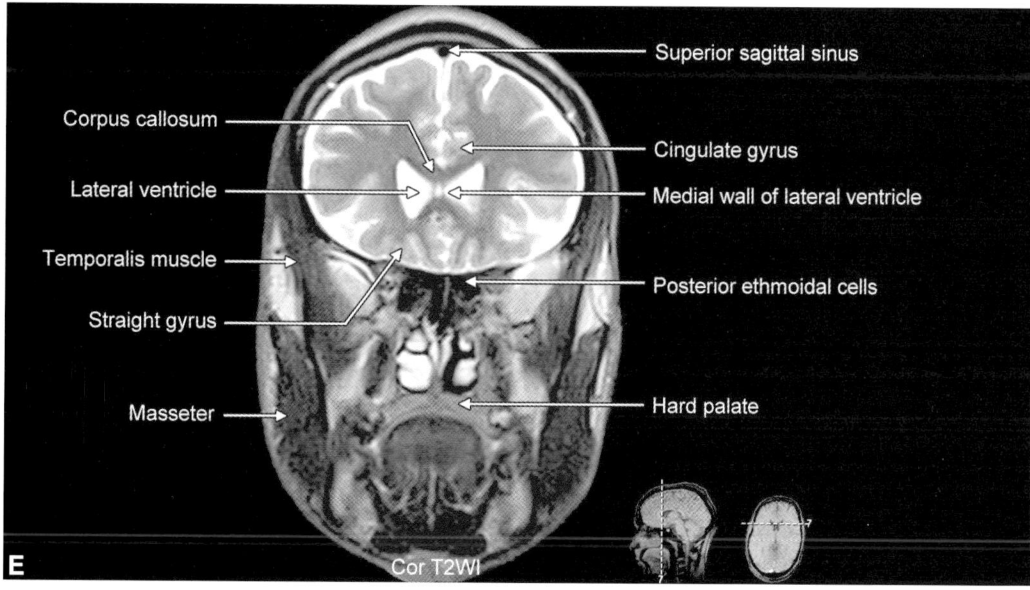

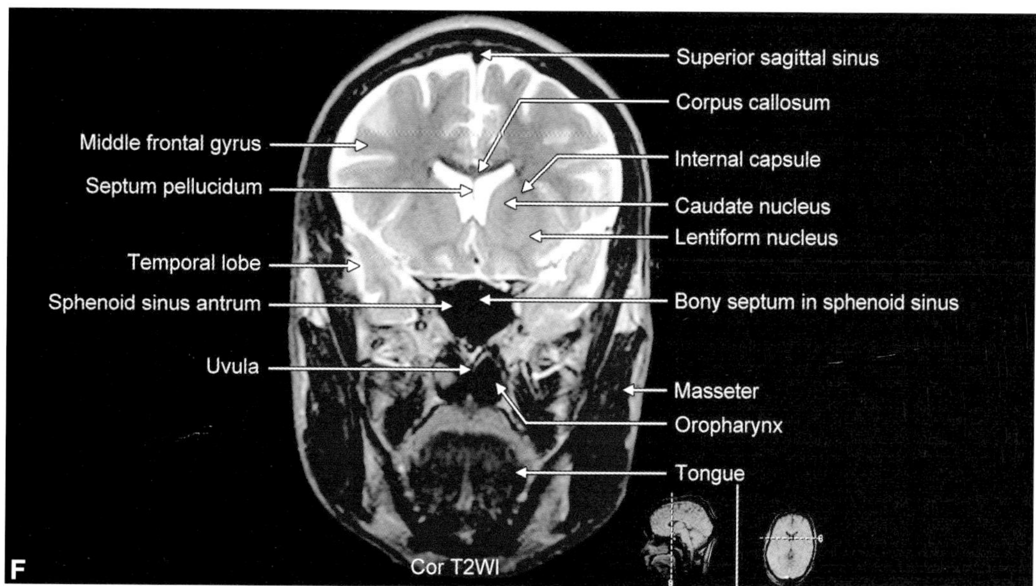

The midbrain contains the trochlear nerve nucleus at the level of the inferior colliculus and the oculomotor nucleus at the level of the superior colliculus. The mesencephalic part of the trigeminal nerve nucleus, responsible for receiving proprioceptive information from the regions of head and neck is located at all levels of midbrain. The pretectal nucleus is seen at the upper levels of the midbrain. It is a relay station in the pupillary light reflex arc. The anterior part is called as the cerebral peduncle and the posterior part is called as the tectum. The tegmentum is further divided into the anterior crus cerebri, a middle layer called the substantia nigra and a posterior tegmentum. The posterior tegmentum contains the superior colliculus at the upper levels, a relay station in the visual pathway and the inferior colliculus at the lower levels of midbrain—a relay station in the auditory pathway.

- *Pons* (Figs 1C to E, 2B, and 3K) means 'bridge' in Latin language, because it is a part of the brainstem which connects the midbrain above to the medulla oblongata below. Pons is visualized as a large ventral protuberance in brainstem on T1W and T2W images in axial,

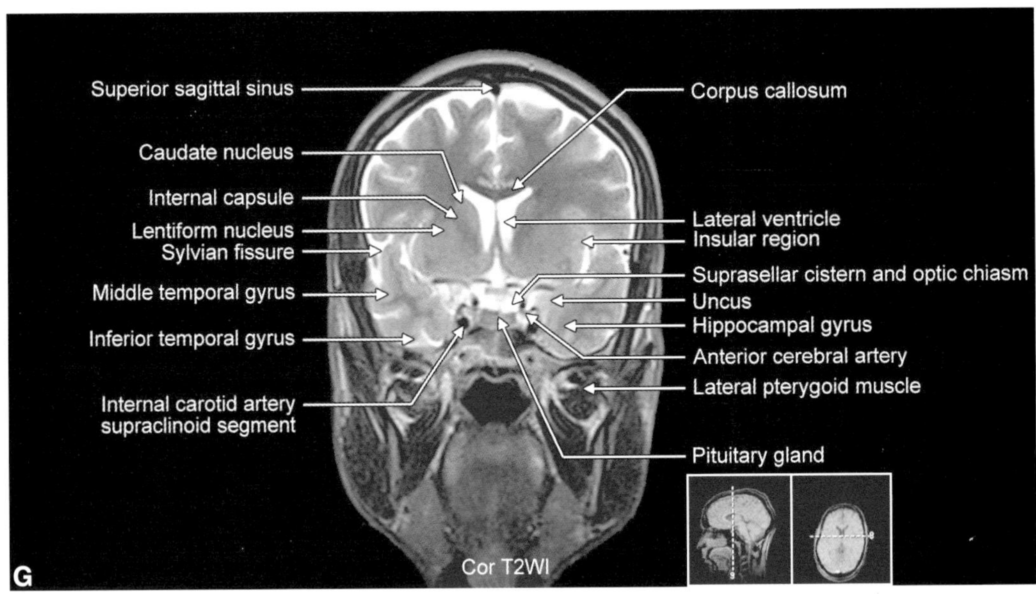

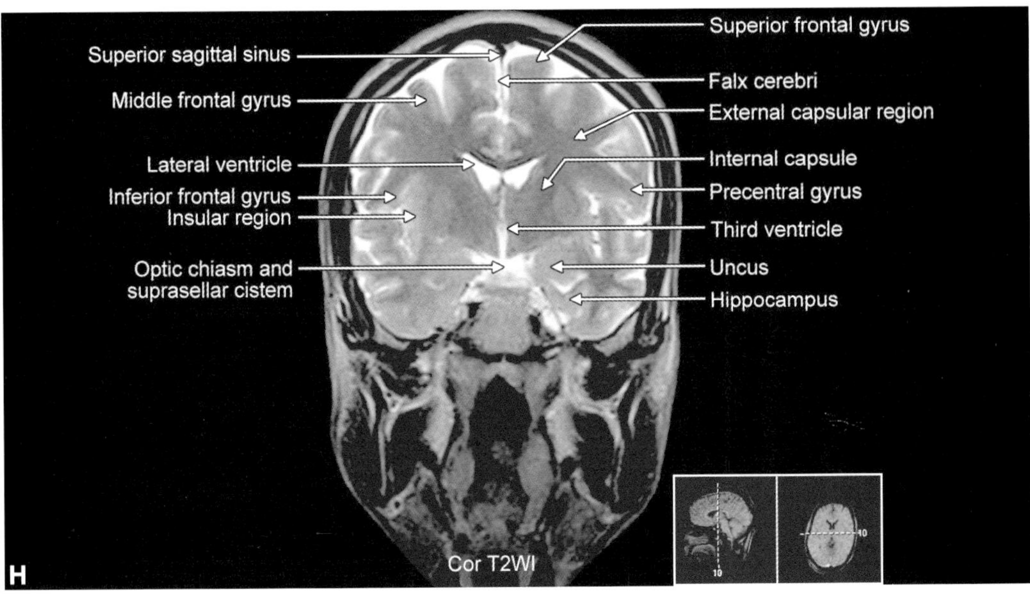

sagittal and coronal sections. The superior pontine sulcus separates the pons from midbrain above. The inferior pontine sulcus separates the pons from medulla oblongata below. The pons consists of an anterior basilar part and a posterior tegmentum. The basilar part shows an anterior midline sulcus called the basilar sulcus which lodges the basilar artery. The basilar part contains pontine nuclei and the descending corticospinal and corticonuclear tracts. The posterior tegmentum contains the pontine reticular formation, the band of lemnisci (medial lemniscus, trigeminal lemniscus, spinal lemniscus, lateral lemniscus) and cranial nerve nuclei. The anterior most part of the tegmentum contains the trapezoid body—formed by the crossing over of fibers from the cochlear nuclei. The lower part of pons has nuclei of the abducent nerve, facial nerve and spinal nucleus of the trigeminal nerve. It also contains the vestibular nuclei and the dorsal and ventral cochlear nuclei. The upper part of pons contains the chief sensory nucleus and the motor nucleus of the trigeminal nerve. The pons is supplied by blood via the pontine

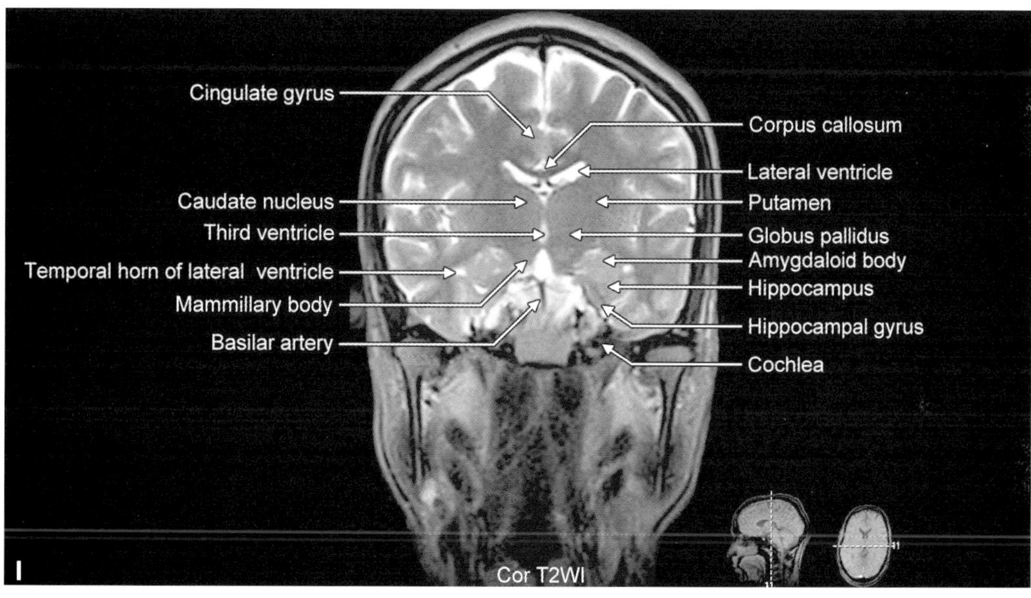

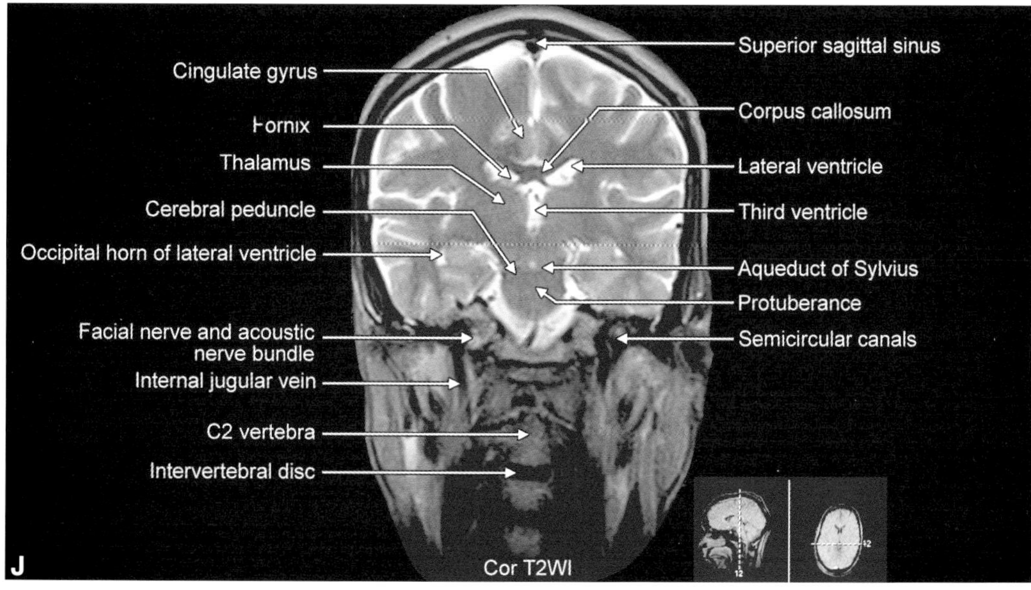

branches of the basilar artery. Bilateral pontine hemorrhages result in pin point pupils, hyperpyrexia, coma, bilateral paralysis of face and limbs. Millard Gubbler syndrome is due to a lesion in the anterior part of the lower pons, which involves the pyramidal tracts, the emerging fibers of the abducent and facial nerves.

- *Medulla oblongata* (Figs 2B, C and 3L) is the lowest part of the brainstem which continues below as the spinal cord and seen on T1W and T2W images in axial, coronal and MRI sagittal sections. The medulla oblongata is 3 cm in length, sagittal diameter is 1.25 cm and width is 2 cm. The medulla contains the vital cardio-respiratory centers in its reticular formation. The medulla contains important cranial nerve nuclei—they are hypoglossal nucleus, dorsal nucleus of vagus, nucleus of tractus solitarius, the nucleus ambigus, the spinal nucleus and tract of the trigeminal nerve, the vestibular nucleus and the cochlear nucleus. The upper part of the medulla contains the inferior olivary nucleus and the medial leminiscus. The posterolateral parts of the medulla are supplied by the posterior inferior cerebellar

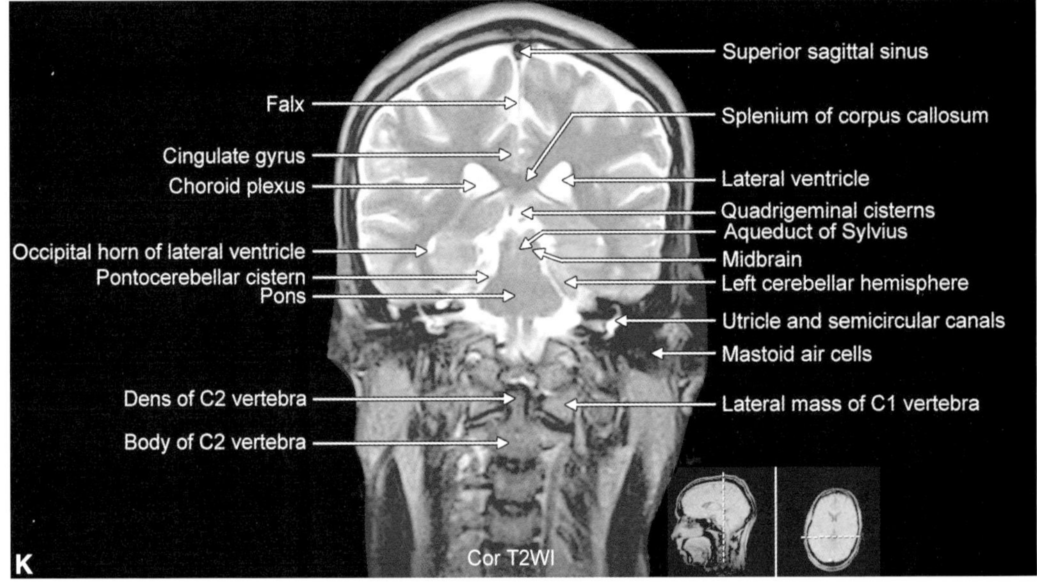

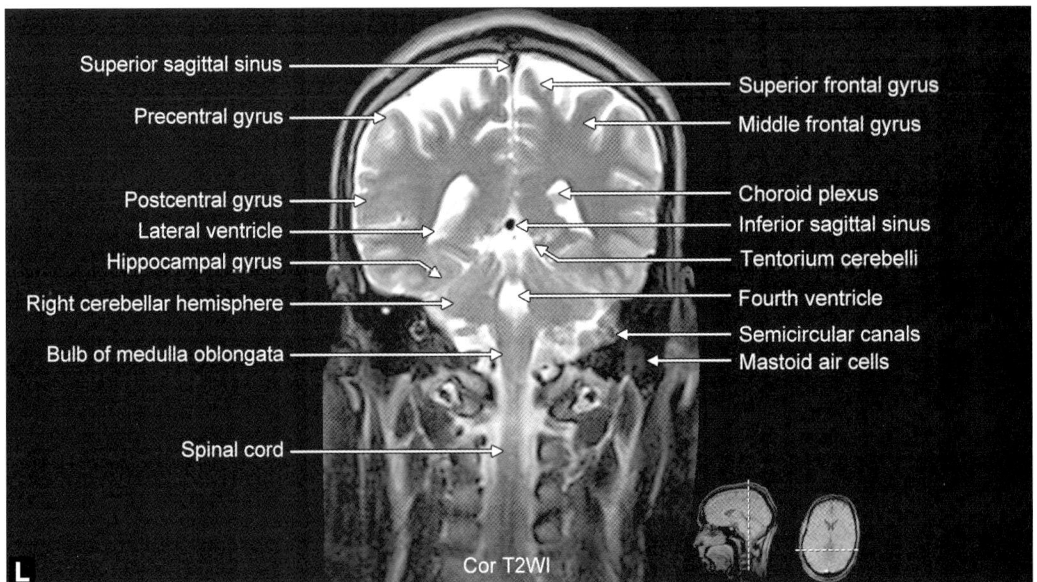

artery, the anteromedial parts are supplied by the anterior spinal artery, the part intervening being supplied by the anterior choroidal artery.

Important Nuclei of Midbrain

- Substantia nigra (Fig. 1I) is a layer of dark semilunar pigmented area located in the ventral part of midbrain, is identified by the hypointense signal on T1W images in axial MRI sections. It is composed of a dorsal pars compacta and a ventral pars reticularis. The pars reticularis is continuous above with the lentiform nucleus. The substantia nigra has important reciprocal connections with the corpus striatum, the pathways are dopaminergic. Parkinsonism is a disorder due to a depletion of dopamine in these pathways.
- Red nucleus (Fig. 1J) is seen at the level of the superior colliculus on T2W images in axial sections as hypointense signals due to pigmentation from iron deposits. It is an oval shaped nucleus, varies from 0.5 to 0.6 cm in diameter. The main afferents of the red nucleus are the dentato-rubro-thalamo-cortical fibers and the cortico-striato-rubral fibers. Efferent fibers from the red nucleus go to various subcortical centers. The rubrospinal or the rubroreticulospinal tract is the main efferent

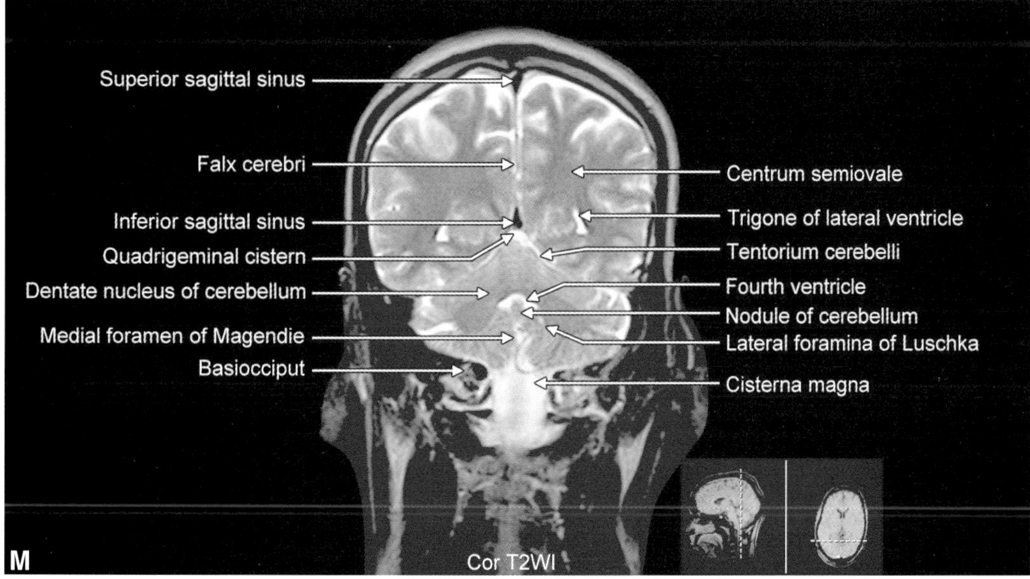

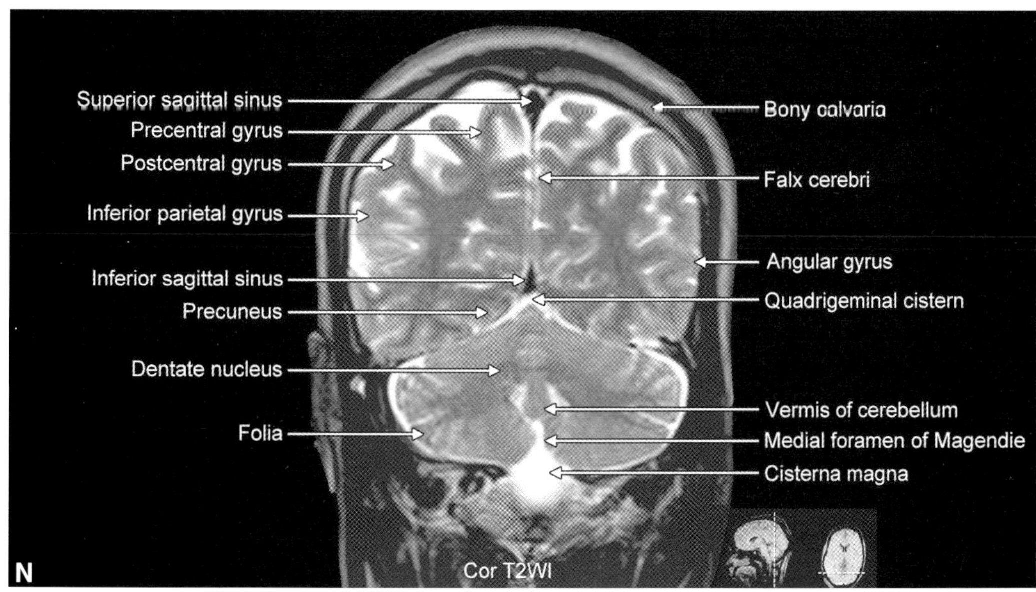

pathway. The red nucleus is considered to be a part of the functional basal ganglia.

Cerebellum

Cerebellum (Figs 1A to D, and 3P to R) is seen on T1W and T2W axial and sagittal MRI sections. The cerebellum is located in the posterior cranial fossa below the tentorium cerebelli. The cerebellum is posterolateral to pons and medulla separated by fourth ventricle in the midline. The posterior surface of cerebellum is related to the inner table of occipital bone. The anterolateral surface of cerebellum is related to the inner table of temporal bone. The cerebellum is connected to the brainstem by the superior, middle and inferior cerebellar peduncles. The cerebellar tonsils are located posterolateral to the medulla and cerebellar hemisphere. Normal range for the cerebellar tonsils below foramen magnum is 2 to 3 mm in adults and 5 mm in infants. When the cerebellar tonsils are more than 4 mm below foramen magnum ectopic position of cerebellar tonsils is considered. The cerebellar hemispheres consist of an outer shell of gray matter and an inner core of white matter. The inner core of white matter contains a collection of gray matter called the cerebellar nuclei. These nuclei are named as nucleus fastigius, nucleus globosus, nucleus emboliformis and dentate nucleus.

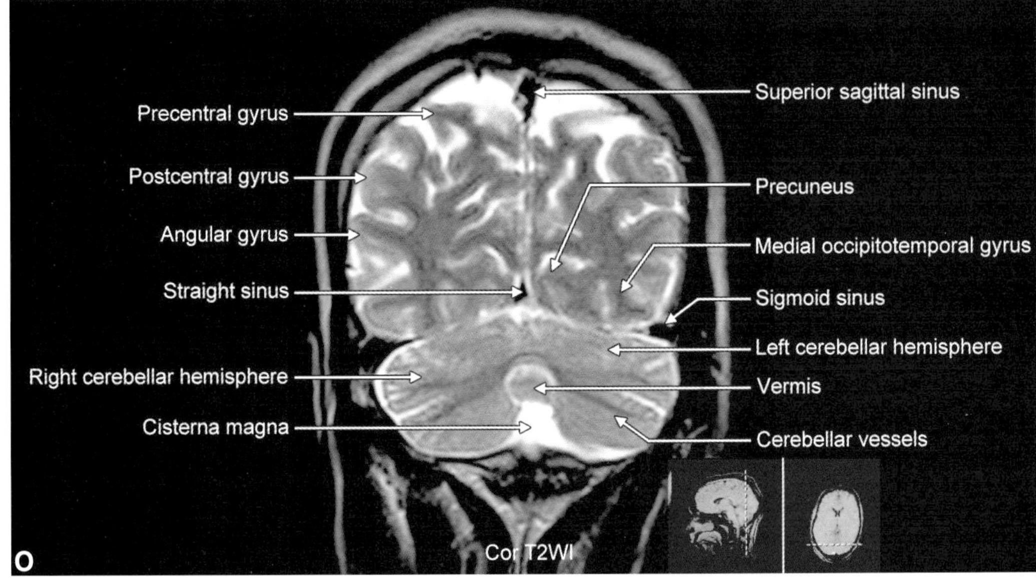

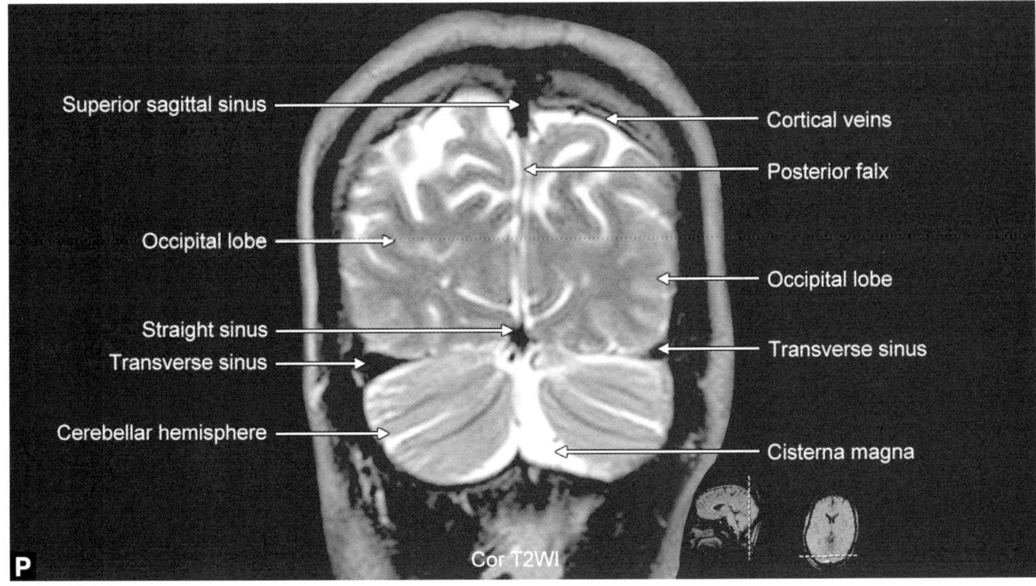

Incoming afferent fibers are essentially of two types. Climbing fibers are those which climb around the dendrites of the Purkinje cells. Olivocerebellar fibers are the only examples of climbing fibers. All other afferent fibers constitute Mossy fibers. These fibers end as synaptic rosettes with whom dendrites of granule cells synapse. Generally, all afferent fibers terminate in the cortex while giving small collaterals to the cerebellar nuclei. Fibers from the cortex end in the cerebellar nuclei. Efferent fibers from the cerebellar nuclei pass through the superior or inferior cerebellar peduncles to reach their destinations in the brainstem, spinal cord and the cerebrum. Morphologically, the cerebellum is divided into archicerebellum-flocculonodular lobe, paleocerebellum-central lobule, culmen, pyramid, uvula and their corresponding hemispherical lobes and neocerebellum-declive, folium, tuber and their corresponding cerebellar hemispheres. The archicerebellum corresponds to vestibulocerebellum the paleocerebellum corresponds to spinocerebellum and the neocerebellum corresponds to corticocerebellum. The cerebellum is supplied by blood from superior cerebellar and anterior inferior and posterior inferior cerebellar arteries. The cerebellum is mainly concerned with maintenance of equilibrium, muscle tone and muscle coordination. Lesions of the cerebellum typically result in ataxia, atonia and motor coordination difficulties.

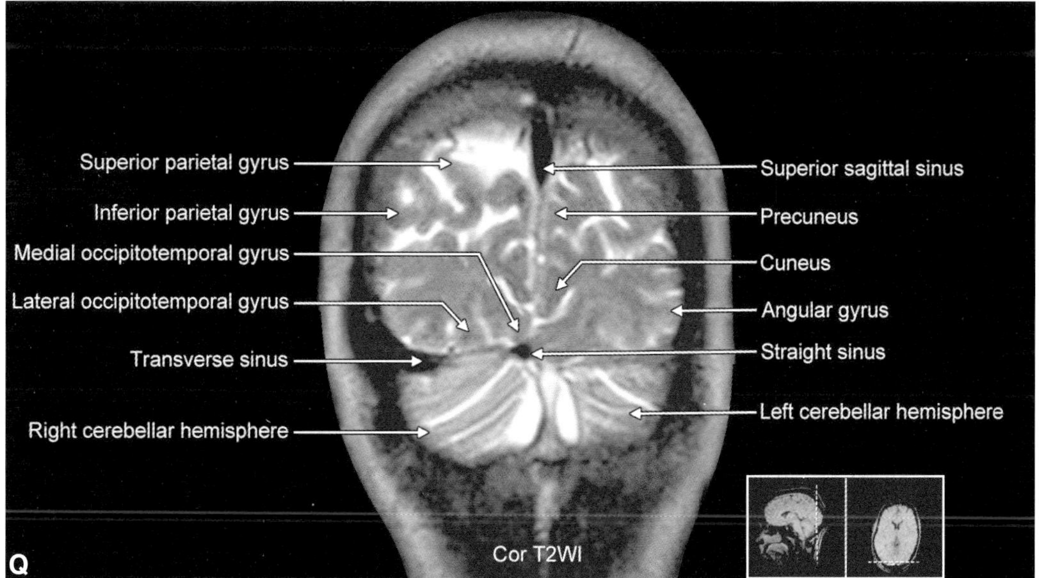

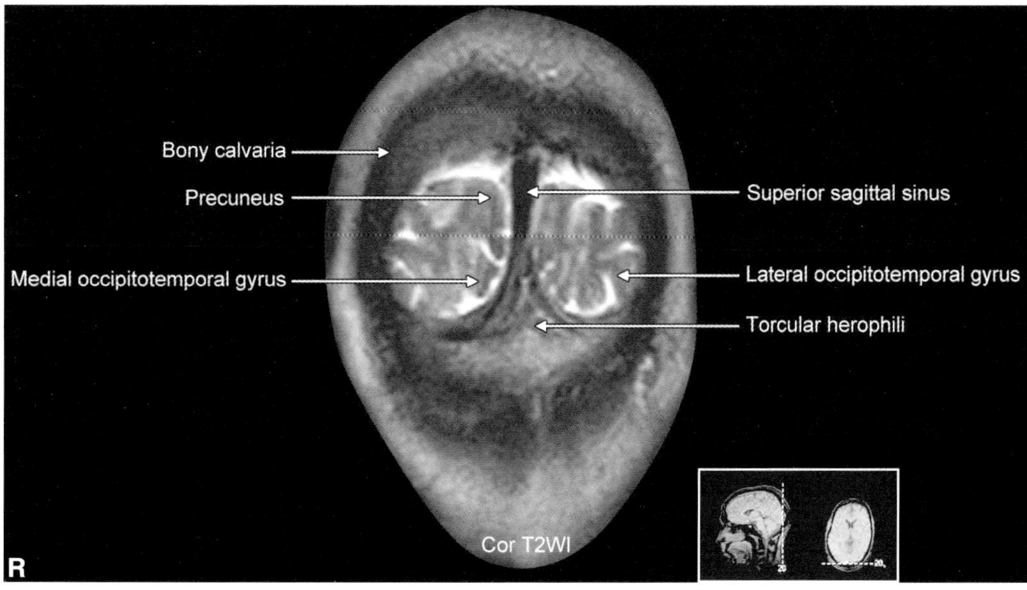

Figs 3A to R: MRI head coronal T2 weighted images

Falx Cerebri

Falx cerebri (Fig. 3M) appears isointense to hypointense on T1W images and hypointense to hyperintense on T2W images due to calcifications. The falx cerebri is the largest fold of dura mater, is seen as a thin membrane between the two cerebral hemispheres in the interhemispheric fissure. It is a double fold of the inner meningeal layer of dura matter. It lies in the longitudinal cerebral fissure. It is attached anteriorly to crista galli and posteriorly to the tentorium cerebelli. The falx cerebri is more wide posteriorly. It contains the superior sagittal sinus in its upper margin and the inferior sagittal sinus in its lower free margin.

Tentorium Cerebelli

Tentorium cerebelli (Fig. 3P) is a dura mater partition which makes a strong membranous roof or superior surface over the cerebellum as an arched lamina, elevated in the middle and supports the occipital lobes. Its anterior border is free and concave, with a large oval opening called incisura tentorii, for the transmission of the cerebral peduncles. It is attached; behind, by its convex border, to the transverse ridges upon the inner surface of the occipital bone, and there encloses the transverse sinuses.

Cerebrospinal Fluid and Ventricular System

- The cerebrospinal fluid (CSF) is hypointense on T1W images and hyperintense on T2W images. Its signal characteristics depend on image acquisition time (TR/TE), relaxation time of the CSF and its constituents, physiological flow factors. The CSF is produced by the choroid plexus of lateral ventricles, third and fourth ventricle. The CSF is in constant motion. In the ventricular system the CSF flow is cephalo-caudal direction. In the subarachnoid cisterns the flow is in the caudal-cephalic direction.
- *Ventricular system:*
  - Lateral ventricles (Figs 1J, L, M, 2G and 3C to F, and I) are large cavities located within the cerebral hemispheres. They contain the CSF and the choroid plexus. The lateral ventricles are seen on axial, coronal and sagittal MRI sections. The CSF within the lateral ventricles appears hypointense on T1W images and hyperintense on T2W images. The lateral ventricle has frontal horn, temporal horn and occipital horn (trigone). The inner lining of the lateral ventricles is formed by ependymal cells. Near the midline on the floor of lateral ventricles lies the interventricular foramen of Monro which allows the flow of CSF to the third ventricle.
  - Choroid plexus of lateral ventricle (Figs 1N and 3K) is seen on axial and coronal MRI images. The choroid plexus is a cluster of vascular glomera with a spongy appearance and is responsible for producing CSF. The glomera measures between 3 mm and 22 mm in size normally. The glomerula of the choroid plexus show hypointense signals on T1W images due to their vascularity or calcium deposits. On T2W images the glomerula of choroid plexus show variable heterogeneous signal intensity due to flow void, cysts, lipid deposits and calcifications.
  - Septum pellucidum (Figs 1M, N and 2C) appears as two thin leaves on the medial side of lateral ventricles in midline on axial and coronal MRI sections. They are isointense to hypointense on both T1W and T2W images. Occasionally, there may be a small cavity with CSF within the leaves of septum pellucidum; this is called cavum septum pellucidum.
  - Interventricular foramen (Fig. 2B) is seen at the floor of each lateral ventricle. This foramen connects the lateral ventricles to the third ventricle and allows the CSF to circulate.
  - Third ventricle (Fig. 3H) is a single midline cavity located between the two thalami on axial and coronal MRI sections. CSF within the third ventricle shows hypointense signal on T1W images and hyperintense signal on T2W images. The third ventricle communicates above with the lateral ventricles via the interventricular foramen of Monro. It communicates below with the fourth ventricle via the aqueduct of Sylvius. Its anterior wall is formed by lamina terminalis. The floor of the third ventricle is related to optic chiasma, infundibulum, mammillary bodies and the

midbrain tegmentum. The choroid plexus is located on the roof of the third ventricle. The lateral walls of the third ventricle are formed by the thalami.

- Aqueduct of Sylvius (Figs 2A and 3J) is a thin slit like tubular hollow structure which connects the third ventricle to the fourth ventricle. It is closely related to the midbrain anteriorly and the colliculi posteriorly. It is well visualized on axial and sagittal T1W images.
- Fourth ventricle (Figs 1C, D, 2A, B and 3L) is seen on T1W axial and sagittal MRI sections. It appears as a diamond shaped cavity on sagittal sections located behind the pons and medulla and in front of the cerebellum. On T1W images it appears as hypointense signal and on T2W images it appears as hyperintense. The fourth ventricle communicates above with the aqueduct of Sylvius. The midsagittal section is useful in evaluating the shape and configuration of the acqueduct of Sylvius. The fourth ventricle communicates below with the central canal of spinal cord.
- The foramina of Magendie and Luschka (Fig. 3O) are openings in the posterior walls of fourth ventricle which allow the cerebrospinal fluid in the ventricular system to enter the subarachnoid space. The lateral openings are called the foramina of Luschka and the midline opening is called the foramina of Magendie. The floor of the fourth ventricle is formed by the pons in its upper part and the medulla in the lower half.

- Subarachnoid space is the space between the arachnoid and the pia mater. Large collections of CSF within the subarachnoid spaces are called cisternal spaces are better seen on T2W images as hyperintense signals around the brain structures they surround. Blood vessels of the brain travel in the subarachnoid space for considerable distances before piercing the pia and entering the substance of the brain. The subarachnoid space contains the CSF. The subarachnoid space is continous with the subarachnoid space of the spinal cord. Subarachnoid hemorrhage is usually an arterial bleed while subdural hemorrhage is usually a venous bleed. Arterial bleeds could be a result of trauma to the bones of skull, rupture of aneurysms, etc. Venous bleeds are usually a result of tearing of the cerebral veins draining into the superior sagittal sinus due to a sudden antero-posterior movement of the brain as a result of severe injuries.
- The cisternal spaces (Figs 2B, 3K and N) are large collections of CSF in subarachnoid space. These cisternal spaces are named according to their location. The cisternal spaces contain the CSF and appear hypointense on T1W images and hyperintense on T2W images. In addition to the CSF, the cisternal spaces contents contain nerves and vessels. The cisternal spaces are:
  - The olfactory sulcal cistern (Figs 2B and 3G) contains olfactory bulb and tract.
  - The suprasellar cistern contains the optic nerve, optic chiasm, optic chiasm tract, pituitary stalk, internal carotid arteries, origins of middle and anterior cerebral arteries and posterior communicating artery.
  - The parasellar and Sylvian cisterns (Figs 2B and 3G) contain the middle cerebral artery, Meckel's cave and trigeminal nerve. The Sylvian cistern is a lateral extension of the suprasellar cistern.
  - The interpeduncular cistern (Fig. 3N) contains oculomotor nerve, basilar artery, posterior cerebral artery and superior cerebellar artery.
  - Mesencephalic cistern contains choroidal arteries, basal vein of Rosenthal, trochlear nerve and abducens nerve.
  - The cerebellopontine angle cistern (Fig. 1D) contains the facial nerve and acoustic nerve.
  - The medullary cistern (Figs 1A and 2B) contains the vertebral artery, the glossopharyngeal nerve, vagus nerve and hypoglossal nerve. The pontomedullary cistern is located in front of pons and medulla, it communicates laterally with the cerebellopontine cistern and posteriorly with the cisterna magna.
- Subdural space is a potential space between the dura mater and the underlying arachnoid mater. It acts like a bursa allowing movement between dura and the structures it encloses. Subdural hemorrhage usually occurs due to rupture of veins as they enter the dural venous sinuses and is identified on GRE recalled sequences.

CONGENITAL

Congenital Aqueductal Stenosis

The cerebral aqueduct of Sylvius is a narrow channel that connects 3rd and 4th ventricles and passes through the midbrain. Aqueductal stenosis is a common cause of obstructive hydrocephalus. Causes of a blockage of the aqueduct are congenital, post-infectious, idiopathic, and tumors.

CT is less effective at delineating the cause of the hydrocephalus. Stenosis of the aqueduct causes enlargement of both lateral and 3rd ventricle with a normal appearing 4th ventricle. MRI is the modality of choice enlargement of the ventricles and possible cause for aqueductal stenosis (Figs 4A to D).

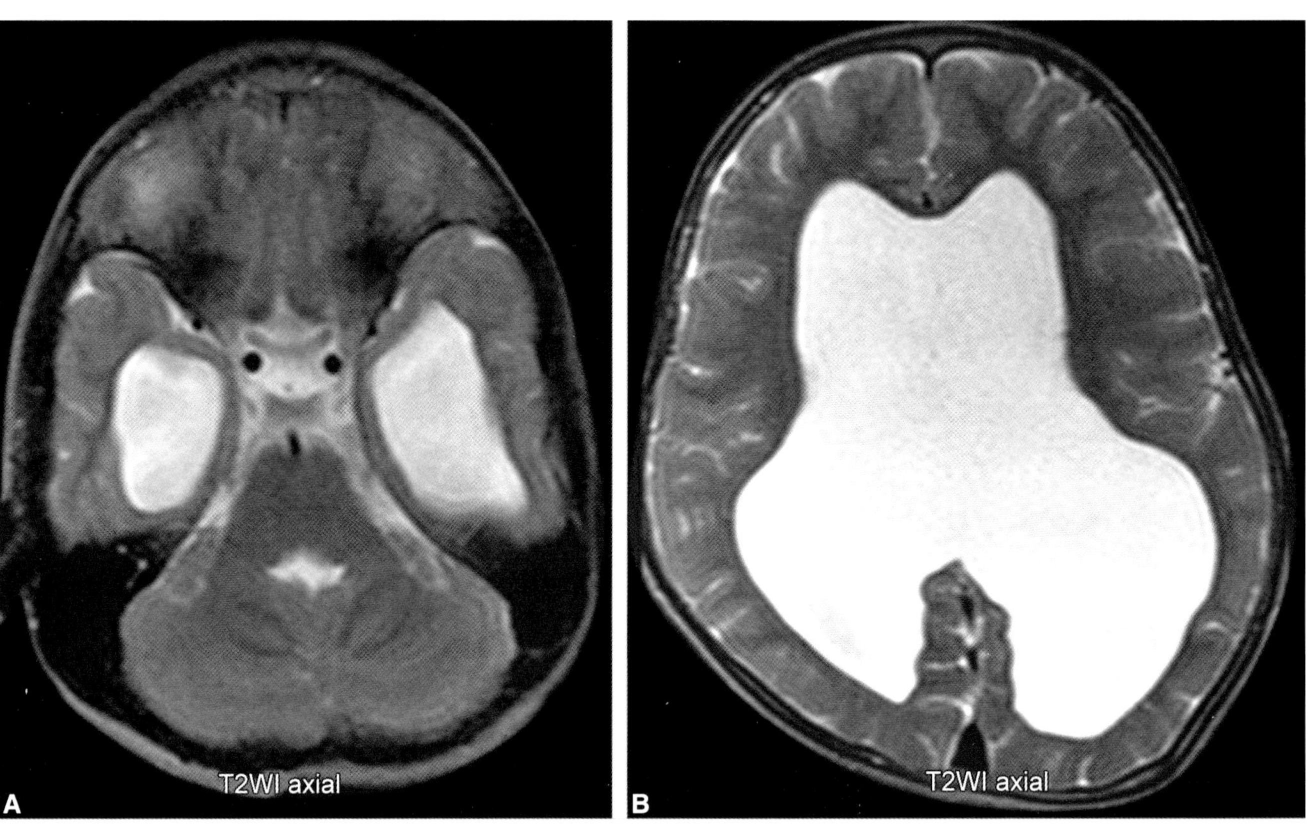

Figs 4A and B

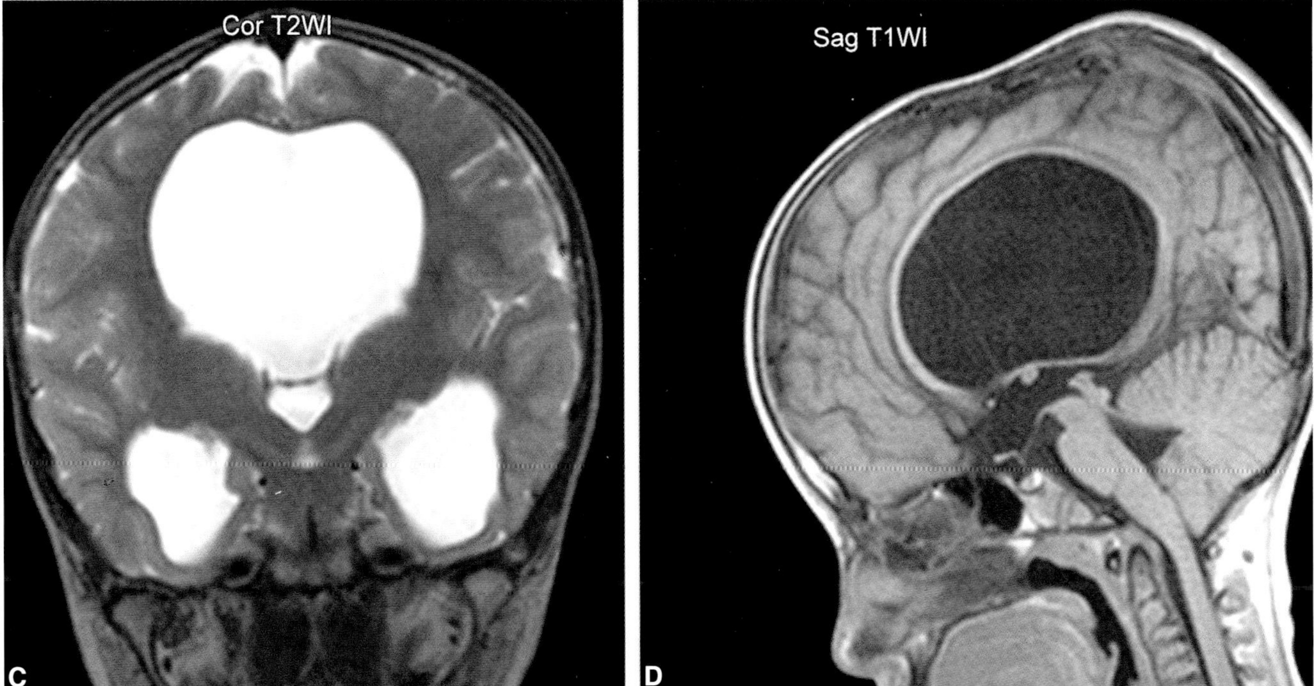

Figs 4C and D

Figs 4A to D: MR in a 2-month-old child, axial T2WI (A and B) shows dilatation leading to ballooning of lateral ventricles including temporal horns. Coronal T2WI (C) shows dilatation of frontal and temporal horns of lateral ventricles. Sagittal T1WI (D) shows dilatation of lateral and 3rd ventricles

Corpus Callosum Agenesis

Corpus callosum consist of rostrum, genu, body and splenium which forms from anterior to posterior except for the rostrum, which is bent downward and backward from genu to front of the septum pellucidum. Corpus callosum agenesis may be complete or partial. In partial agenesis, splenium and rostrum commonly undergo agenesis.

Imaging of complete callosal agenesis shows high riding third ventricle with spoke-like orientation of gyri around it, lateral ventricles are widely separated, parallel and non-converging (Figs 5A to D). Colpocephaly is commonly seen, lateral ventricles are indented superomedially by the longitudinal white matter bundles (Probst bundles).

Anomalies associated with corpus callosum agenesis are Chiari malformations, heterotopias, lissencephaly, schizencephaly, Dandy-Walker malformation, holoprosencephaly and lipomas.

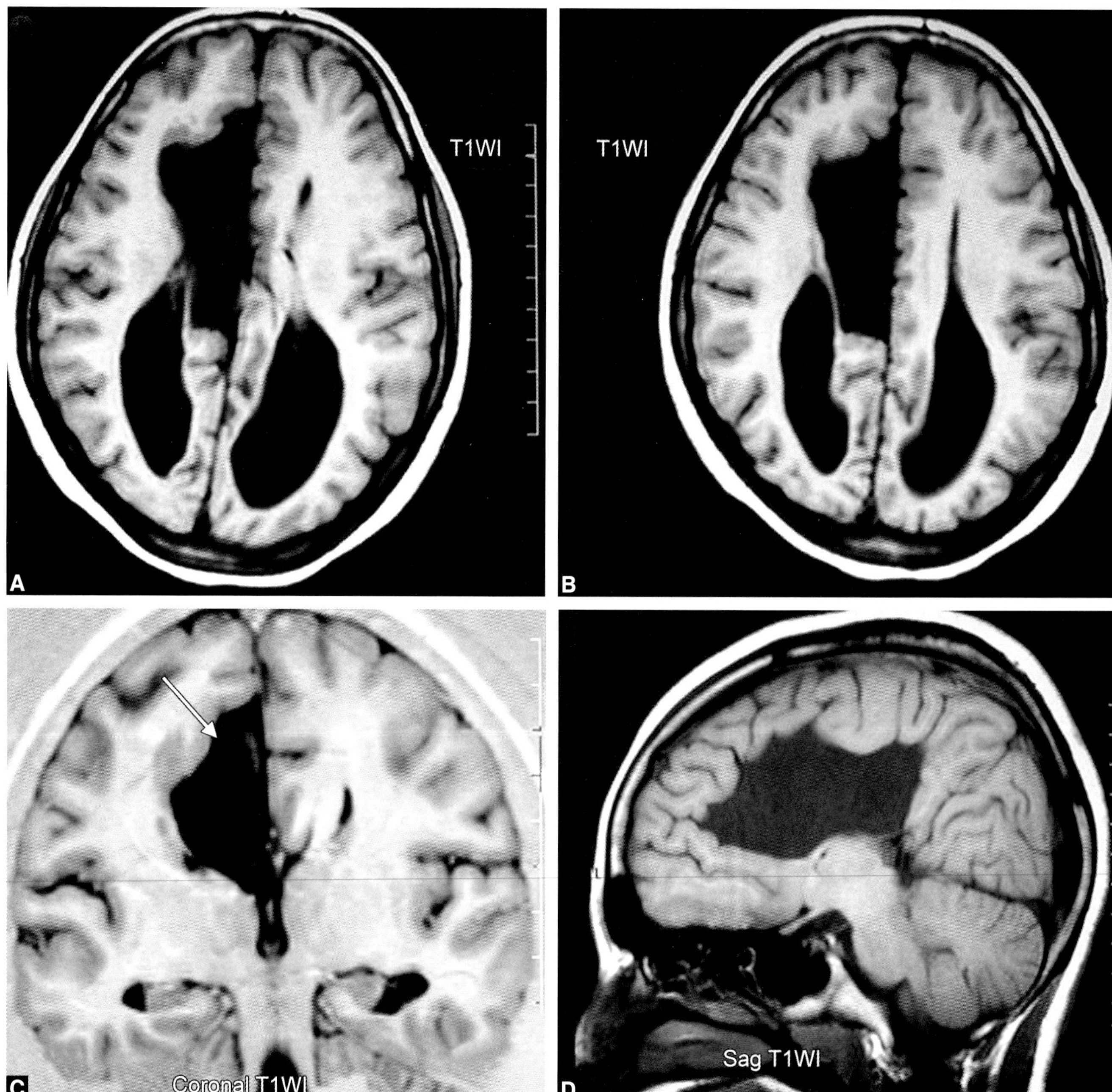

Figs 5A to D: T1W axial (A and B), coronal T1W (C) and sagittal T1W (D) images show agenesis of corpus callosum with a paramidline dorsal interhemispheric cyst lined by dysplastic cortex

Heterotopia

Heterotopia is collection of normal neurons in abnormal locations. It is caused by arrested migration of neurons from periventricular germinal zone to cortex. It can be inherited or acquired, where causes are maternal trauma, infection or toxins. It can be band-like (laminar) or nodular.

Subependymal heterotopias are most common, seen as nodules indenting the ventricles. On CT and MRI heterotopic gray matter is isodense with gray matter. Band heterotopias resemble double cortex (Figs 6A and B). Calcification is rarely seen in the heterotopic gray matter.

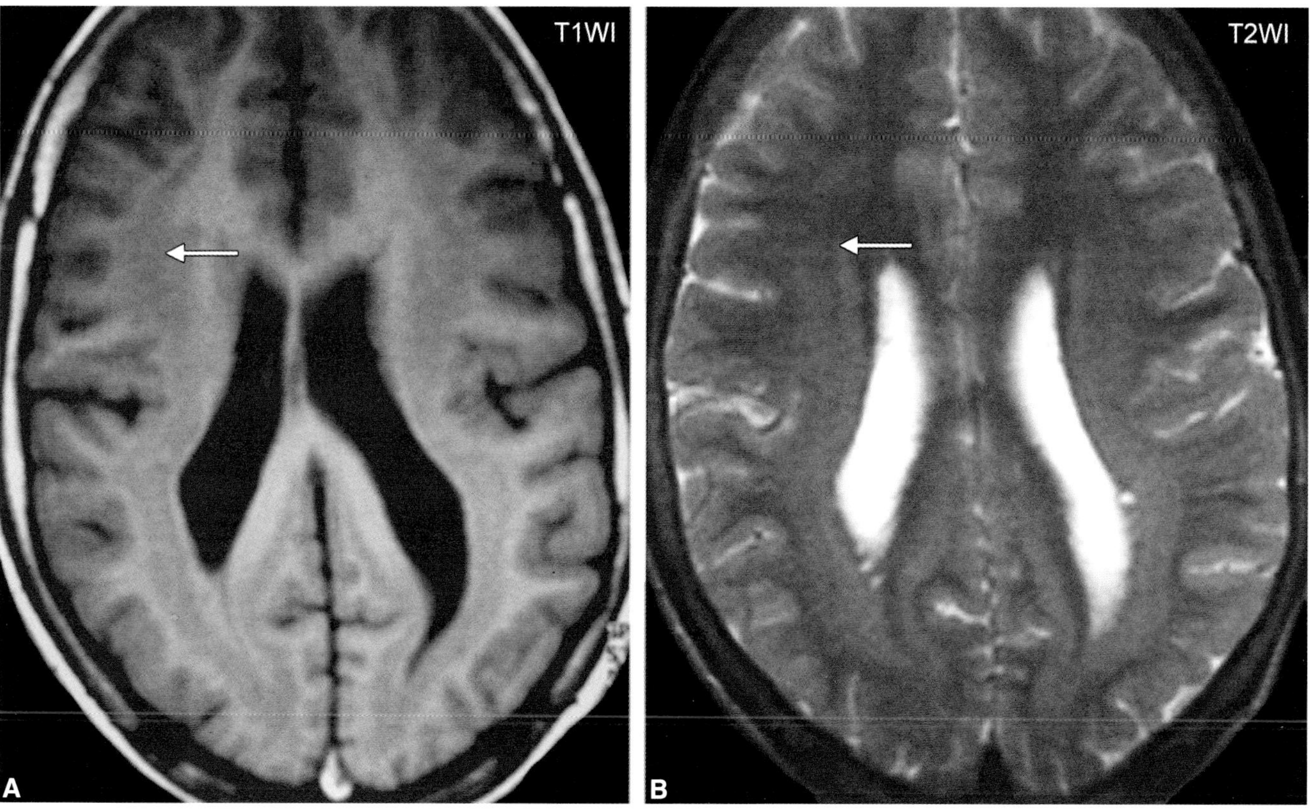

Figs 6A and B: Axial T1WI (A) shows band-like isointense gray matter seen in bilaterally in white matter (arrow). Axial T2WI (B) shows bilateral band heterotopia

Focal Cortical Dysplasia

Focal cortical dysplasia is a potent epileptic foci in children and leads to disorganization of the normal structure of the cerebral cortex resulting in intractable seizures, however they are amenable to surgical excision. The presence of ectopic neurons and bizarre glial cells, dysmyelination and a reduction in the number of myelinated fibers are likely responsible for the MR imaging characteristics (Figs 7A and B).

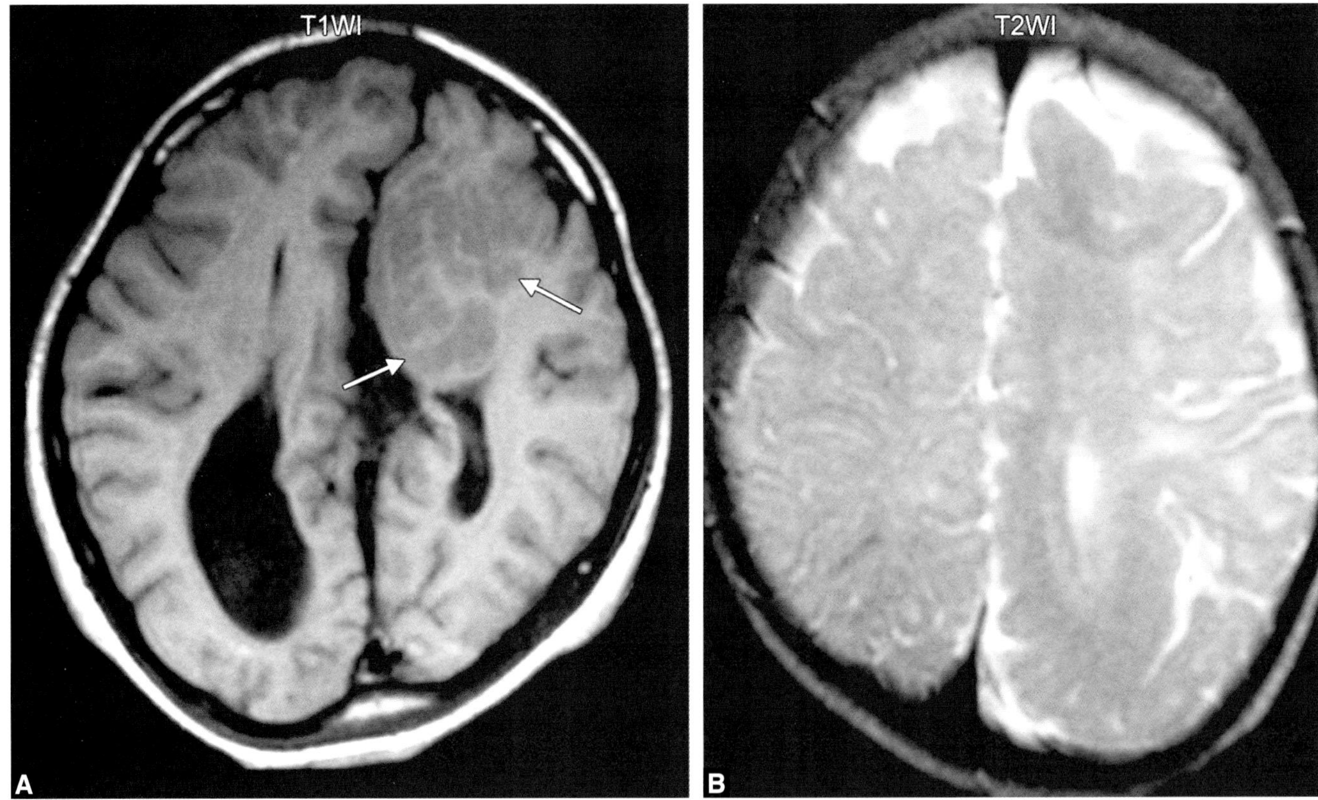

Figs 7A and B: MR T1WI (A) shows focal cortical enlargement in which sulci and gyri are appreciated (arrows) with resultant mass effect on the ipsilateral lateral ventricle and falx, there is dilatation of contralateral lateral ventricle. T2-weighted (B) image shows blurring of the gray and white matter junction and abnormal signal intensity in the white matter in left cerebral hemisphere

Chiari Malformation

Hans Chiari described congenital hindbrain anomalies in 1891 in which cerebellar tissue descends into cervical canal. He divided the malformation into four types.

Type I Consist of elongated peg-like cerebellar tonsils displaced into the upper cervical canal.

Type II Consist of vermis, pons, medulla and an elongated fourth ventricle displaced inferiorly into the cervical canal.

Type III Consist of hindbrain herniation into a low occipital or high cervical encephalocele in combination with features of the Chiari II malformation.

Type IV Consist of severe cerebellar hypoplasia and Chiari II signs with lumbosacral myelomeningocele.

Chiari Type I Malformation

Chiari type I malformation also known as cerebellar tonsil ectopia, this condition can be defined as a caudal protrusion of the cerebellar tonsils below the foramen magnum.

Main imaging features include low-lying peg-shaped cerebellar tonsils, more vertical appearance of the tonsillar sulci (Figs 8A and B) along with compression of cistern magna.

Position of cerebellar tonsils is measured with respect to the "opisthion-basion line", which is the line joining the anterior and posterior margins of the foramen magnum.

Cerebellar tonsils protruding more than 6 mm below this line is abnormal in the first decade and 5 mm in 2nd and 3rd decades. It is most pronounced at 4 years of age.

On radiography, features such as short clivus, atlas assimilation, craniovertebral segmentation, fusion anomalies or absence of cervical lordosis may be present. CT or MRI may reveal small posterior fossa. On MRI, one should look for presence of upper cervical cord edema and syrinx, which show correlation with the symptomatology.

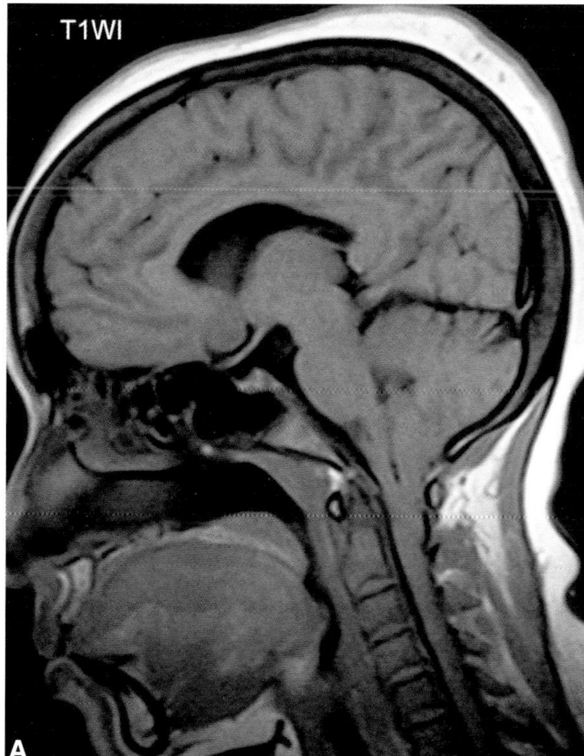

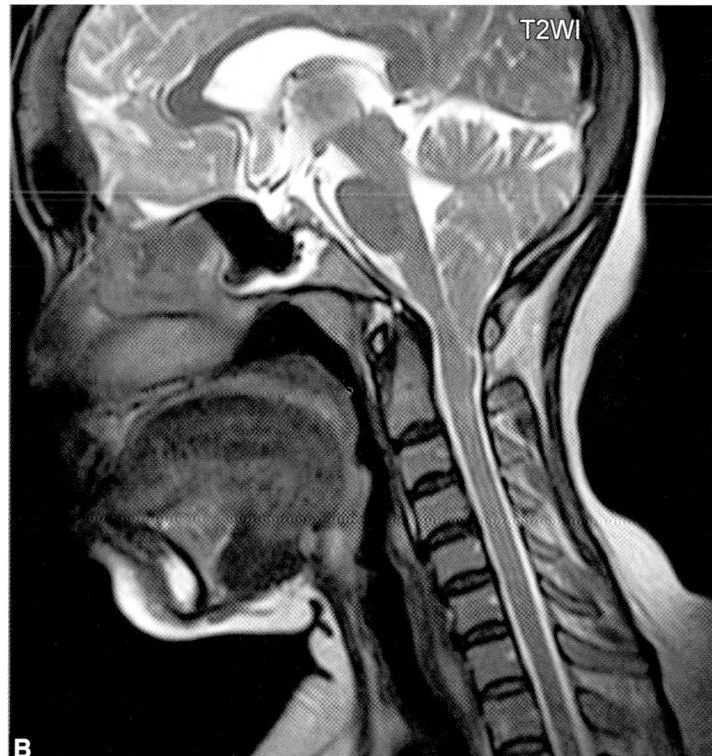

Figs 8A and B: Sagittal T1WI and T2WI show herination of peg-like tonsil in upper cervical region below the foramen magnum in the upper cervical region

Chiari Type II Malformation

Chiari type II malformation is a complex hindbrain malformation and is characterized by small posterior fossa herniation of cerebellar vermis, choroid plexus of fourth ventricle and part of medulla through foramen magnum (Figs 9A to E). It is associated with lacunar skull; neural tube closure defects such as myelomeningocele are present in almost all cases.

Tentorium is hypoplastic and falx may be fenestrated. It is best appreciated on sagittal MRI image, which shows cascading protrusions of vermian nodulus and uvula, fourth ventricle, medulla, and cervical cord into the spinal canal. Cervicomedullary "kinking" is characteristic. Tectum appears inferiorly beaked. Axial images show cerebellar hemispheres extending anteriorly surrounding the brainstem. Cerebellum may also herniate upward through the tentorial incisura. Hydrocephalus is present in majority of the cases. Other associated malformations include callosal

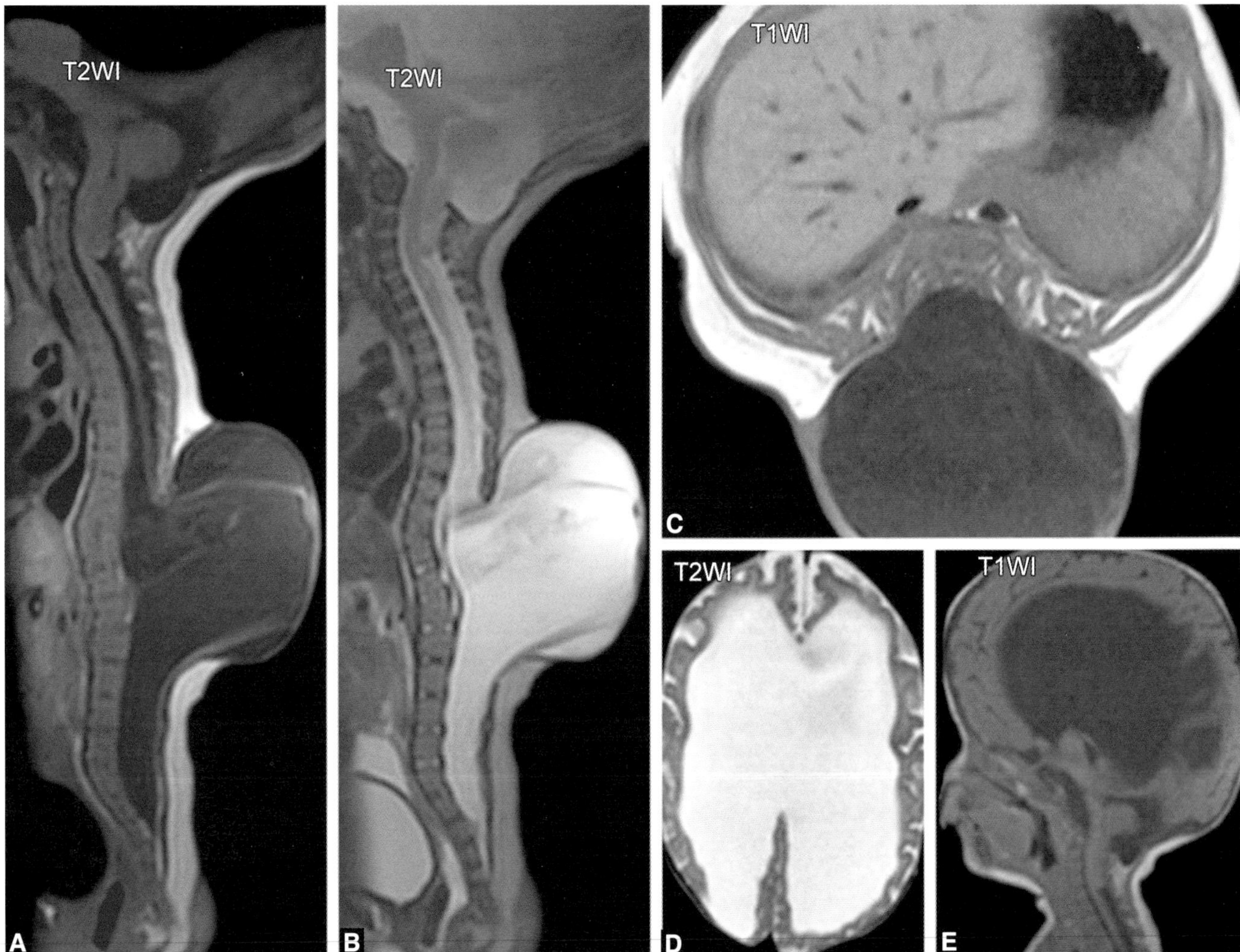

Figs 9A to E: In 1-day-old male neonate with Chiari type II malformation presented with swelling on back, no head holding with widely open sutures. MR sagittal T1W (A), sagittal T2W (B), axial T1W (C), axial T2W (D) and sagittal T1W (E) images show midline defect in the posterior elements of D9 to L2 vertebrae. A CSF filled sac is seen protruding through this defect beyond the plane of the back. It is not covered with skin. The spinal cord continues into the sac and the neural placode is adherent to the posterior aspect of the sac. Nerve roots are seen traversing through it. Segmentation anomalies are seen in the vertebral bodies at this level. No evidence of lipoma, dermoid or diastematomyelia. Small syrnix is seen in cervical cord. Cerebellar tonsils are peg shaped and low lying. Posterior fossa structures are small. There is severe dilatation of third and both lateral ventricles

dysgenesis, heterotopias, polymicrogyria and diastematomyelia. Syrinx is associated in about 70 to 90 percent of cases. Most of the imaging features are result of very small posterior fossa.

Chiari Type III Malformation

Chiari type III malformation may be defined as Chiari II malformation with high cervical or occipital meningoencephalocele. The herniated sac may contain meninges, cerebellum, occipital lobe or brainstem. Features of Chiari II malformation are present.

Chiari Type IV Malformation

In Chiari type IV malformation there is severe cerebellar hypoplasia and with Chiari II signs found in small subset of patients with lumbosacral meningomyelocele.

Findings in this entity include absent or severely hypoplastic cerebellum, small brainstem, and large posterior fossa cerebrospinal fluid spaces (Figs 10A and B).

Associated abnormalities with Chiari IV malformation are Dandy-Walker malformation and obstructive hydrocephalus.

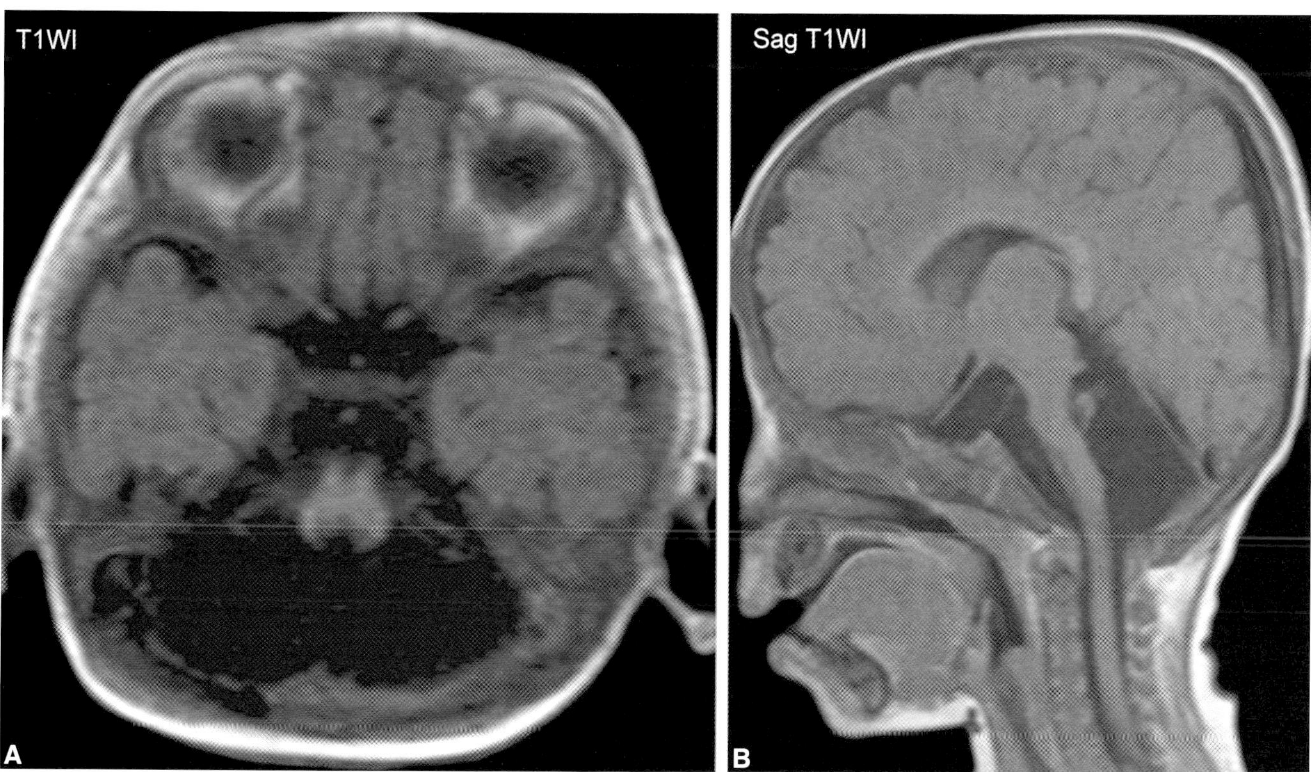

Figs 10A and B: A 2-year-boy, who presented with developmental delay. Axial (A) and sagittal (B) T1W images reveal near complete aplasia of the cerebellum. Only a small superior portion of vermis is seen. The posterior fossa is filled with CSF. The brainstem is small in size

Vermian Hypoplasia

Malformations of the posterior fossa have been recognized more frequently during the past few decades as the result of recent advances in imaging technology. With the advent of magnetic resonance imaging (MRI), the resolution of cranial structures including the mid-hind brain regions has improved dramatically.

The following conditions are associated with vermian hypoplasia (Figs 11A and B):

- Joubert syndrome (JS) is one of the most commonly diagnosed syndromes associated with the molar tooth sign (MTS), or hypoplasia/dysplasia of the cerebellar vermis accompanied by brainstem abnormalities. JS is defined clinically by features of hypotonia in infancy later development of ataxia, developmental delays, mental retardation abnormal breathing patterns, abnormal eye movements specific to oculomotor apraxia or the presence of the MTS on the cranial MRI. JS is an autosomal recessive condition with an estimated prevalence of 1: 100,000.
- Dandy-Walker malformation (DWM) is a relatively common congenital brain malformation with a prevalence of 1:5,000 live births. DWM is characterized by enlarged posterior fossa and in which the cerebellar vermis is completely absent, or present in a rudimentary form, sometimes rotated accompanied by elevation of the fourth ventricle. It is also commonly associated with dysplasias of brainstem nuclei. DWM has been reported to be in association with a wide array of chromosomal anomalies, including trisomy 18, trisomy 9, and trisomy 13. Prenatal exposure to teratogens such as, rubella or alcohol, are correlated with development of Dandy-Walker malformation.
- Rhombencephalosynapsis is a rare anomaly characterized by the absence or severe dysgenesis of the cerebellar vermis (Figs 11C and D) with fusion of the cerebellar hemispheres, peduncles, and dentate nuclei. Diagnostic features include fusion of the midbrain colliculi, hydrocephalus, absence of the corpus callosum and other midline structural brain malformations.

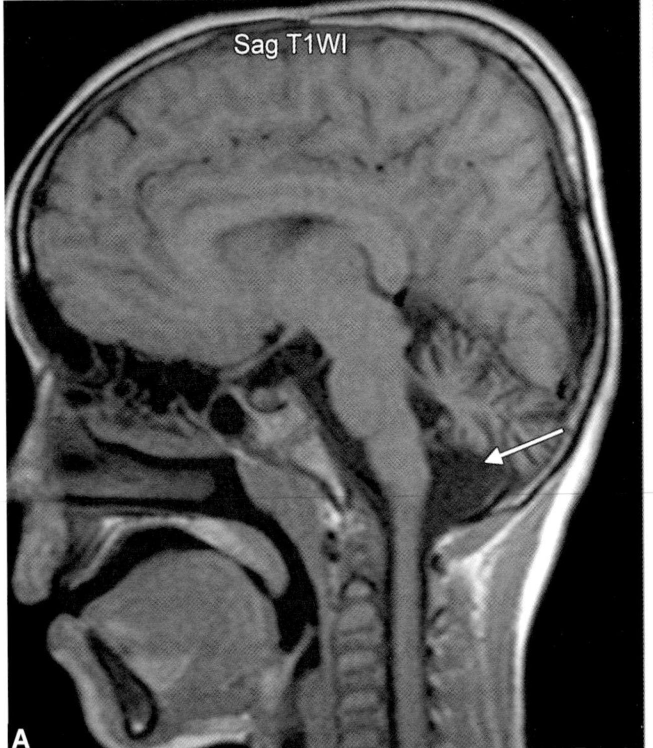

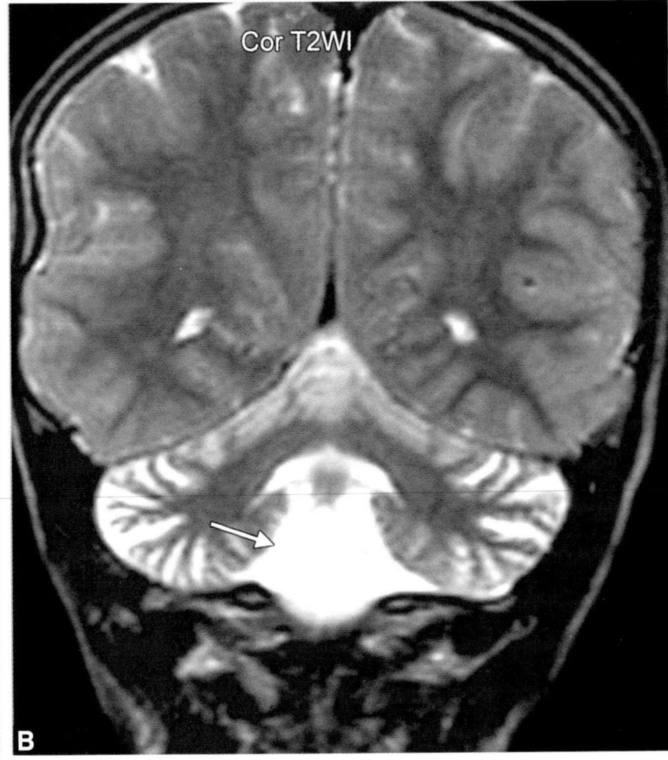

Figs 11A and B

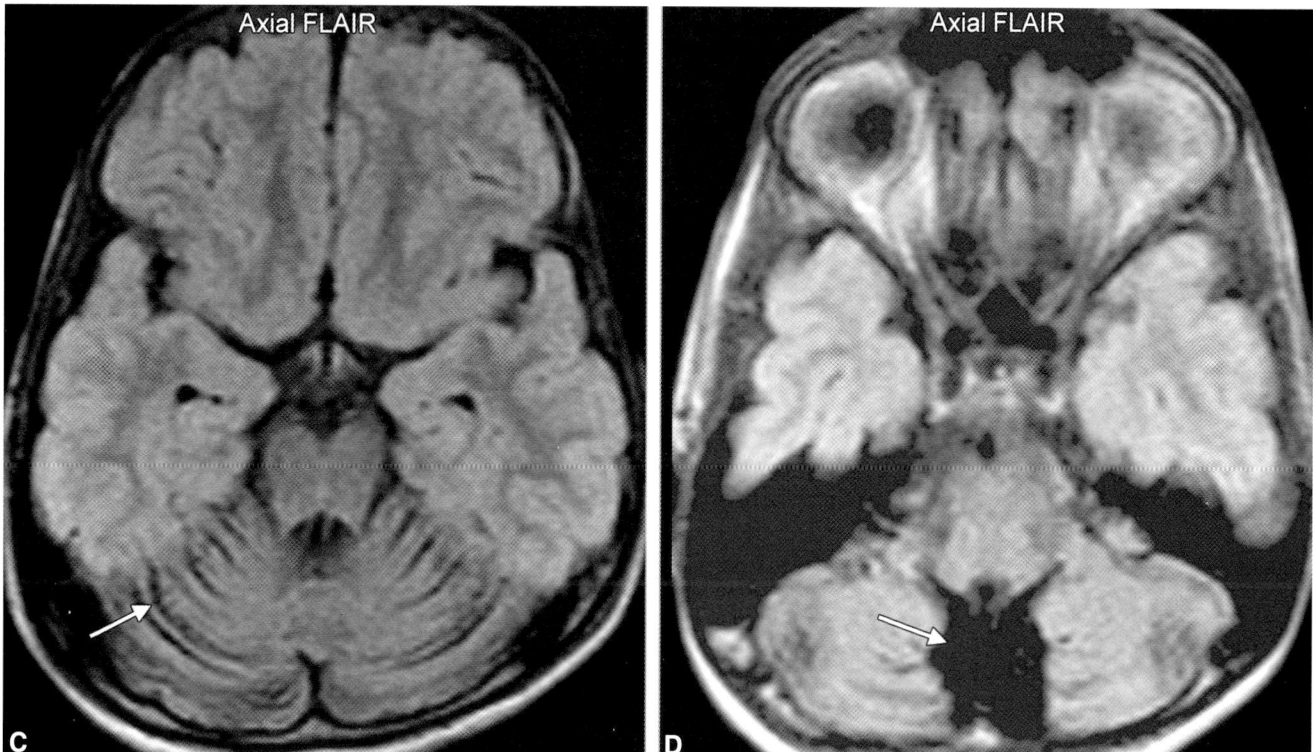

Figs 11C and D

Figs 11A to D: Sagittal T1W (A) and coronal T2W (B) images show inferior vermian hypoplasia (arrow). FLAIR axial images show cerebellar atrophy (C) and inferior vermian hypoplasia (D)

Joubert's Syndrome

Joubert's syndrome is inherited hypoplasia or aplasia of cerebellar vermis. Fourth ventricle is enlarged and has a typical "bat-wing" or "umbrella" appearance, isthmus is narrow and midbrain has the typical "molar tooth" (Figs 12A and B) appearance (arrow). Abnormal signal may be noted in periventricular white matter. Associated abnormalities include holoprosencephaly, frontonasal dysplasia and pituitary hypoplasia.

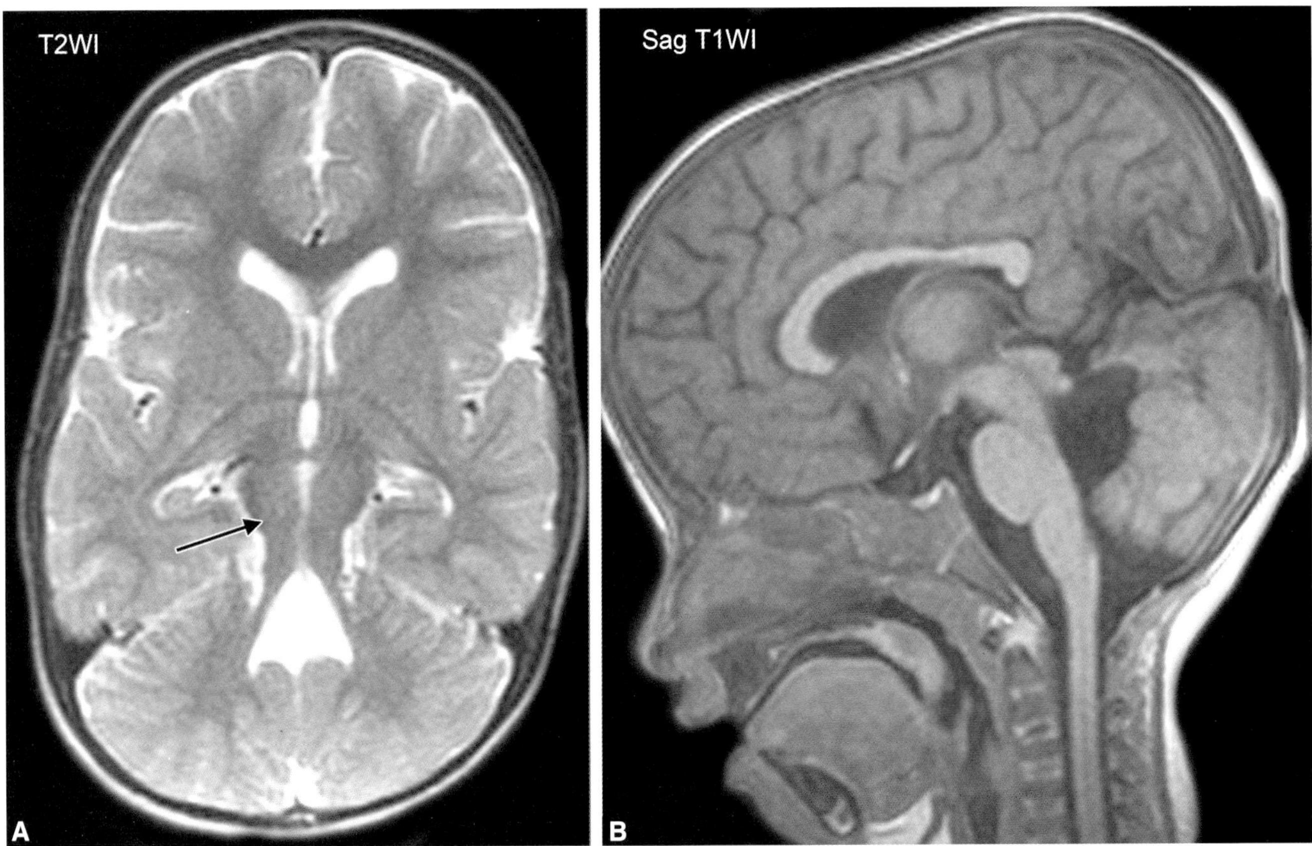

Figs 12A and B: In a 3-year-old girl axial T2W (A) and sagittal T1W (B) images reveal dysgenetic superior vermis, elongated bat wing shaped fourth ventricle with superior convex margin and hypoplastic superior cerebellar peduncles seen as molar tooth sign (arrow)

Temporal Choroidal Fissure Cyst

The temporal portion of the choroidal fissure is a cleft, in a C-shaped arc, between the fornix and the thalamus, where the choroid plexuses join. The tela choroidea invaginates into the temporal horn and forms the choroid plexus. The development of the choroidal fissure and choroid plexus can lead to errors that may result in a cyst.

In temporal choroidal fissure cyst the patients often present with complex partial seizure and medical treatment generally provides seizure control

On MR (Figs 13A and B) the signal intensity of the choroidal fissure cyst is identical to that of the cerebrospinal fluid. The choroid plexus cyst and choroidal fissure cyst are similar. Both are neuroepithelial cysts, probably due to sequestration of neuroectoderm and vascular pia mater or ependymal diverticulum formation and both are lined by epithelium.

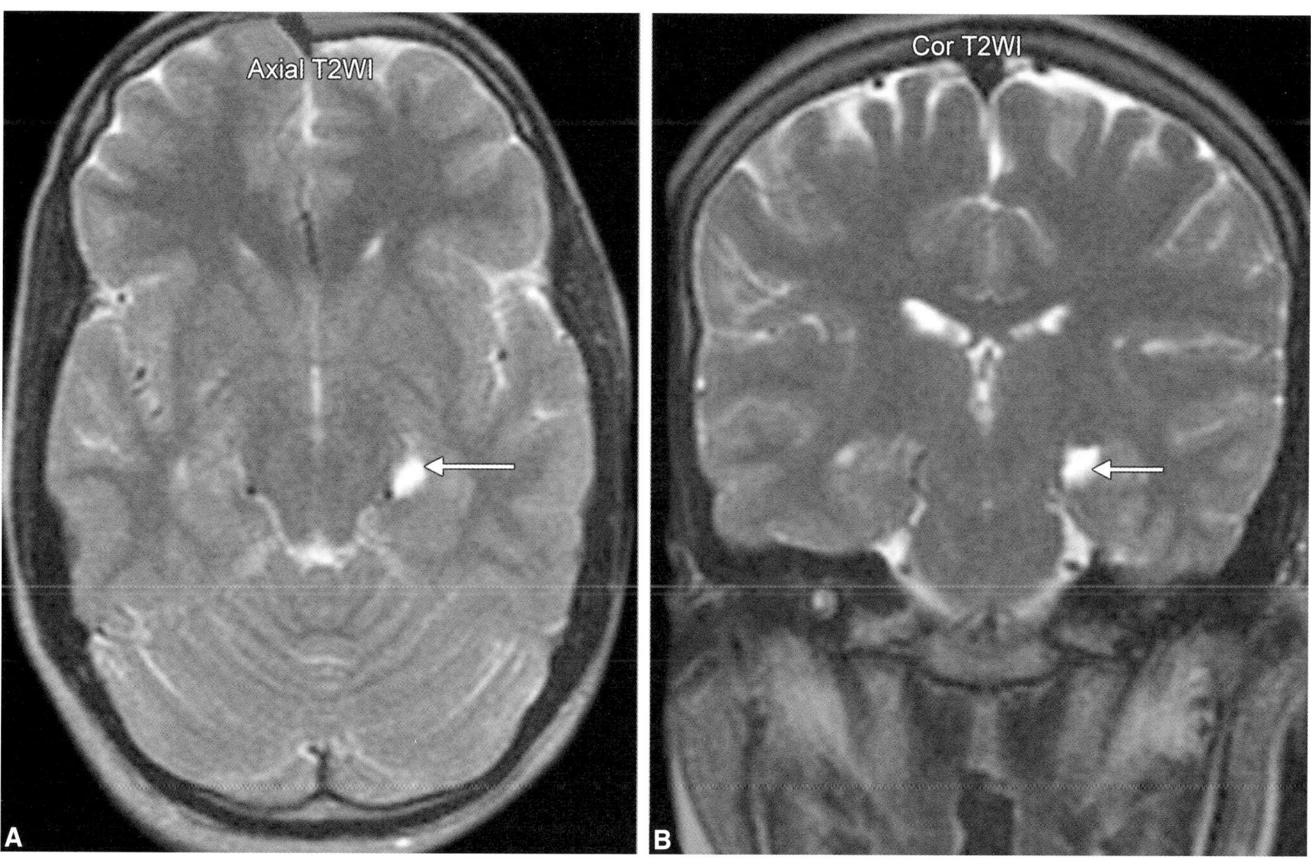

Figs 13A and B: Axial (A) and coronal (B) T2W images reveal an approximately 8 × 6 mm hyperintense lesion (arrow) in the left temporal lobe abutting the hippocampus. MR findings are consistant with temporal choroidal fissure cyst

INFECTIONS

Tuberculoma

Tuberculoma is nodular space-occupying lesion of size from one to several centimeter, frequently with a central caseous necrotic core surrounded by epitheloid cells, lymphocytes and Langerhans giant cells.

CNS tuberculomas present with a slow progressing mass lesion syndrome with focal seizures or neurological deficits. Fever and other signs of systemic infection are rarely present.

CT and MRI show one or more lesions with uniform or ring-like enhancement. Most common sites are the cortical, subcortical regions and the basal ganglia. On CT the lesion is hypodense to brain parenchyma and may be missed if the scan is performed without contrast. On MRI it is isointense to brain parenchyma on T1-weighted images and shows a central hyperintensity surrounded by a hypointense rim on T2-weighted images. The hypointense component is believed to correspond to gliosis, macrophage infiltration and fibrosis. Post-contrast T1W image shows ring enhancing lesions (Figs 14 to 16). It is important to differentiation between tuberculoma and neurocysticercosis (Table 1).

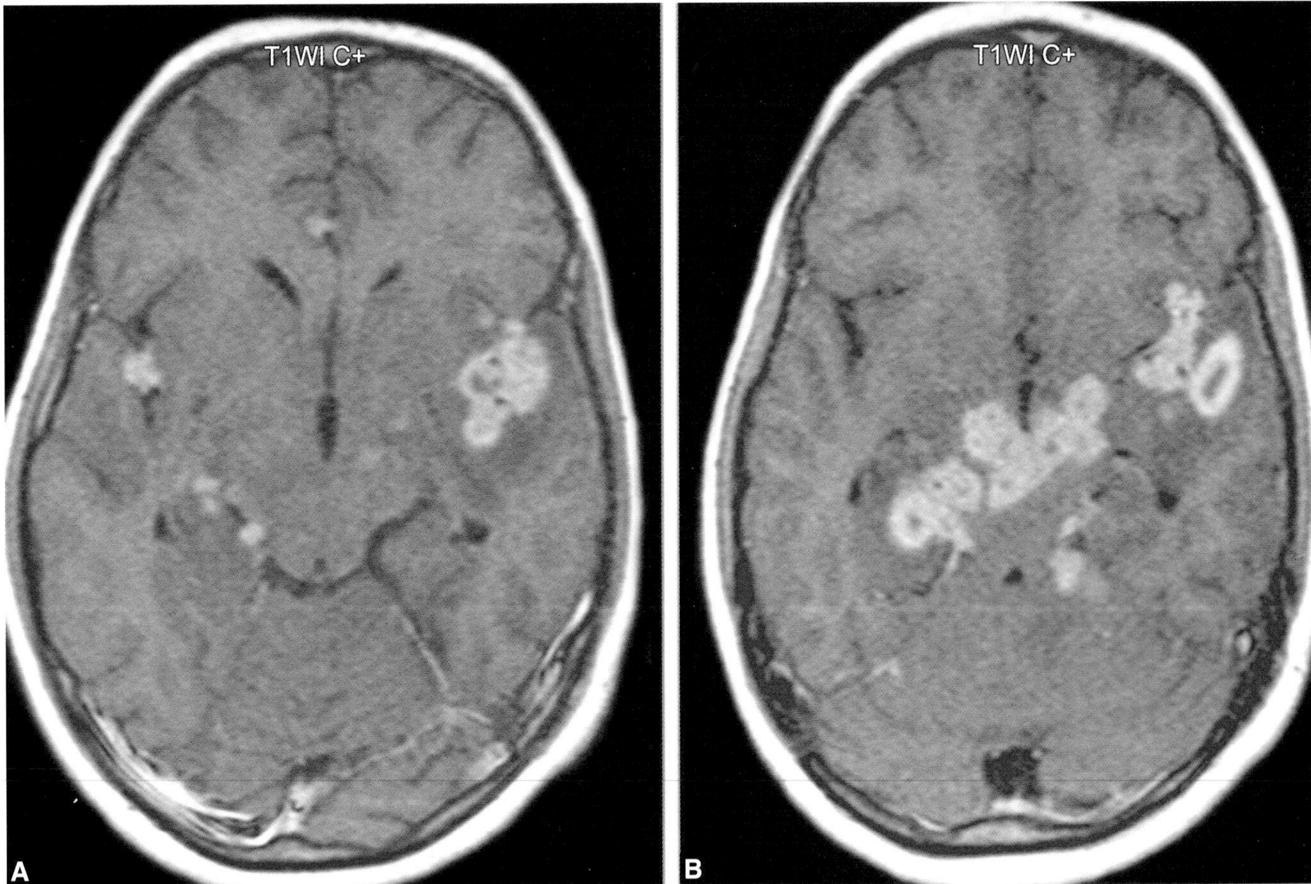

Figs 14A and B: Post-contrast T1W image axial images shows conglomerate ring enhancing lesions seen in basal, Sylvian cisterns and left temporal region

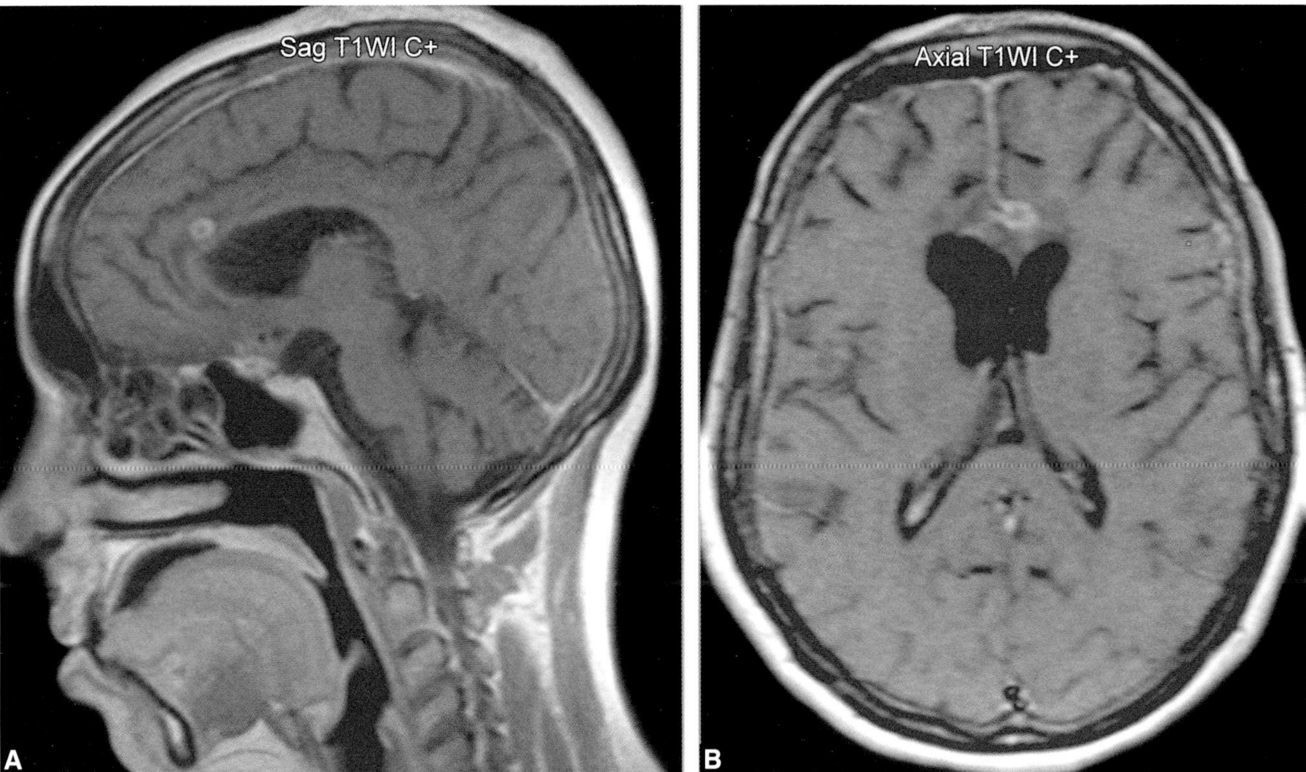

Figs 15A and B: In another case (A) Sag T1WI post-contrast shows ring enhancing lesion seen in pericallosal region; (B) Axial T1W contrast image shows ring enhancing lesion seen in the parafalcine region on left side with mild prominence of right lateral ventricle

Table 1: Differentiation between tuberculoma and neurocysticercosis

S. No.	*Features*	*Tuberculoma*	*Neurocysticercosis*
1.	Size	> 2 cm	< 2 cm
2.	Scolex	Absent	Present
3.	Stages	Not seen	Four stages
4.	MR spectroscopy	Increased choline peak	Increased lipid peak
5.	Meningitis	Associated	Not associated
6.	MR appearance	Central hyperintensity surrounded by a hypointense rim on T2-weighted images	Hyperintense on T2WI
7.	Conglomerated lesion	Seen	Not seen
8.	Number	Mostly single	Mostly multiple

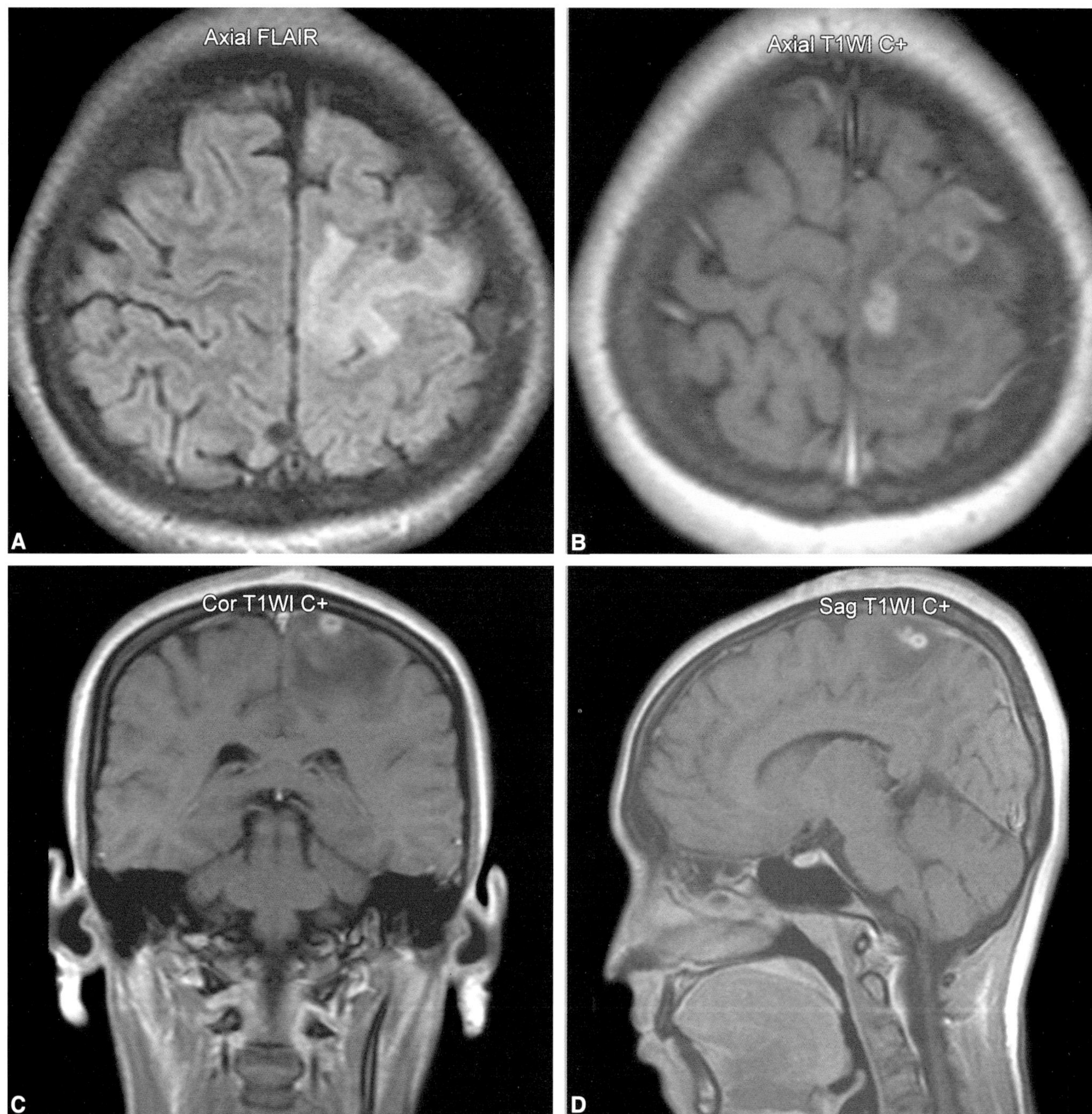

Figs 16A to D: In another case (A) Axial FLAIR image shows hypointense lesion seen in left high parietal region with edema extending up to left high parafalcine region; (B to D) Axial, coronal and sagittal post-contrast T1WI show ring enhancing lesions seen in left high parietal region with perilesional edema suggestive of active granuloma

Neurocysticercosis

Cysticercosis is the most common central nervous system parasitic infection. The causative agent is the larval form of the intestinal tapeworm *Taenia solium*. *Taenia* lives in the intestine of infected humans as an asymptomatic infestation. The worms release the eggs in the feces. The eggs may be ingested from contaminated food and water. Both humans and pigs are susceptible to egg infection. Once in the intestine of their host the eggs develop into oncospheres, the primary larvae. These larvae penetrate the intestinal mucosa, enter the circulatory system and seed into the neural, muscular and ocular tissues.

The symptoms depend principally on the degree of inflammatory response of the host to the dying larvae. The location of the cyst may be parenchymal, subarachnoid or intraventricular. Parenchymal cysts most often present with seizures and subarachnoid or intraventricular cysts with meningismus or hydrocephalus.

On MR, the signal of the lesions appear hypointense on T1WI and hyperintense on T2WI (Figs 17 and 18) seen in vesicular stage. On colloidal stage the cyst appear hyperintense on T1WI and isointense to hypointense on T2WI. Sometimes, these parasites are so numerous that the brain resembles a swiss cheese.

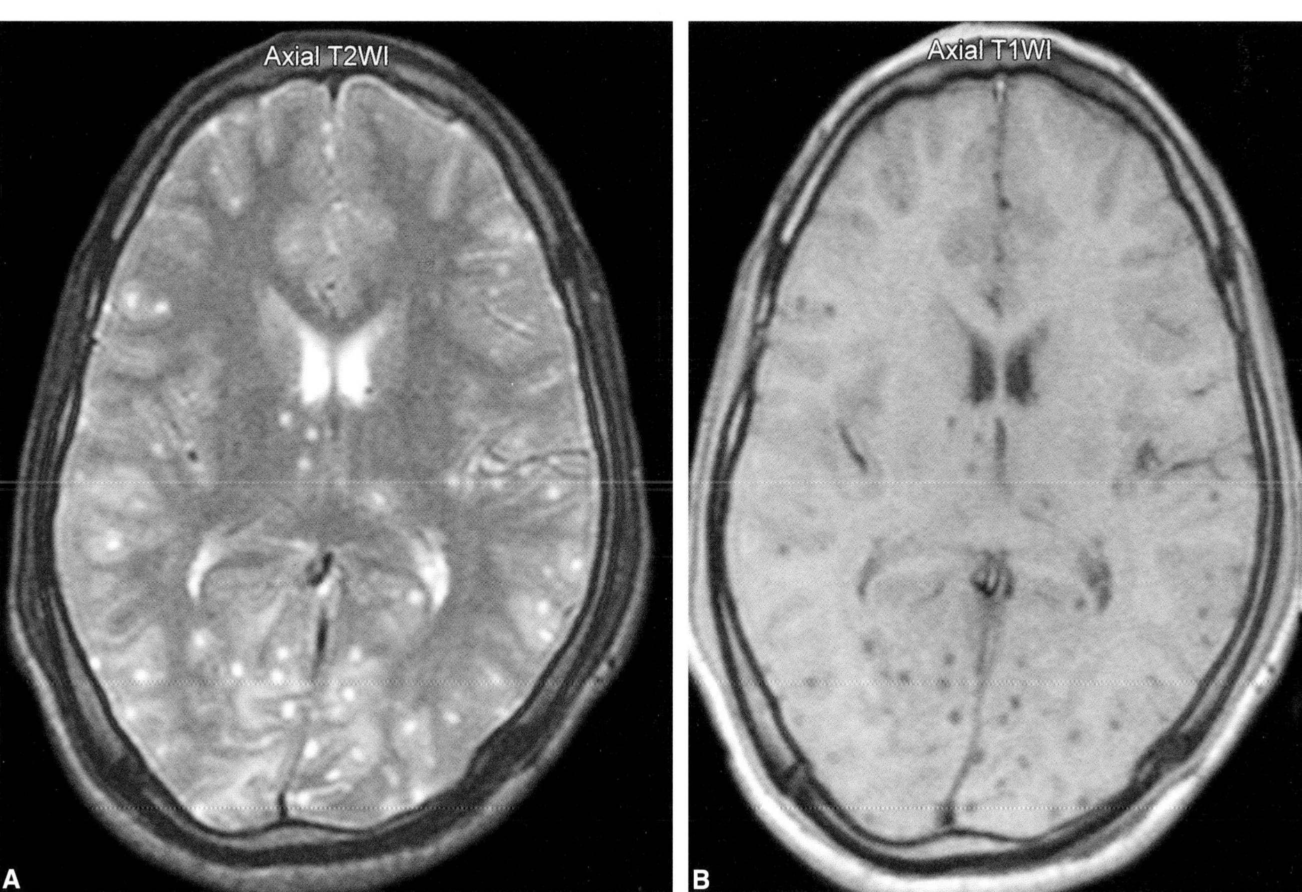

Figs 17A and B

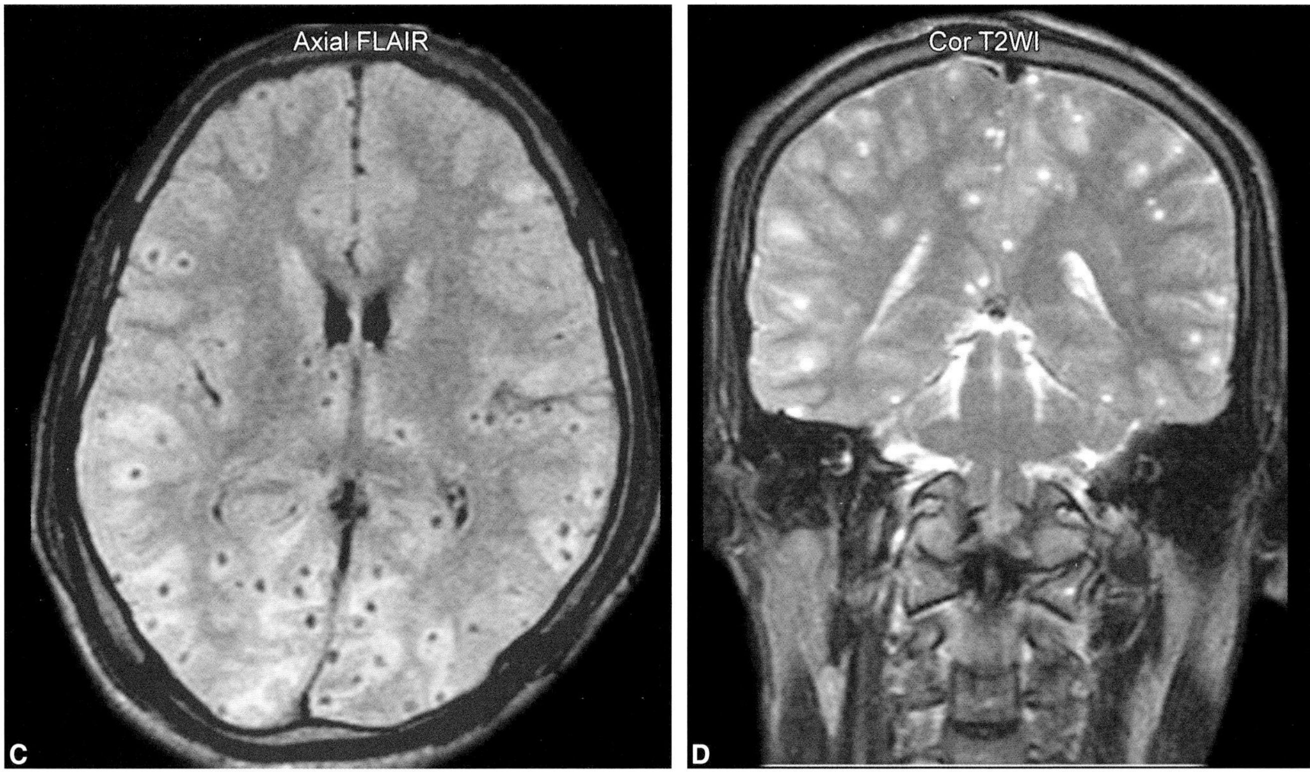

Figs 17C and D

Figs 17A to D: T2WI axial (A) show multiple tiny hyperintense lesions scattered throughout brain parenchyma, appearing hypointense on T1WI (B) seen predominantly in occipital lobe. Axial FLAIR image (C) and coronal T2WI (D) shows multiple hyperintense lesions scattered throughout the brain parenchyma

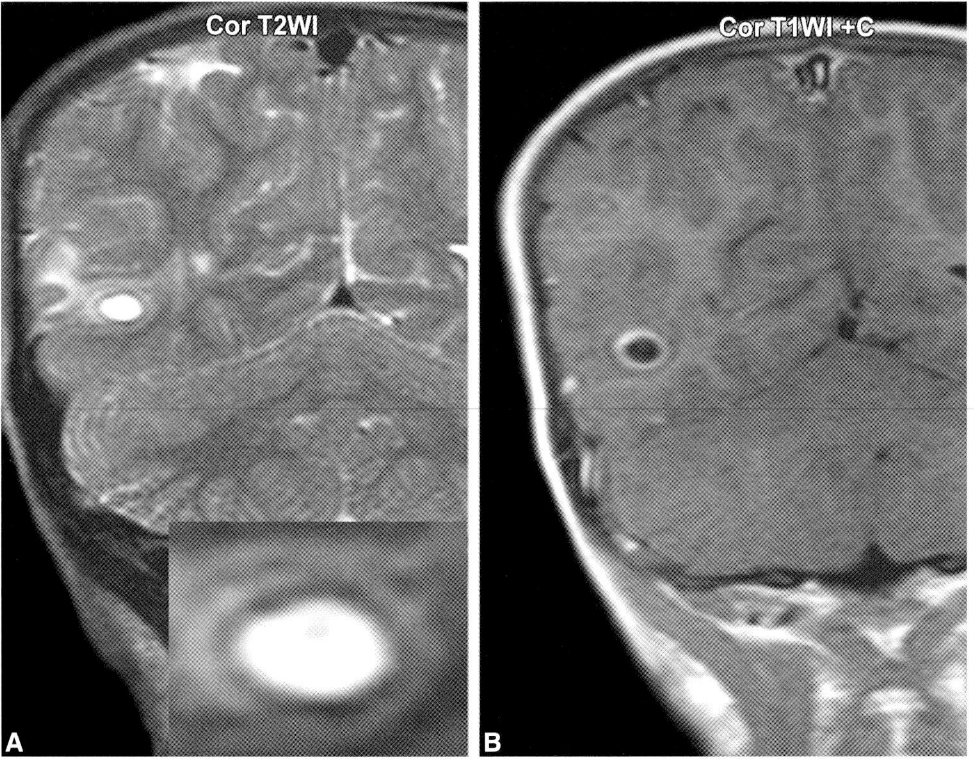

Figs 18A and B: Another case T2W coronal image (A) in 6-year-old male shows a small cystic lesion with hypointense rim and eccentric hypointense nodule (inset) the scolex, surrounding white matter hyperintensity is due to perilesional edema. Post-contrast coronal T1W images reveal smooth peripheral enhancement with mild enhancement of the nodule (B)

Brain Abscess

Cerebral abscess is an infectious process in which a phase of inflammation involving vessels and brain tissue develops into organized pus collection surrounded by a capsule. Patient presents with headache and focal neurological deficit. This may progress to a raised intracranial pressure syndrome with nausea, vomiting and impairment of consciousness with fever.

Extensions of infection from an otologic infection (30%), sinusitis (15%) are the most frequent causes. Hematogenous seeding from a distant focus of infection accounts for about 25 percent of cases. Endocarditis is the most frequent source of hematogenous infection. Other causes of brain abscess are dental and facial infections, trauma with penetrating injuries and surgery.

On CT there is focal, usually round or oval expanding lesion. Lesion shows a hypodense center with an outlying uniform ring surrounded by a variable hypodense region of brain edema. Ring like contrast enhancement is seen. Ring-enhancing lesions are not diagnostic of abscess. Tumors, granulomas and resolving hematomas may have the same appearance. As compared to tumors abscesses usually exhibit thinner, more regular and more homogeneously enhancing rings. On MRI, the three regions (necrotic central region, surrounding rim and edema) may be seen clearly (Figs 19A to E). The necrotic central region shows a different signal as compared to CSF, higher on both T2- and T1-weighted images.

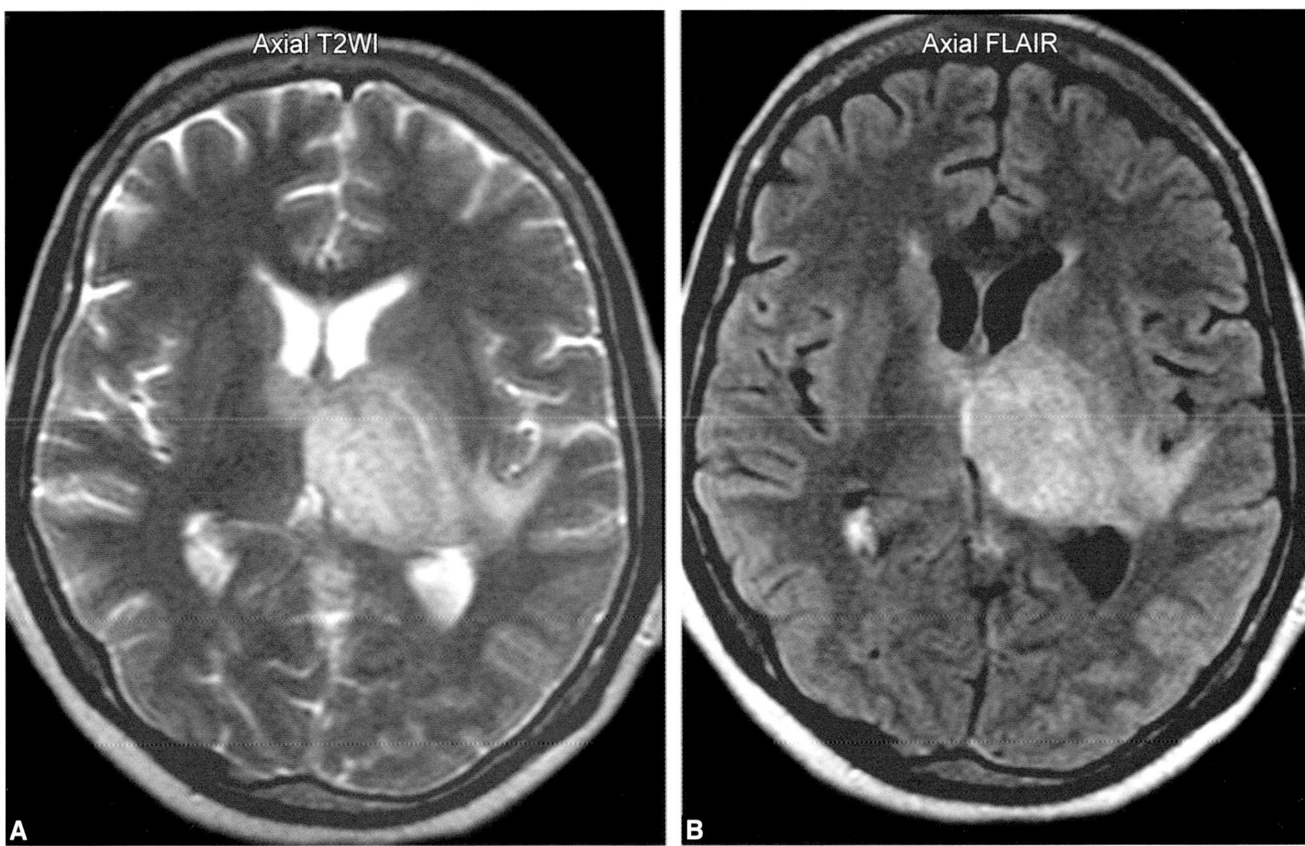

Figs 19A and B

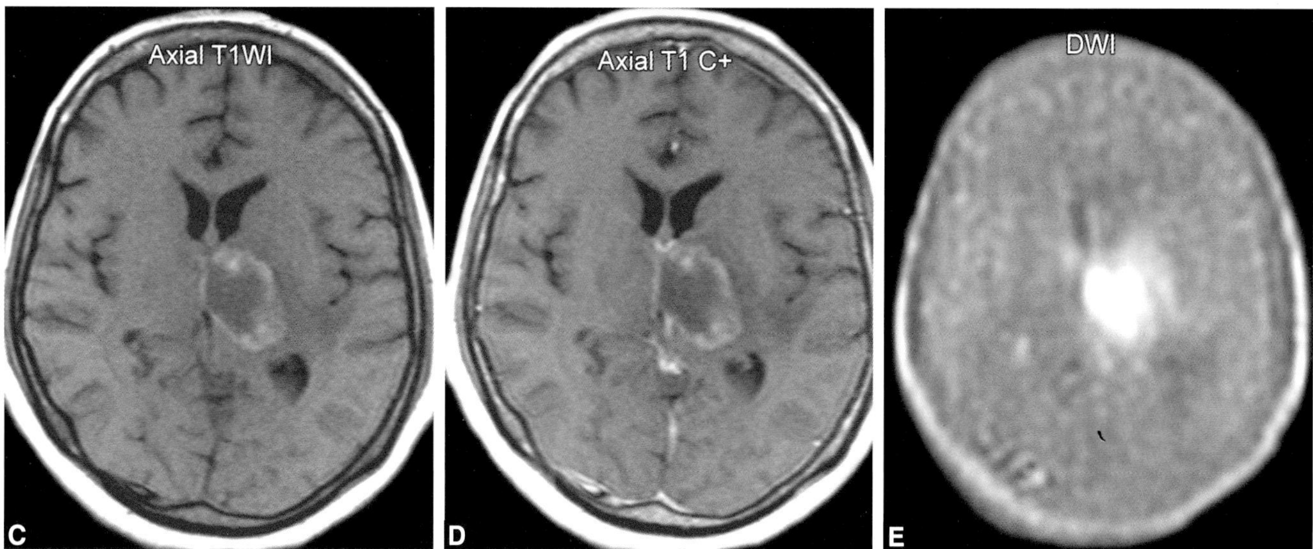

Figs 19C to E

Figs 19A to E: Left thalamus shows a well-defined T2 and FLAIR hyperintense lesion (A and B) with peripheral hyperintense rim on T1WI (C), showing mild peripheral post-contrast enhancement (D) and restricted diffusion on DWI (E) suggesting abscess

Rasmussen Encephalitis

Rasmussen encephalitis (RE) is a chronic, progressive inflammation of the brain of unknown origin. The onset is in childhood and is characterized by an abrupt appearance of focal, persistent motor seizure activity, i.e. epilepsia partialis continua (EPC) followed by hemiplegia and progressive cognitive deterioration. Early diagnosis and treatment with immunoactive agents or hemispherectomy are sought to prevent the cognitive decline. A hypothesis of the pathogenesis is glutamate receptor autoimmunity associated with persistent viral infection. This receptor activation may trigger seizures in these patients.

Histopathologic examination of biopsy material reveals a characteristic triad of findings: perivascular lymphocytic cuffing of round cells, gliosis and microglial nodules. CT and MRI demonstrate progressive destruction of a single cerebral hemisphere. Decreased (N-acetylaspartate) NAA and elevation of glutamate/glutamine levels on MR spectroscopy are reported.

Progressive cerebral hemiatrophy associated with clinical deterioration and focal EEG features, is the key to the diagnosis of RE, avoiding brain biopsy.

Seizures are focal, involving exclusively one hemibody, and refractory to antiepileptic drugs. In the initial phase the diagnosis of chronic encephalitis may be difficult, particularly in the absence of EPC. There is a progressive increase in seizure frequency and severity and patients develop permanent neurological deficits contralateral to the affected cerebral hemisphere. The initial MRI scans shows the inflammatory lesion (hyperintense T2/FLAIR signal). The next phase of disease is marked by

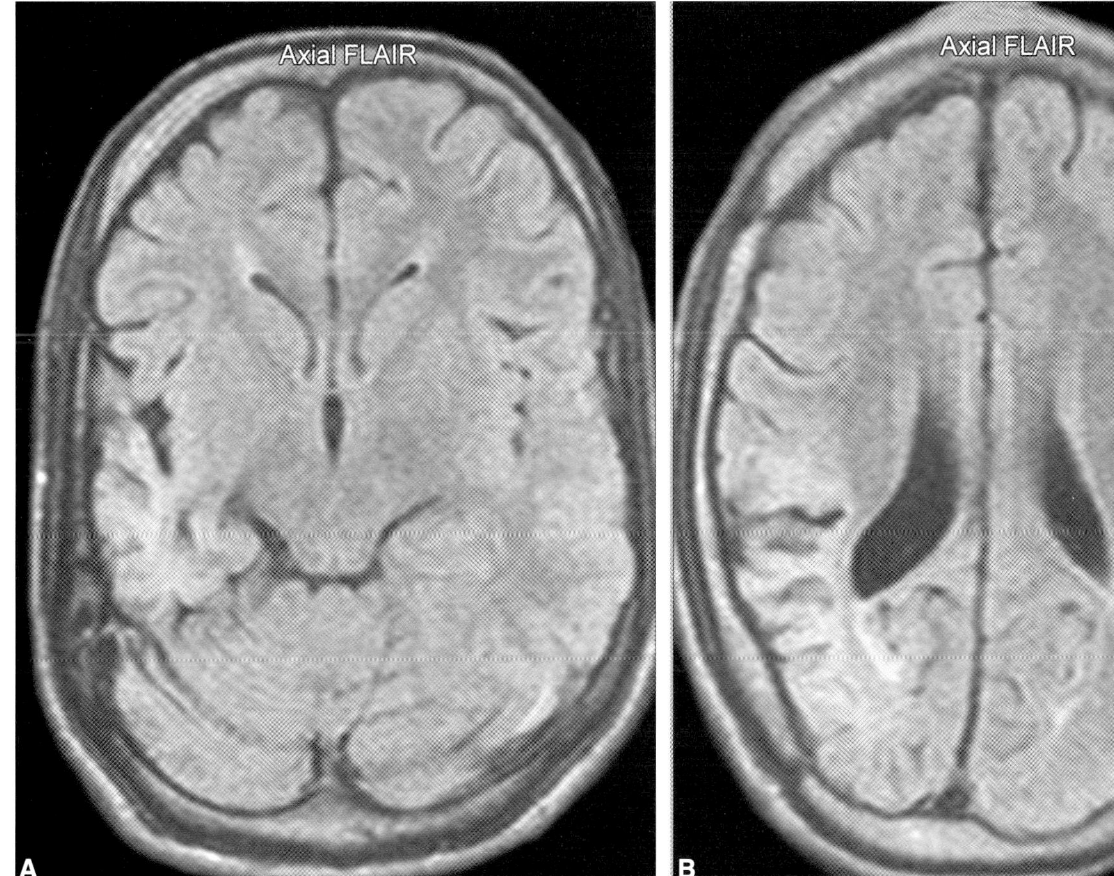

Figs 20A and B

neurological deterioration and may persist for more than 10 years. In the last phase, characterized by hemiparesis, seizures are not so frequent but motor and mental deterioration continues sometimes in spite of surgery.

MRI typically shows hemiatrophy with enlargement of ipsilateral ventricles and subarachnoid spaces. Cortical atrophy occurs, probably secondary to the long course of disease, proportional to the severity of symptoms, most likely reflecting the severity of disease. However, even patients without hemiparesis present diffuse hemispheric atrophy. Caudate atrophy has been rarely reported.

Patients with hemiparesis and more frequent seizures also present gray and focal white matter hyperintensity in T2-weighted images (Figs 20A to F). MRS contributes to evaluation and progression of metabolic changes in RE. Although the patterns of metabolites observed are nonspecific, compared with normal hemisphere, the atrophic regions showed increased lactate, a consequence of repetitive focal epileptic neuronal activity, as well as increased choline related to gliosis, microglial proliferation and elevated membrane turnover and reduced NAA. As NAA plays a role as neuron-glia signaling system, this reduction reflects neuronal loss and axonal dysfunction/depletion and possibly also changes in neurotransmitter system, altered in RE. This reduction in NAA suggests ongoing neuronal and axonal damage and loss in RE.

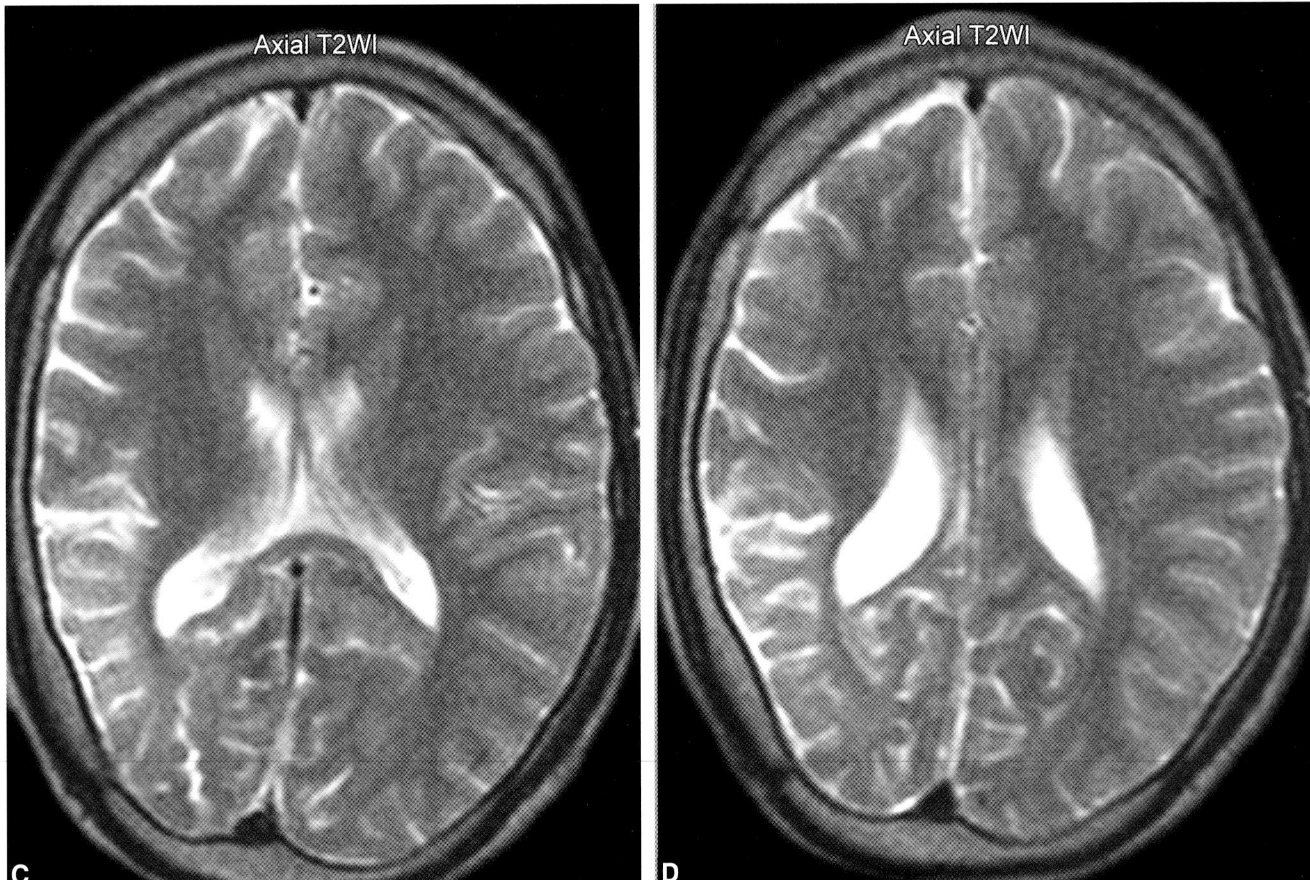

Figs 20C and D

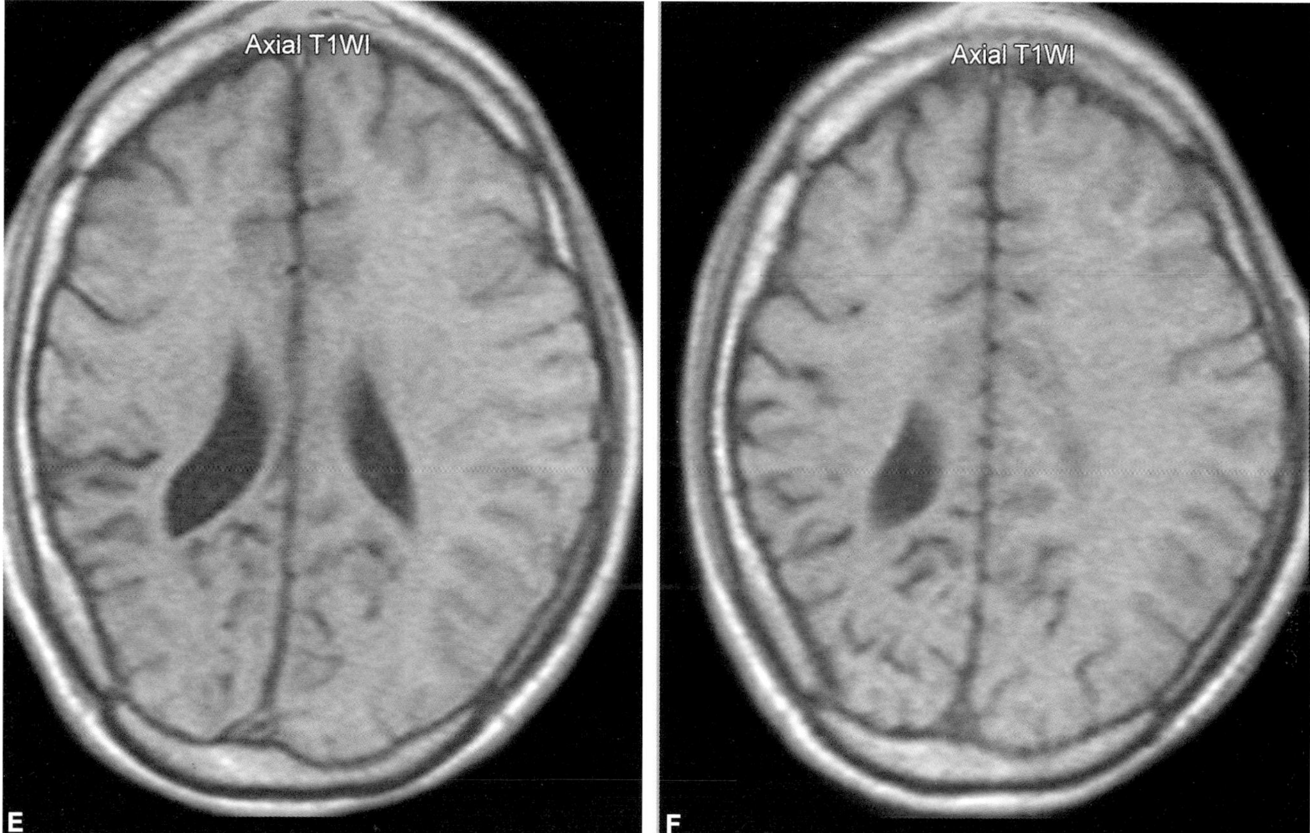

Figs 20E and F

Figs 20A to F: Axial FLAIR (A and B), T2W (C and D), and T1W (E and F) images reveal atrophy of right cerebral hemisphere with hyperintense signal in the subcortical white matter (prominent in temporoparietal region) with mild prominence of the right lateral ventricle

Japanese Encephalitis

Japanese encephalitis (JE) is an acute viral encephalitis which is caused by JE virus. It belongs to the Flaviviridae family, which also includes St Louis encephalitis virus, Murray Valley encephalitis virus, Tick-borne encephalitis virus, Russian spring-summer encephalitis virus. The age distribution and incidence depend on the target population for vaccination, the amount and distribution of the vector, the vaccination availability for the amplifying host, and the social and financial lifestyle and preventive healthcare changes.

The clinical symptoms include high fever, headache, impaired consciousness and seizure. JE also presents with extrapyramidal symptoms similar to parkinsonism, with incidence of up to 30 percent. The bilateral thalamic involvement in JE is the most frequent and characteristic finding and was present in almost all patients on MRI scan. Common sites of involvement include basal ganglia, substantia nigra, red nucleus, pons, hippocampus, cerebral cortex, and cerebellum.

Classically MR imaging demonstrates hyperintense lesions on the T2WI (Fig. 21A) and FLAIR image and hypointense lesions on the T1WI (Fig. 21B). Hemorrhagic transformations in the lesions of JE is not uncommon, with corresponding expected T1 and T2 changes. No or minimal effect of enhancement was noticed on contrast-enhanced study.

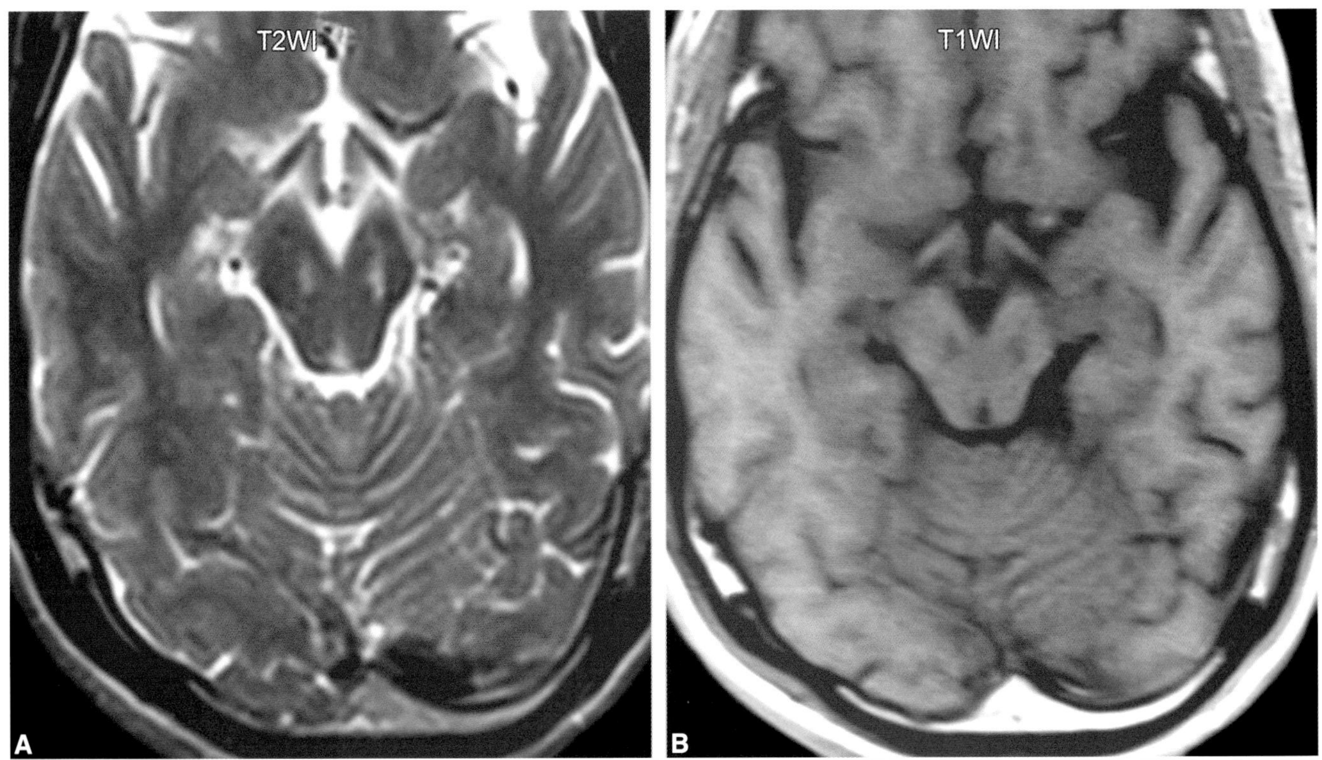

Figs 21A and B: Axial T2W (A) image shows symmetrical hyperintensities seen in bilateral substantia nigra and hypointensities in axial T1W image (B)

STROKE

Acute Infarct

The goal of imaging in a patient with acute stroke is to exclude hemorrhage, differentiate between irreversibly affected brain tissue and reversibly impaired tissue, and identify stenosis or occlusion of major extra or intracranial arteries.

Although conventional CT imaging and MR imaging (Figs 22A to C) are excellent modalities for detecting and characterizing cerebral ischemia or infarction, they may fail to depict acute ischemia reliably at its earliest stage. One of the most useful methods currently available is MR diffusion-weighted imaging (Fig. 22C), which may also underestimate the final size of the infarct when performed within the first day. In the acute stage of stroke, therefore, it has been shown that DWI combined with measures of cerebral hemodynamics, may be beneficial in the estimation of the surrounding area of ischemic tissue at risk, the so-called ischemic penumbra.

On CT early signs of ischemia are hypo attenuating brain tissue, obscuration of the lentiform nucleus, insular Ribbon sign, dense MCA sign and presence of hemorrhagic areas within the hypo attenuating brain tissue.

On MRI, PD-T2WI and FLAIR infarction is seen as high SI (Figs 22A and B). These sequences detect 80 percent of infarctions before 24 hours. High signal on conventional MR-sequences is comparable to hypodensity on CT. DWI is the most sensitive sequence for stroke imaging. High intensity on DWI (Fig. 22C) indicates restriction of the ability of water protons to diffuse extracellularly. DWI is positive in the acute phase and then becomes brighter with a maximum at 7 days.

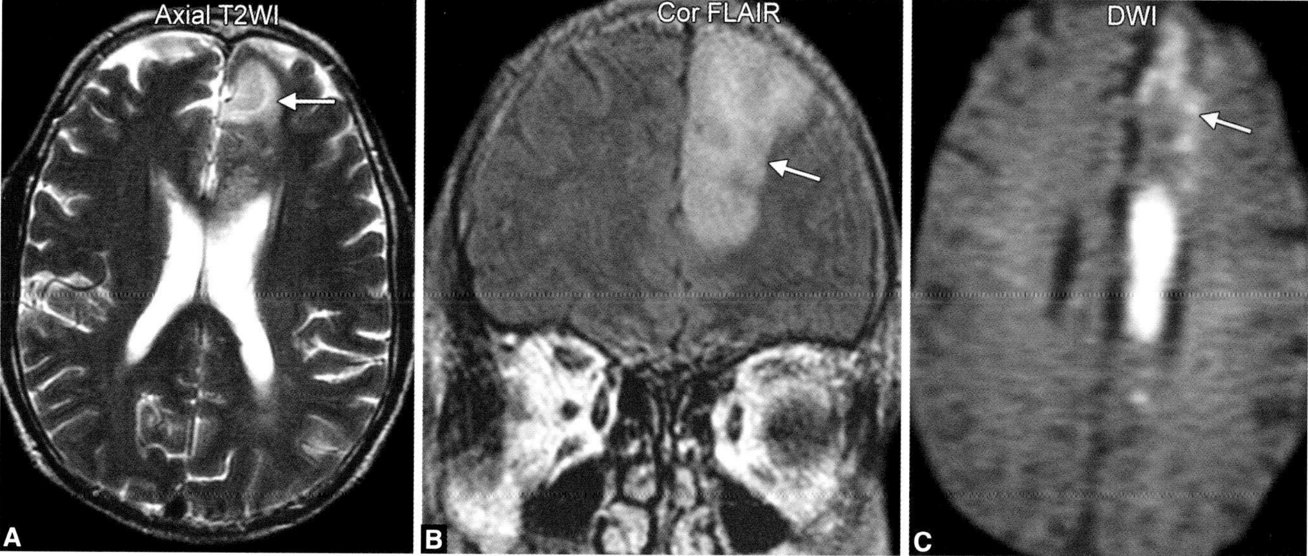

Figs 22A to C: Wedge shaped hyperintensity on T2W (A) and (B) FLAIR images with restricted diffusion, high intensity on DWI (C) indicates restriction

Lacunar Infarct

Lacunar infarcts are small infarcts in the deeper parts of the brain (basal ganglia, thalamus, white matter) and in the brainstem. Lacunar infarcts are caused by occlusion of a single deep penetrating artery. Lacunar infarcts account for 25 percent of all ischemic strokes. Atherosclerosis is the most common cause of lacunar infarcts followed by emboli. Around 25 percent of patients with clinical and radiologically defined lacunar infarct had a potential cardiac cause for their strokes. On the FLAIR (Fig. 23) the infarct is seen as hyperintensity, T1W image shows foci of decreased signal and T2W image shows foci of increased signal.

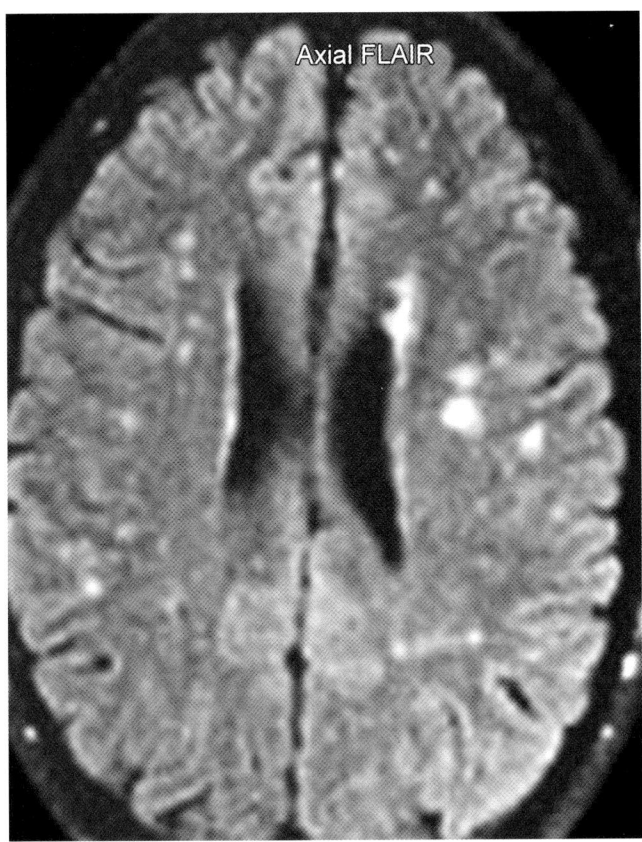

Fig. 23: Shows multiple lacunar infarcts seen in white matter bilaterally

Cystic Encephalomalacia

Cystic encephalomalacia is a cystic area in the brain parenchyma with presence of multiple glial septations. They result from infarction, infection or trauma and may be focal or diffuse depending on cause and severity. The presence of glial septations distinguishes cystic encephalomalacia from an area of porencephaly and indicates that the injury occurred after birth. On imaging the cavities and septations are best seen on MRI, both on T1WI and T2WI (Figs 24A and B) than on CT scan images. Calcification may be present and is best seen on CT.

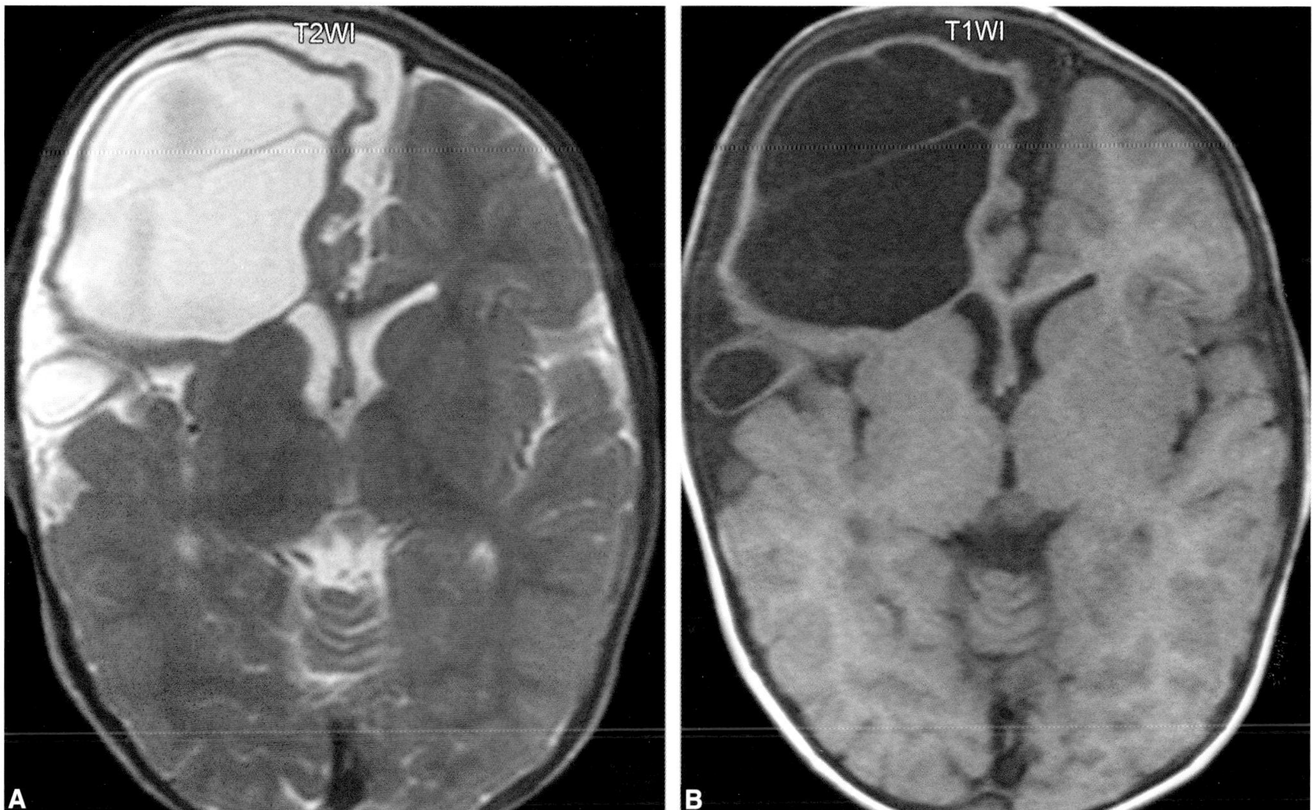

Figs 24A and B: CSF intensity lesions with thin walls and few internal septae are seen in the right frontal parenchyma. These lesions appear hyperintense on T2W image (A) and hypointense on T1W image (B). The CSF spaces in this region are prominent. There is loss of white matter with resultant minimal dilatation of the right frontal horn

Hypoxic Ischemic Encephalopathy

Hypoxic ischemic encephalopathy (HIE) is a condition in which the brain does not receive enough oxygen. This particular condition refers to an oxygen deficiency to the brain as a whole, rather than a part of the brain. Although the term most often refers to injury sustained by newborns. The disease can also cause long-term damage, including intellectual disability, delayed development, seizures, and cerebral palsy.

There are a variety of causes of HIE. Any injury and many health conditions can potentially cause oxygen deprivation to the brain. Some common causes are: injury or complication during birth, respiratory failure, blocked or ruptured blood vessel, carbon monoxide or cyanide poisoning, drug overdose, drowning, lack of oxygen due to smoke inhalation, extremely low blood pressure, strangulation, cardiac arrest, carbon monoxide poisoning, high altitudes, choking, compression or injury, to the trachea that reduces or stops breathing, complications from general anesthesia.

Symptoms of HIE are difficulty concentrating or paying attention, poor judgment euphoria, extreme lethargy, seizures, coma.

US findings may include hyperechogenicity of involved structures and/or abnormal resistivity index on duplex Doppler images. Changes on CT scans may be subtle, with mild hypoattenuation of the thalami and basal ganglia, which appear isoattenuated compared with the surrounding white matter. On MR images, abnormal T2 and FLAIR hyperintensity (Figs 25A and B) are noted. Diffusion-weighted imaging is more sensitive and shows restricted diffusion in the affected areas. MR spectroscopy reveals an elevation of lactate concentration in the basal ganglia and thalami.

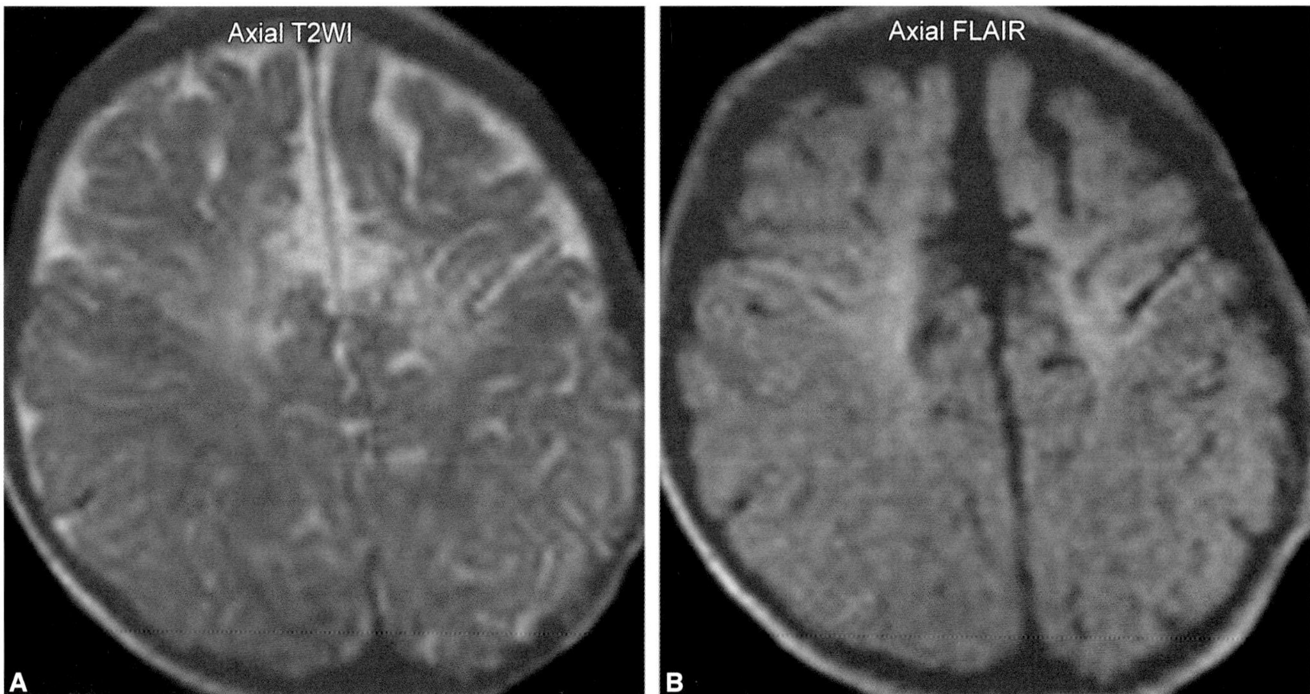

Figs 25A and B: A 4-month-old child with history of full term delivery and birth asphyxia shows hypoxic ischemic encephalopathy with involvement in form of hyperintensity in perirolandic region on T2W and FLAIR images

Global Hypoxia

Global hypoxic-ischemic injury to the brain is a significant cause of mortality and severe neurologic disability. In adults and children who are not candidates for cranial US owing to closure of the anterior fontanelle, CT Brain is the initial screening test of choice

MR imaging to assess the overall extent of injury.

MR imaging is an accurate modality for evaluating neonatal hypoxic ischemic insult. Diffusion-weighted imaging is sensitive for the detection of injury in the first 24 hours, during which time conventional T1- and T2-weighted images may appear normal. Diffusion-weighted images will demonstrate increased signal intensity in the region of the ventrolateral thalami and basal ganglia in the perirolandic regions, and along the corticospinal tracts. FLAIR image shows hyperintense signal and ADC (Figs 26A to D) demonstrate lower values.

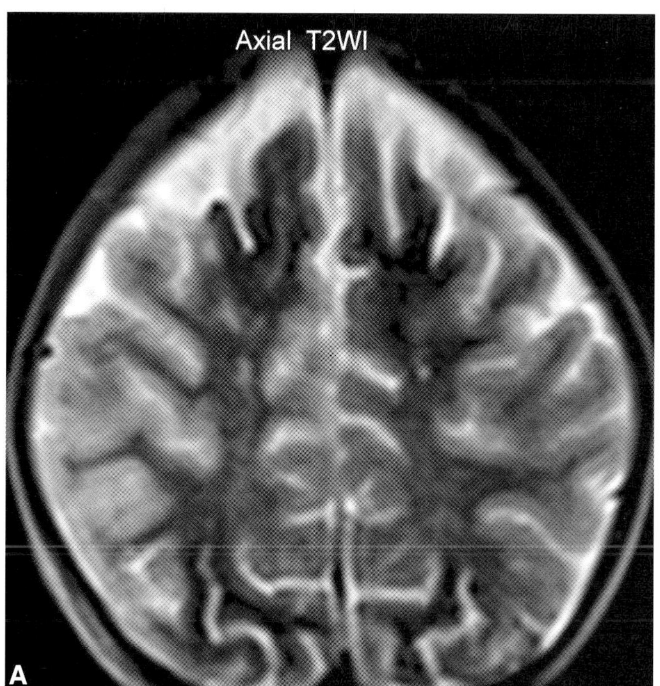

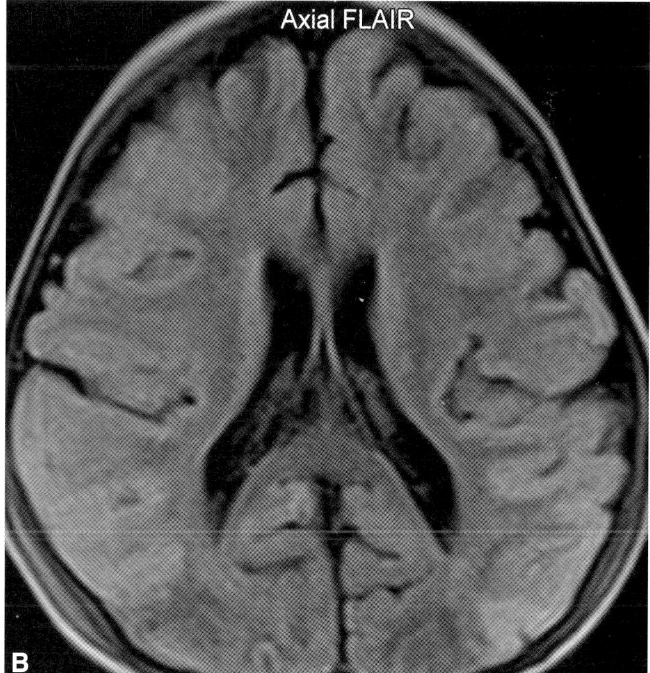

Figs 26A and B

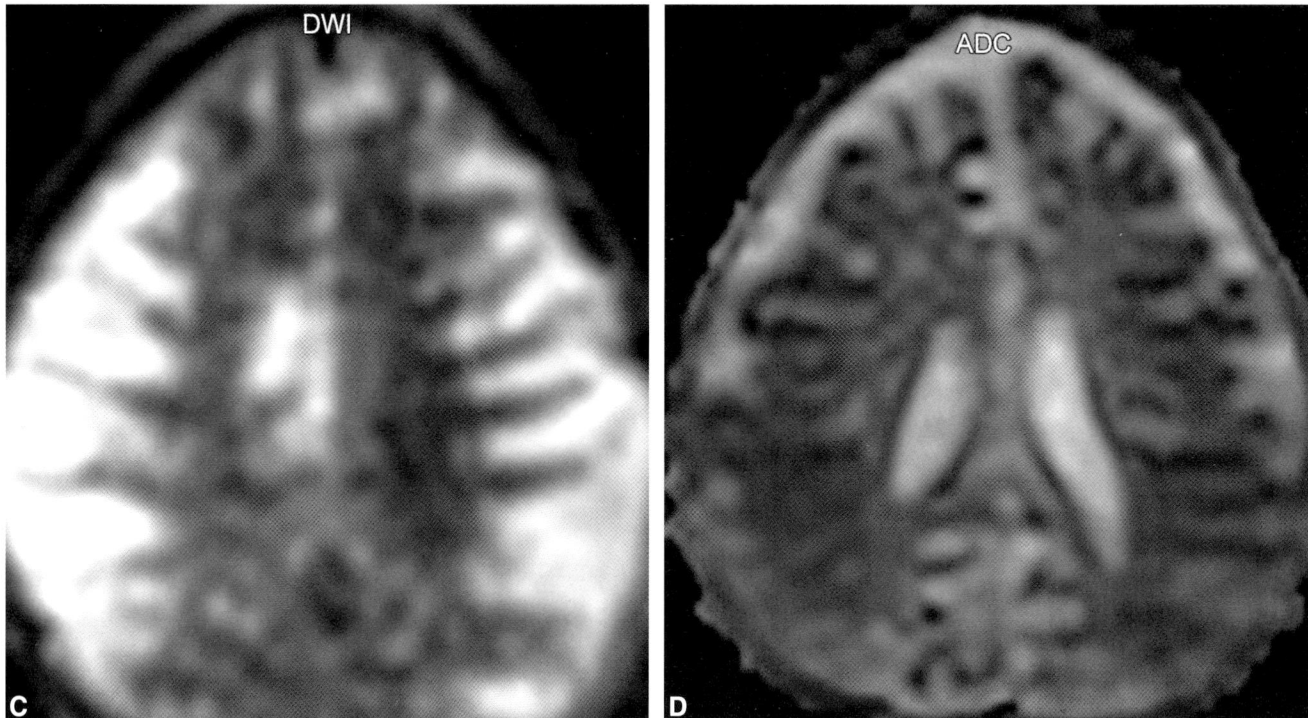

Figs 26C and D

Figs 26A to D: Global hypoxic insult in a 2-year-old girl who presented with status epilepticus. T2W (A), FLAIR (B) images reveal hyperintense signal in the bilateral cortical and subcortical regions with restriction of diffusion on DW and ADC images (C and D). This represents cytotoxic edema and is suggestive of prolonged global hypoxia

WHITE MATTER DISEASE

Adrenoleukodystrophy

X-linked adrenoleukodystrophy (ALD) is a peroxisomal disorder that affects the white matter of the central nervous system, adrenal cortex, and testes. It is caused by a deficiency of acyl-CoA synthetaze. This deficiency prevents the breakdown of very long chain fatty acids, which then accumulate in tissue and plasma.

Patient presents with symptoms of adrenal insufficiency and neurological deterioration, with gait disturbances, loss of vision, spastic diplegia, epileptic seizures and progressive dementia.

On MRI, in T2-weighted images white matter hyperintensity is seen involving the occipital area and splenium of the corpus callosum (Fig. 27A). The lesions are symmetrical and demyelination progresses anteriorly. Late in the disease the brainstem and cerebellum may be involved. Post-contrast image shows peripheral enhancement (Fig. 27B).

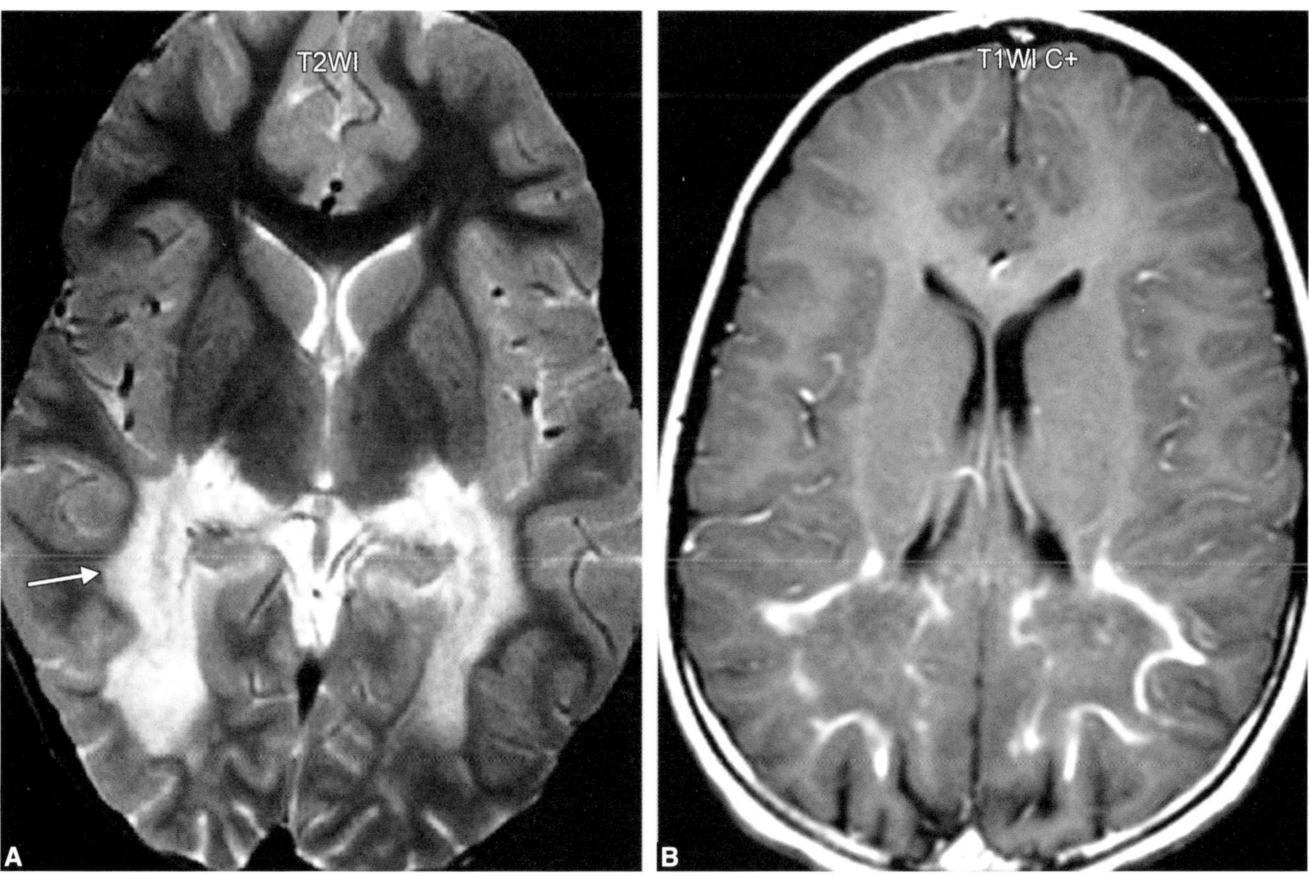

Figs 27A and B: X-linked adrenoleukodystrophy symmetrical hyperintense signal is seen in the bilateral peritrigonal white matter on T2W images (A). The subcortical white matter is spared. There is no mass effect. On post-contrast T1W image (B) Bilateral peripheral enhancement of the lesion is noted, representing active demyelination. These findings are suggestive of X-linked adrenoleukodystrophy

Canavan's Disease

Canavan's disease is a leukodystrophy inherited as autosomal recessive disease. There is deficiency of N-acetylaspartase, which is a key enzyme in the myelin synthesis pathway, that results in accumulation of N-acetylaspartic acid in the urine, plasma and brain. The disease manifests as decreased motor activity, hypotonia, visual loss and increased skull growth. Patient generally dies within first few years of life.

On MRI, there is diffuse increased signal throughout the white matter symmetrically on T2-weighted images (Figs 28A to C), with relative sparing of the internal capsules and early involvement of the subcortical arcuate fibers. T1-weighted images sometime shows involvement of white matter.

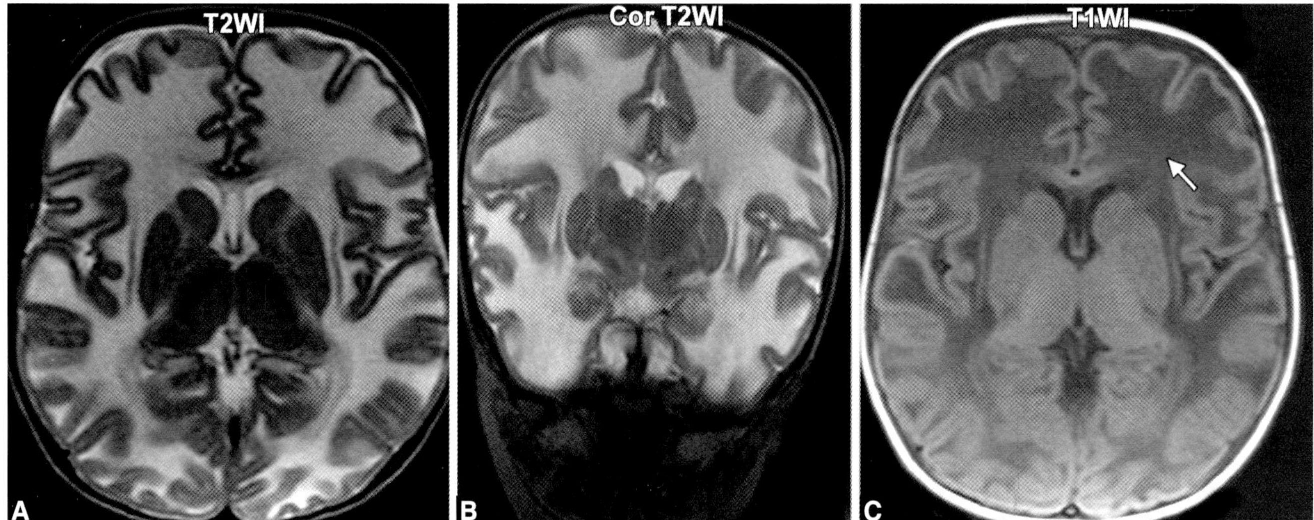

Figs 28A to C: Axial T2WI (A) and coronal T2WI (B) shows macrocephaly, complete lack of myelination, extensive demyelination in frontal lobe with involement of whole white matter, abnormal hyperintense signal is also noted in bilateral internal and external capsule. Axial T1WI (C) shows involvement of frontal white matter with macrocephaly

Alexander's Disease

It is a dysmyelinating leukodystrophy. There are three clinical subgroups according to age of onset: infantile, juvenile and adult. Infantile form is the most common and presents with macrocephaly with developmental delay, spasticity and seizures. In juvenile form the onset is between 7 and 14 years, and presents with spasticity and bulbar symptoms. In the adult form onset of symptoms is variable. Clinical manifestation may have an intermittent course and resemble multiple sclerosis.

On CT and MR, there is involvement of the white matter, starting bilaterally first in the frontal lobes (Fig. 29) and subsequently involving the peritrigonal temporoparietal regions.

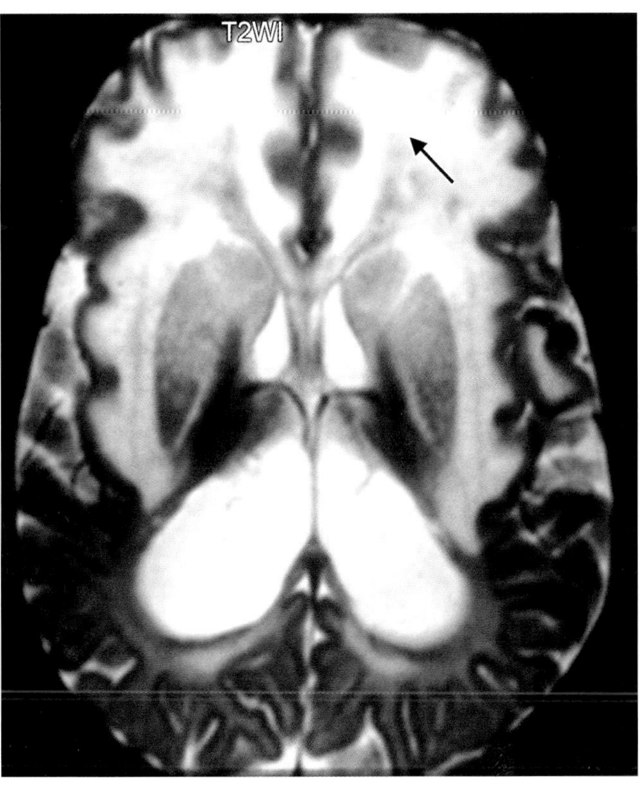

Fig. 29: T2W axial image reveals extensive hyperintense signal suggestive of demyelination in the bilateral frontal white matter (black arrow) and external capsules

Metachromatic Leukodystrophy

Metachromatic leukodystrophy is an autosomal recessive disorder caused by a deficiency of the lysosomal enzyme arylsulfatase A. This enzyme is necessary for the normal metabolism of sulfatides, which are important constituents of the myelin sheath. In metachromatic leukodystrophy, sulfatides accumulate in various tissues, including the brain, peripheral nerves, kidneys, liver, and gallbladder. The accumulation of sulfatides within glial cells and neurons causes the characteristic metachromatic reaction. Metachromatic leukodystrophy is diagnosed biochemically on the basis of an abnormally low level of arylsulfatase A in peripheral blood leukocytes and in urine.

Three different types of metachromatic leukodystrophy are recognized according to patient age at onset: late infantile, juvenile, and adult. The most common type is late infantile metachromatic leukodystrophy, which usually manifests in children between 12 and 18 months of age and is characterized by motor signs of peripheral neuropathy followed by deterioration in intellect, speech, and coordination. Within 2 years of onset, gait disturbance, quadriplegia, blindness, and decerebrate posturing may be seen.

At T2-weighted MR imaging, metachromatic leukodystrophy manifests as symmetric confluent areas of high signal intensity in the periventricular white matter (Fig. 30) with sparing of the subcortical U fibers. No enhancement is evident at computed tomography (CT) or MR imaging. The tigroid and "leopard skin" patterns of demyelination, which suggest sparing of the perivascular white matter, can be seen in the periventricular white matter and centrum semiovale. The corpus callosum, internal capsule, and corticospinal tracts are also frequently involved. The cerebellar white matter may appear hyperintense at T2-weighted MR imaging. In the later stage of metachromatic leukodystrophy, corticosubcortical atrophy often occurs, particularly when the subcortical white matter is involved.

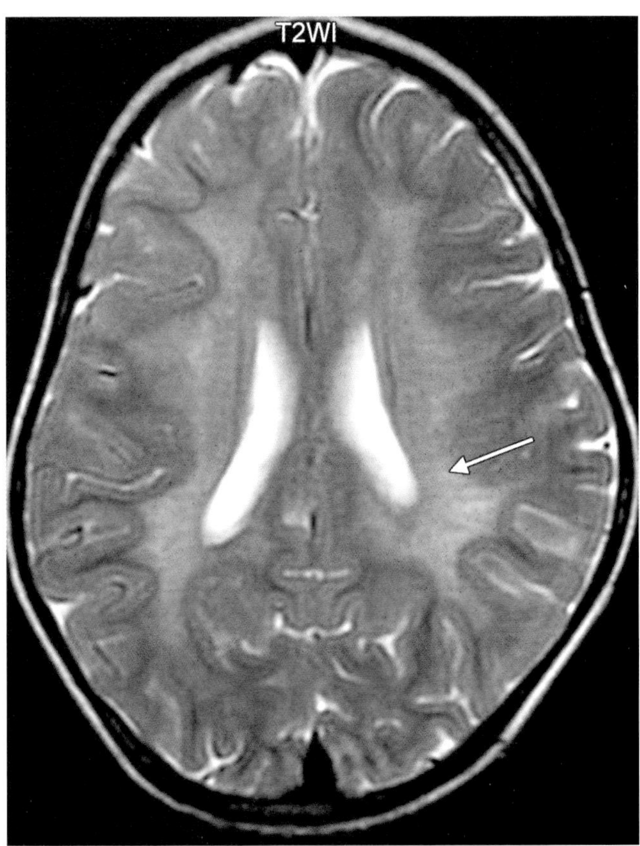

Fig. 30: T2W image reveals diffuse hyperintense signal (arrow) in corona radiate both sides. There is sparing of the sub-cortical white matter. No evidence of mass effect

Mucopolysaccharidosis

Mucopolysaccharidosis is a group of disorders which are closely related and characterized by dwarfism and presence of certain mucopolysaccharides in the urine. These syndromes have common clinical and radiographic features.

Radiographically patients have large and dolichocephalic skulls, poorly developed mastoids and paranasal sinuses, an elongated J-shaped sella turcica, flattened mandibular condyles, a thick diploic space and hook-shaped vertebrae. There is underdevelopment of the superior acetabular region, which results in a widened acetabular roof and wide acetabular index. The ribs are widened but taper near their vertebral margins, and the clavicles are short and widened. Long tubular bones show diaphyseal and metaphyseal expansion. Abnormalities in the hands include diffuse osteopenia, cortical thinning, proximal tapering of the second to fifth metacarpal bones, and small and deformed carpal bones. The distal portions of the radius and ulna taper, thus altering the carpal angle.

MRI shows thickening of dura mater at the craniocervical junction, causing narrowing of the subarachnoid space. Other findings are white matter alterations, mild to severe hydrocephalus, skull dysplasia and odontoid dysplasia. Reduced gray/ white matter contrast is seen on T2-weighted MRI and dilated Virchow-Robin spaces (Figs 31A and B).

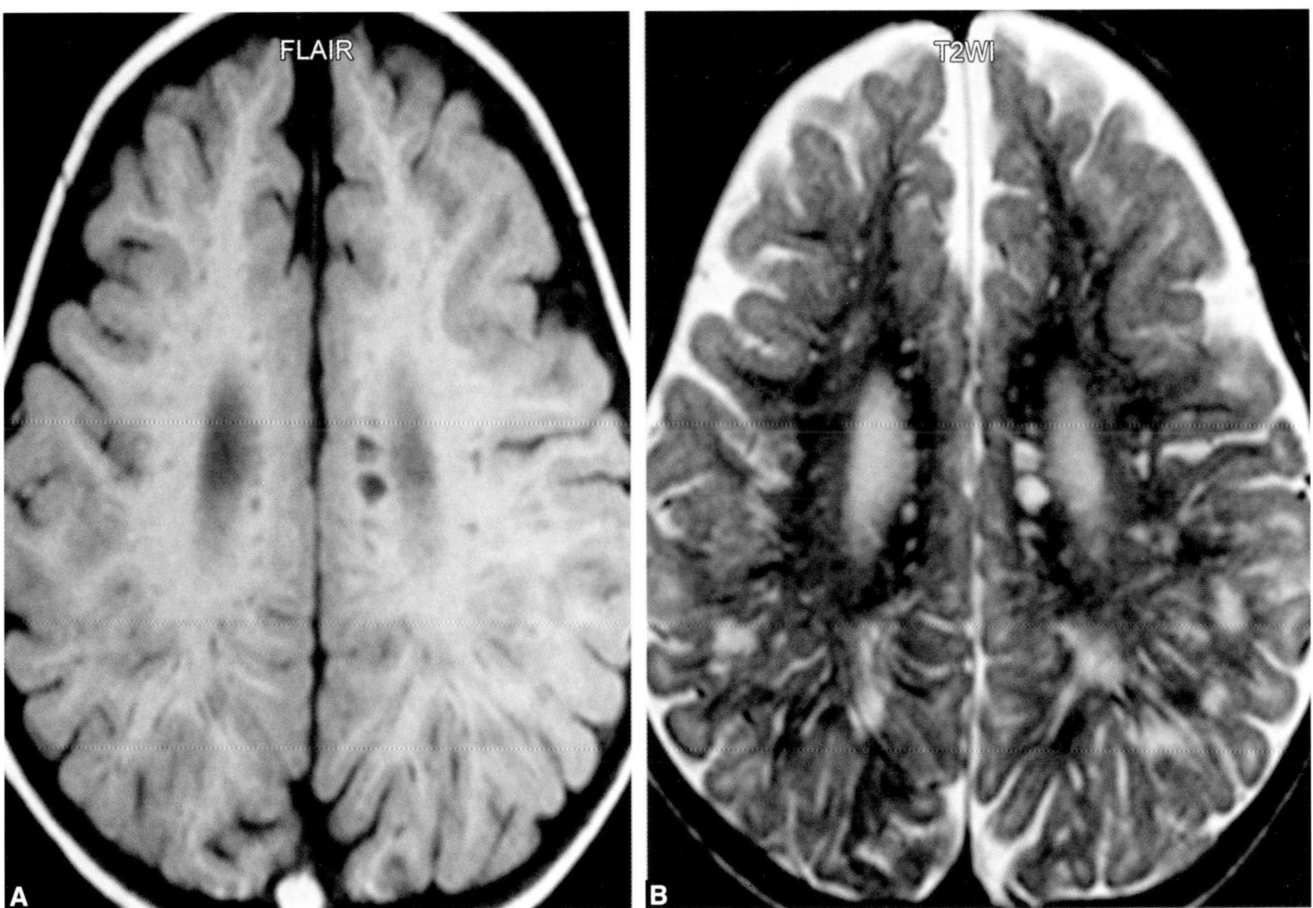

Figs 31A and B: Flair and T2WI axial MRI in mucopolysaccharidosis shows dilated Virchow-Robin spaces seen bilateral in the periventricular white matter

Periventricular Leukomalacia

Periventricular leukomalacia (PVL) is the result of hypoxic ischemic encephalopathy in premature infants. It is due to selective damage to the periventricular white matter. It is the second most common central nervous system complication in preterm infants, after periventricular hemorrhage.

On MRI, there are peritrigonal hyperintensities on T2-weighted images, focal ventricular enlargement (Figs 32A and B), and irregular ventricular contours. White matter volume is reduced, and the posterior part of corpus callosum atrophies. PVL is usually bilateral but is often asymmetrical.

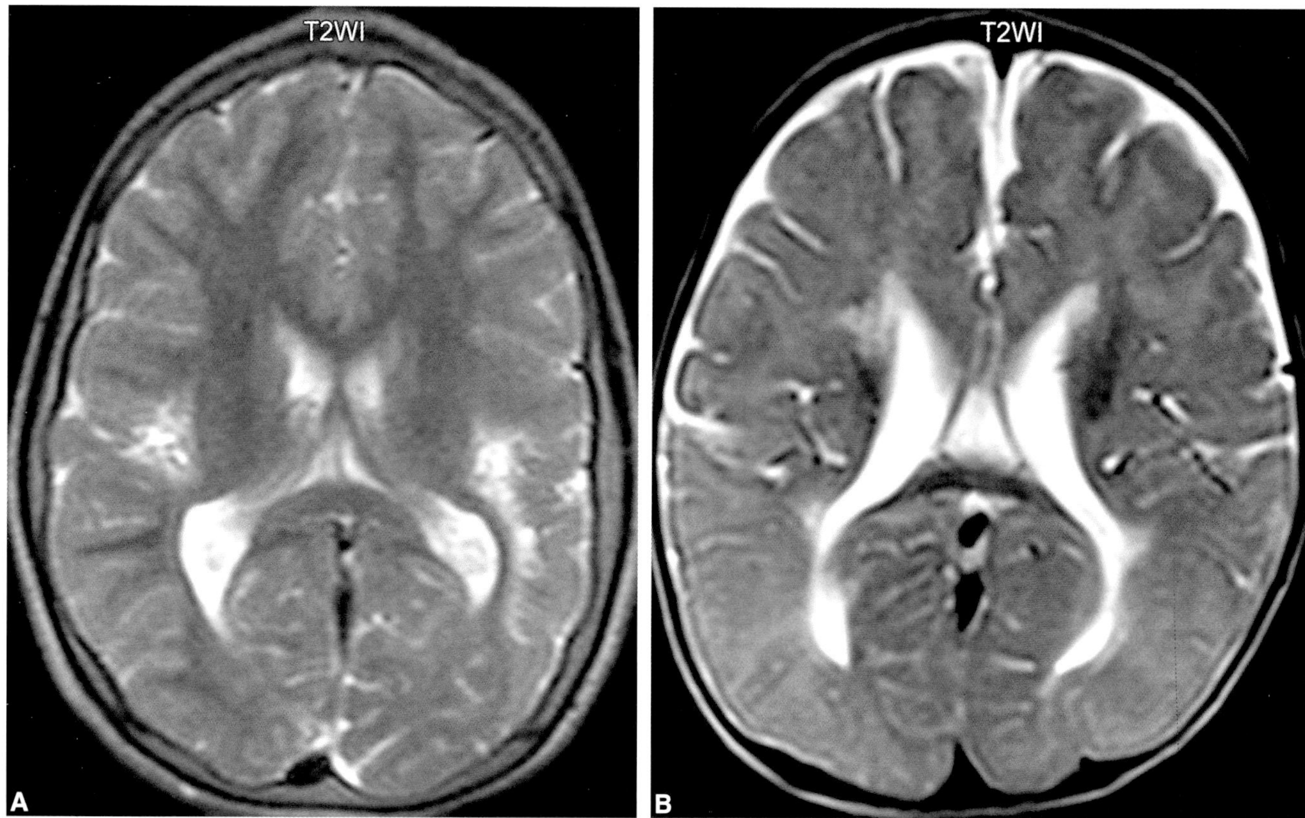

Figs 32A and B: (A) Axial T2WI shows peritrigonal hyperintensity with white matter volume loss and crowding of gyri in bilateral perirolandic region with enlargement of occipital horn; (B) Another case, axial T2WI shows peritrigonal hyperintensities within white matter with irregular ventricular contour and ventricular enlargement

NEUROCUTANEOUS SYNDROME

Neurofibromatosis

Neurofibromatosis is inherited nerve sheath disorder with two distinct types, neurofibromatosis type 1 (NF1) and neurofibromatosis type 2 (NF2). NF1 is von Recklinghausen disease. It is 10 times more common than NF2. NF1 has prominent superficial tumors (neurofibromas), macular hyperpigmentation (café-au-lait spots) and CNS abnormalities that include true neoplasms usually optic nerve gliomas, dysplastic and hamartomatous lesions. Multifocal increased signal intensiy is seen on T2WI in brainstem, cerebellar white matter, dentate nucleus, basal ganglia, periventricular white matter, optic nerve and optic pathways. These hyperintensities represent either abnormal myelination or hamartomatous change. The presence of bilateral optic nerve gliomas is considered diagnostic for NF1 (Figs 33 and 34).

NF2 develops bilateral acoustic schwannomas with trigeminal nerve being next in frequency. They are predisposed to intracranial or intraspinal meningiomas.

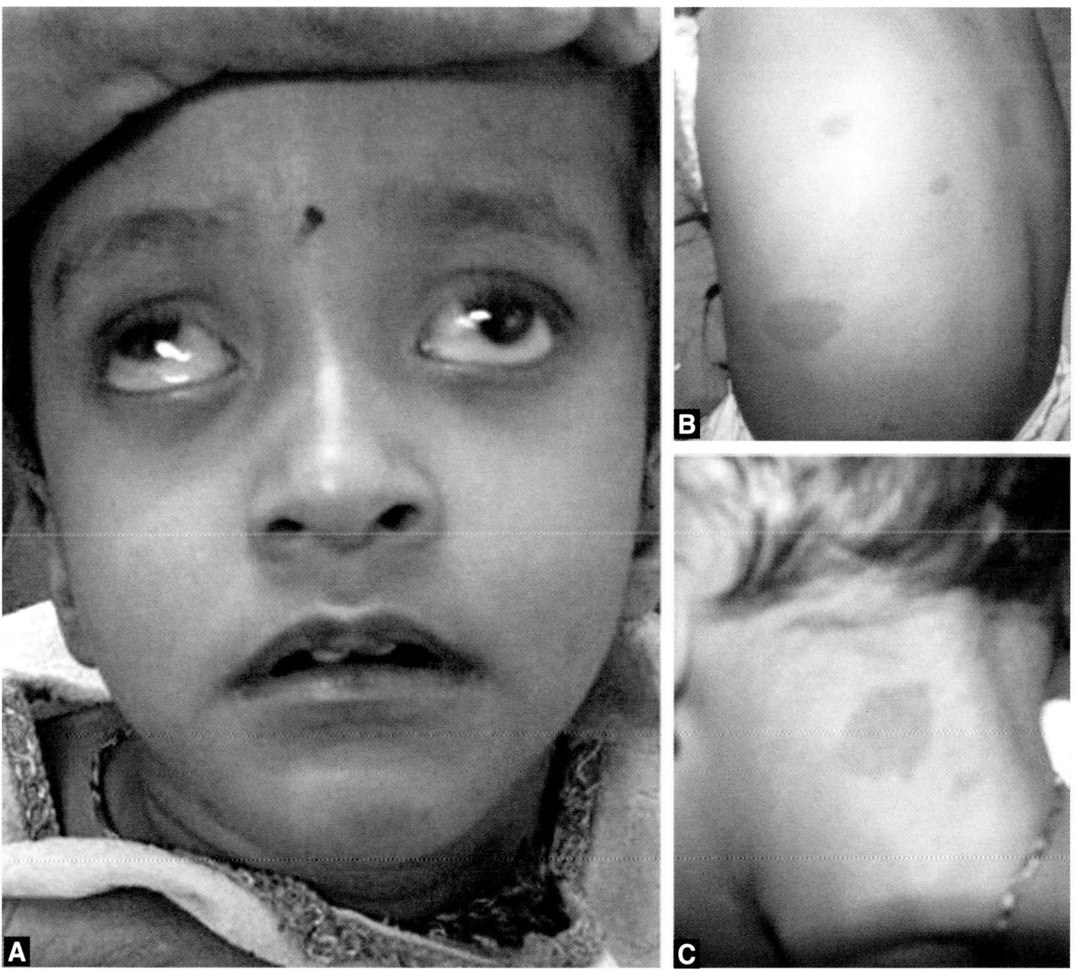

Figs 33A to C: Photographs of patient showing squint (A) and café-au-lait spots (B and C) *(For color version, see Plate 1)*

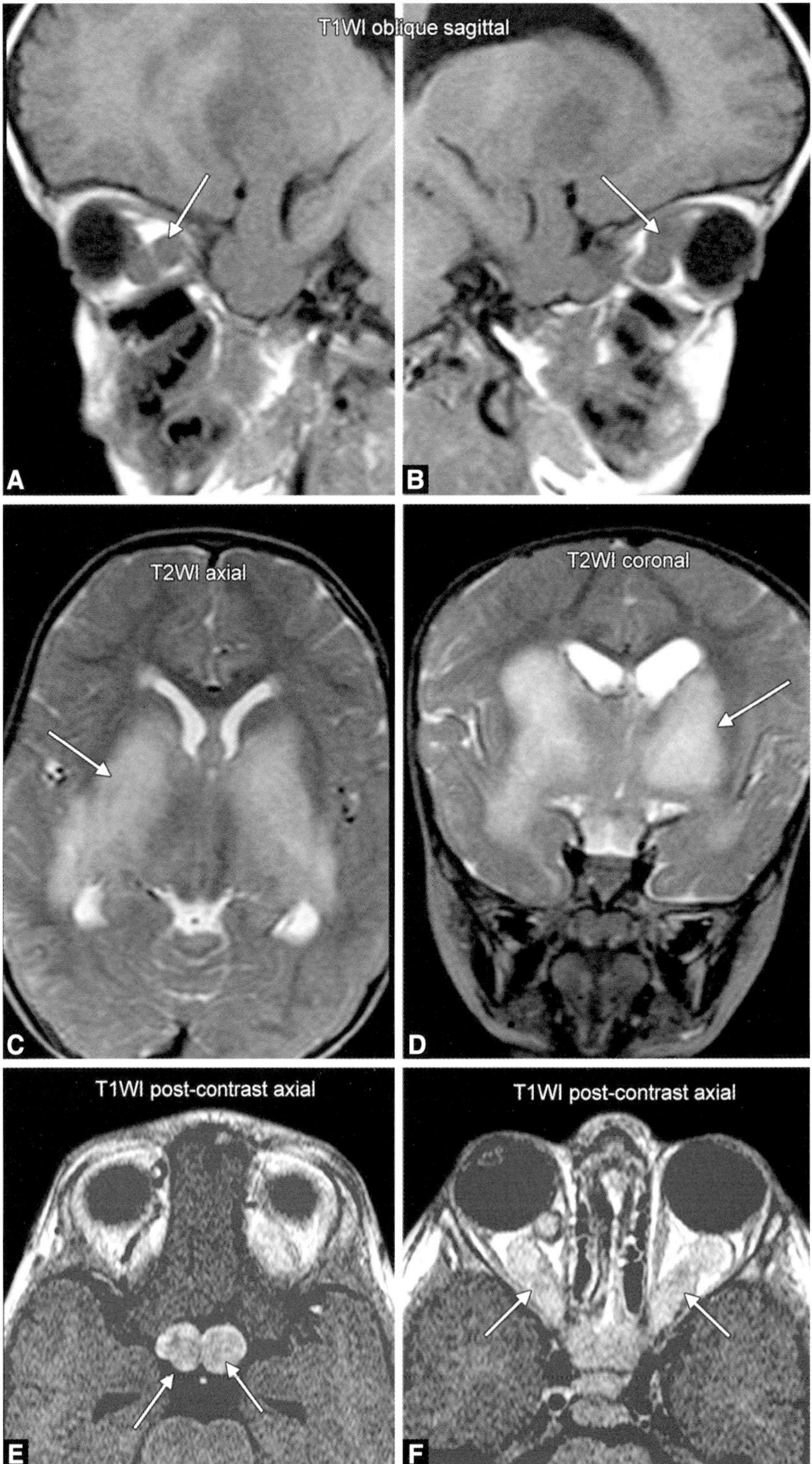

Figs 34A to F: Oblique sagittal T1W images show (A) right and (B) left tortuous and enlarged optic nerves (arrow). T2WI (C) axial and (D) coronal images show abnormal hyperintense signal in both gangliocapsular region and along optic tracts. Axial post-contrast T1WI shows (E) enlarged enhancing optic chiasma and (F) bilateral tortuous and enlarged enhancing optic nerves

Tuberous Sclerosis

Tuberous sclerosis is an autosomal dominant disease with high peneterance that demonstrate widespread potential for hamartomatous growths in multiple organ systems. Tuberous sclerosis presents as a classical triad of papular facial lesions, seizures and mental retardation, this triad is seen in more than 50 percent of patients. CT and MRI (Figs 35A to C) findings in tuberous sclerosis include subependymal nodules, subependymal giant cell astrocytoma, and cortical tubers, retinal phakomas, aneurysms, facial angiofibromas, shagreen patches, subungual fibromas, renal cyst, cardiac rhabdomyomas, leiomyomas, bone islands, and periosteal new bone formation.

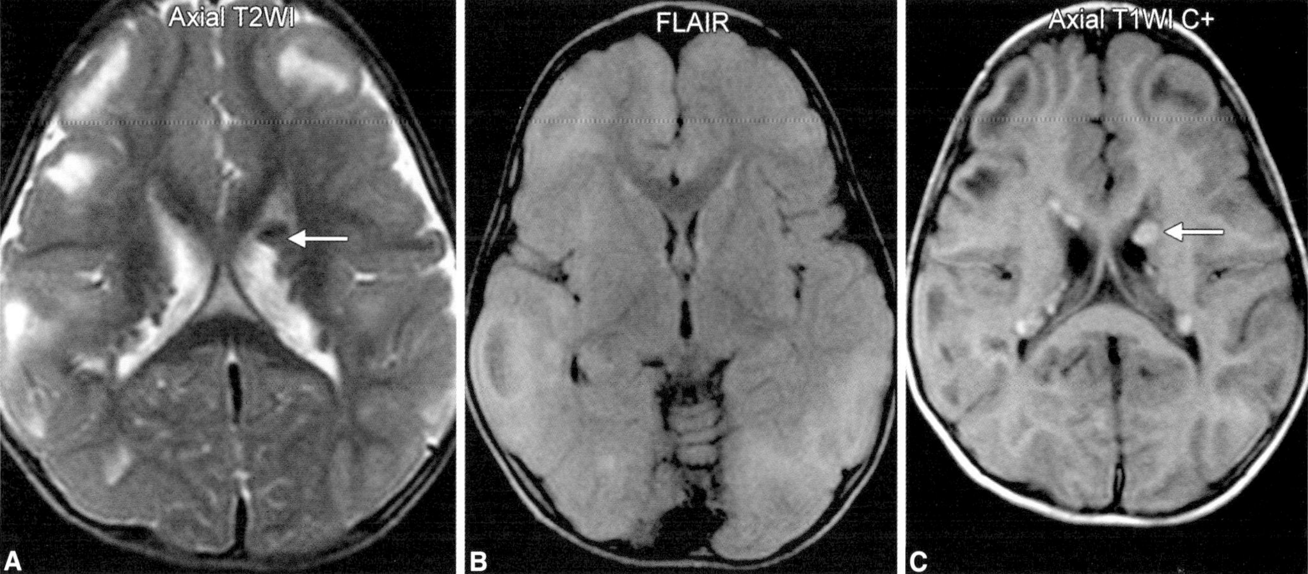

Figs 35A to C: Axial T2WI (A) brain shows hypointense subependymal nodules (arrow) with hyperintense cortical tubers in a 3-years-old child. Axial FLAIR demonstrates cortical hyperintense tubers (B) and post-contrast axial section (C) demonstrates enhancement of subependymal tubers (arrow)

Sturge-Weber Syndrome

Sturge-Weber syndrome is one of the neurophakomatosis, it is a sporadic disease, with no racial or sex predilection, characterized by angiomatosis involving the face, the choroid of the eye and the leptomeninges. The clinical components of this syndrome are the "port-wine" vascular nevus flammeus in the trigeminal nerve distribution, seizure (90%), hemiparesia, hemianopsia (30%), buphthalmos, glaucoma and mental retardation.

Plain skull radiographs and computed tomography (CT) scans may show the tramline gyriform patterns of intracranial calcifications. The CT and magnetic resonance features of cortical calcifications and meningeal angiomatosis are typical of Sturge-Weber syndrome, but unusual in children younger than one year. The calcifications occur in areas of the brain subjacent to the leptomeningeal vascular malformation (angioma). They begin in the subcortical white matter and latter develop in the cortex. They are most frequently seen in the temporo-parieto-occipital region of the brain, but can be located anywhere in the cerebrum. Enhancement of the leptomeningeal angioma can sometimes be seen by CT if patient is imaged in infancy, before the appearance of cortical calcifications.

MR is superior to CT in the demonstration of leptomeningeal enhancement (Fig. 36), particularly in the presence of dense cortical calcifications, which mask enhancement as determined by CT. Enlarged vessels are seen on CT and MR (Fig. 36) studies in the subependymal and periventricular region of the involved cerebral hemisphere and are frequently associated with an enlarged choroid plexus. The overlying superficial cortical veins are reduced in size and number, with a prominent deep collateral venous system. Cranial asymmetry often results from cerebral hemitrophy. CT scan may show ipsilateral skull-table and orbital thickening, enlarged ipsilateral paranasal sinuses and mastoid air cells, as well as elevation of the sphenoid wing and petrous ridge because of the lack of brain growth on the affected side. Midline structures are often displaced towards the side of the leptomeningeal angioma. As might be expected atrophy is bilateral in those patients with bilateral angiomas.

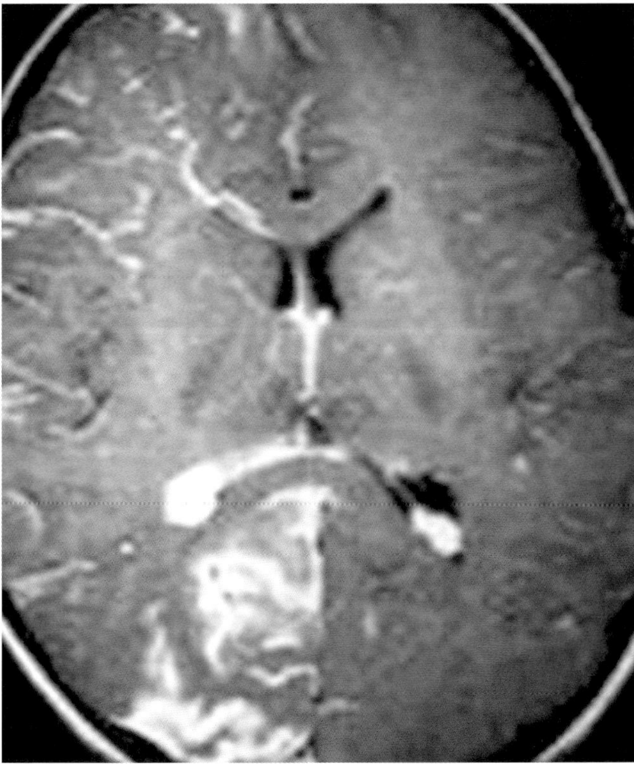

Fig. 36: Gyriform enhancement shows the pial angiomas and adjacent ischemic occipital cortex on post-contrast axial T1 weighted image

NEOPLASM

Meningioma

Meningiomas are the most common nonglial primary tumors of the central nervous system and the most common extra-axial neoplasms, accounting for approximately 15 percent of all intracranial tumors. The typical meningioma is a homogeneous, hemispheric, markedly enhancing extra-axial mass located over the cerebral convexity, in the parasagittal region, or arising from the sphenoid wing.

CT demonstrates sharply circumscribed unilobular mass with a broad based dural attachment.

On plain CT scan the mass appears as an area of homogeneous hyperattenuation and after administration of contrast the mass homogeneously enhances.

Magnetic resonance images of meningiomas shows sharply circumscribed mass characteristically hypointense to isointense on T1W images, isointense to hyperintense on T2-weighted pulse sequence and on post-contrast scans show homogeneously enhancing mass (Figs 37A to C).

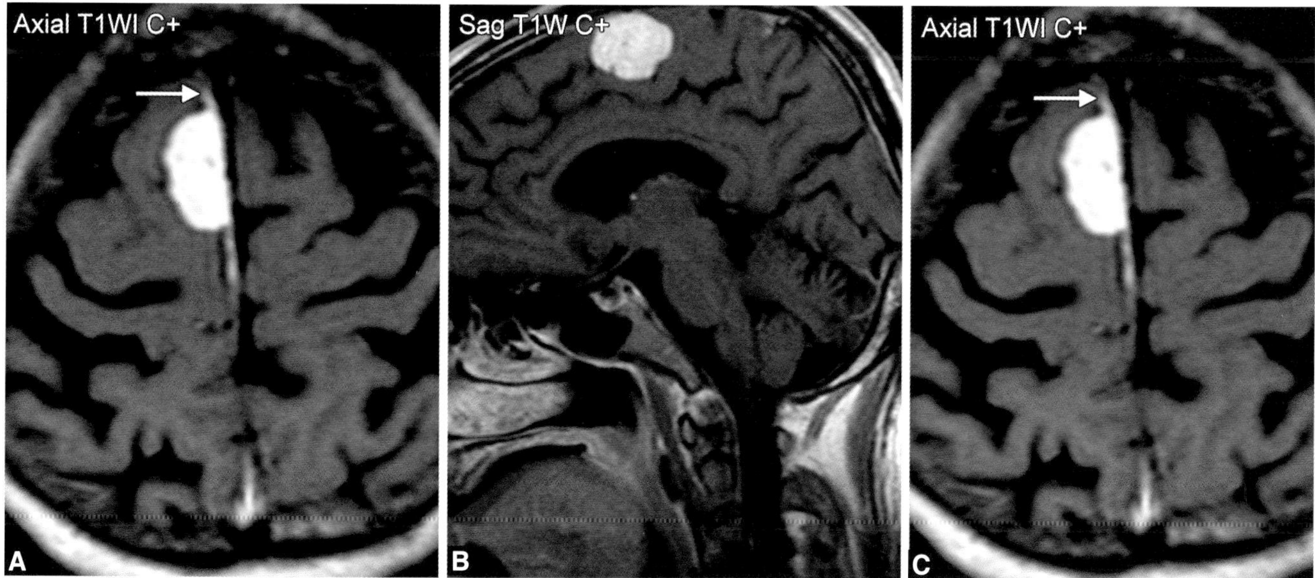

Figs 37A to C: Axial, sagittal and coronal T1W post-contrast images shows well-defined intensely enhancing lesion is seen in the right high frontal parafalcine region. It is abutting the falx and small dural tail seen anteriorly (arrow)

Arachnoid Cysts

Arachnoid cysts represent congenital malformations of the arachnoid membrane. They account for 1 percent of all intracranial tumors. Arachnoid cysts are fluid filled cavities, situated entirely within the arachnoid membrane. They either communicate freely with or are separated from the subarachnoid space. The majority of arachnoid cysts remain constant in size, but slow expansion is possible. They occur in decreasing order of frequency in the middle cranial fossa, suprasellar region, quadrigerminal cistern, convexity and posterior fossa. Arachnoid cysts can be an incidental finding or can be found in patients with nonspecific complaints such as headache, seizures or behavioral problems. Larger cysts can cause increased intracranial pressure.

On CT, it shows a low density, non-enhancing cyst, with the same density as CSF. On MRI the intensity of the cyst is identical to CSF (Figs 38A to C), with evidence of long T1 and long T2 relaxation times. They are sharply demarcated and frequently quadrangular in shape. In case of middle cranial fossa cysts which are often large in size the temporal lobe can be hypoplastic. Posterior fossa cysts are frequently associated with hydrocephalus.

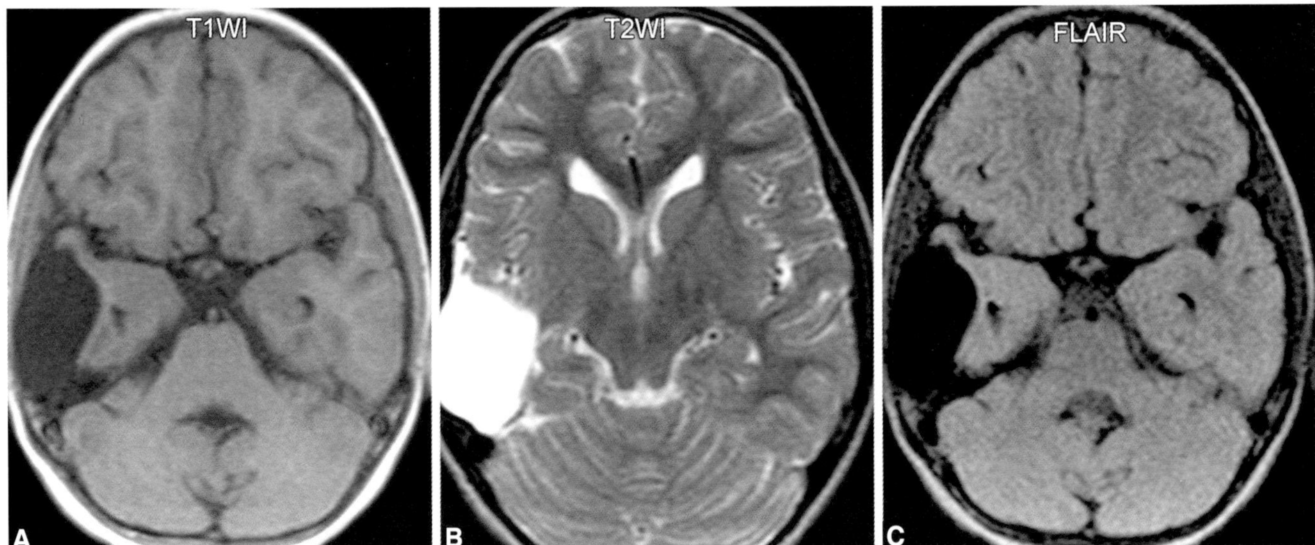

Figs 38A to C: A large well-defined CSF intensity extra-axial lesion is seen in the right temporal region. It appears hypointense on T1W, hyperintense on T2W images and gets suppressed on FLAIR images

Epidermoid

Epidermoid cysts are benign congenital lesions of ectodermal origin and account for approximately 1 percent of all intracranial tumors. It is a benign extracerebral intradural lesion and in about 40 percent of cases is located in the cerebellopontine angle. Although these lesions are congenital, patients are usually not symptomatic until they are aged 20 to 40 years.

On CT, scans, epidermoids show decreased attenuation are most often extra-axial in location (Figs 44A and B). They usually have the same attenuation as that of cerebrospinal fluid (CSF); this characteristic makes their differentiation from arachnoid cysts difficult on CT scans, but they are easily differentiated by MRI. Enhancement is rare but can sometimes be seen around the margin of the tumor. Calcification occurs in only 15 to 20 percent of cases. Rarely, epidermoids can appear hyperdense on CT scans secondary to high protein content.

On T1-weighted images, these lesions are generally slightly hyperintense or isointense relative to gray matter. More specifically, the T1-weighted signal intensity tends to vary with the lipid content, with the signal intensity being increased in lesions with a high lipid content and decreased in those with a low lipid content. The lesions are usually isointense relative to CSF on T2-weighted images, but they may be slightly hyperintense. Enhancement of portions of the rim may be seen after the administration of contrast.

Proton density-weighted and then fluid-attenuated inversion recovery (FLAIR) images demonstrate epidermoids as being hyperintense

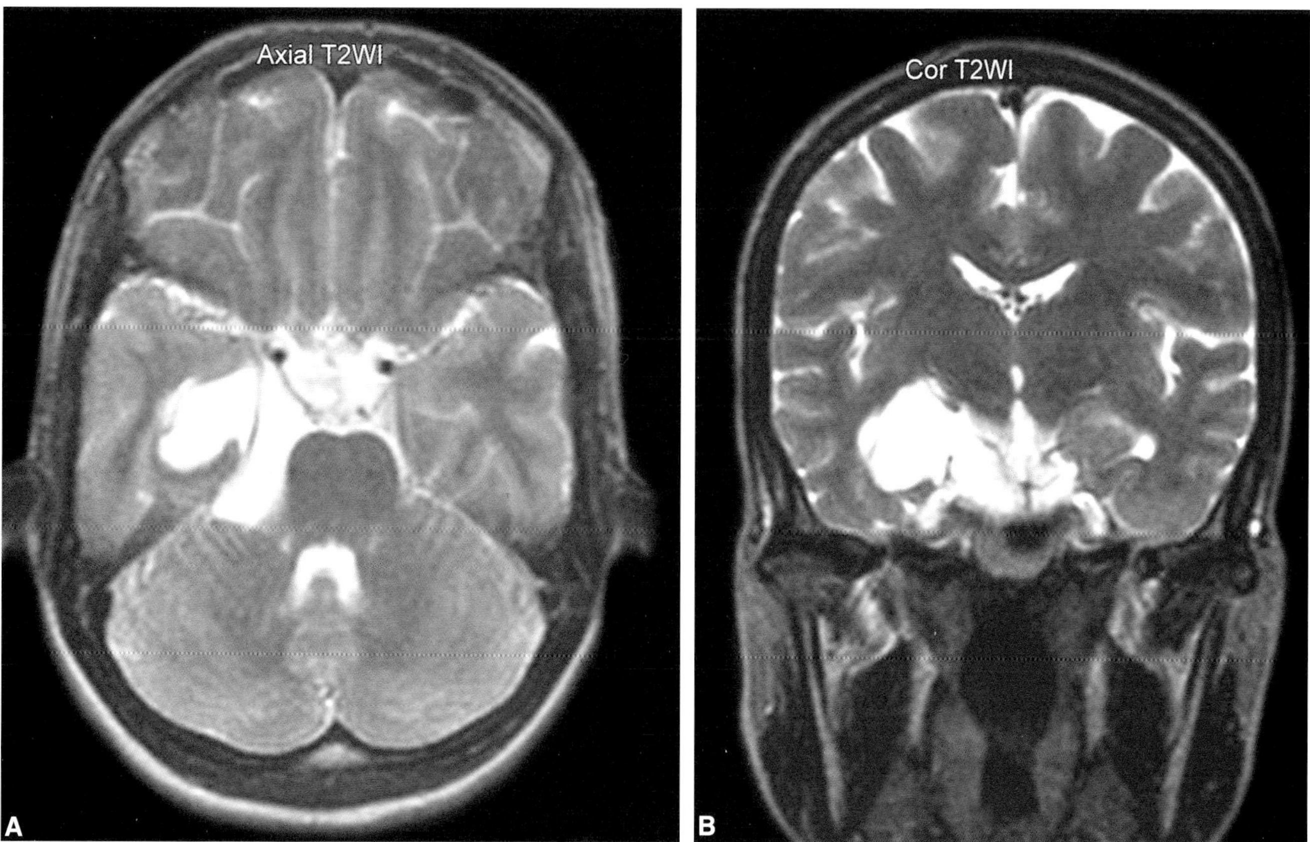

Figs 39A and B: Axial and coronal T2 weighted images reveals well-defined CSF intensity extra-axial lesion in right medial temporal region insinuating in suprasellar cistern, right ambient cistern and inferiorly in right CP angle cistern. It shows some internal inhomogeneity

(Figs 40A and B) relative to CSF (Figs 39A and B) and are useful to differentiate epidermoids from arachnoid cysts. Diffusion-weighted imaging can now be used to differentiate these entities (Figs 42A and B), because epidermoids have markedly restricted diffusion and, therefore, high signal intensity on the diffusion-weighted images. The free water in arachnoid cysts has low signal intensity. Diffusion-weighted images are helpful in assessing residual epidermoid tumors after surgical resection. In rare cases, epidermoids with high protein content can appear hyperintense on T1-weighted images and hypointense on T2-weighted images. Epidermoids can also occur in unusual locations, such as the parenchyma or ventricle.

The major differential consideration for the epidermoid cyst is an arachnoid cyst. Arachnoid cysts are isointense to CSF at all sequences, including FLAIR. They displace rather than invade structures such as the epidermoid. Finally, arachnoid cysts do not show restricted diffusion on DWI. Epidermoid cysts typically show undulating margins and have a tendency to insinuate around the nerves and blood vessels cisterns. Epidermoids reveal no significant enhancement on contrast (Figs 41 and 43).

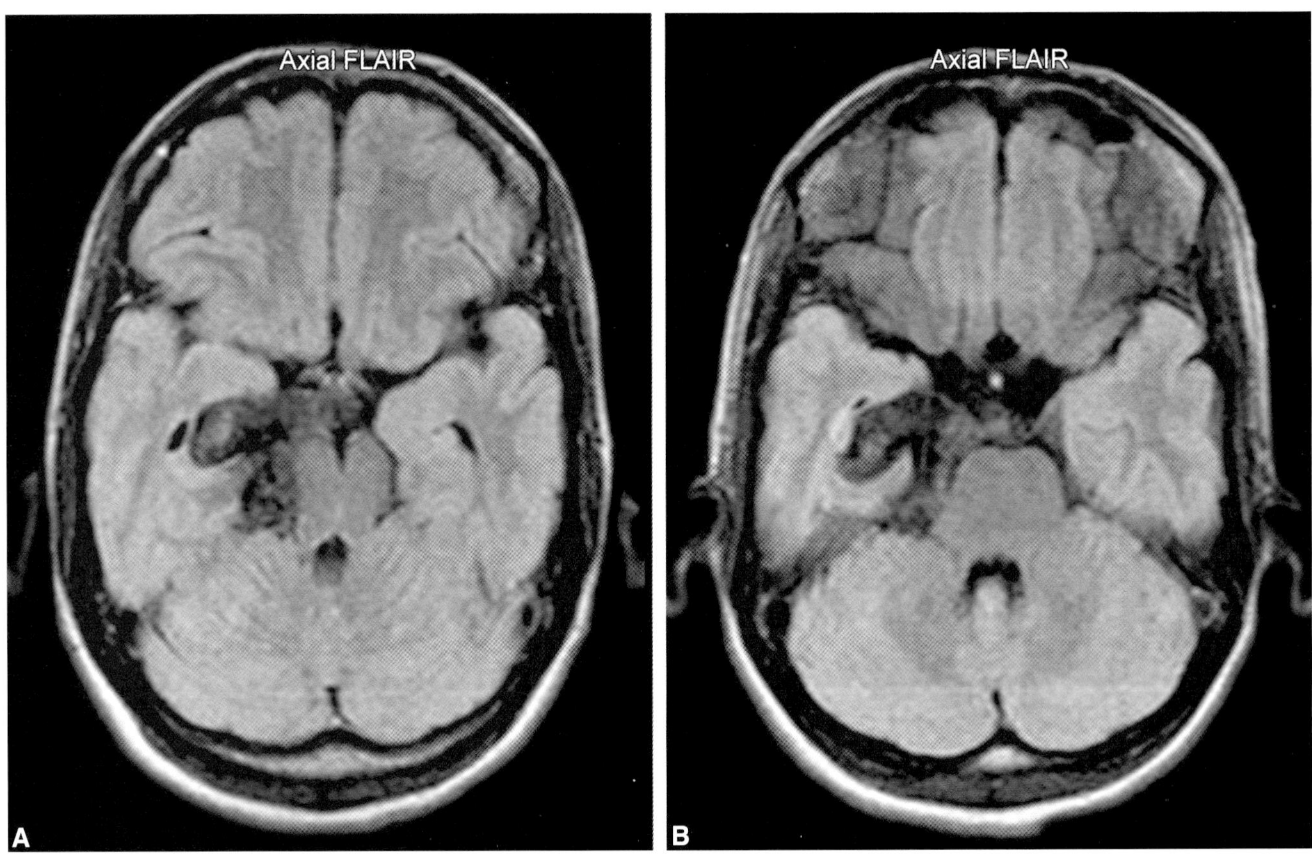

Figs 40A and B: The lesion is mildly hyperintense to CSF on FLAIR images with internal heterogeneity and is causing mass effect on the brainstem and right medial temporal lobe

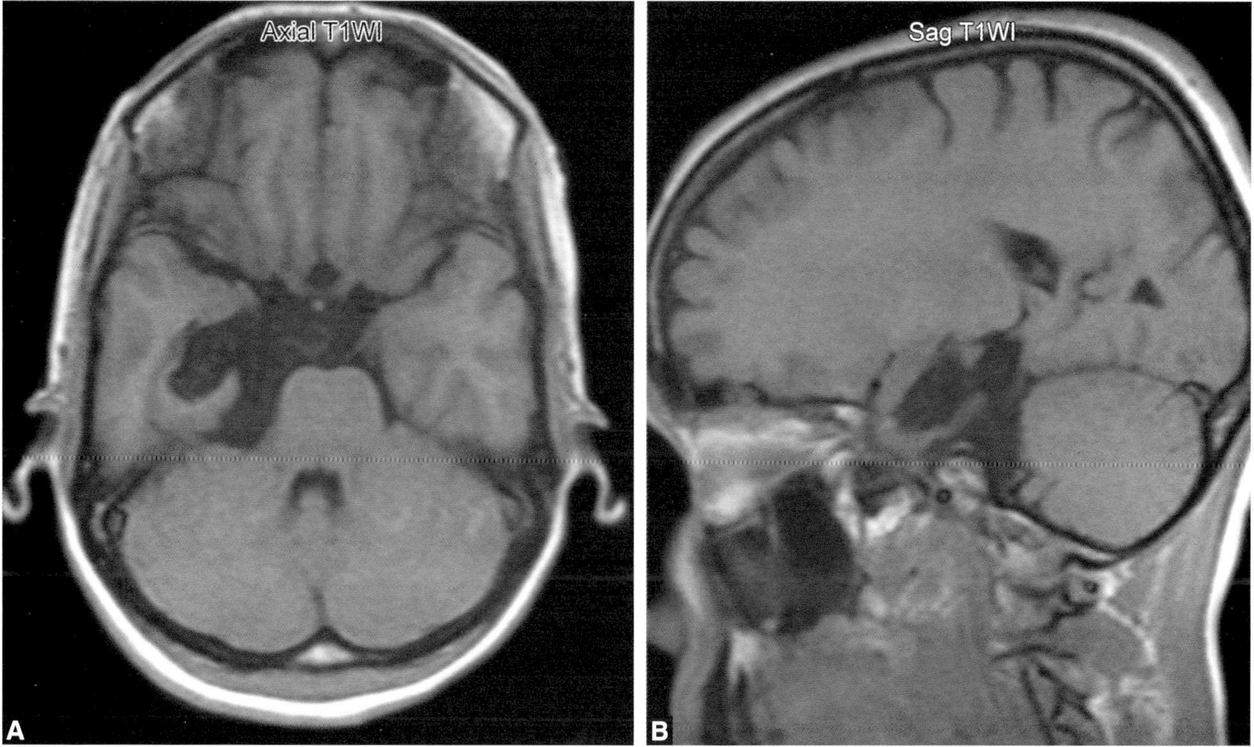

Figs 41A and B: Axial and sagittal T1 weighted images show lesion to be hypointense

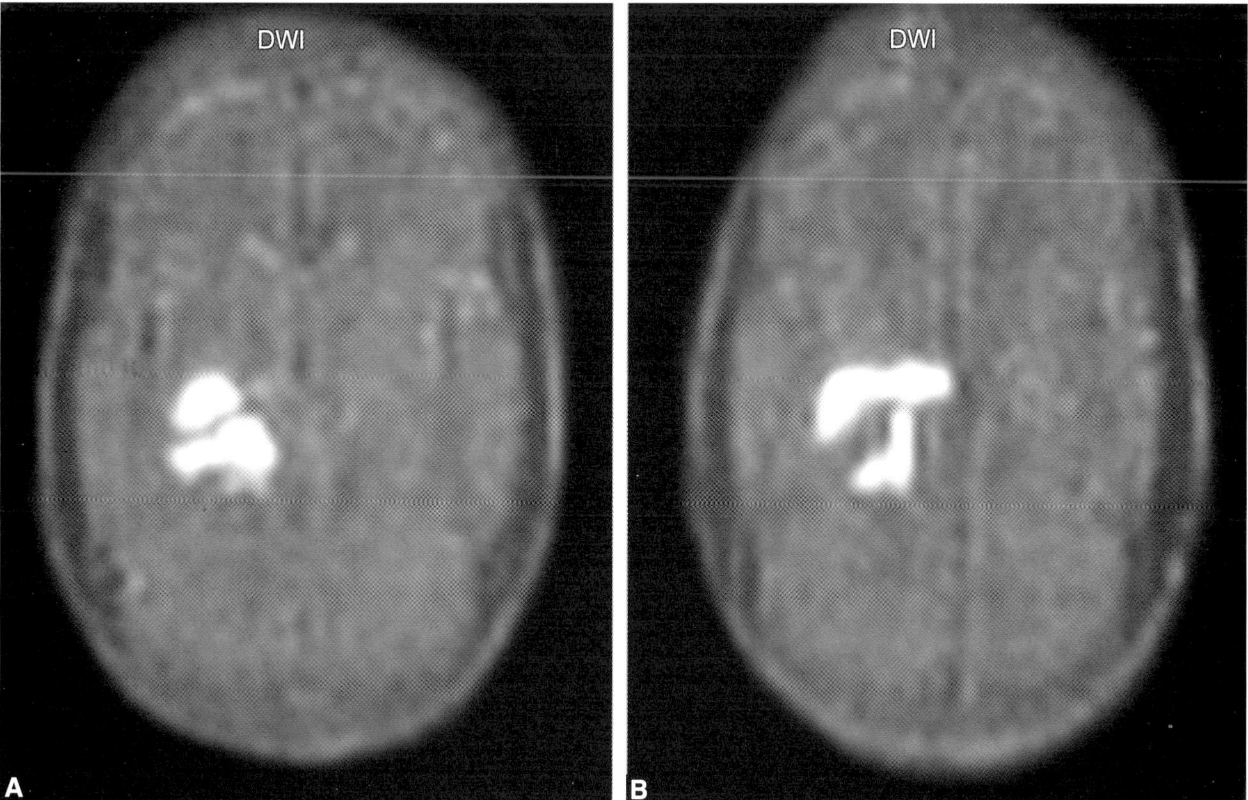

Figs 42A and B: Significant restricted diffusion of the lesion is seen on diffusion weighted images

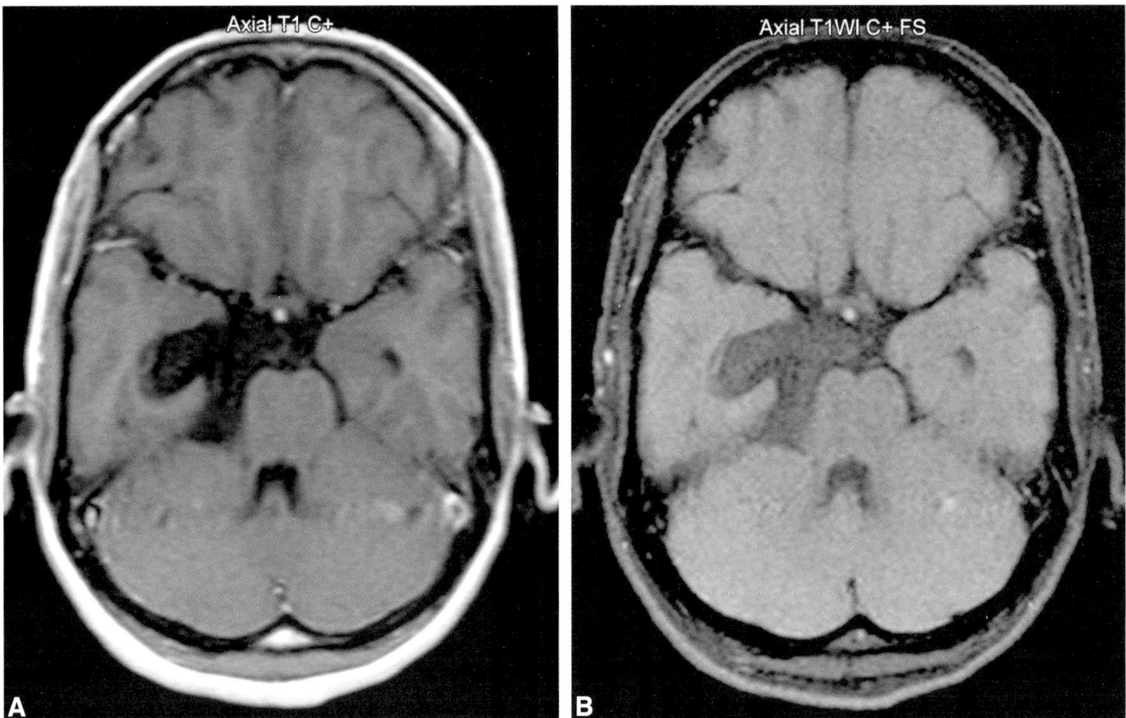

Figs 43A and B: Post-contrast axial T1W and T1FS images reveal no significant enhancement of the lesion

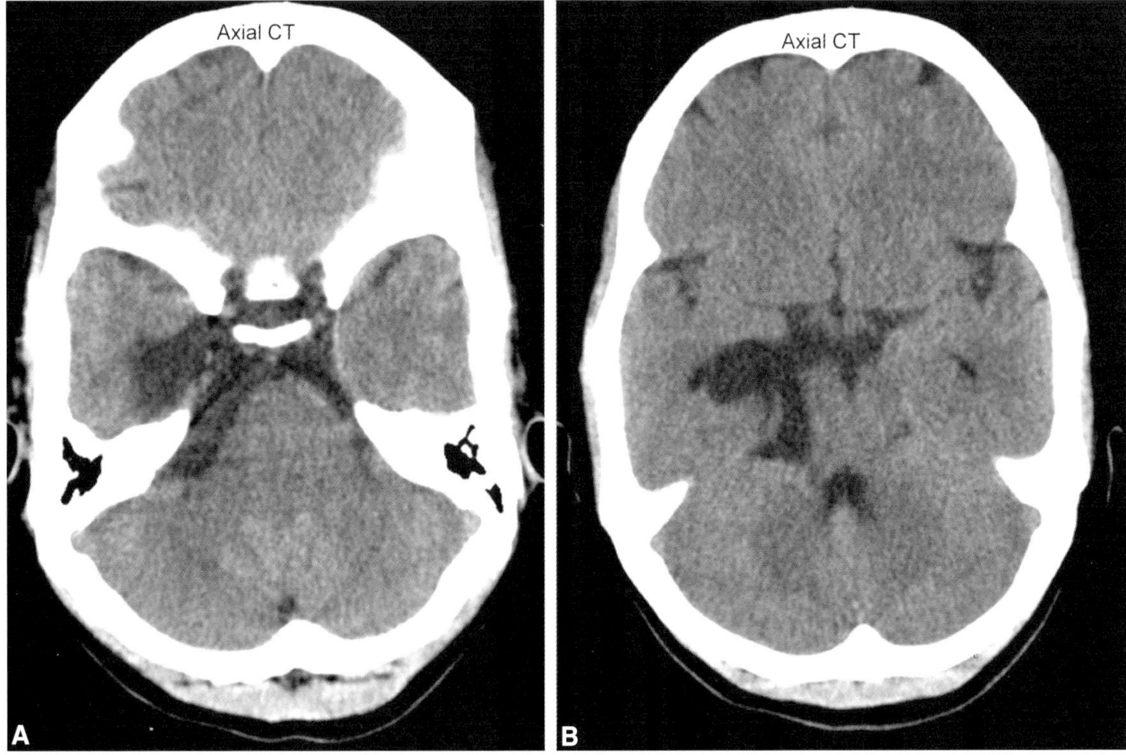

Figs 44A and B: Axial CT images reveals hypodense near CSF attenuation lesion in the right CP angle and ambient cistern, extending into suprasellar cistern and medial to the right temporal lobe with mass effect on the brainstem and the right temporal lobe

Pineal Epidermoid Cyst

Epidermoid cyst is a developmental lesion which arises from abnormal rests of tissue that remain in the intracranial and spinal cavities as a result of incomplete separation of the neuroectoderm from cutaneous ectoderm. In the skull the location of an epidermoid is typically away from the midline, the most common location being the cerebellopontine angle followed by the suprasellar cistern, pineal region and middle cranial fossa. Those in the pineal region may present with hydrocephalus.

On conventional CT and MRI epidermoids have the same density and signal as CSF (Figs 45A to D). They are space-occupying and may mimic an arachnoid cyst. However, the margins of these lesions are typically lobulated and may contain fine linear strands. They may also envelope rather than displace surrounding structures such as cranial nerves. Differentiation from CSF-filled lesions can be on diffusion weighted MRI because these lesions have diffusion characteristics of solid tissue whereas the diffusion characteristics of an arachnoid cyst are similar to CSF.

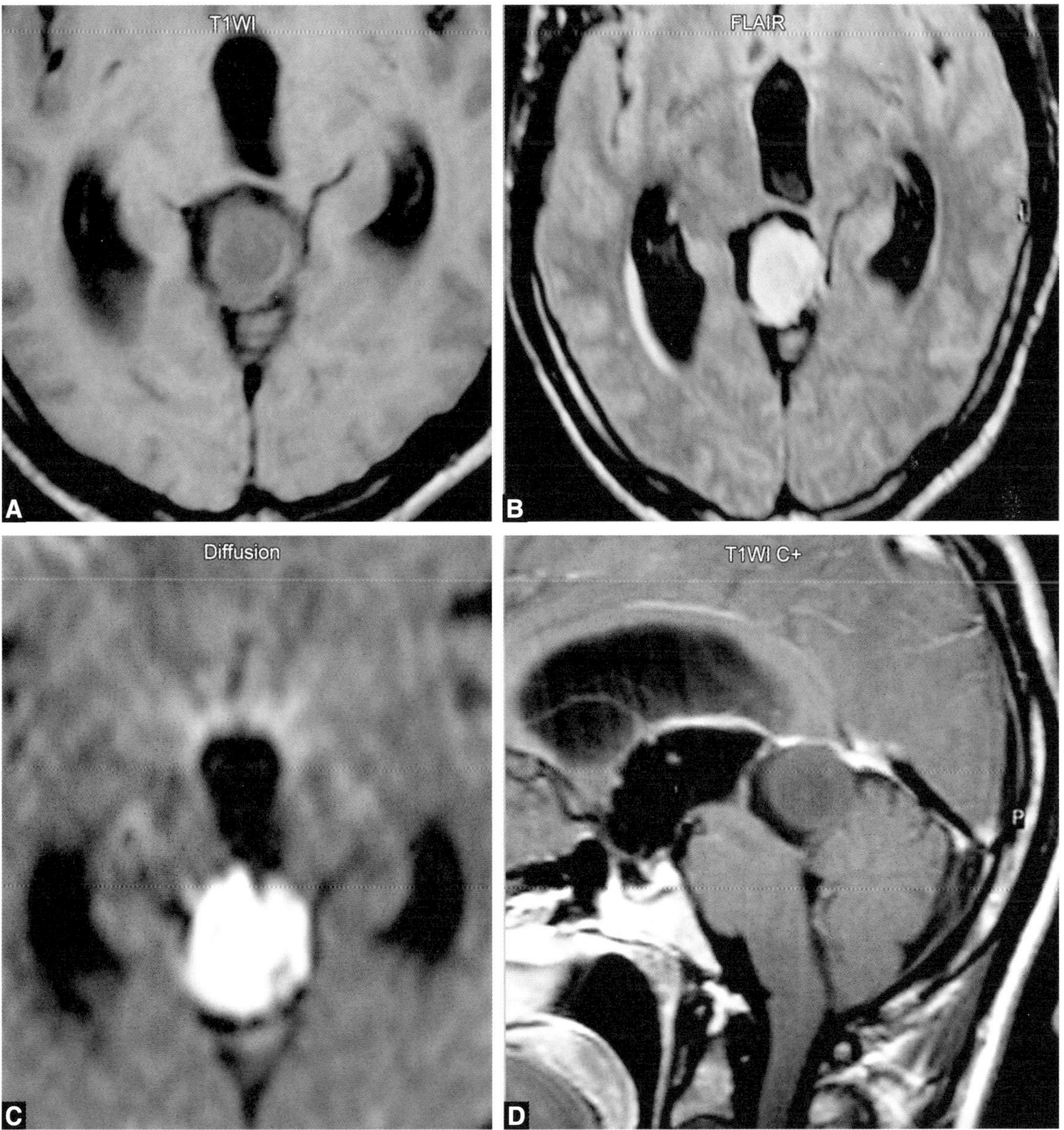

Figs 45A to D: A well-defined extra-axial mass is seen in the quadrigeminal plate cistern. It is hypointense on T1W, hyperintense on FLAIR and diffusion images and does not enhance on contrast image. It compresses the posterior third ventricle leading to moderate hydrocephalus

Gliomas

Gloimas are the largest single group of all intracranial tumors; they are derived from glial cell or stromal cells of the brain and spinal cord. Major types of gliomas are astrocytomas, ependymomas, oligodendrogliomas and choroid plexus tumors. Astrocytomas are the most common among gliomas, they are subdivided into Grade I pilocytic astrocytomas, Grade II diffuse infiltrating astrocytomas, Grade III anaplastic astrocytomas and Grade IV glioblastoma multiforme the most aggressive subtype. On MRI astrocytomas appear as hypo or isointense cysts on T1W1, and hyperintense on T2W, the solid component is isointense or hyperintense to brain parenchyma. Oligodendrogliomas on MRI appear as heterogeneous lesions on all pulse sequences, hyperintensity from a previous hemorrhage may be seen on T1WI, calcification may be hypointense on all spin echo sequences. Choroid plexus tumors on MRI appear as hypo or isointense to the brain on most pulse sequences, they may occasionally be hyperintense on T1WI, and hydrostatic edema may show as hyperintense signals on T2W images (Figs 46A to D). Ependymomas on MRI show marked heterogeneous signals and variable contrast enhancement.

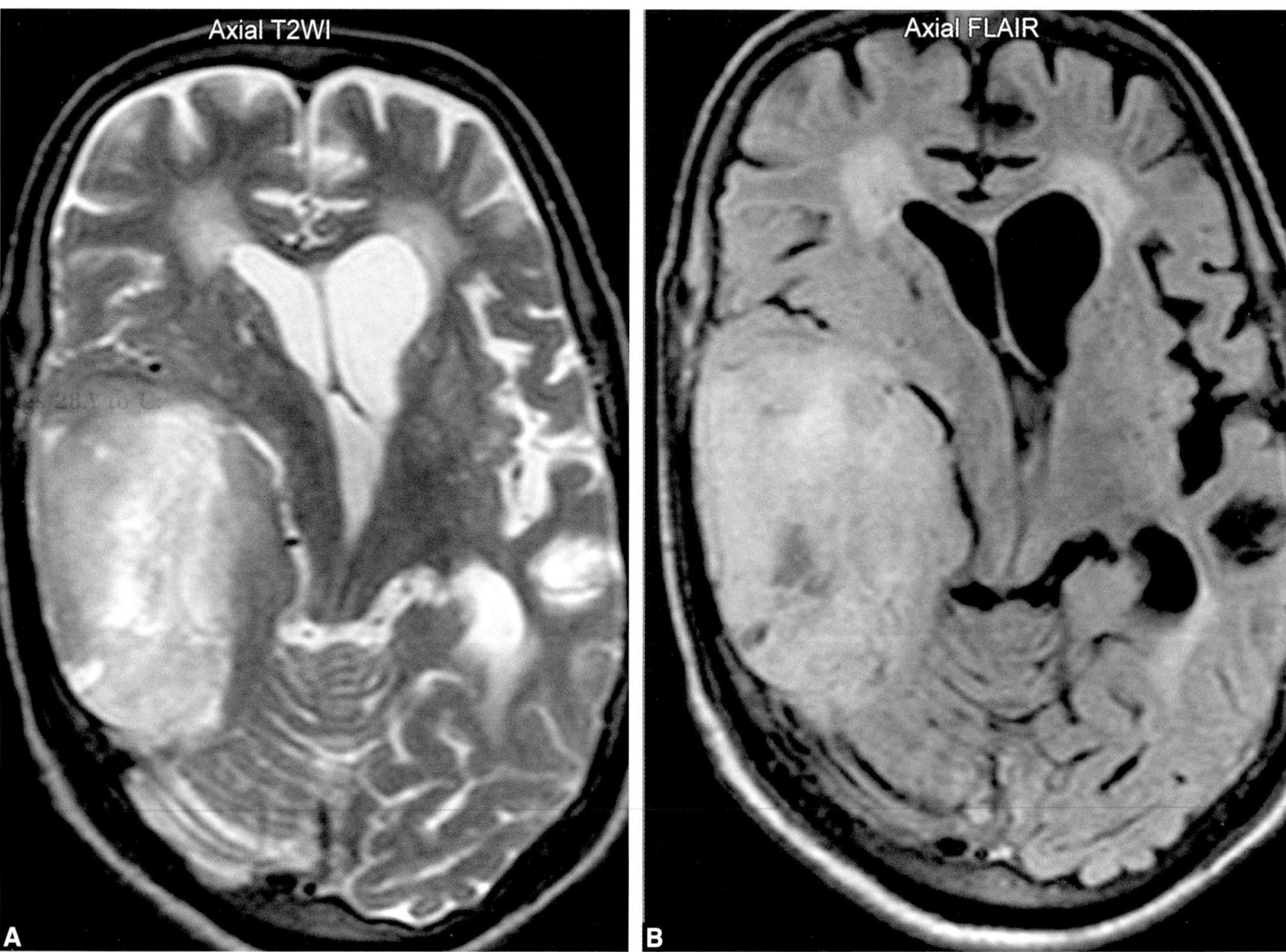

Figs 46A and B

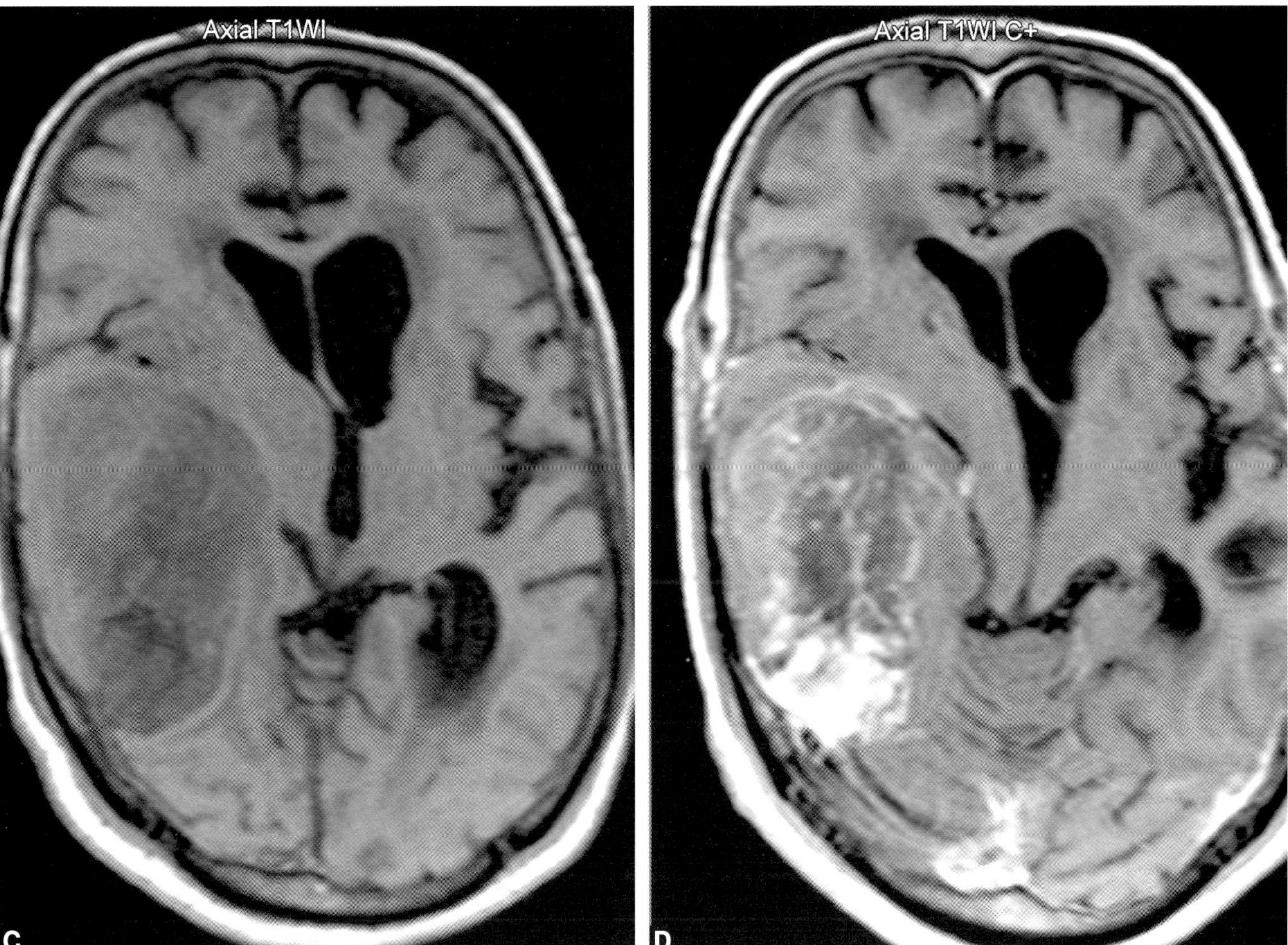

Figs 46C and D

Figs 46A to D: A 85-year-old male diagnosed as glioma shows a heterogeneously hyperintense lesion on T2WI and FLAIR images (A and B) and appears hypointense on T1W image in right temporal lobe on T1W image (C) shows heterogeneous enhancement on post-contrast T1W image (D)

Pontine Glioma

Brainstem gliomas are tumors arising within the region of the brain between the aqueduct of Sylvius and the 4th ventricle. This includes the midbrain, pons, and medulla. The majority of brainstem tumors occur within the pons although the midbrain and medulla may also be involved. Brainstem gliomas are highly aggressive tumors classified as Grade III anaplastic astrocytomas and carry a grave prognosis. Brainstem gliomas are usually nonpilocytic, low grade astrocytomas.

Tumors intrinsic to the brainstem are biologically more aggressive than pilocytic astrocytomas arising in the optic pathways or cerebellar hemispheres, with most patients dying within two years. The incidence of brainstem gliomas has a bimodal distribution with a peak incidence in the second half of the first decade of life and a second peak in the fourth decade. The median age of diagnosis is 5 to 9 years. In adults, the incidence is lower than that in children and the tumor tends to be of lower grade. Clinically, patients present with rapidly progressive cranial nerve and long tract signs. These include double vision, drooping of one side of the face, dysphagia, weakness in the arms and legs. CT can assess tumor density and establish mass effect, the appearance of brainstem gliomas is variable on CT scan and so the diagnostic test of choice is MRI. A round mass expanding the pons is typical. The tumor appears as a hypointense lesion on T1-weighted imaging and hyperintense on T2-weighted imaging. The tumor is often seen locally infiltrating surrounding structures and the leptomeninges. Gadolinium administration frequently displays ring-enhancement (Figs 47A and B).

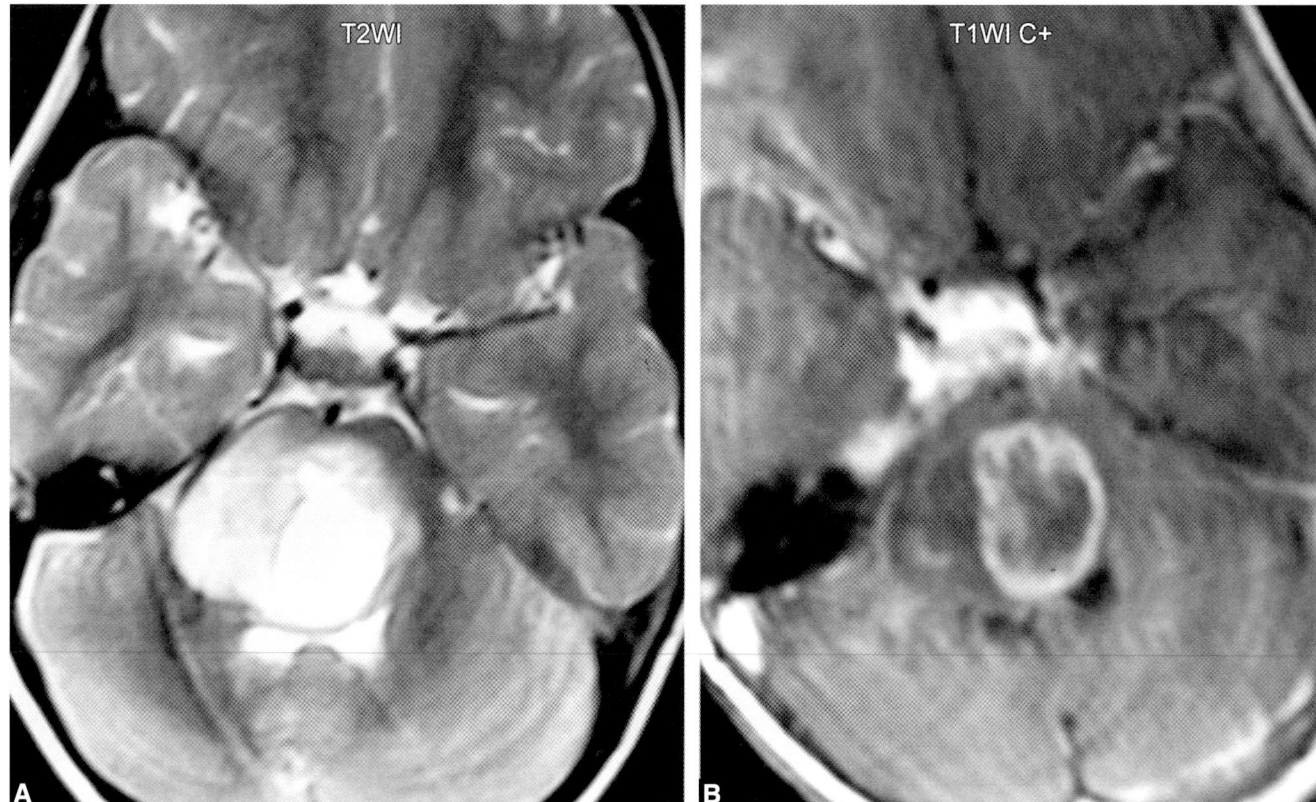

Figs 47A and B: Axial T2W and post-contrast axial images reveal a large heterogeneous lesion in the pons. A part of it shows ring enhancement and rest of it shows mild patchy enhancement with mild perilesional edema, the fourth ventricle is compressed

Glioblastoma Multiforme

The term "multiforme" refers to the highly variable appearance both macroscopically as well as microscopically. Glioblastoma multiforme is the most common of all the primary intracranial tumors of the CNS accounting for about 25 percent of all tumors and 50 percent of all gliomas.

The tumor occurs in adult life, with a peak incidence between 45 and 60 years. They are typically located in the cerebral hemisphere, most frequently frontotemporal. Origin of the tumor in the corpus callosum with bihemispheric extension to the frontal or parieto-occipital lobes is common.

On non-contrast CT the tumor is very inhomogeneous with evidence of a large area of central necrosis with cyst- or pseudocyst formation. The tumor can be hemorrhagic and is surrounded by extensive edema with finger-like infiltration of the white matter tracts. Enhancement is typically multifocal and ring-like with asymmetry of the thickness of the enhancing rim and focal nodular enhancing formations.

On MRI the tumor is strikingly inhomogeneous with foci of cyst formation, necrosis and hemorrhage. Enhancement is inhomogeneous and pronounced with large areas of inhomogeneous diffuse enhancement, alternating with multifocal-ring (Figs 48A to D) enhancement with wall irregularities and nodular enhancing formations.

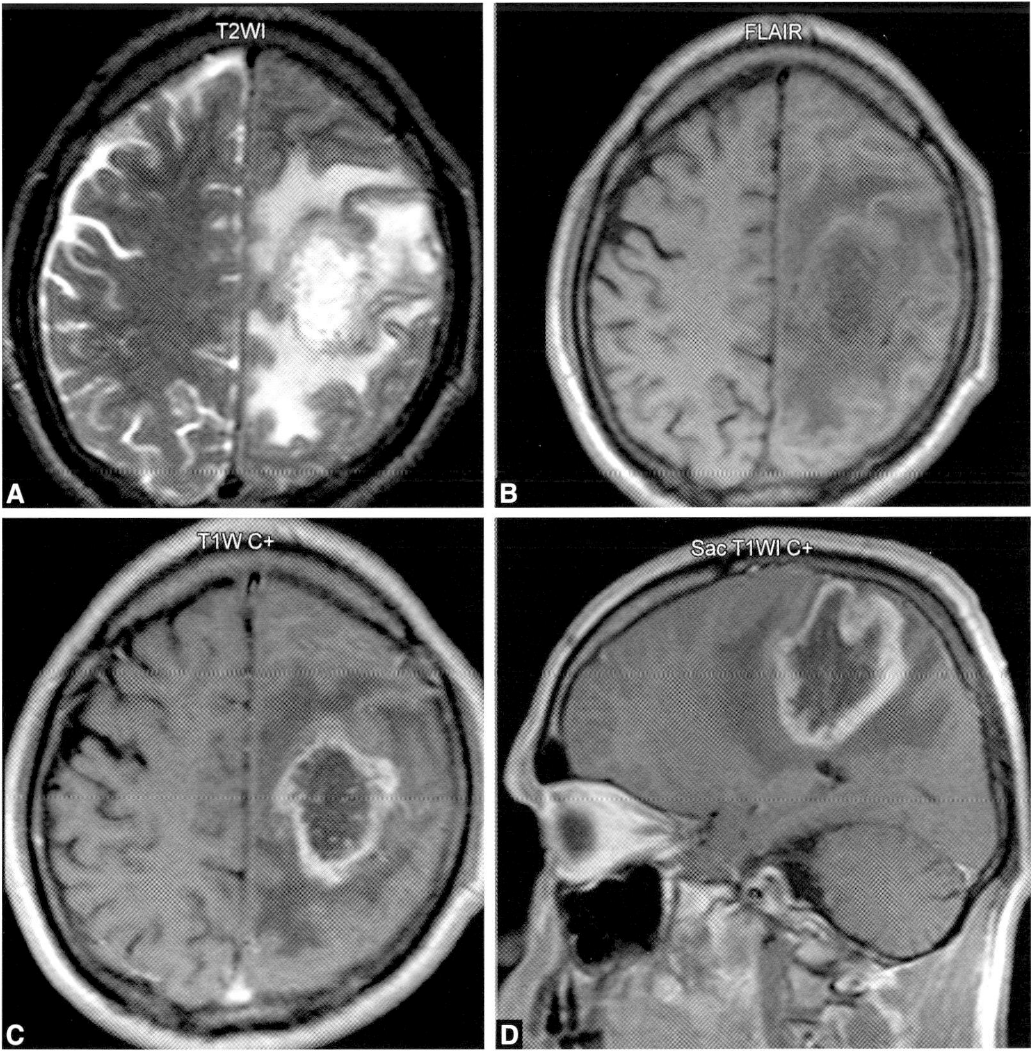

Figs 48A to D: T2WI, FLAIR, post-contrast T1W axial and sagittal image shows a large ring enhancing lesion with central necrosis in left frontoparietal parenchyma. There is moderate perilesional edema and mass effect

Pituitary Macroadenoma

Pituitary macroadenoma is the most common intrasellar tumor. Size is more than 1 cm and they are associated with pituitary insufficiency or visual impairment due to compression of the optic chiasma from suprasellar extension of the mass. It may be associated with cranial nerve deficit. Enlarged sella may also be evident. Macroadenomas are usually solid encapsulated tumors that may have necrotic, cystic, hemorrhagic or sometimes calcified areas. On MRI, they appear isointense with brain on both T1W and T2W images, enhance moderately with intravenous contrast, cystic components within the tumor has a signal intensity intermediate between that of the CSF and the tumor in T1WI and have high signal on T2WI images (Figs 49A to D).

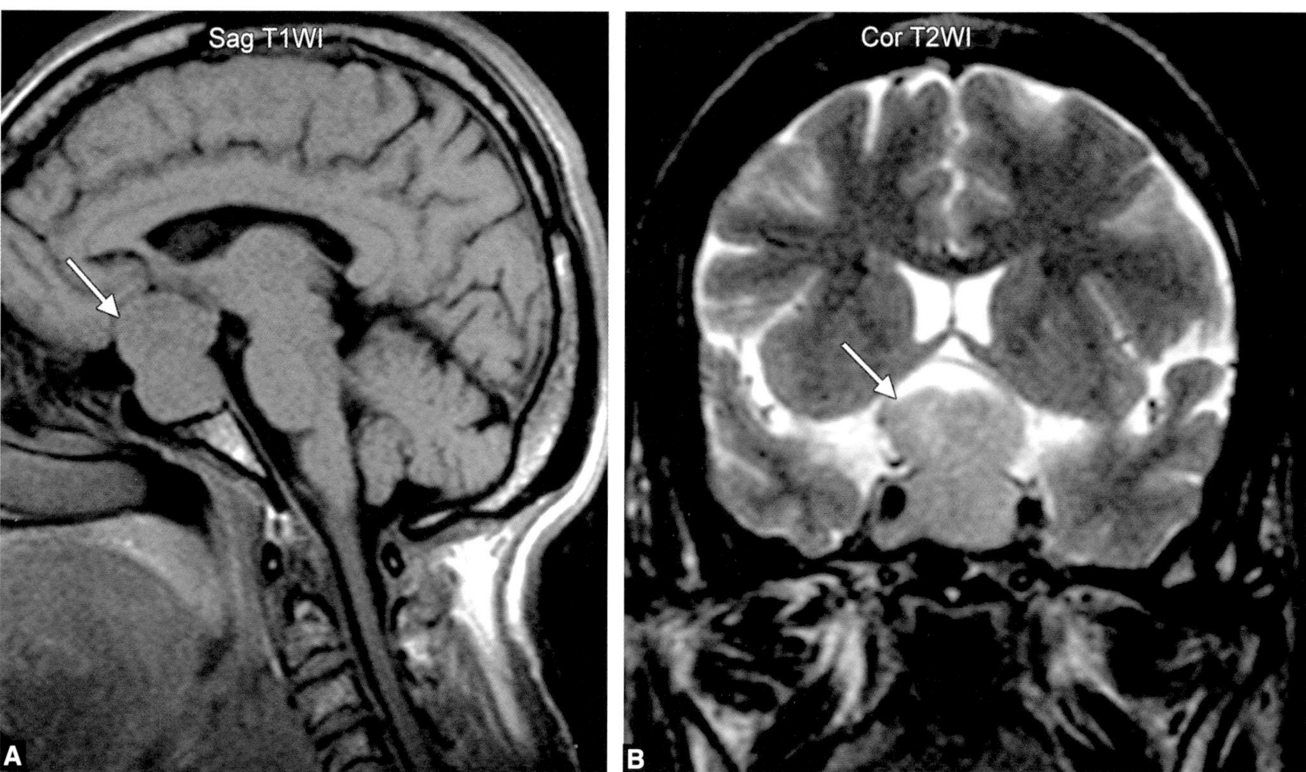

Figs 49A and B

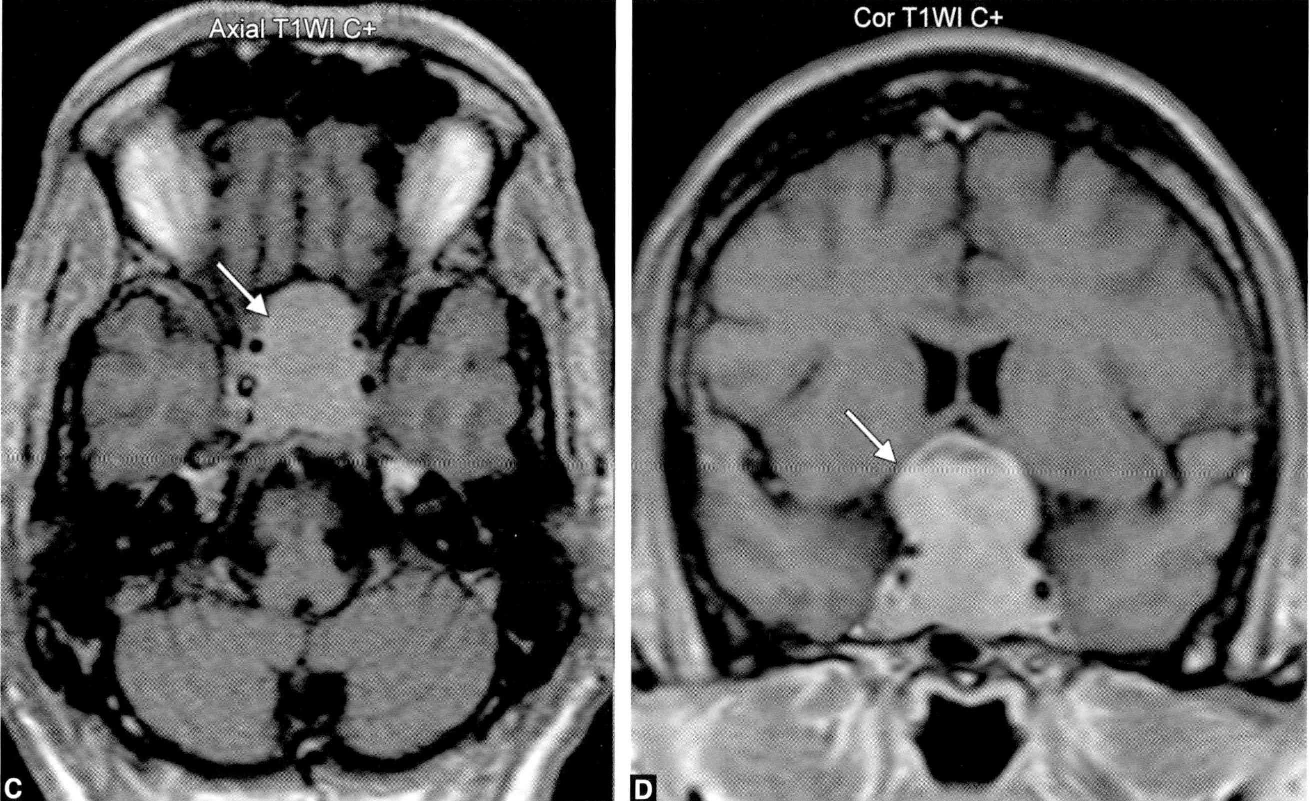

Figs 49C and D

Figs 49A to D: Sagittal T1 (A), coronal T2 (B) images reveal a large isointense lesion in the sella, extending into suprasellar region. Post-contrast axial T1W (C) and coronal T1W (D) images reveals intense homogeneous enhancement in a 55-year-old male patient

Craniopharyngioma

Craniopharyngioma accounts for 3 to 5 percent of all primary brain tumors. They are epithelial neoplasms arising from squamous epithelial nests of Rathke's pouch. Craniopharyngioma is a supra and/or intrasellar mass with cystic and solid components. The cysts have a content of brown cholesterol containing "machinery oil" like fluid. Calcification is common and can be nodular or curvilinear. The majority of craniopharyngiomas are suprasellar.

On CT, craniopharyngioma is seen as a heterogenous mass with cystic and solid components. Calcification is extremely frequent and is nodular or curvilinear. Enhancement can be confined to the solid part of the tumor or can be rim-like.

On MR, the signal intensity of craniopharyngioma is highly variable. The cysts can be hypointense to hyperintense on T1 weighted spin echo images. Increased signal intensity on T1 weighted MR images are due to higher protein concentration and the presence of free methemoglobin, or both. Post-contrast image shows well defined heterogeneously enhancing lesion with enhancing mural nodule (Figs 50A and B).

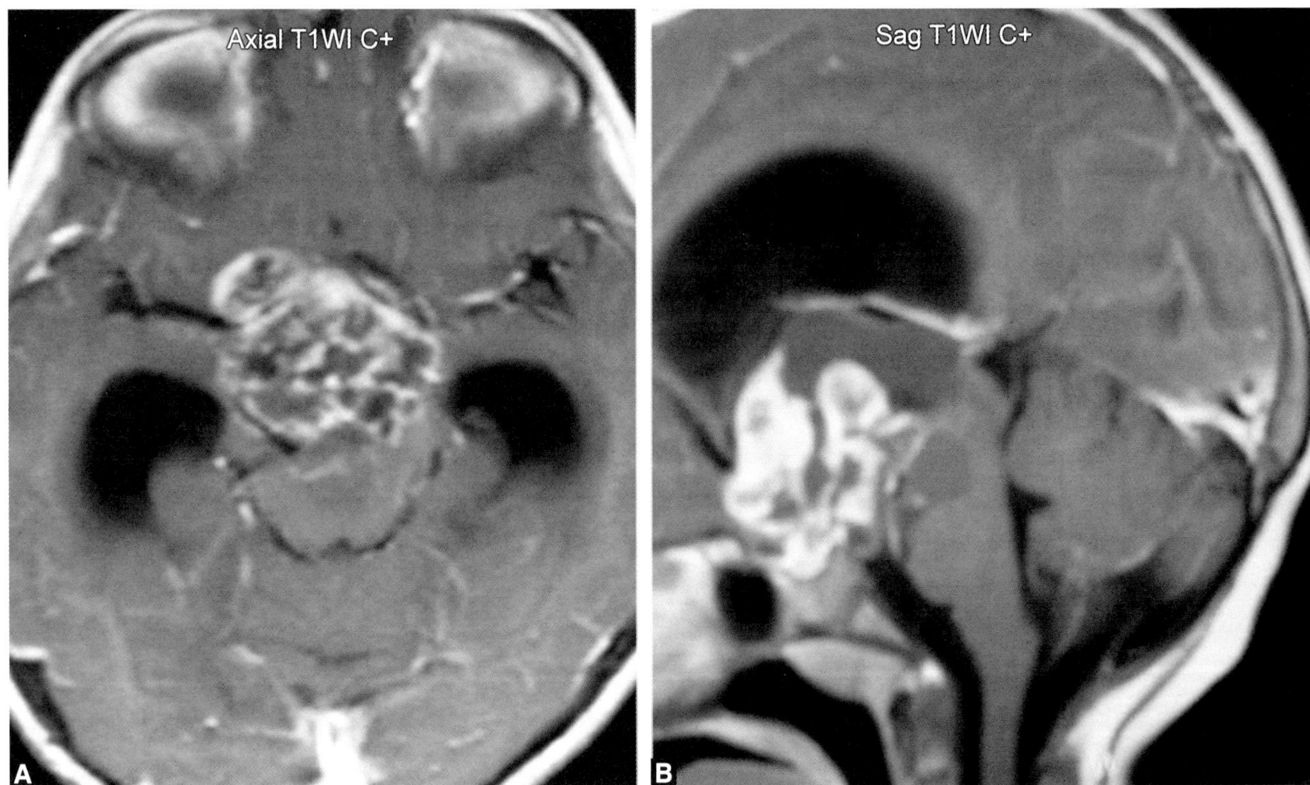

Figs 50A and B: Post-contrast axial T1W and sagittal images shows a well-defined heterogeneously enhancing lesion in the sellar and suprasellar region with enhancing solid component and nonenhancing cystic component. The ventricular dilatation is due to compression of third ventricle

Acoustic Schwannoma

Acoustic schwannoma accounts for 5 to 8 percent of all intracranial tumors. They constitute 70 to 90 percent of all cerebellopontine angle masses. Acoustic neuromas originate from Schwann cells. The most common site of origin is the superior vestibular nerve. These are slowly growing, encapsulated tumors. Intratumoral bleeding and cyst formation is frequent. The tumor erodes and widens the internal auditory canal and shows extra-axial growth in the cerebellopontine angle cistern. Compression of the cerebellum and brainstem is possible.

Patient presents with slowly progressive sensorineural hearing loss and tinnitus. Later gait disturbance and dizziness reflect vestibular symptoms. Acoustic schwannomas can be part of neurofibromatosis type 2 when it usually presents earlier and are predominantly bilateral.

On CT, acoustic schwannomas appear mostly iso to hypodense, with intense and homogeneous enhancement. Funnel shape widening of the internal auditory canal is evident on bone window settings. On MR intracanalicular acoustic neuromas enhance brightly and stand out clearly against the absent signal from the cortical bone of the internal auditory meatus. On T1 weighted images the tumor is iso to hypointense (Figs 52A to C) and on T2 weighted sequences the tumor can be hyperintense. Hyperintense cystic components are common. Enhancement is intense and homogeneous (Figs 51 and 52).

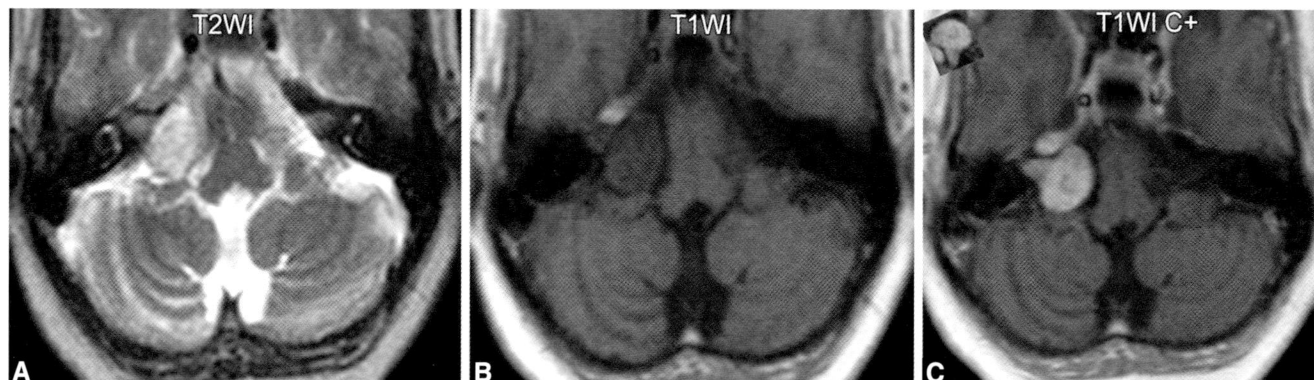

Figs 51A to C: Axial T2W image shows a hyperintense mass in right CP angle causing compression of the pons (A) on axial T1W image mass in right CP angle is hypointense (B) axial post-contrast T1W image (C) shows the mass intensely enhancing giving "icecream cone" appearance having cisternal and canalicular component (inset)

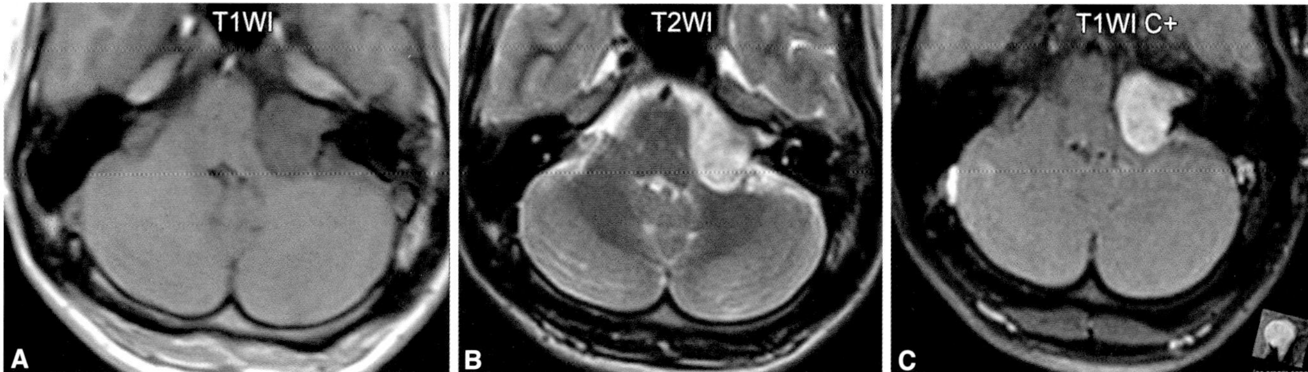

Figs 52A to C: T2W shows hyperintense and T1W shows hypointense mass lesion in the region of left VII-VIII nerve complex, on post-contrast T1W image shows intense enhancement of the mass, it extends into the left internal acoustic meatus giving "icecream cone" appearence (inset) with mass effect noted on pons and fourth ventricle

Cerebellar Astrocytoma

Cerebellar astrocytoma accounts for about 11 to 30 percent of primary CNS tumors in children and constitutes about one-third of childhood posterior fossa tumors. These present late in the first decade or in the early second decade. Cerebellar astrocytoma tends to involve the hemispheres, although extension into or origin within the vermis or even the fourth ventricle have been described infrequently. It may be predominantly cystic with a mural nodule, multicystic, or predominantly solid (diffuse) on CT or MR. Radiographically, cerebellar astrocytoma arises within the cerebellar hemisphere and less often in the vermis, and displaces the fourth ventricle without invading it.

On CT, 10 to 25 percent contains foci of calcification. The mass is hypointense on T1-weighted (Fig. 53A) and hyperintense on T2 weighted MR (Fig. 53B), with one or more cystic components. After contrast administration, the mural nodule and/or solid components enhance, rendering nonenhancing cysts more conspicuous (Fig. 53C).

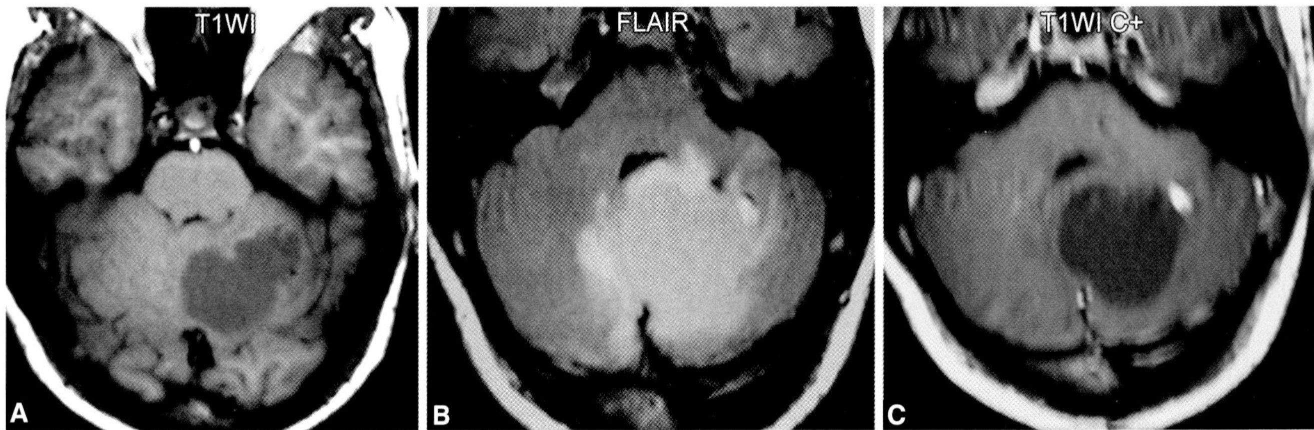

Figs 53A to C: Axial T1W image (A) shows a cystic lesion in the left cerebellar hemisphere with a small isointense mural nodule. Small flow voids are seen due to high velocity blood flow in the vessels that supply the nidus. The cyst is hyperintense on FLAIR image (B) and the mural nodule remains isointense. Post-contrast T1W axial image (C) reveals intense enhancement of the mural nodule

Medulloblastoma

Medulloblastoma accounts for 4 to 8 percent of primitive intracranial tumors of neuroepithelial origin. It represents 15 to 30 percent of all pediatric brain tumors and it is a rare entity in the adult age accounting to less than 1 percent of brain tumors in this age group. The peak of occurrence is between 5 and 7 years of age, with 70 percent of them occurring under 16 years. At the presentation truncal ataxia, intracranial hypertension syndrome, lethargy, headache, and morning vomiting are the most frequent symptoms.

On CT scans, these tumors are described as a well-defined hyperdense and homogeneous midline mass with marked enhancement after contrast injection.

The MRI frequently shows a well-defined posterior fossa tumor, which presents low signal on T1 and high signal on T2 weighted images, with marked enhancement after gadolinium injection (Figs 54A to C).

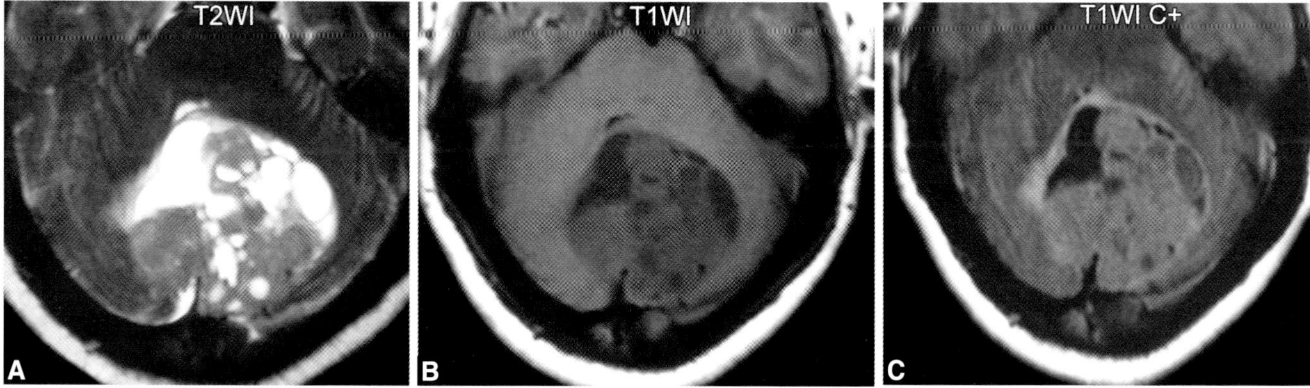

Figs 54A to C: Well-defined heterogeneous lesion with solid and cystic components is seen in the posterior fossa involving the vermis. The solid component is isointense to mildly hyperintense on T2W image (A) isointense on T1W image (B), and reveals moderate enhancement on post-contrast image (C). The cystic component is hypointense on T1W image and hyperintense on T2W image

Metastases

Metastases are probably the most common brain tumor. They occur in all age groups. The most common primary malignancies to metastasize to the brain in adults are breast, lung, melanoma, kidney, and GI, and in children are neuroblastoma, lymphoma/leukemia, and sarcoma. Metastases may be solitary in 30 to 50 percent of cases. Classically, metastases occur at the gray-white matter junction, although they may be seen anywhere. They tend to be round but can be multilobulated and confluent. They have a highly variable appearance on imaging studies. Lesions with cystic centers may demonstrate ring-enhancement.

The pre-contrast CT may identify hemorrhage within a mass that would be masked if only post-contrast images were obtained. The presence of hemorrhage may narrow the differential considerations. Hemorrhagic metastases are commonly caused by melanoma, breast carcinoma, lung carcinoma, renal cell carcinoma, and colon carcinoma. Choriocarcinoma metastases are also known to bleed, but they are very rare tumors. On T1WI the metastasis are hypointense with perilesional edema (Fig. 55A) and on contrast T1WI it may show ring enhancement (Fig. 55B)/ heterogeneous enhancement.

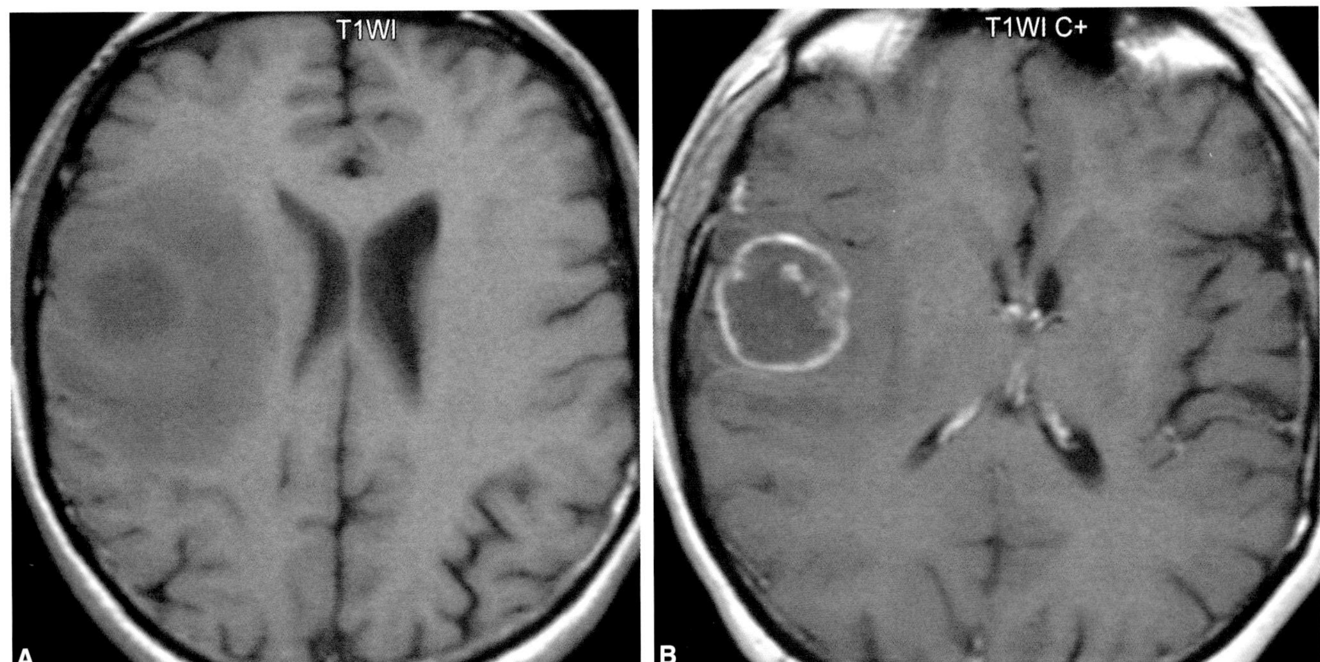

Figs 55A and B: T1WI (A) shows a solitary well-defined hypointense lesion at gray-white matter interface seen in right temporal region with perilesional edema. The post-contrast image (B) shows peripheral ring enhancement of the lesion

MISCELLANEOUS

Empty Sella

In empty sella the content of the sella is mainly composed of CSF-filled subarachnoid space. The pituitary gland is present but usually flattened over the sella floor and the pituitary stalk is slightly stretched. The bony sellar cavity may be of normal volume or slightly enlarged. It may be asymptomatic or accompanied by headache, blurred vision, visual field defects and mild endocrinopathies like obesity, hypopituitarism and hyperprolactinemia.

Plain film may show a slightly enlarged sella without significant floor erosion. CT shows a hypodense content. MR demonstration is superior and shows the CSF signal within the sella on both sagittal and coronal T1 and T2 weighted images, the pituitary gland may be flattened and thinned and stalk is generally stretched (Fig. 56).

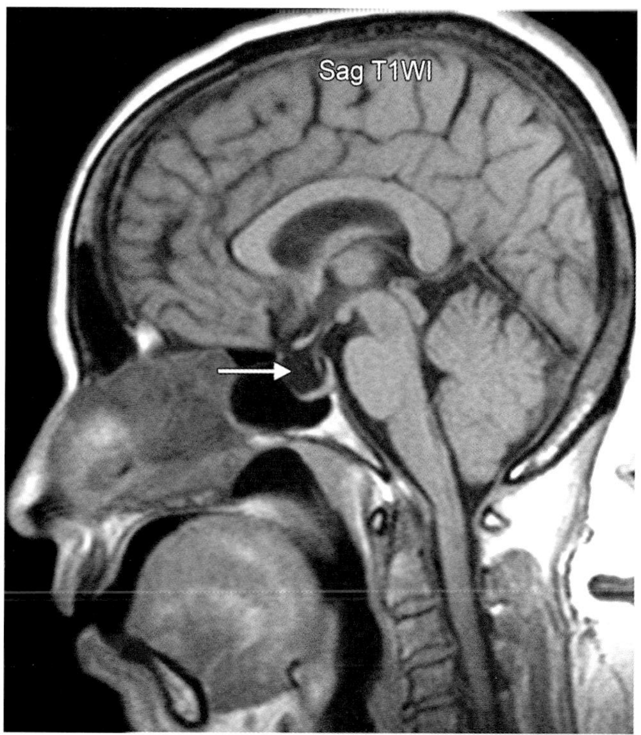

Fig. 56: Sagittal T1WI image shows that the sella is filled with CSF as a result appears hypointense. and is called empty sella, the pituitary gland is flattened

Cerebral Venous Thrombosis

Cerebral venous thrombosis is a relatively uncommon disorder. Causal factors may be classified as local (related to intrinsic or mechanical conditions of the cerebral veins and dural sinuses) or systemic (related to clinical conditions that promote thrombosis). Local processes that alter the venous flow (e.g. sinus trauma, regional infection such as that in mastoiditis, and neoplastic invasion or compression) may potentiate the development of thrombosis. Systemic causes include protein S and protein C deficiencies, a peripartum state, oral contraceptive use, and hypercoagulable states secondary to malignancy. In as many as 25 percent of cases, no cause is identified.

Generalized neurologic symptoms like headache is experienced by 75 to 95 percent of patients and focal neurologic deficits, including seizure, may result.

The pathophysiology of brain parenchymal involvement in venous occlusion differs from that in arterial occlusion. Parenchymal changes may be secondary to cytotoxic edema, vasogenic edema, or intracranial hemorrhage. The primary underlying mechanism is likely to be increased venous pressure. If collateral pathways of venous drainage are insufficient, especially in the presence of cortical venous involvement, subsequent parenchymal changes may occur. If venous pressure continues to increase, with a consequent diminishment in arterial perfusion pressure, cell death may ensue. If adequate collateral pathways develop or recanalization occurs before cell death or intracranial hemorrhage, the parenchymal changes may resolve partly or completely.

On MRI venous sinus thrombosis vary with clot age. Acute thrombus is isointense with cortex on T1WI, whereas subacute clots are hyperintense on T1W scans and hypointense on T2WI. T2WI shows loss of normal flow void (Fig. 57A). Subacute thrombi are typically hyperintense on all pulse sequences,

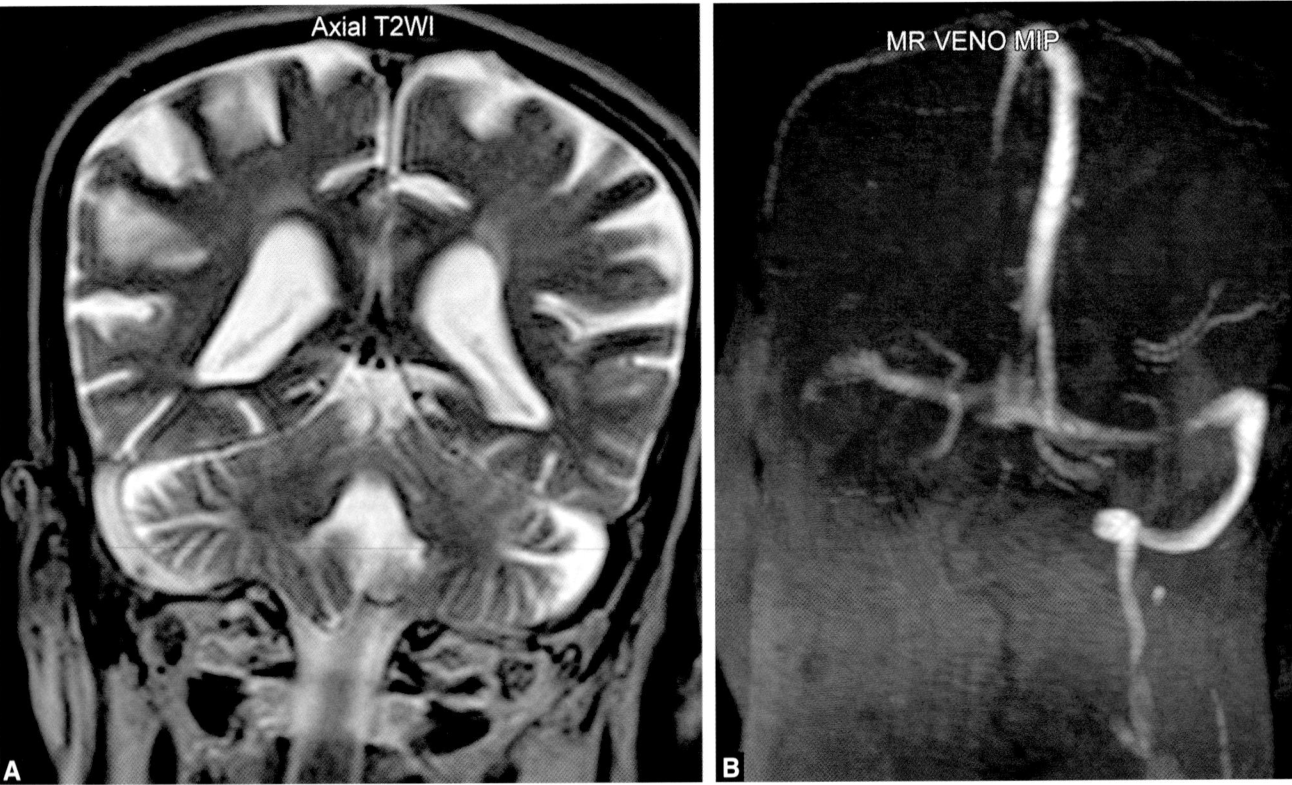

Figs 57A and B: Coronal T2W image shows loss of normal flow void of right sigmoid sinus (A) and MIP MR venogram (B) shows nonvisualization of right sigmoid sinus

chronic thrombosed sinuses often undergo fibrosis. MR venography (Fig. 57B) is the method most commonly used for the diagnosis of cerebral venous thrombosis. Two-dimensional TOF techniques are used to evaluate the intracranial venous system because of their excellent sensitivity to slow flow and their diminished sensitivity to signal loss from saturation effects compared with the sensitivities of three-dimensional TOF techniques.

Hypoplasia and aplasia of the right or left transverse sinus is a common finding. It can easily be mistaken for sinus thrombosis, because on the MRV one of the transverse sinuses is missing. In case of hypoplastic transverse sinus, one should look at the size of the jugular foramen (Fig. 58).

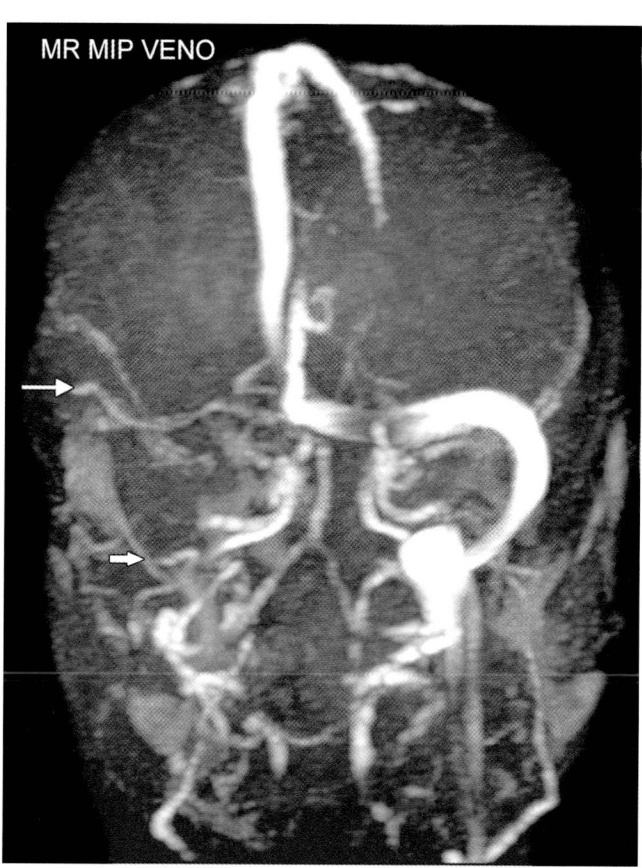

Fig. 58: Another case MR venogram MIP image shows hypoplastic left transverse sinus

Germinal Matrix Hemorrhage

The germinal matrix is the most common site of intracranial hemorrhages in preterm infants. The blood vessels within the germinal matrix are very fragile and consist of a single layer of endothelial cells. In addition there is a poor supporting stroma. Therefore are vulnerable to damage and rupture when exposed to the stress suffered in preterm neonates during the perinatal period.

Ultrasound can easily detect germinal matrix-related hemorrhage, and is used for grading the severity of hemorrhage and in follow-up.

CT scan generally shows the hyperdensity of extravasated blood laterally to the lateral wall of the frontal horns, involving the head of the caudate nucleus and within the lateral ventricles.

MR is also highly informative (Figs 59A and B) but difficult to perform because of the poor clinical condition of these babies, particularly in the acute phase. In the chronic phase MR is helpful in determining the extent of brain damage.

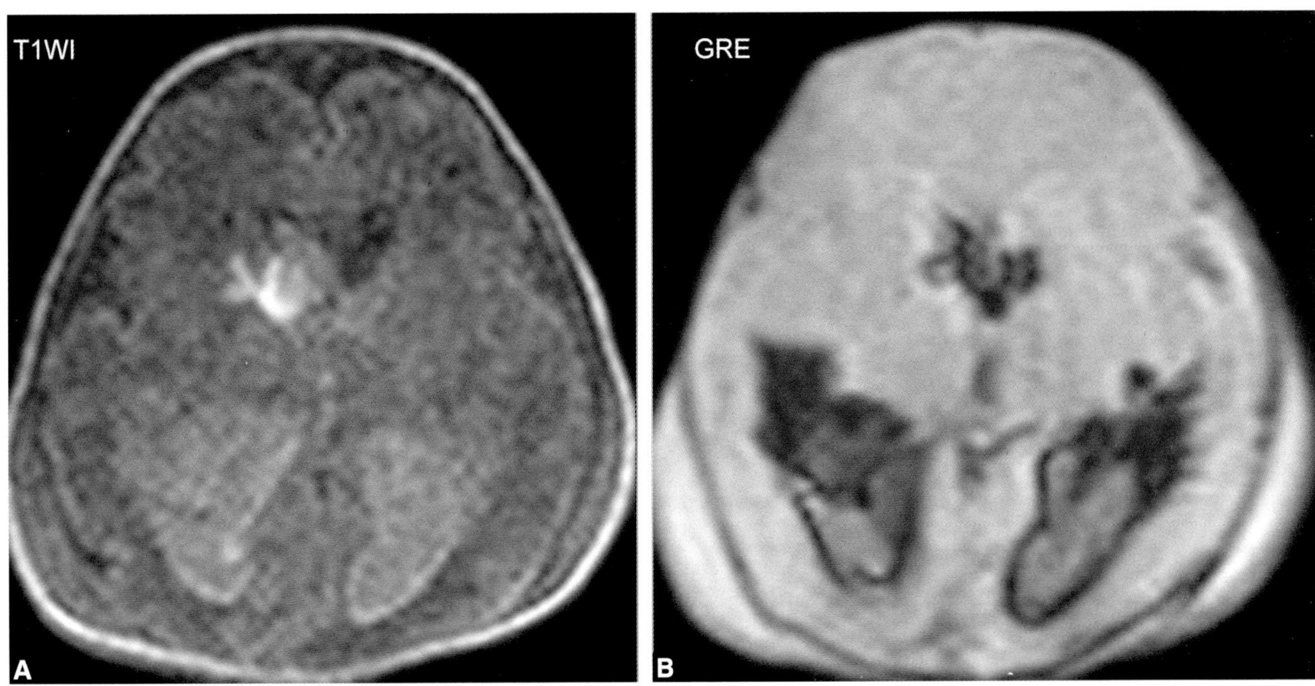

Figs 59A and B: Axial T1W and GRE images reveal hemorrhage in the right germinal matrix with intraventricular extension

Basal Ganglia Hyperintensities

The causes of isolated bilateral basal ganglia hyperintensity in T2 sequence (Figs 60A to C) is possibly due ischemia is seen in:

- *Toxins:* Acute carbon monoxide poisoning, cyanide, hypoglycemia and methanol
- Lymphoma
- *Ischemia:* Hypoxia and venous infarction (internal cerebral vein thrombosis).
- *Neurodegenerative or metabolic diseases:* Wilson disease, Huntington disease (specially caudate heads), methylmalonic acidemia, mitochondrial diseases (Leigh disease) and extrapontine myelinolysis.

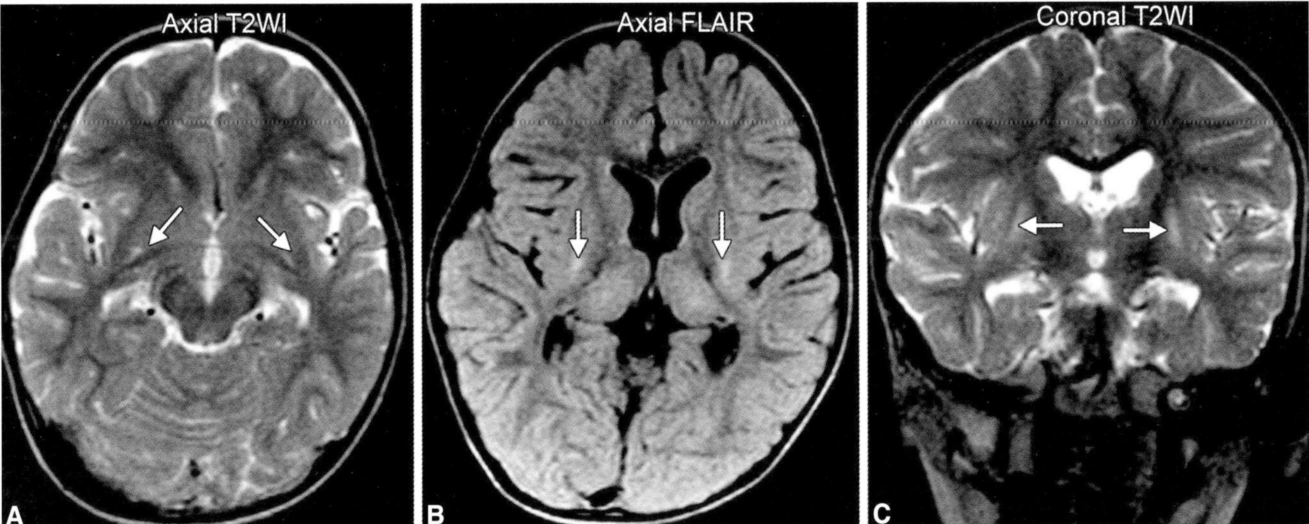

Figs 60A to C: MR 2-year-old male presented with developmental delay hypertonia on axial T2W (A) FLAIR (B) and coronal T2W (C) images show bilateral basal ganglia hyperintensities

Fibrous Dysplasia

Fibrous dysplasia is an uncommon, benign disorder characterized by a tumor-like proliferation of fibro-osseous tissue. The cause of fibrous dysplasia is unknown. Fibrous dysplasia is usually found in the proximal femur, tibia, humerus, ribs, and craniofacial bones in decreasing order of incidence. Usually, only one bone is involved (monostotic fibrous dysplasia). Less often, multiple bones are involved (polyostotic fibrous dysplasia). The polyostotic form is generally more severe and is discovered earlier. This form can involve as few as two bones in the same limb or multiple bones throughout the skeleton. Males and females are equally affected by the disorder. Cases are usually diagnosed within the first three decades of life. It is usually asymptomatic, though pain and swelling may accompany the lesion.

Polyostotic fibrous dysplasia is known to have multiple associations with other disorders. The combination of polyostotic fibrous dysplasia, precocious puberty, and café-au-lait spots is called McCune Albright's syndrome. The association of fibrous dysplasia and soft tissue tumors has been given the name Mazabraud's syndrome. Other endocrine abnormalities including hyperthyroidism, Cushing's disease, thyromegaly, hypophosphatemia, and hyperprolactinemia have been associated with fibrous dysplasia.

Radiographically, fibrous dysplasia appears as a well-circumscribed lesion in a long bone with a ground glass or hazy appearance of the matrix. There is a narrow zone of transition and no periosteal reaction or soft tissue mass. The lesions are normally located in the metaphysis or diaphysis with occasional focal thinning of the overlying cortex due to scalloping from within. The radiological appearance can also be cystic, pagetoid, or dense and sclerotic. Repeated fractures through lesions in the proximal femur can result in the formation of a shepherd's crook deformity. CT scan (Figs 61 and 62) and MRI (Fig. 63) can be helpful in delineating the extent of the lesion and identifying possible pathological fractures and also sarcomatous change within the lesion.

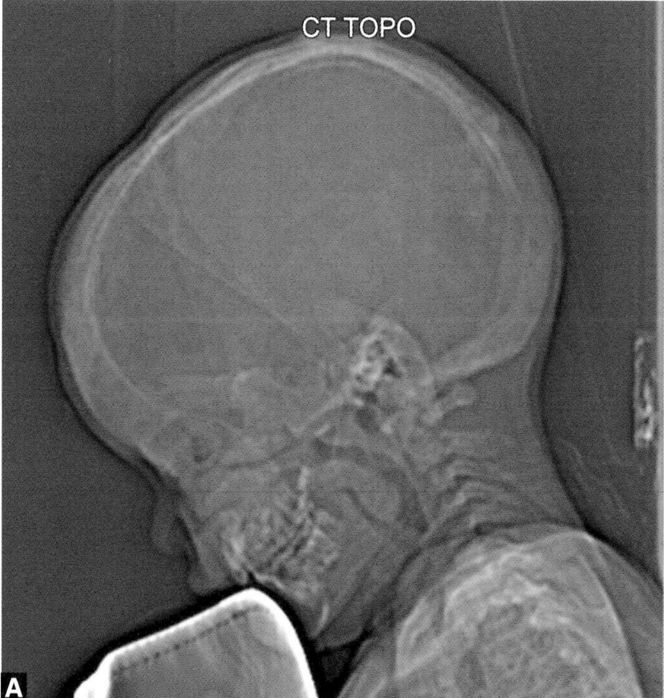

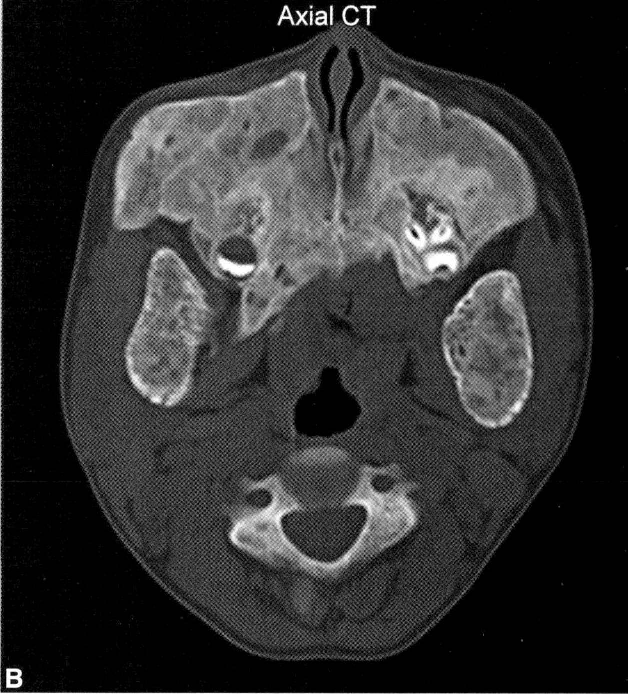

Figs 61A and B: CT topogram (A) and axial CT images reveals diffuse thickening of calvarium, skull base and maxillofacial bones with ground glass appearance

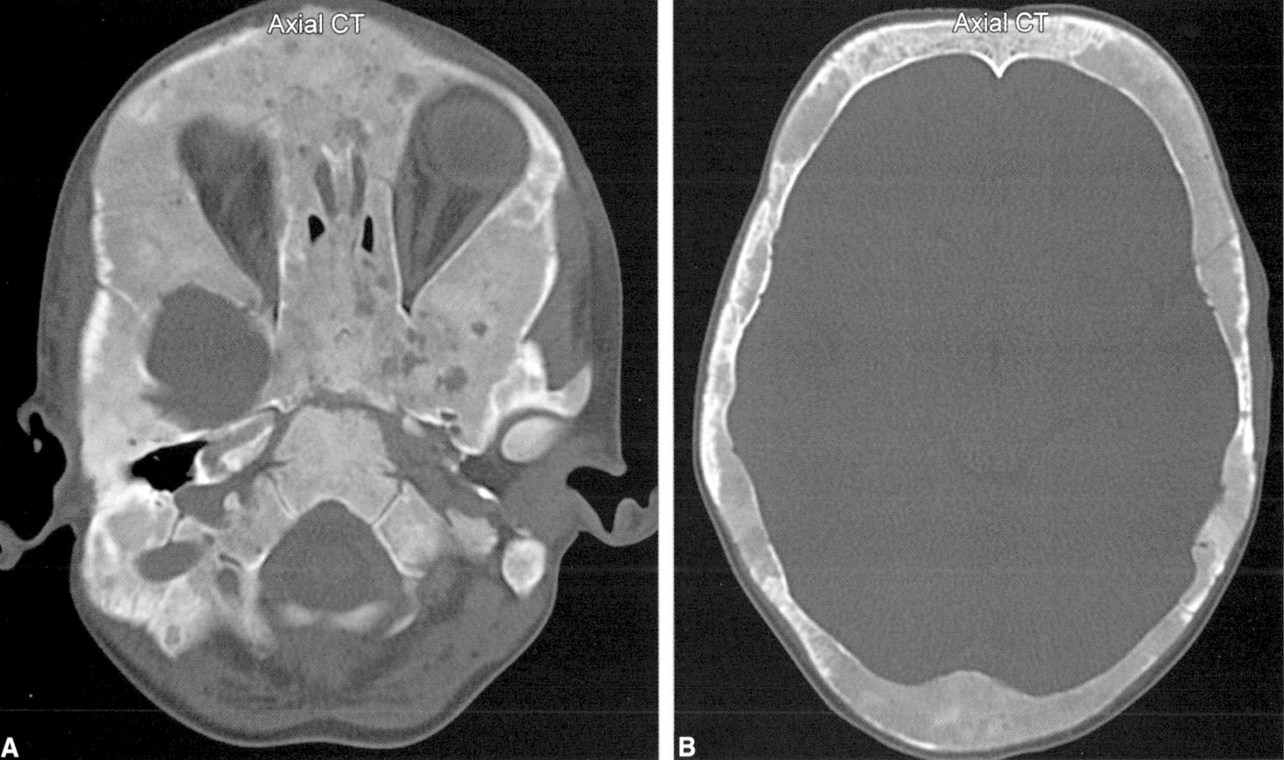

Figs 62A and B: Axial CT base of skull (A) and skull vault (B) reveal diffuse thickening of skull base and maxillofacial bones, and calvarium, with ground glass appearance

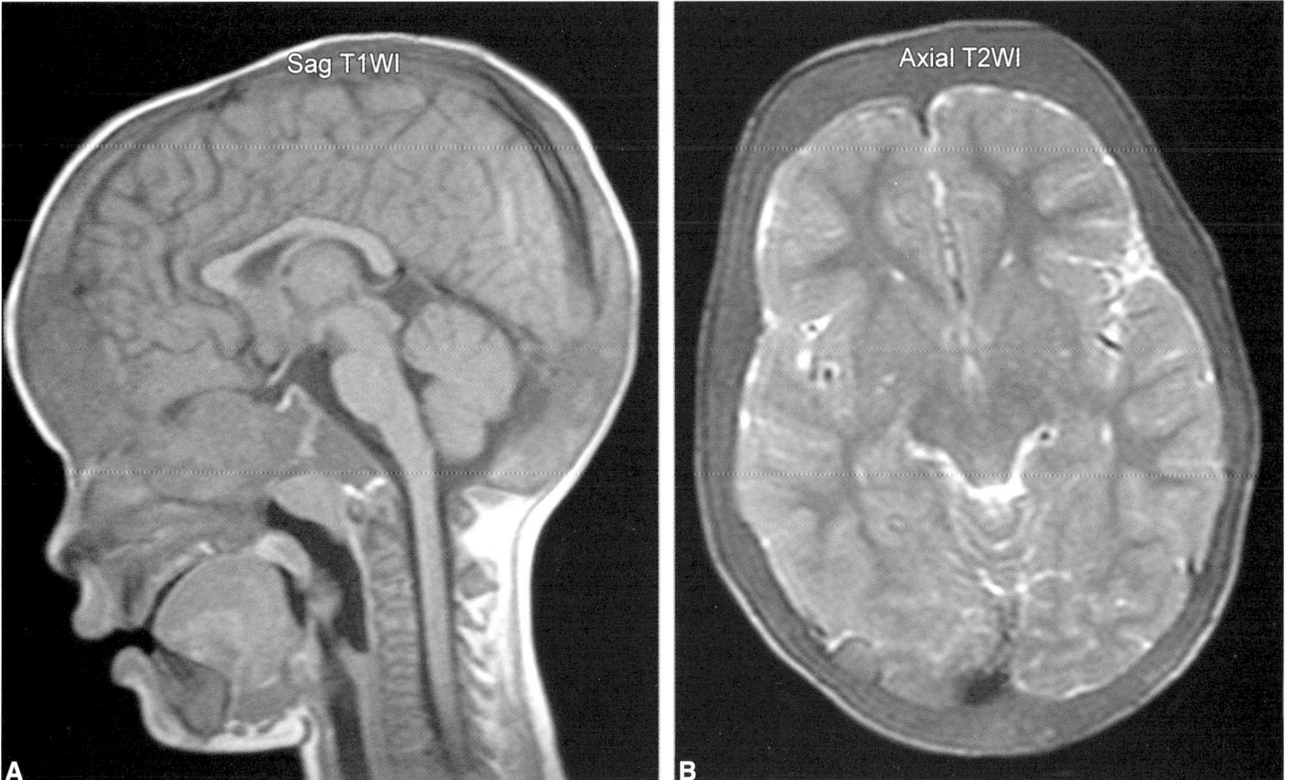

Figs 63A and B: Sagittal T1 (A) and axial T2 (B) weighted images reveal diffuse calvarial thickening

Cerebellar Atrophy

Cerebellar atrophy is wasting or decrease in size of cerebellum with decrease in size of cerebellar folia. Isolated atrophy of cerebellum is either age related or related to metabolic or systemic disorders. Common causes include alcoholic encephalopathy, chronic phenytoin use, radiation and chemotherapy, lithium intoxication and hypothyroidism. Cerebellar atrophy on MRI shows decrease in size of cerebellar folia with hyperintense signal on T2WI around the folia (Figs 64A to D), because of excessive space made available for CSF to collect.

MR signal characteristics of cerebellar atrophy in specific conditions are:

Disease	*MR signal changes*
Chronic alcoholism	Involves superior vermis and associated cerebral atrophy
Chronic phenytoin use	Mild to moderate changes in vermis and cerebellum
Olivopontocerebellar atrophy	Severe changes in vermis and cerebellum
Trienreich's ataxia	Atrophy of spinal cord with cerebellum

Cerebellar hypoplasia is small or incompletely formed but otherwise normal appearing cerebellum. It occurs as a result of reduction or premature cessation of cell production or excessive apoptosis in developing cerebellum. On imaging hypoplasia is classified either as general hypoplasia or focal hypoplasia. Focal hypoplasia may be isolated hypoplasia of one hemisphere or vermis, it is appreciated on MR imaging. Generalized hypoplasia may occur with either enlarged IV ventricle as in Dandy-Walker syndrome or with normal IV ventricle as in mega cistern magna.

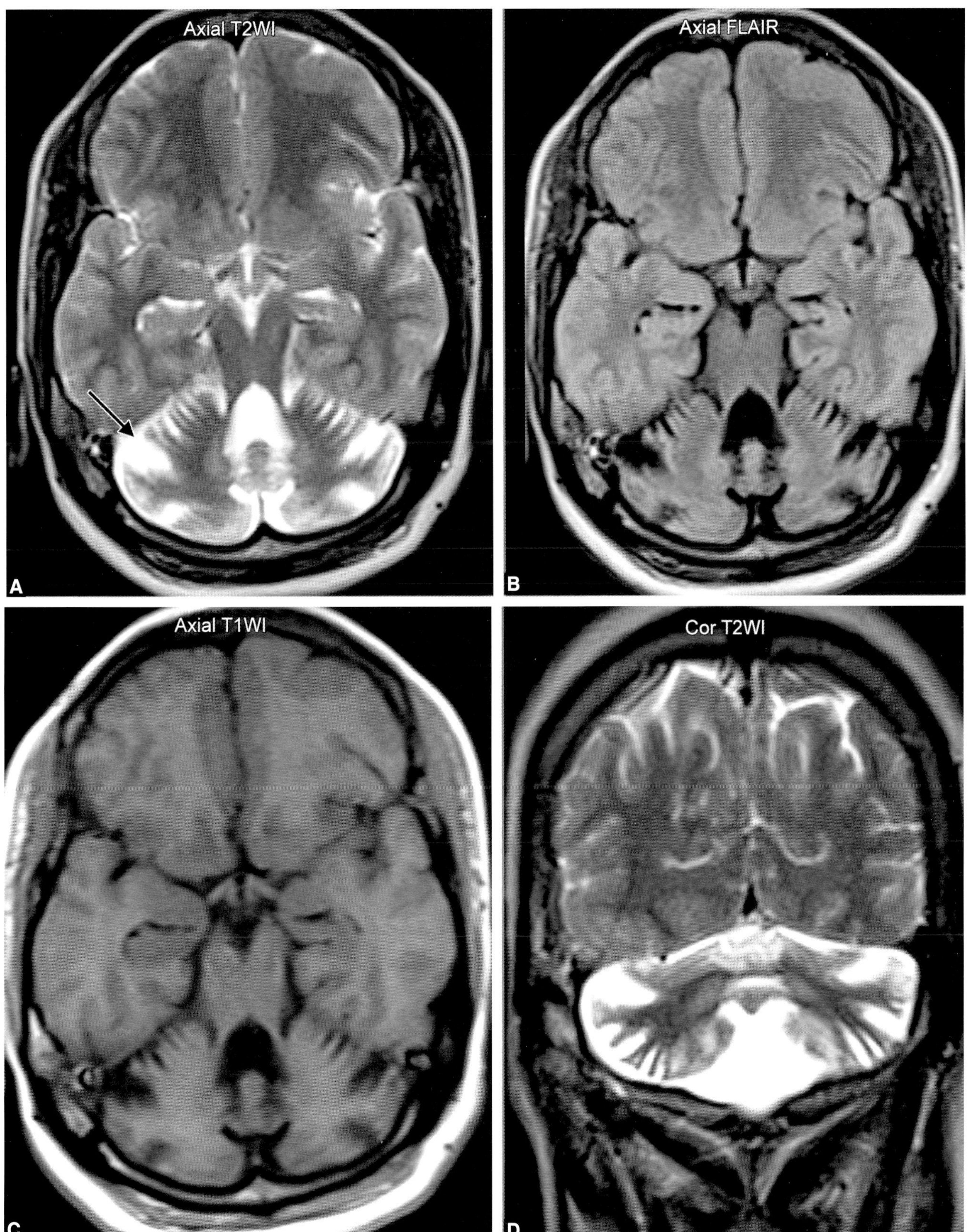

Figs 64A to D: Axial T2 (A), FLAIR (B), axial T1W (C), coronal T2W (D) and sagittal T1W images reveal marked prominence of cerebellar folia, this is the feature of cerebellar atrophy

Marchiafava-Bignami Disease

Marchiafava-Bignami (MB) disease or syndrome is a primary degeneration of the corpus callosum associated with chronic alcohol consumption, mainly due to a deficiency in the vitamin B complex. It presents mostly in males, between 40 and 60 years of age with history of chronic alcoholism and malnutrition. The disease typically affects the body of the corpus callosum, followed by the genu, and finally the splenium and sometimes entire corpus callosum. Other white matter tracts such as the anterior and posterior commissures and the corticospinal tracts, the hemispheric white matter and in the middle cerebellar peduncles may be involved. The corpus callosum degenerates and splits into three layers with the middle layer being most affected. This layered necrosis may lead to cystic cavities formation.

Diagnosis is made on the basis of clinical findings in combination with imaging features. In acute form, acutely patients present with mental confusion, disorientation, neurocognitive deficits, and seizures. The chronic form of MB is characterized by a chronic dementia.

On MR images, patients with MB show areas of low T1 signal intensity and high T2 and FLAIR signal intensity in the body of the corpus callosum (Figs 66 to 68), extending into the genu and the adjacent white matter without any mass effect and may show peripheral contrast enhancement during the acute phase. Later on the lesions cavitate and become well marginated. In a recent report, the initial MR spectra showed a mildly increased choline level (probably secondary to acute demyelination), low N-acetyl aspartate (probably secondary to neuronal damage), and the presence of lactate. On long-term follow-up after treatment, the spectra showed nearly complete normalization of the peak heights. On CT scans (Figs 65A and B), these lesions appear as hypoattenuated areas. Other lesions involving the corpus callosum that may have a similar appearance include infarctions, shearing injuries, and demyelination process.

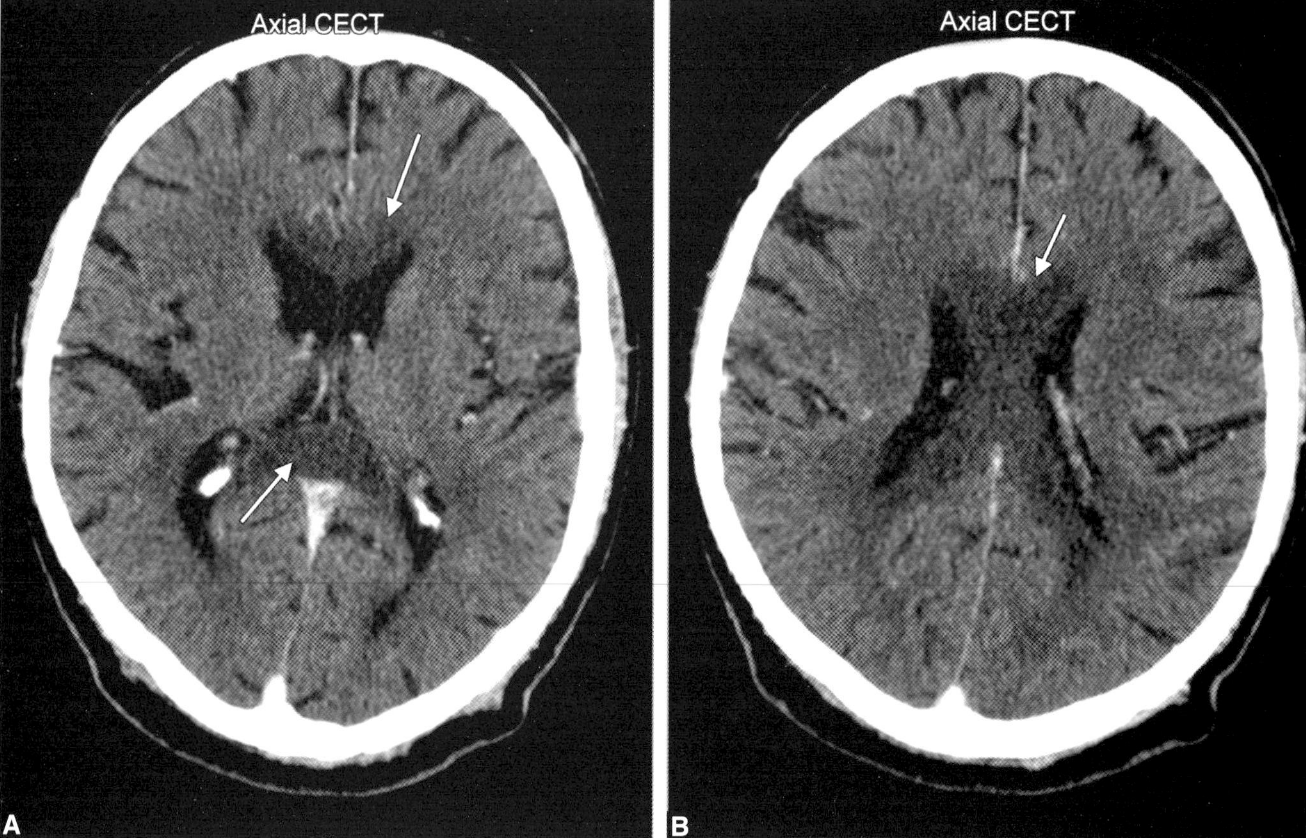

Figs 65A and B: CECT shows nonenhancing hypodensity (arrows) involving the genu, splenium (A) and body (B) of corpus callosum

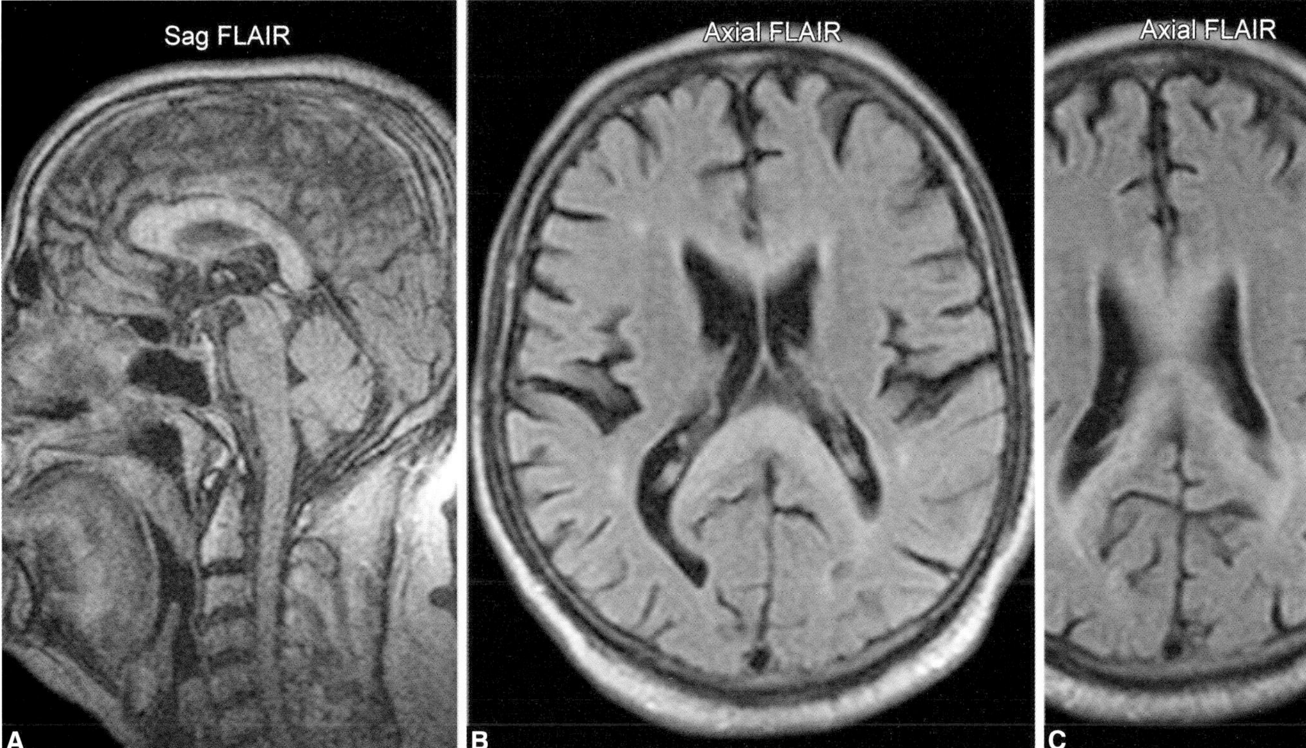

Figs 66A to C: Sagittal (A) and axial (B and C) FLAIR images show hyperintense signals in corpus callosum

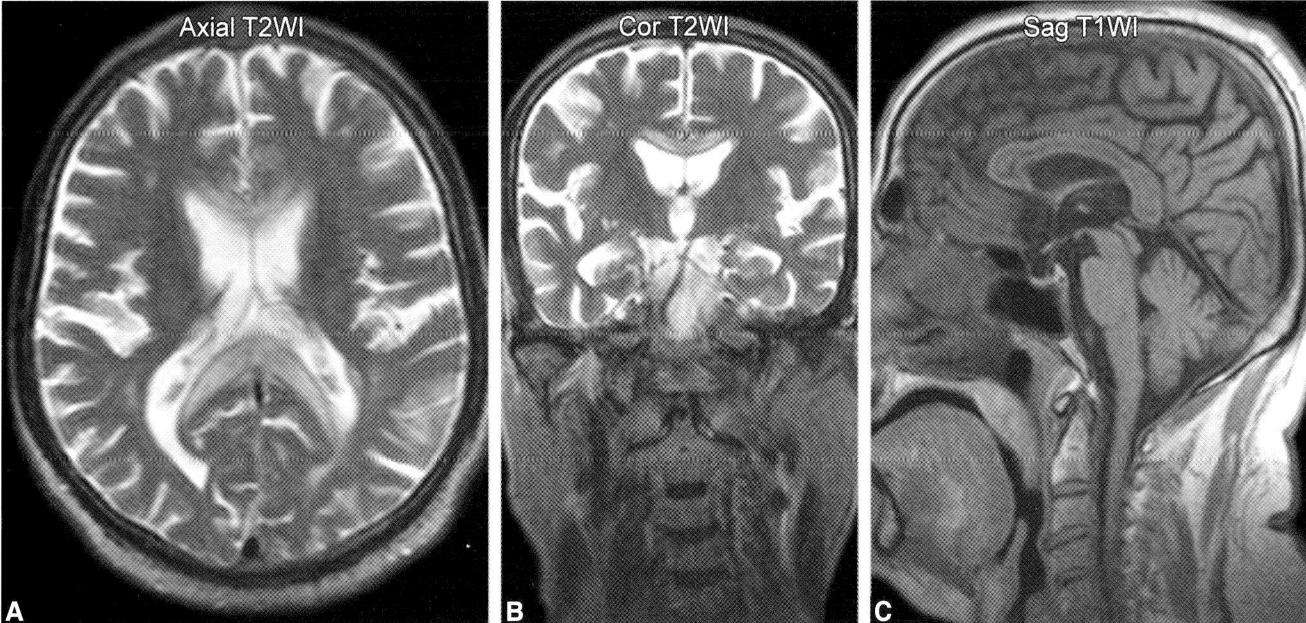

Figs 67A to C: Axial and coronal T2W images (A and B) show hyperintense signals in corpus callosum, sagittal T1W image (C) show hypointense signals in corpus callosum

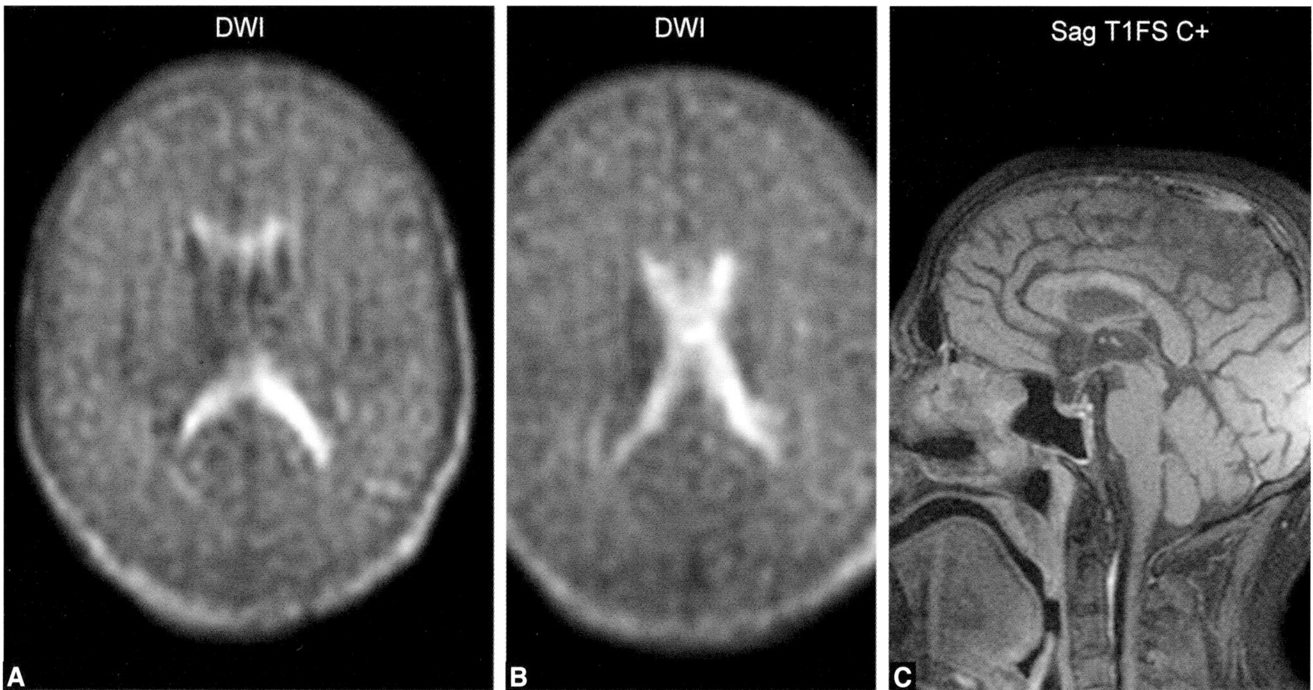

Figs 68A to C: DW images (A and B) showing restriction of diffusion in corpus callosum. Post-contrast sagittal T1FS image (C) showing enhancement in corpus callosum

Acquired Hepatocerebral Degeneration

Acquired hepatocerebral degeneration (AHD) is a chronic encephalopathy with predominant motor signs seen in severe liver disease. Its clinical picture is not well-defined, and risk factors are not well known. Its prevalence is about 1 percent of patients with cirrhosis. AHD seems to be related to presence of portosystemic shunts. Hepatic damage leads to buildup of ammonia and other toxic materials in the body leading to damage of brain tissue precisely the basal ganglia which control the movement is damaged. Movement disorders, especially a combination of Parkinsonism and cerebellar signs are seen in most patients. AHD cases shows on T1 weighted images hyperintensities in the globus pallidus (Figs 69A and B), and 75 percent show extrapallidal involvement as well. This condition is 'Non-Wilsonian' as the liver damage is not caused by copper deposits, which is the key feature of Wilson's.

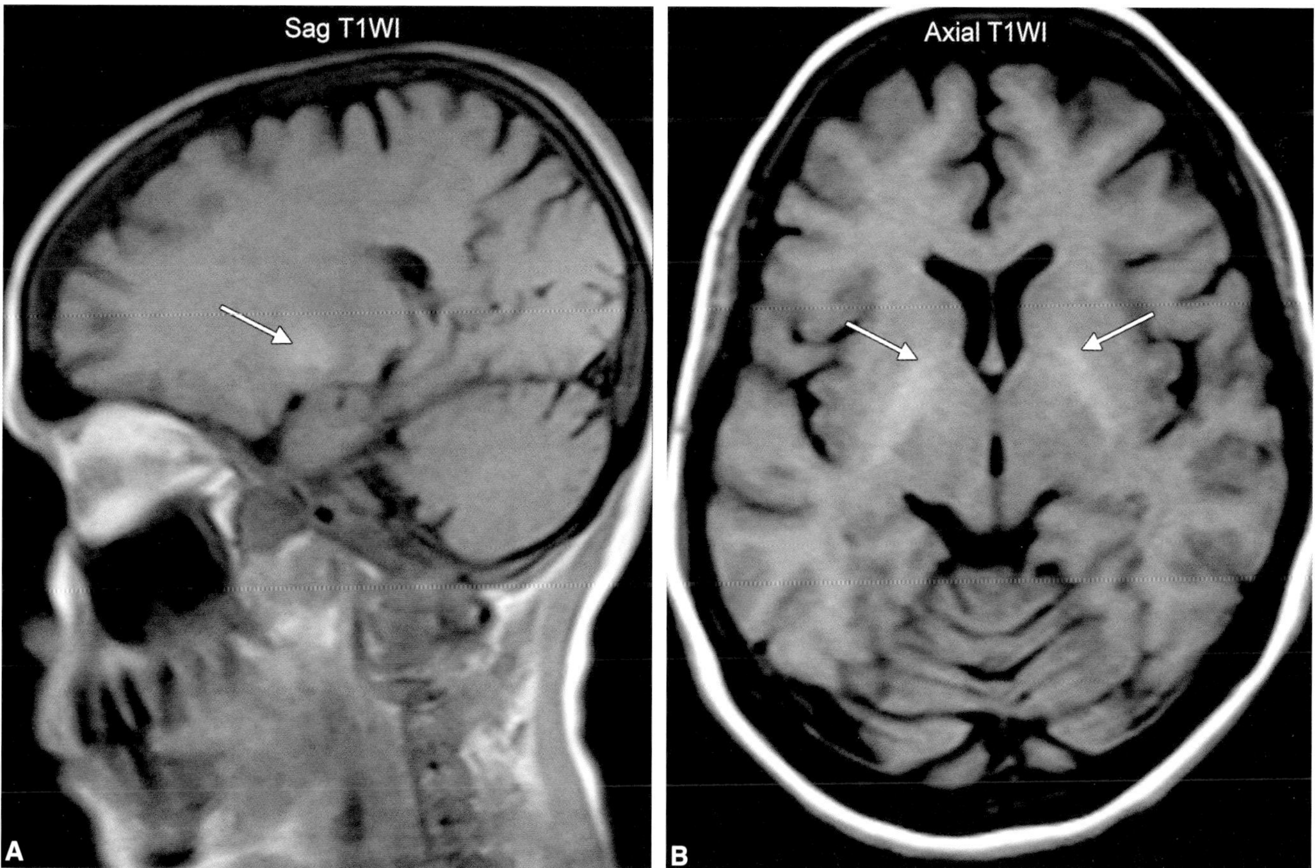

Figs 69A and B: Axial and sagittal T1 weighted images show hyperintensities in the globus pallidus

3 Orbit

Aditi Dongre

DACRYOCYSTOCELE

A dacryocystocele forms when tears accumulate within the lacrimal sac as a result of an obstruction more distally in the lacrimal drainage apparatus, which may occur as a complication of sinonasal surgery. The lacrimal drainage apparatus begins in the medial aspect of the orbit with two orifices known as the superior and inferior puncta. These orifices drain into canaliculi, superior and inferior, which then form a common canaliculus. The valve of Rosenmuller, which lies at the junction of the common canaliculus and the lacrimal sac, prevents the reflux of tears back into the canaliculus. The lacrimal sac is located within the inferomedial wall of the orbit known as the lacrimal fossa. The lacrimal sac is oval and measures 12 to 15 mm. The nasolacrimal duct is a membranous canal extending inferiorly for about 18 mm from the nasolacrimal sac to the inferior meatus of the nasal cavity.

Patients with dacryocystocele may present clinically with a pink or blue mass in the medial canthal region. Obstruction of the nasolacrimal duct may lead to epiphora. Secondary infection of a dilated lacrimal sac may lead to dacryocystitis and mucopurulent discharge and/or periorbital or facial cellulitis. Unless there are imaging findings such as preseptal soft tissue swelling or adjacent bone destruction, the diagnosis of dacryocystitis is generally made on a clinical basis.

The findings on magnetic resonance imaging (MRI) are similar to those reported in several case reports of prenatal and childhood dacryocystoceles. Dacryocystocele on T2WI images appear as homogeneous, hyperintense cystic mass within the medial canthal region (Figs 1A to E). The mass is centered in the region of the medial canthus and may extend inferiorly into the nasal cavity, elevating the inferior turbinate.

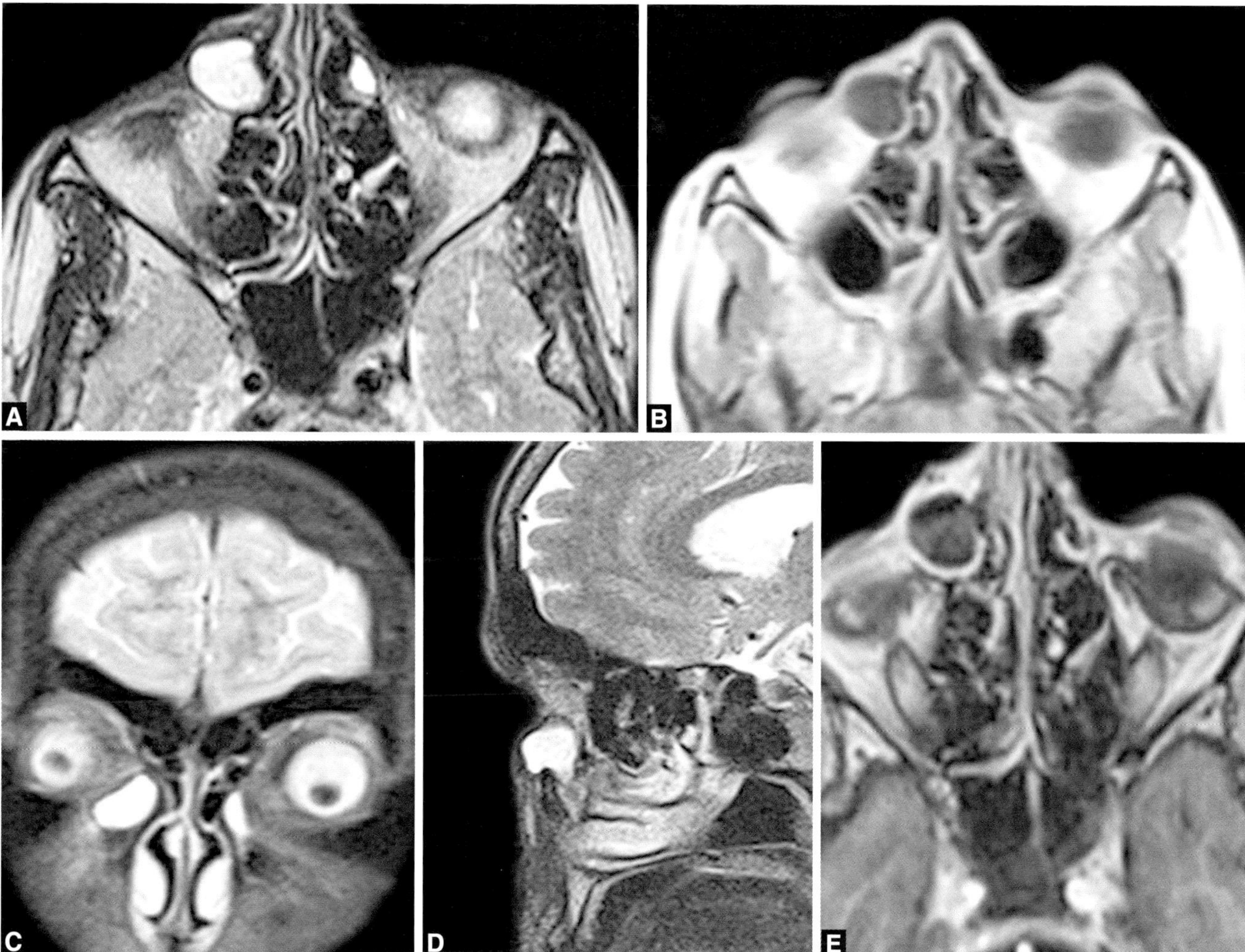

Figs 1A to E: STIR (A and D) and T2 (C) images show hyperintense lesion appearing hypointense to isointense on T1W (B) image is seen in the region of right lacrimal sac with minimal peripheral enhancement in postcontrast image (E)

GRAVE'S OPHTHALMOPATHY

Thyroid ophthalmopathy is currently recognized as the most common cause of proptosis in adults. Clinical features include upper and or lower eyelid retraction, restrictive myopathy causing diplopia, compressive optic neuropathy, and exposure keratopathy. Although most patients are clinically hyperthyroid, signs of thyroid ophthalmopathy can be present regardless of thyroid function.

Imaging demonstrates enlargement confined to the muscle belly (Figs 2A and B) sparing the tendinous insertion. CT density measurements of affected muscles may not vary from normal, but areas of increased T2W signal intensity are often seen on MR. Patients with these findings have a more favorable response to treatment. Enhancement of the affected muscle takes place in acute stage but may be diminished in the chronic phase.

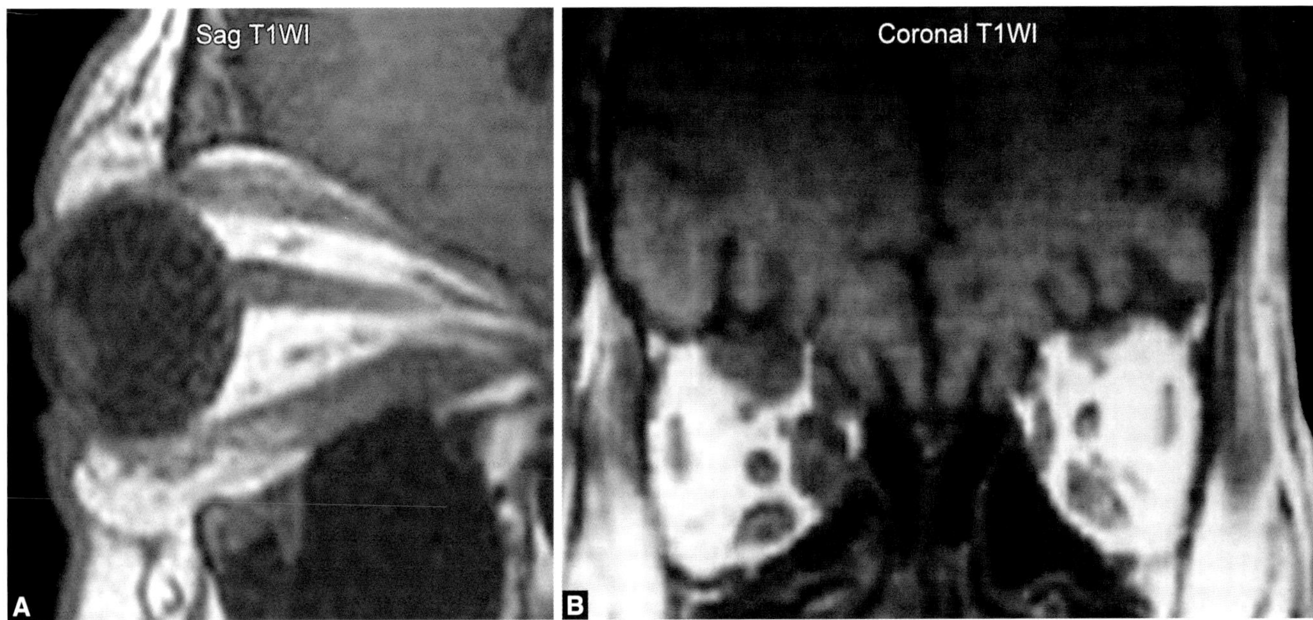

Figs 2A and B: Sagittal and coronal T1W images reveal the enlargement of superior, medial and inferior rectus muscles with proptosis and accumulation of fat tissue in the eyelids

DERMOID

Dermoids are examples of choristomas, tumors that originate from aberrant primordial tissue. These tumors contain normal appearing tissue in an abnormal location. As two suture lines of the skull close during embryonic development, dermal or epidermal elements may be pinched off and form cysts, which are adjacent to the suture line. Approximately 50 percent of dermoids that involve the head are found in or adjacent to the orbit.

Dermoid cysts are generally thought to be congenital lesions of childhood with the vast majority presenting in the first few years of life. However, deep lesions can go undiagnosed for years and may present for the first time in late adulthood.

Magnetic resonance imaging (MRI) is often used imaging modality for dermoid cysts, and has the added advantage of not exposing the patient to radiation. This is especially important in the pediatric population. The lesions are generally hyperintense on T1-weighted imaging (Figs 3B to D) with respect to fat and diagnosis can be confirmed using fat suppression techniques. The lesions tend to be hyperintense on T2-weighted imaging (Fig. 3A).

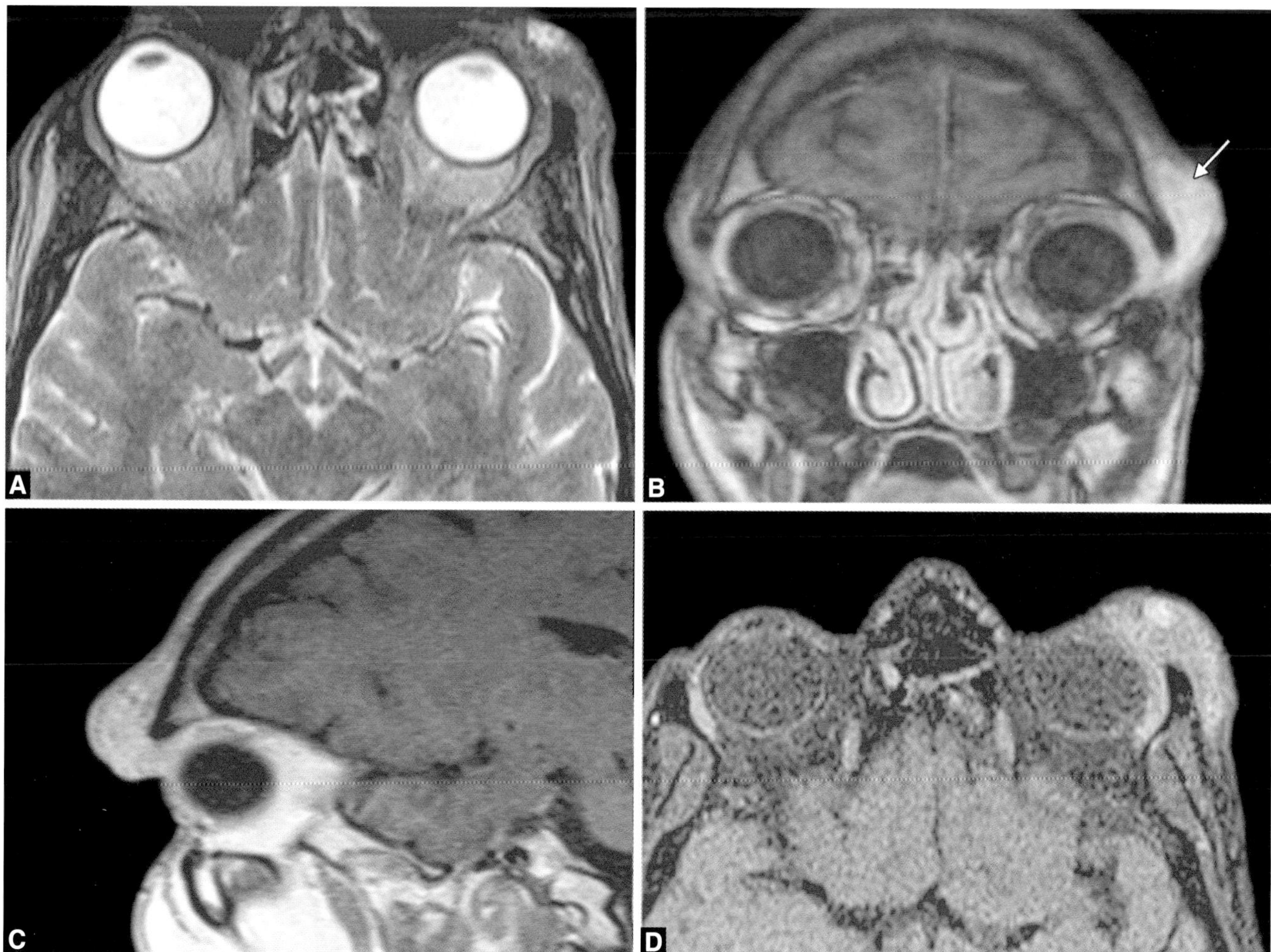

Figs 3A to D: Axial T2W, coronal T1W, sagittal T1W and axial post-contrast fat saturated T1W images showing heterogeneous lesion (arrow) with areas of T1 hyperintensity with mild postcontrast enhancement in the left lateral orbital preseptal region in the subcutaneous region

ORBITAL HEMATOMA

The most common symptoms of orbital hemorrhage include pain, pressure and loss of vision, other symptoms are diplopia, nausea and vomiting. Signs of hemorrhage are tense or expanding proptosis, ophthalmoplegia, increased intraocular pressure, loss of pupillary reflexes and optic disc or retinal pallor.

Computed tomography (CT) is preferred because of its fast acquisition time and better visualization of the bony anatomy, where as MR scans provide better visualization of the soft tissues of the orbit (Figs 4A and B).

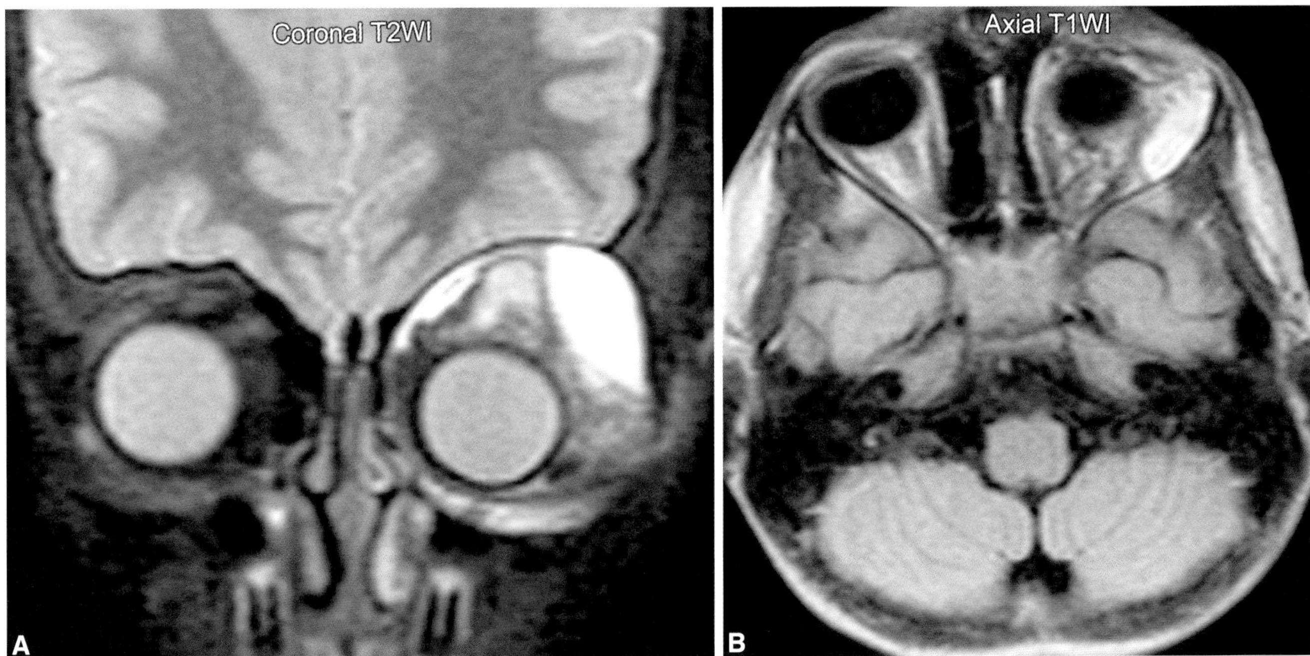

Figs 4A and B: (A) Fat suppressed T2W coronal image reveals localized hyperintense collection in the extraconal compartment of left orbit along the lateral and superior aspect; (B) Flair axial images reveal localized hyperintense collection in the extraconal compartment of left orbit along the lateral and superior aspect. It appears hyperintense on T1W axial image suggestive of hematoma in subacute stage

ORBITAL HYDATID CYST

Orbital hydatid can be differentiated as primary, where cyst or cysts are solely located in orbital cavity (Figs 5A to C) and secondary when orbital lesions represent a component of disseminated multi-organ systemic disease. The incidence of orbital hydatid disease varies from 0.8 to 1.0 percent, however in highly endemic areas, it has been reported up to 25.8 percent of all cystic orbital lesions. The usual strains responsible for orbital cysts are *E. granulosus* and *E. multilocularis.*

The most common presenting clinical symptoms and signs of orbital echinococcosis are nonpulsatile, nontender exophthalmos, visual disturbances, papilledema, diplopia, chemosis, eyelid edema, conjunctivitis and hypopyon. The duration of symptoms has been reported to vary between 3 months and 2 years.

There is a predilection for the superomedial and superolateral orbital areas. Left-sided lesions were more common, due to the fact that left common carotid artery arises directly from the summit of the aortic arch.

The early diagnosis of orbital hydatidosis and its prompt surgical management have excellent results in the vast majority of these patients. This makes the importance of its appropriate diagnosis even more crucial. The clinician should always include the

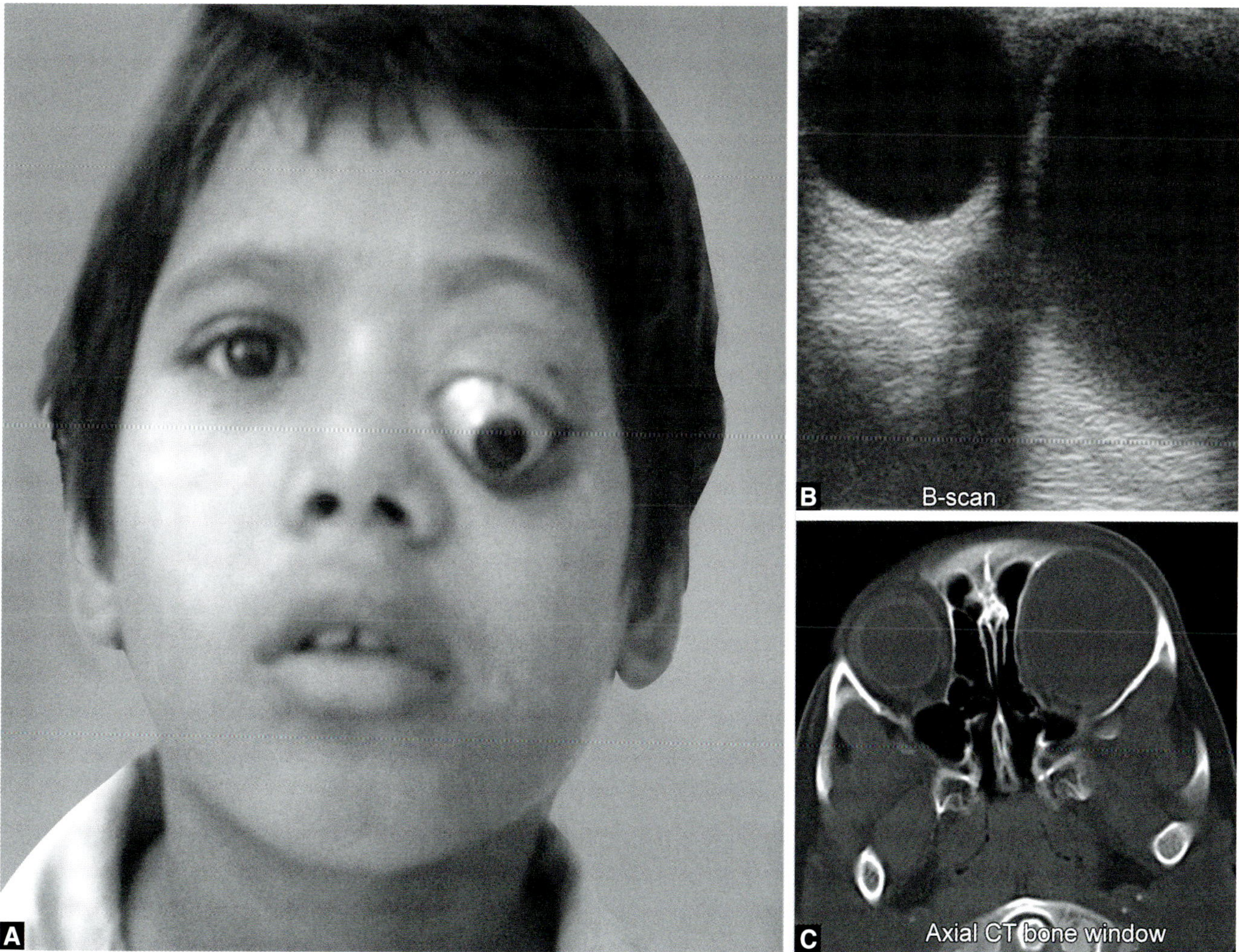

Figs 5A to C: (A) Photograph of the patient with proptosis of the eyeball downwards and medially; (B) B-scan image of left eyes show large cystic lesion in left orbit; (C) Orbital CT shows a large cystic lesion in left orbit causing expansion and scalloping of adjacent bones *(For color version, see Plate 1)*

diagnosis of hydatid cyst in the differential diagnosis list of orbital masses, especially in children.

Magnetic resonance imaging demonstrates a cystic lesion which appears hypointense on T1WI and hyperintense on T2W (Figs 6A and B). Flair sequence shows hyperintense lesion causing displacements of adjacent structures (Fig. 6C).

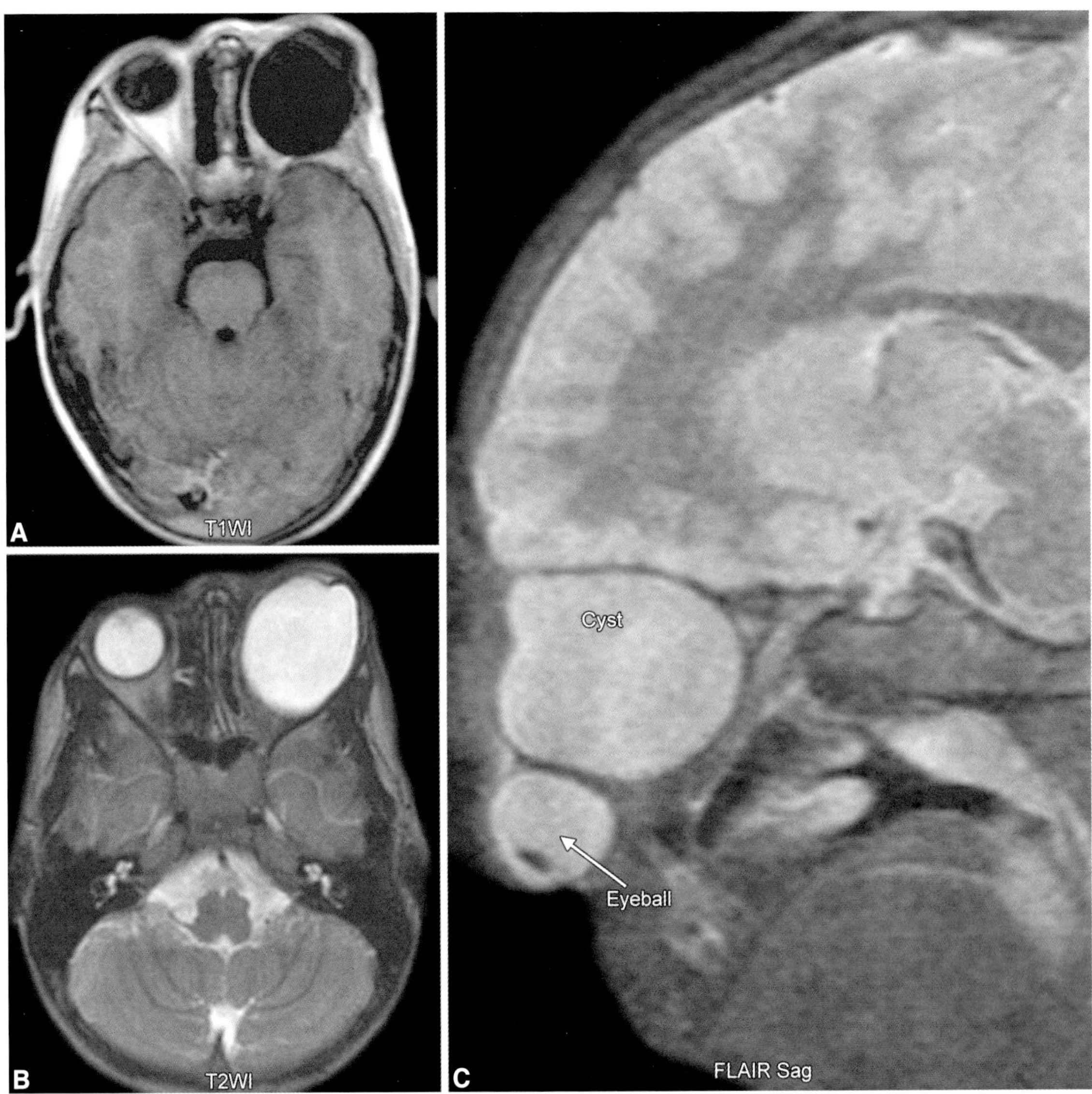

Figs 6A to C: MRI demonstrates a large extraconal cystic lesion in left globe causing pressure effect on lamina papyracea, it appears hypointense on T1WI and hyperintense on T2WI. FLAIR sagittal image shows hyperintense lesion in left orbit, in the superior aspect, displacing the eyeball inferiorly and resulting in scalloping of adjacent bones

ORBITAL RHABDOMYOSARCOMA

Rhabdomyosarcomas are the most common soft tissue sarcomas in childhood accounting for approximately 8 percent of all childhood cancers. Ten percent of pediatric rhabdomyosarcomas occur in the orbit and it is most common primary orbital malignancy of childhood. An average age of presentation is about 7 to 8 years. The lesions typically present with unilateral proptosis. Within the orbit, the superonasal quadrant is the most common location for the tumor. The tumor can cross the muscle cone and may be intra- or extraconal in location.

On both CT and MRI the masses show variable enhancement after contrast administration (Fig. 7D). Calcification may be seen. Bone destruction and skull base erosion must be searched for. On T1 images, the tumor appears isointense to extraocular muscles but hypointense to orbital fat (Figs 7A to C). On T2 images, the tumor shows hypointensity, isointensity or even hyperintensity to extraocular muscles and orbital fat. On postcontrast images (Fig. 7D), the tumor shows moderate to marked contrast enhancement.

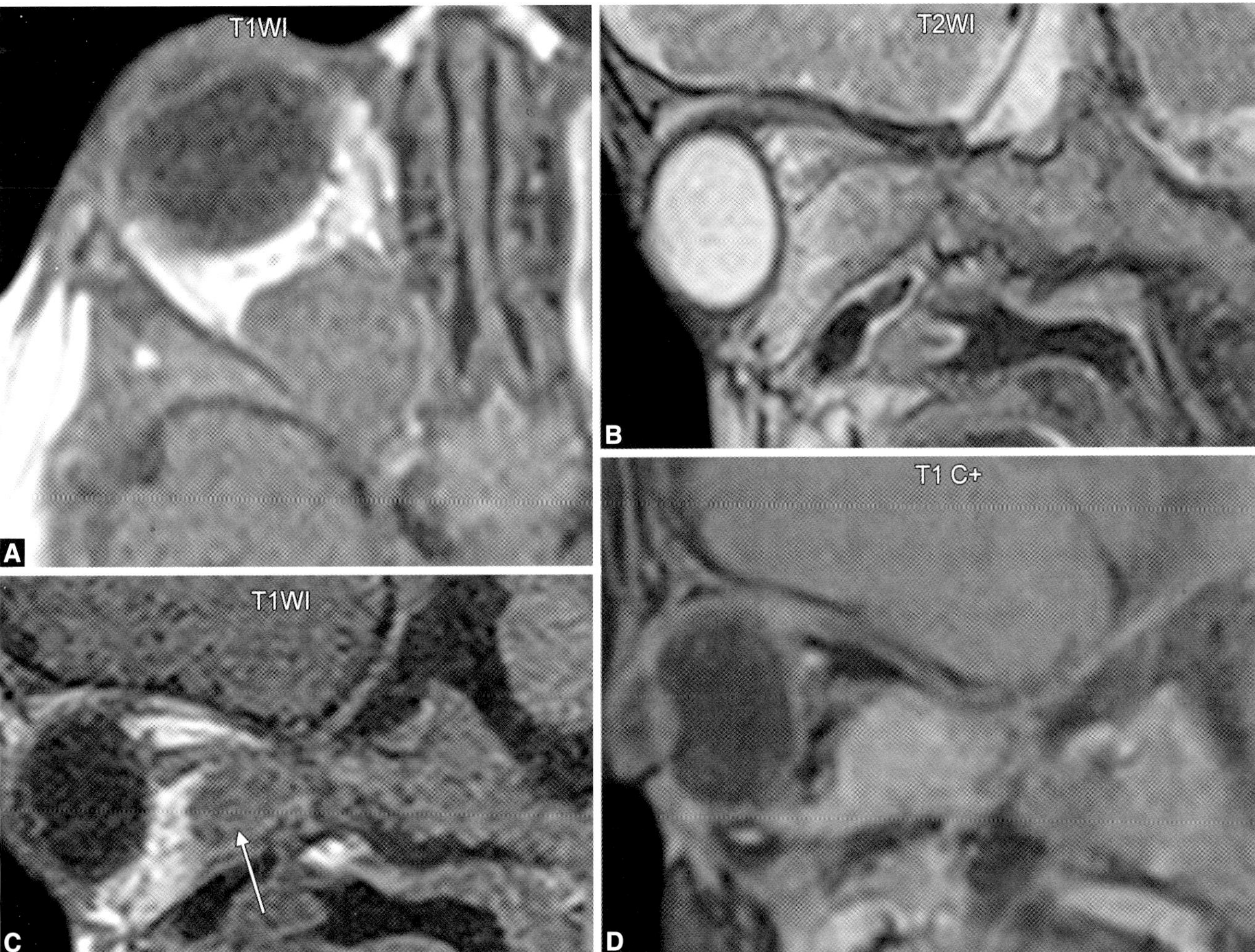

Figs 7A to D: Well-defined intraconal lesion is seen in the right retro-orbital space abutting the inferior rectus muscle and the optic nerve. The optic nerve is mildly displaced superiorly. The lesion is isointense on T1W axial image and iso to mildly hyperintense on T2W coronal image. On postcontrast T1W coronal it shows moderate homogeneous enhancement

Spine 4

Varsha Rangankar

ANATOMY OF SPINE

The spine is made up of five groups of vertebrae. The portion of spine in the neck region is cervical spine. It is formed by first seven vertebrae which are referred as C1 to C7, followed by twelve thoracic vertebrae, i.e. T1 to T12 and subsequently five lumbar vertebrae L1 to L5 in the low back area. The sacrum is a big triangular bone at the base, its broad upper part joins the L5 vertebra and its narrow lower part joins the coccyx or tail bone.

Cervical spine (Figs 1 to 19): It starts with first cervical vertebra (C1) attached to the base of the skull. First vertebra or C1 is called, atlas as it supports and balances the weight of the skull. It has practically no body or spinous process, and appears as two thickened bony arches to form a large hole with two transverse processes. On its upper surface, the atlas has two facets that unite with the occipital condyles of the skull. Structure of atlas is unique and has a large opening which accommodates spinal cord which is widest at this level.

The second vertebra is the "axis", it lies directly beneath the atlas vertebra. It bears large bony tooth-like protrusion on its summit, the odontoid process or the dens. This process projects upward and lies

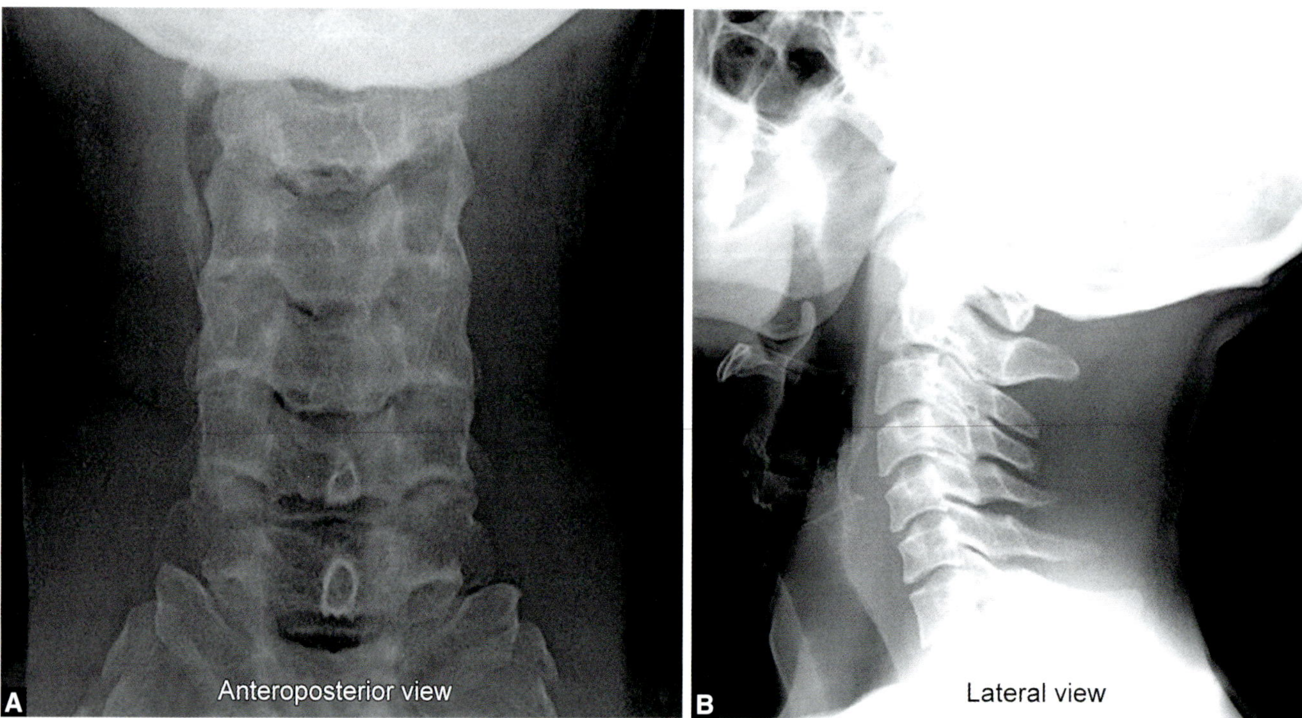

Figs 1A and B: Cervical spine

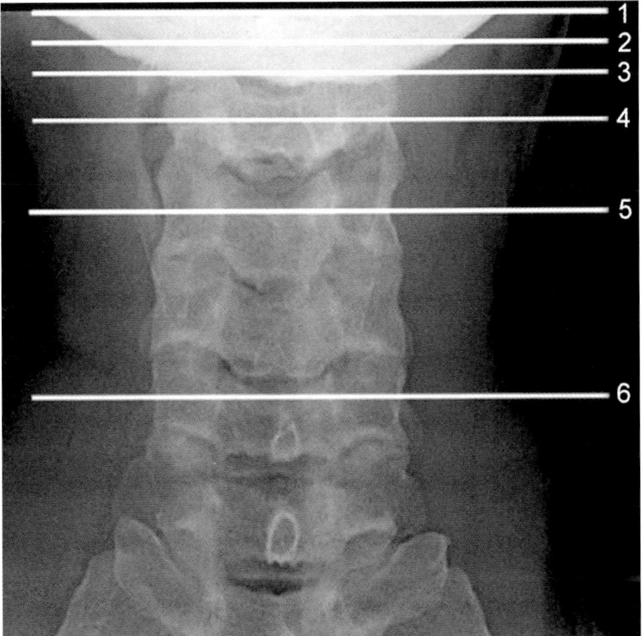

Fig. 2: Cervical spine MRI: Axial section plan

in the ring of the atlas. The joints of the axis give the neck its ability to turn from side to side, i.e. left and right, as the head is turned, the atlas pivots around the odontoid process.

The transverse processes of the cervical vertebrae are distinctive because they have transverse foramina, which serve as passageways for vertebral arteries leading to the brain. Also, the spinous processes of the second to fifth cervical vertebrae are forked providing attachments for various muscles.

C3 to C6 vertebrae have a typical structure. C7 vertebra is called vertebra prominens because of a long prominent thick nearly horizontal non bifurcated spinous process which is palpable from the skin.

Neural foramina of cervical spine allow way out to cervical spinal nerves which are eight in number and are named as C1 to C8.

Thoracic spine (Figs 19 to 35): It consists of twelve vertebrae in the chest area, the first thoracic vertebra articulates with the C7 vertebra above and the last thoracic vertebra articulates with the first lumbar vertebra below. The thoracic vertebrae are larger in size than those in the cervical region. They have long, pointed spinous processes that slope downward, and have facets on the sides of their bodies that join with ribs. From the third thoracic vertebra onwards to the last thoracic vertebra, the bodies of these bones increases in size gradually. This reflects the stress placed on them by the increasing amounts of body weight they bear.

Lumbar spine (Figs 36 to 54): There are five "lumbar vertebrae" in the lower back. They have larger and stronger bodies to provide support. The transverse processes of these vertebrae project backward at sharp angles, while their short, thick spinous processes are directed nearly horizontally.

Sacrum: The sacrum is a large triangular bone at the base of the lower spine. Its broad upper part joins the lowest lumbar vertebrae and its narrow

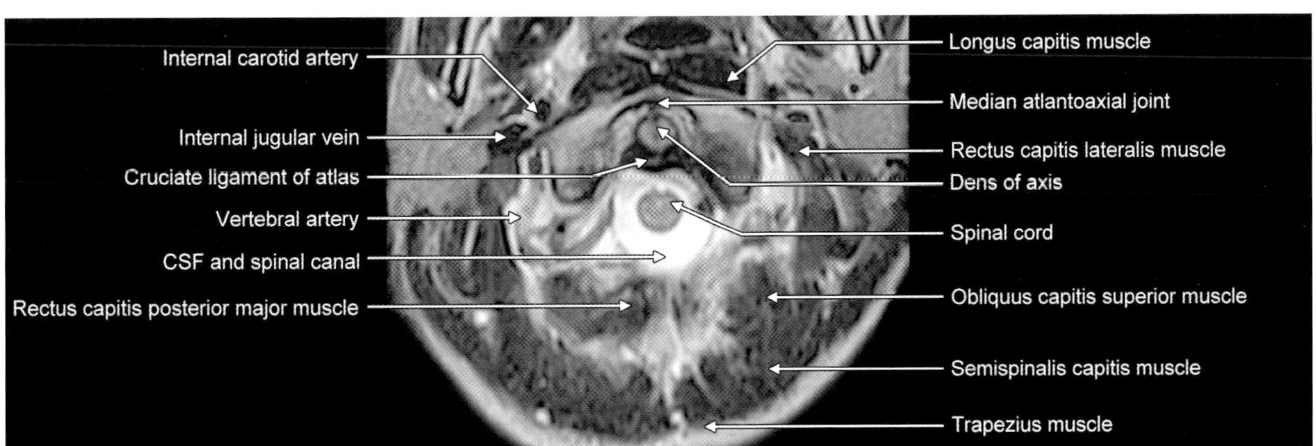

Fig. 3: Cervical spine MRI: Axial T2WI level at C1 (corresponds to level 1 in Fig. 2)

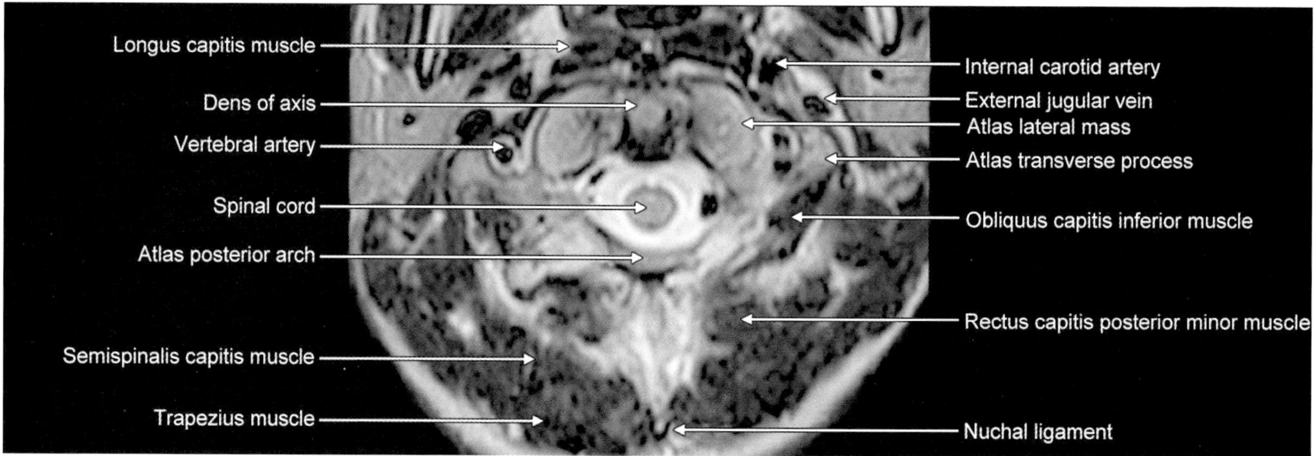

Fig. 4: Cervical spine MRI: Axial T2WI at level upper part of C2 vertebra (corresponds to level 2 in Fig. 2)

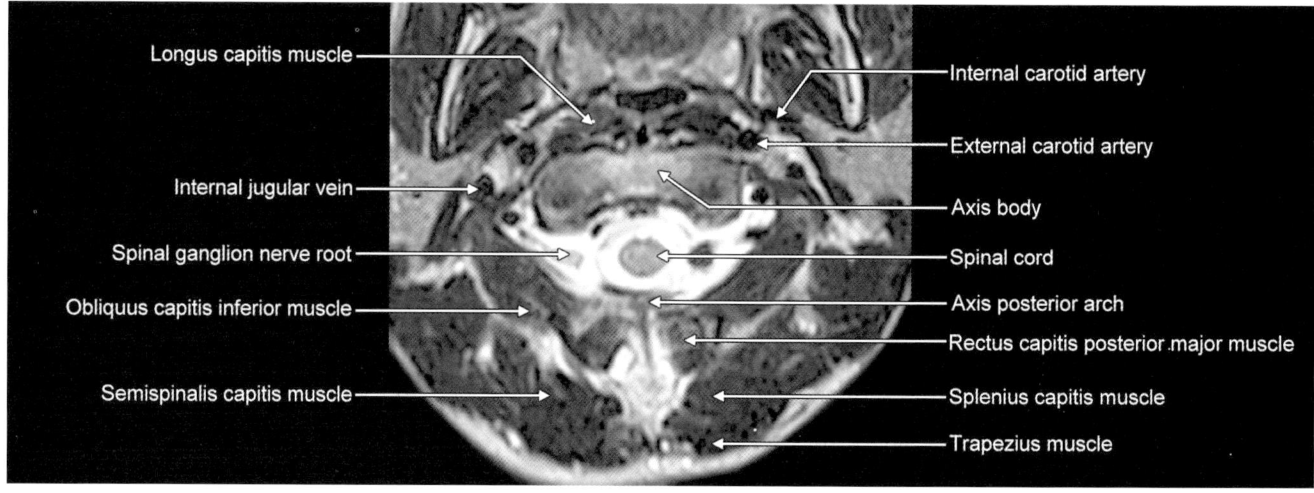

Fig. 5: Cervical spine MRI: Axial T2WI level at C2 body (corresponds to level 3 in Fig. 2)

lower part joins the coccyx or "tail bone". The sides are connected to the iliac bones (the largest bones forming the pelvis). The sacrum is a strong bone and rarely fractures. The five vertebrae that make up the sacrum are separate in early life, but gradually become fused between the eighteenth and thirtieth years. The spinous processes of these fused bones are represented by a ridge of tubercles. The weight of the body is transmitted to the legs through the pelvic girdle at these joints.

Coccyx: It is the lowest part of the vertebral column and is attached by ligaments to the margins of the sacral hiatus. When a person is sitting, pressure is exerted on the coccyx, and it moves forward, acting like a shock absorber. Sitting down with force may cause the coccyx to be fractured or dislocated.

General features of spine: The vertebral body is shaped like an hourglass, thinner in the center with thicker ends. Outer cortical bone extends above and below the superior and inferior ends of the vertebrae to form rims. The superior and inferior endplates are contained within these rims of bone. The bodies of adjacent vertebrae are joined on the front surfaces by "anterior ligaments" and on the back by "posterior

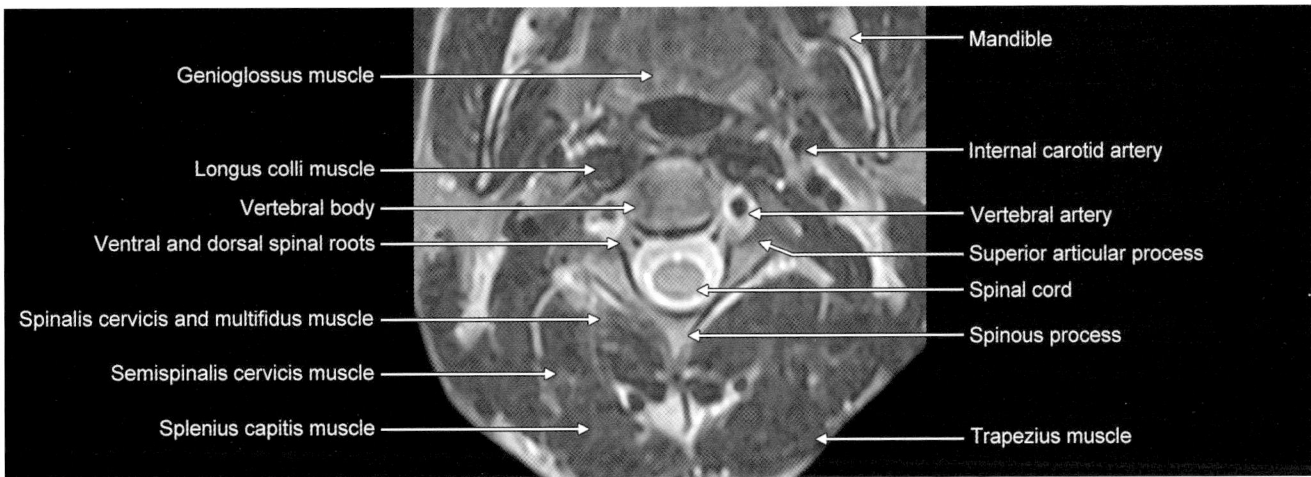

Fig. 6: Cervical spine MRI: Axial T2WI at C3 level (corresponds to level 4 in Fig. 2)

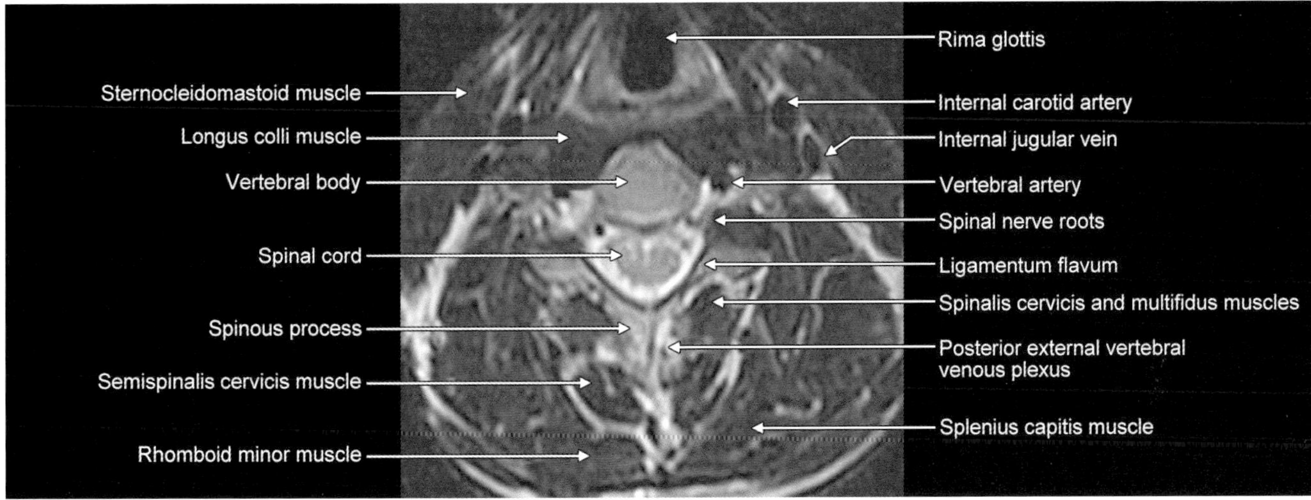

Fig. 7: Cervical spine MRI: Axial T2WI at C4 level (corresponds to level 5 in Fig. 2)

ligaments". A longitudinal row of the bodies supports the weight of the head and trunk.

The anterior longitudinal ligament is a flat band that extends from the basiocciput of the skull and the anterior tubercle of the atlas to the front of the upper part of the sacrum. It is attached to the periosteum of the underlying vertebral bodies.

The posterior longitudinal ligament extends from the back of the body of axis to the anterior wall of the upper sacral canal.

Intervertebral discs are found between each vertebra. Intervertebral discs make up about one-third of the length of the spine and constitute the largest organ in the body without its own blood supply. The discs are flat, round structures about a quarter to three quarters of an inch thick with tough outer rings of tissue called the annulus fibrosis that contain a soft, white, jelly-like center called the nucleus pulposus. Flat, circular plates of cartilage connect to the vertebrae above and below each disc. Intervertebral discs separate the vertebrae, but they act as shock absorbers for the spine.

Projecting from the back of each body of the vertebra are two short rounded stalks called

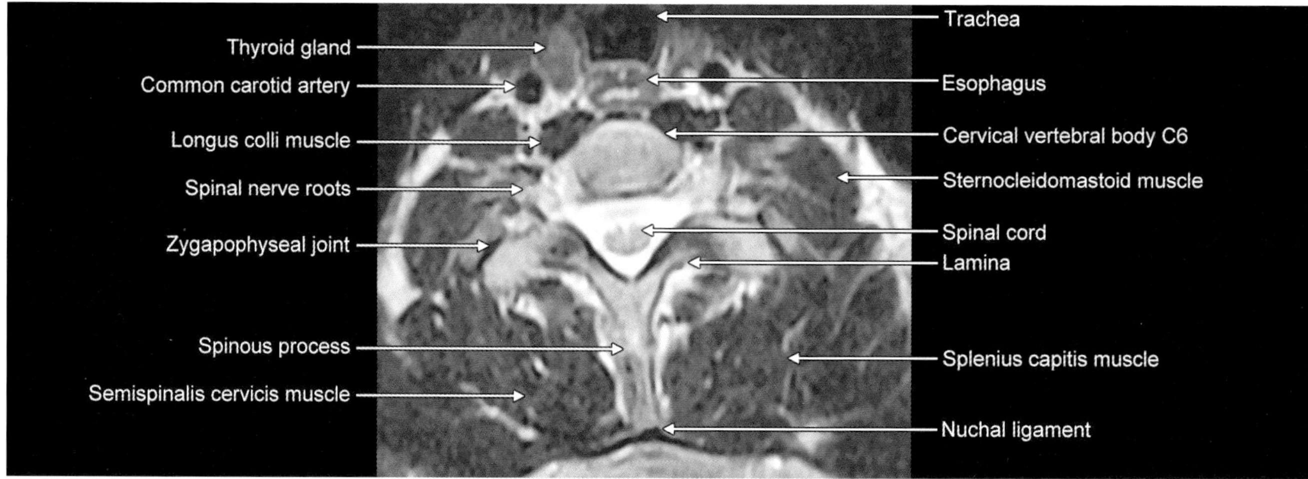

Fig. 8: Cervical spine MRI: Axial at T2WI C6 level (corresponds to level 6 in Fig. 2)

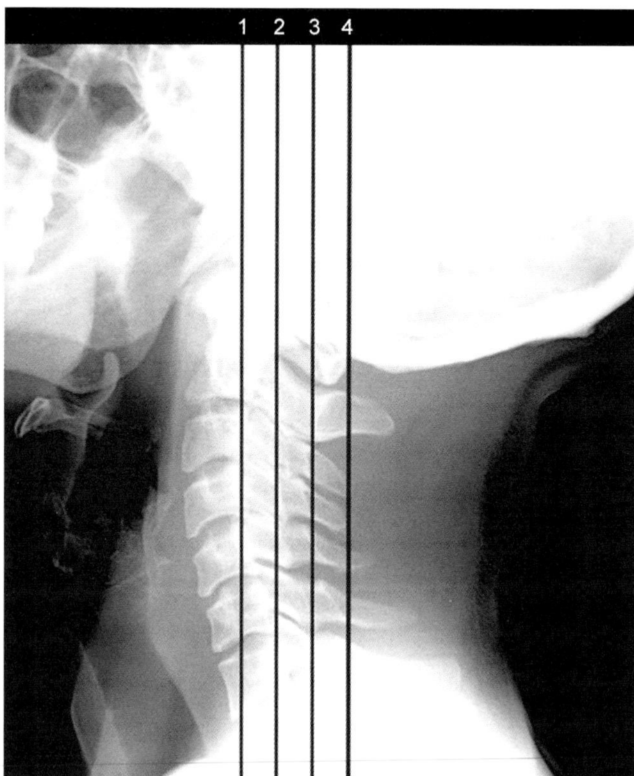

Fig. 9: Cervical spine MRI: Coronal section plan

"pedicles". They form the sides of the "vertebral foramen". They extend posteriorly from the lateral margin of the dorsal surface of the vertebral body.

The laminae are two flattened plates of bone extending medially from the pedicles to form the posterior wall of the vertebral foramen. They fuse in the back to become spinous process. The pars interarticularis is a special region of the lamina between the superior and inferior articular processes. A fracture or congenital anomaly of the pars may result in a spondylolisthesis.

The pedicles, laminae, and spinous process together complete a bony vertebral arch around the vertebral opening, through which the spinal cord passes. Between the pedicles and laminae of a typical vertebra is a "transverse process" that projects laterally and toward the back. Various ligaments and muscles are attached to the transverse process. Projecting upward and downward from each vertebral arch are "superior" and "inferior" articulating processes. These processes bear cartilage-covered facets by which each vertebra is joined to the one above and the one below it. These facet joints facilitate smooth gliding movement of one vertebra on another to produce twisting motions and rotation of the spine. Facet joints are also called as zygapophyseal joints.

On the surfaces of the vertebral pedicles are notches that align to create openings, called "intervertebral foramina". These openings provide passageways for spinal nerves that exit out of the spinal cord.

The ligamentum flavum is a strong ligament that connects the laminae of the vertebrae. The ligamentum flavum serves to protect the neural elements and the spinal cord and stabilize the spine

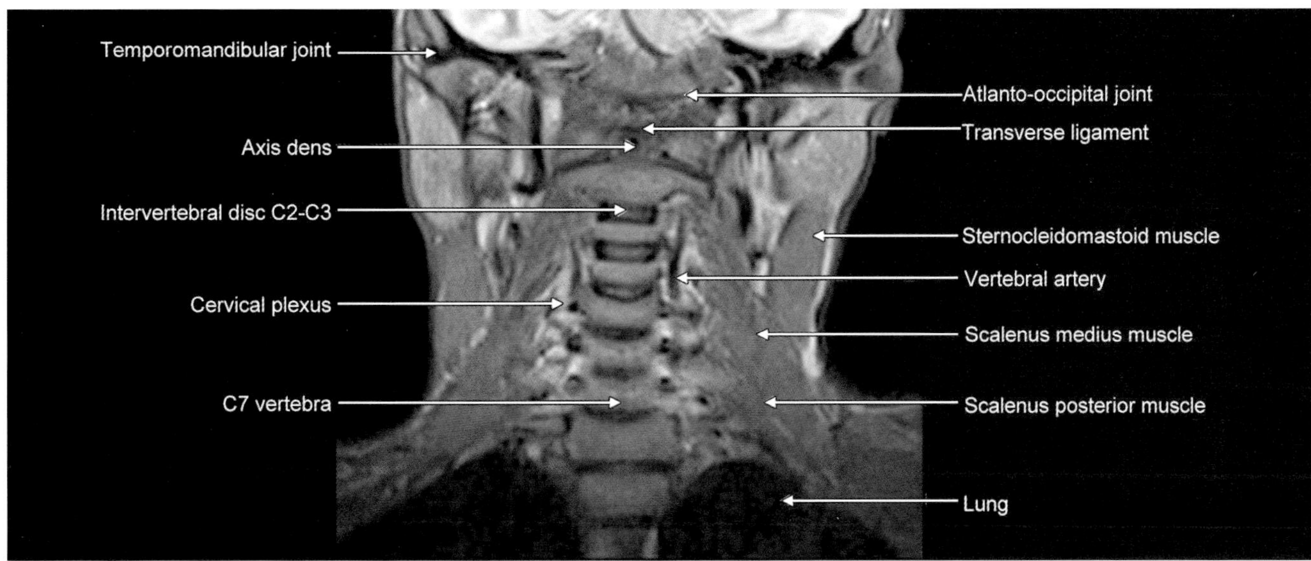

Fig. 10: Cervical spine MRI: Coronal T2WI (corresponds to level 1 in Fig. 9)

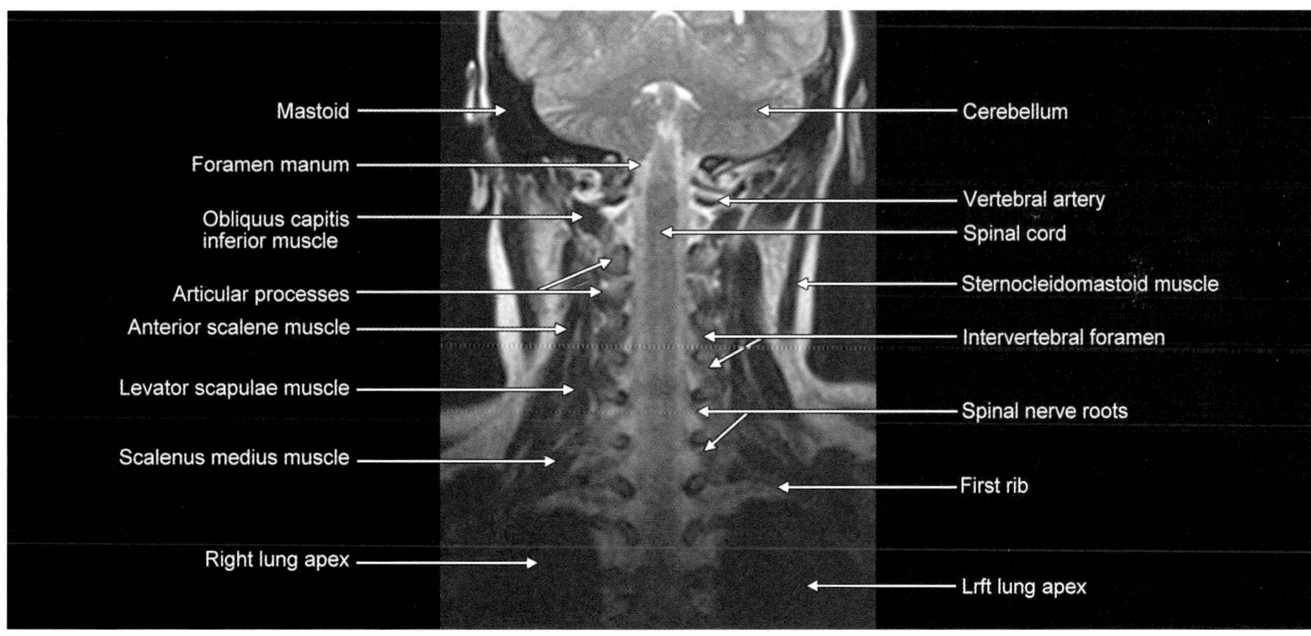

Fig. 11: Cervical spine MRI: Coronal T2WI (corresponds to level 2 in Fig. 9)

so that excessive motion between the vertebral bodies does not occur. It is the strongest of the spinal ligaments and often has a thinner middle section. Together with the laminae, it forms the posterior wall of the spinal canal.

Supraspinous ligaments join the tips of adjacent spinous process in the dorsal spine. In the neck they are replaced by the ligamentum nuchae and they are poorly developed in the lumbar region. During full flexion these ligaments are taut and support the

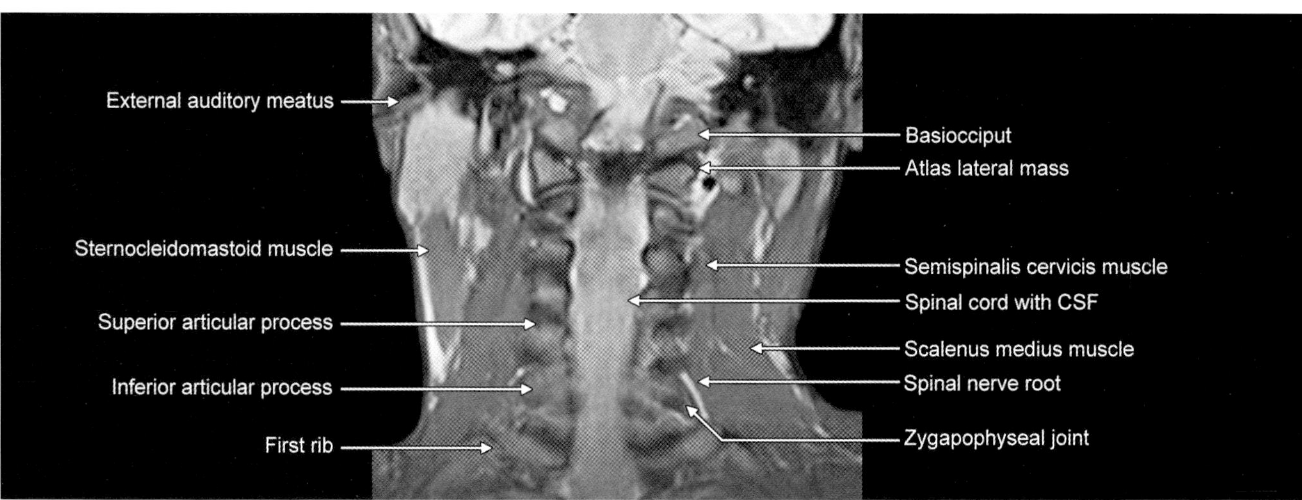

Fig. 12: Cervical spine MRI: Coronal T2WI (corresponds to level 3 in Fig. 9)

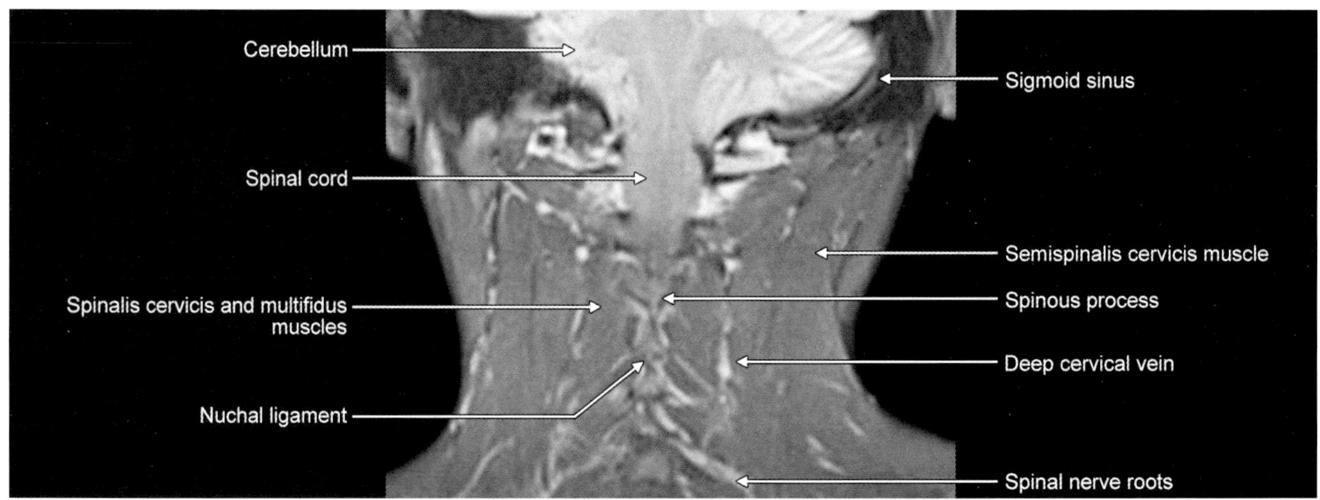

Fig. 13: Cervical spine MRI: Coronal T2WI (corresponds to level 4 in Fig. 9)

spine. Interspinous ligaments are well developed only in the lumbar region, uniting the spinous process along their adjacent borders. Intertransverse ligaments join the tranverse processes along their adjacent borders.

Accessory ligaments: These connect the axis to the occiput, bypassing the atlas. They are the tectorial membrane, cruciform ligament, apical ligament and the paired alar ligaments.

Spinal canal: It is closed anteriorly by the vertebral bodies, the intervertebral discs, posterior longitudinal ligament. Posteriorly it is related to the lamina and ligamentum flavum. Laterally on either sides it is related to the pedicles. The intervertebral foramina contain the spinal nerves, posterior root ganglia spinal arteries and veins. The vertebral canal contains the spinal cord.

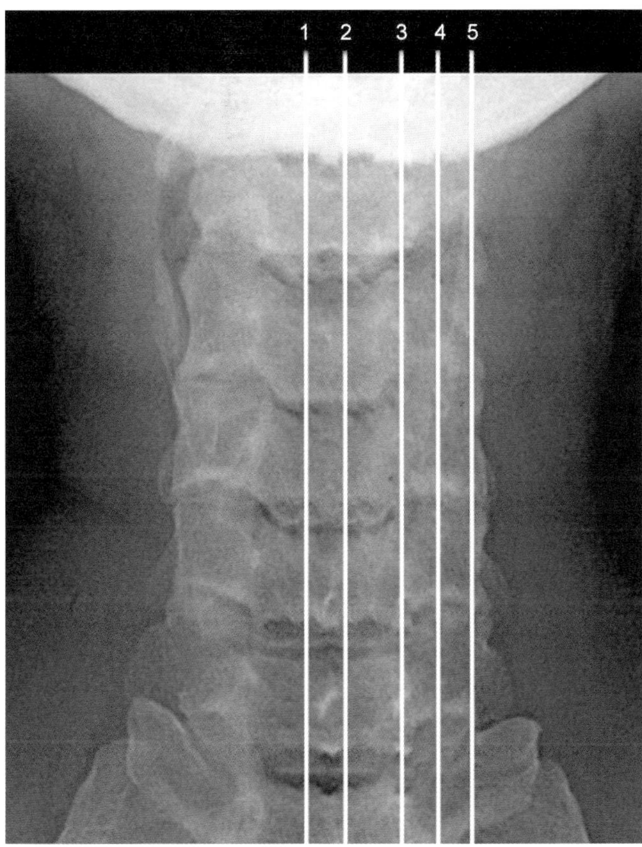

Fig. 14: Cervical spine: Sagittal section plan

Spinal cord: The spinal canal encases the spinal cord. The bones and ligaments of the spinal column are aligned in such a manner to create a column that provides protection and support for the spinal cord. The outermost layer that surround the spinal cord is the dura mater, which is a tough membrane that encloses the spinal cord and prevents cerebrospinal fluid from leaking out. The space between the dura and the spinal canal is called the epidural space. This space is filled with fatty tissue, vessels and large veins. The spinal cord is derived from the ectodermal neural groove, which eventually closes to form a tube during fetal development. From this neural tube, the entire central nervous system, eventually develops. Up to the 3rd months of fetal life, the spinal cord is about the same length as the canal. The growth of the canal outpaces that of the cord from the 3rd months onwards. In an adult the lower end of the spinal cord usually ends at approximately the first lumbar vertebra, where it divides into many individual nerve roots that travel to the lower body and legs. This collection of group of nerve roots is called the "cauda equina".

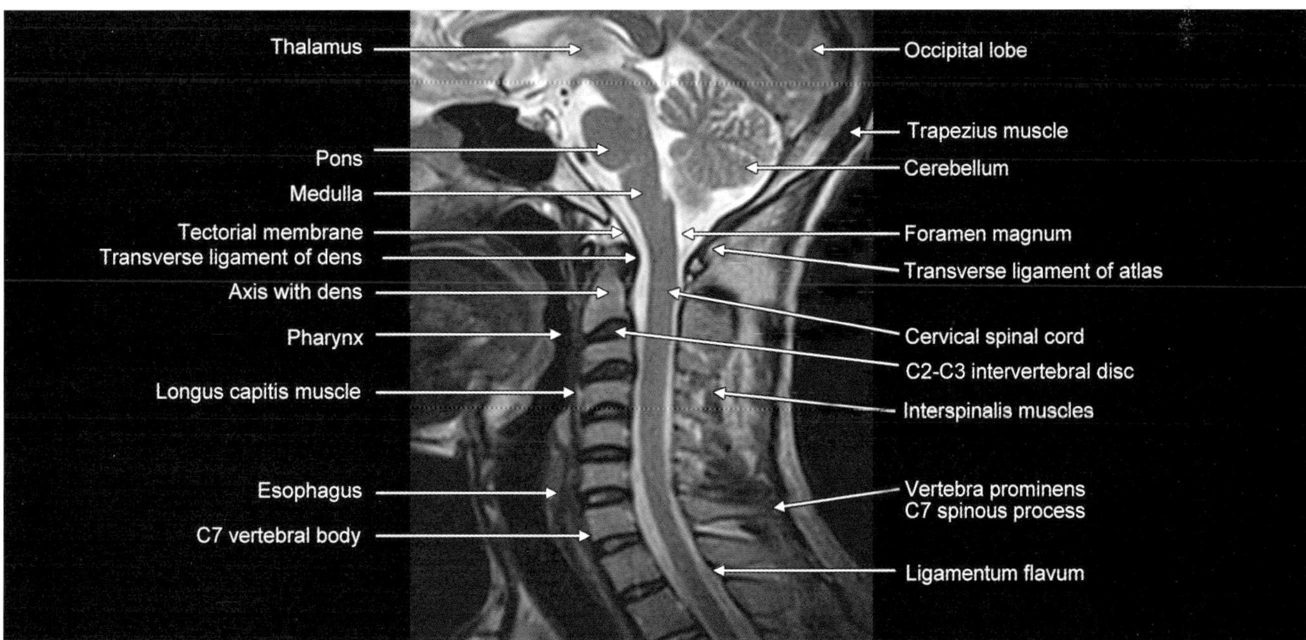

Fig. 15: Cervical spine MRI: Sagittal T2WI (corresponds to level 1 in Fig. 14)

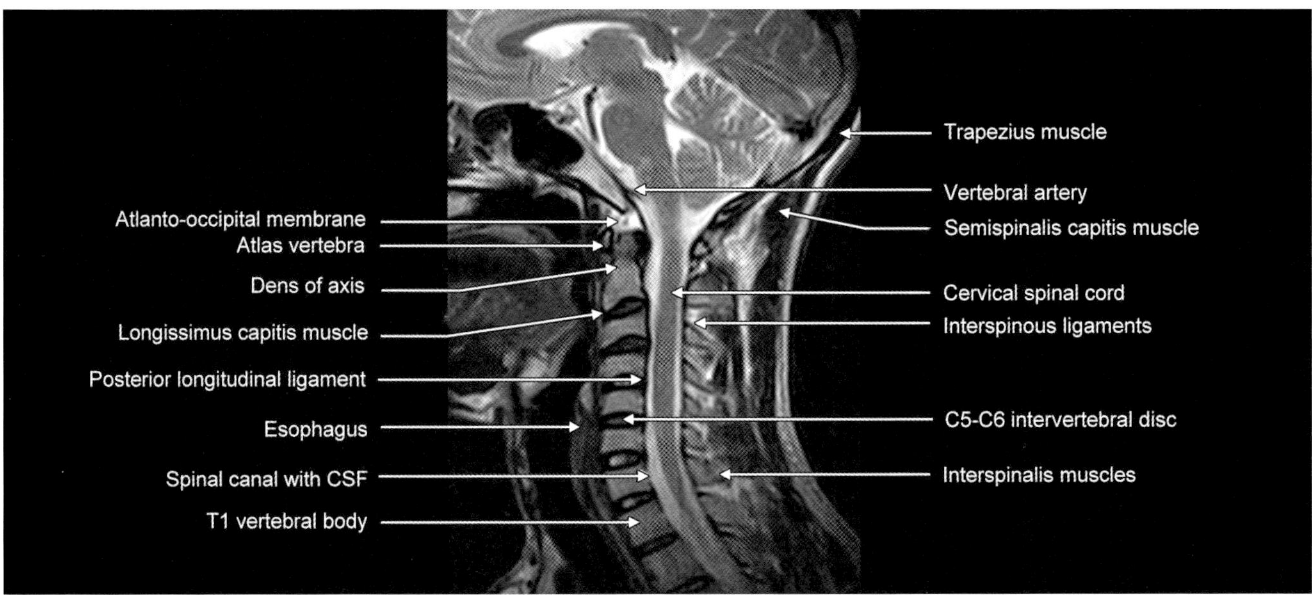

Fig. 16: Cervical spine MRI: Sagittal T2WI (corresponds to level 2 in Fig. 14)

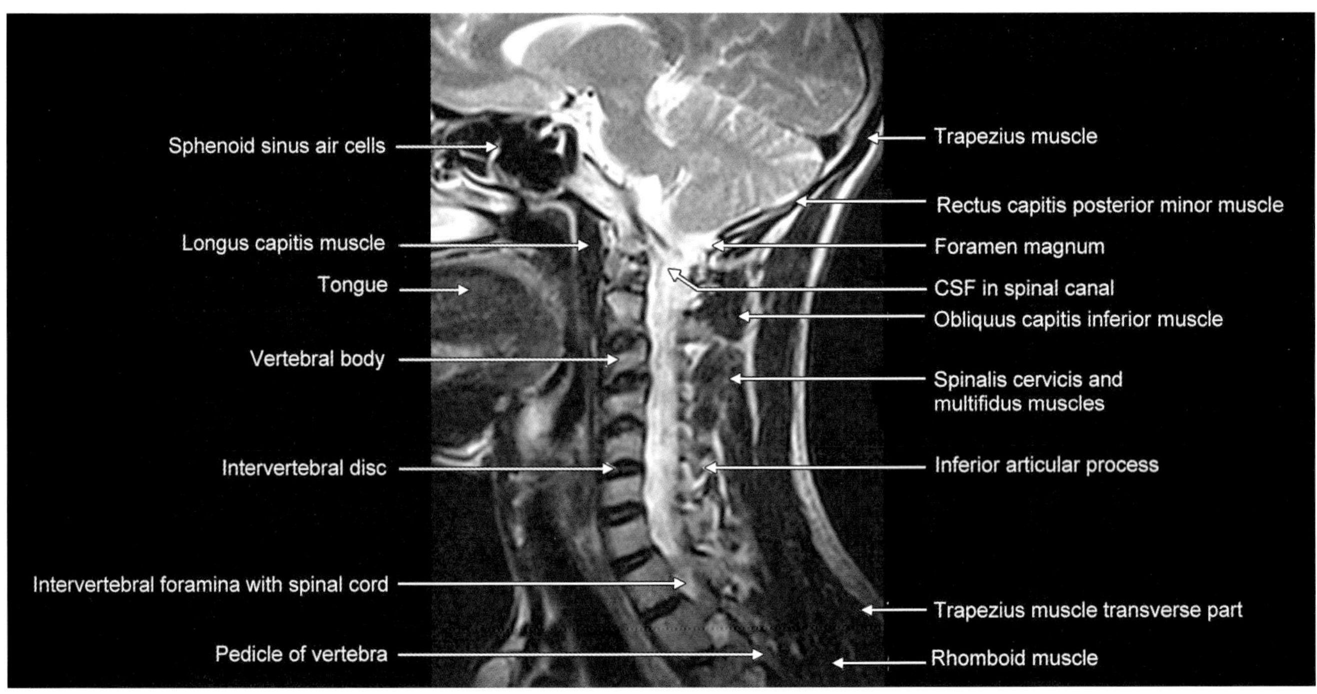

Fig. 17: Cervical spine MRI: Sagittal T2WI (corresponds to level 3 in Fig. 14)

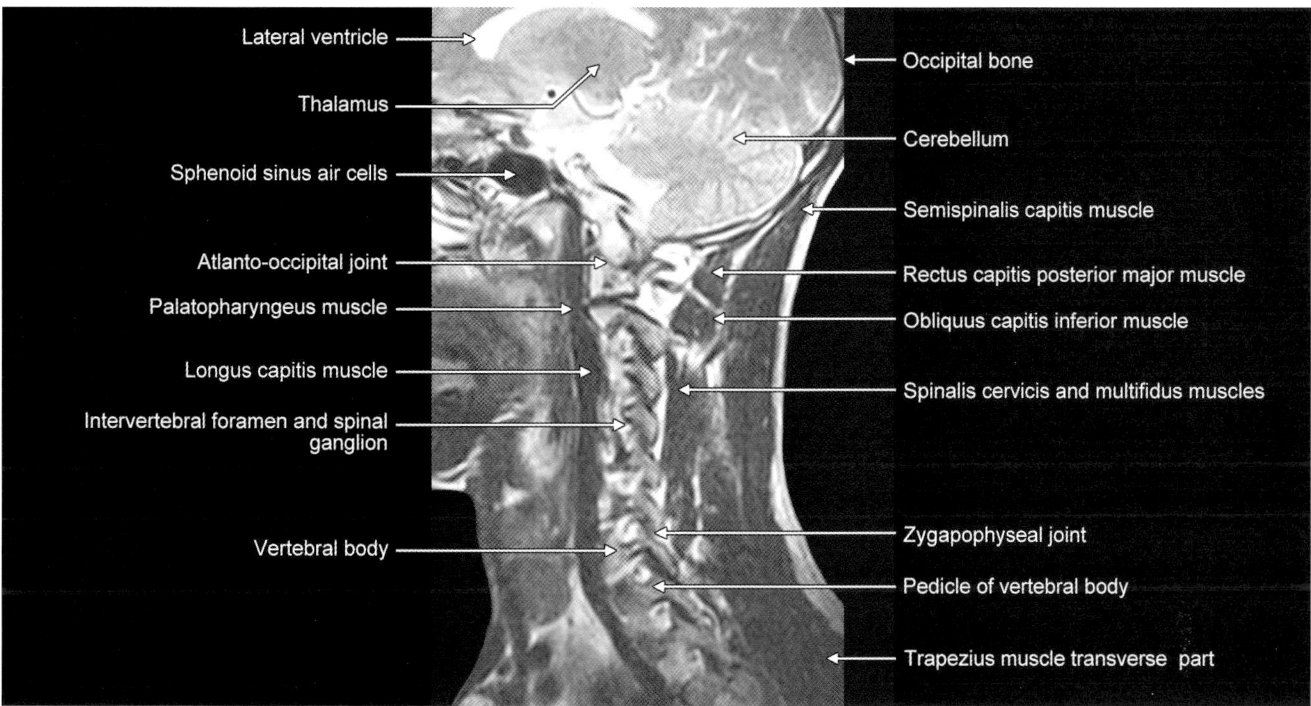

Fig. 18: Cervical spine MRI: Sagittal T2WI (corresponds to level 4 in Fig. 14)

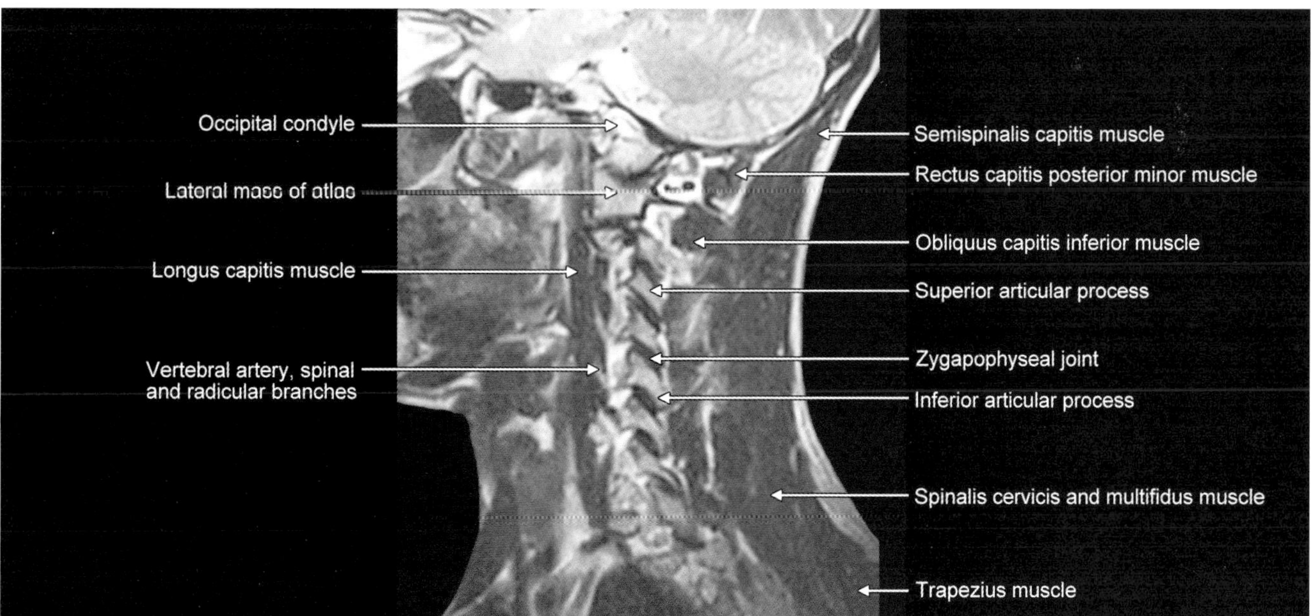

Fig. 19: Cervical spine MRI: Sagittal T2WI (corresponds to level 5 in Fig. 14)

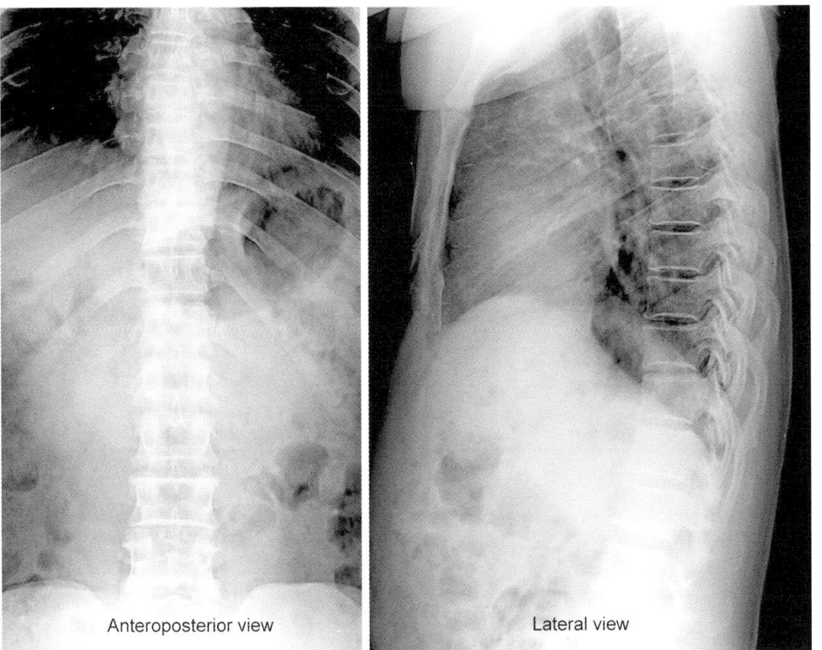

Fig. 20: Dorsal spine

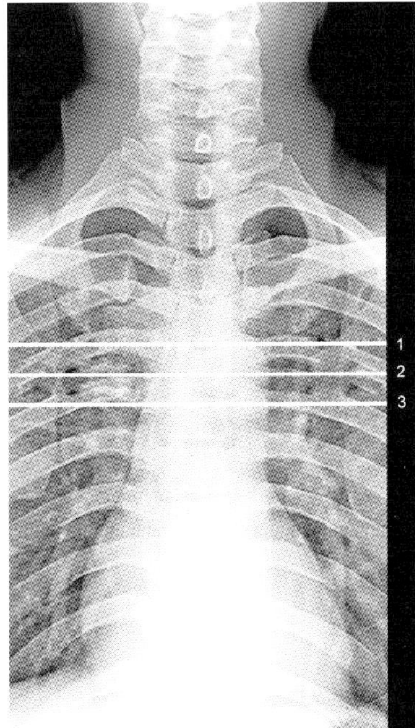

Fig. 21: Dorsal spine: Axial section plan

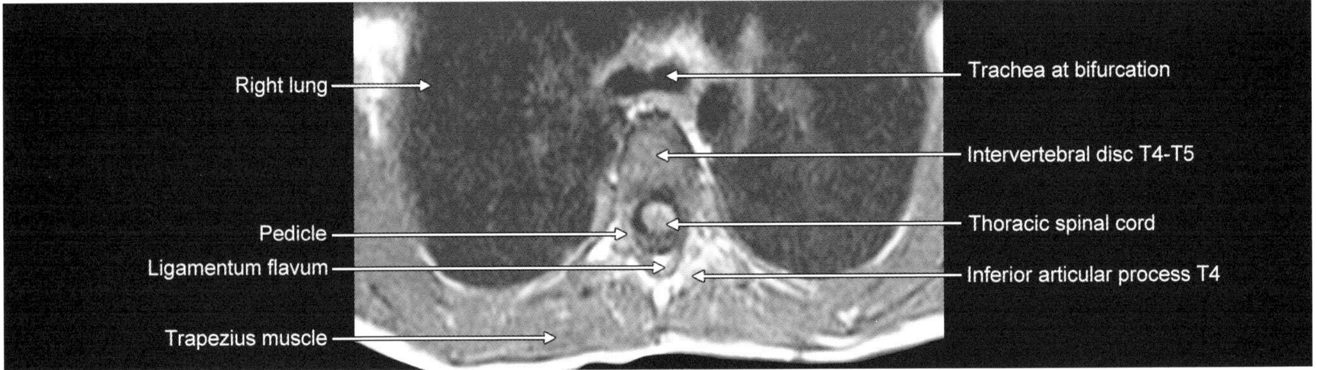

Fig. 22: Dorsal spine MRI: Axial T1WI at level D4-D5 disc (corresponds to level 1 in Fig. 21)

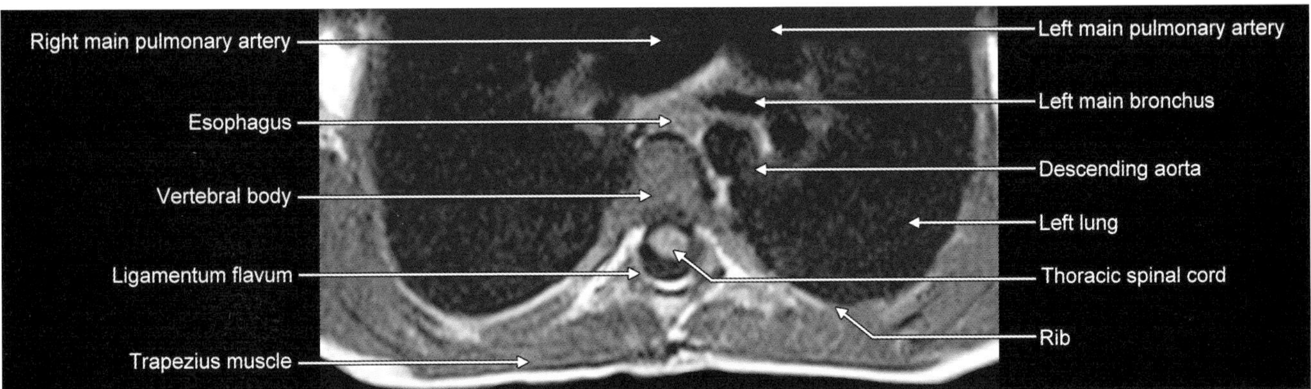

Fig. 23: Dorsal spine MRI: Axial T1WI at level D5 lower part vertebral body (corresponds to level 3 in Fig. 21)

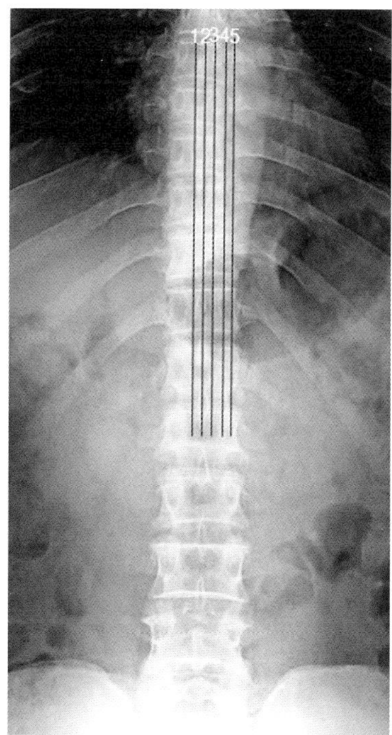

Fig. 24: Dorsal spine: Sagittal section plan

Some differentiating features between cervical, thoracic and lumbar vertebrae: C3-C6 vertebrae have atypical features. The body of these four vertebrae is small and broader from side-to-side than from front-to-back. The pedicles are directed laterally and backward. The laminae are narrow, and thinner above than below. The vertebral foramen is large and has a triangular shape. The spinous process is short and bifid. Superior articular facets face backward, upward, and slightly medially and inferior face forward, downward, and slightly laterally. The foramen transversarium is the opening in the transverse processes of the seven cervical vertebrae. It gives passage to the vertebral artery, vein and plexus of sympathetic nerves in each of the vertebrae except the seventh, which lacks the artery. C7 has enlarged spinous process called the vertebral prominence.

The thoracic vertebrae have costal facets for ribs on either sides of the vertebral body. They increase in size gradually from T3 vertebra downwards.

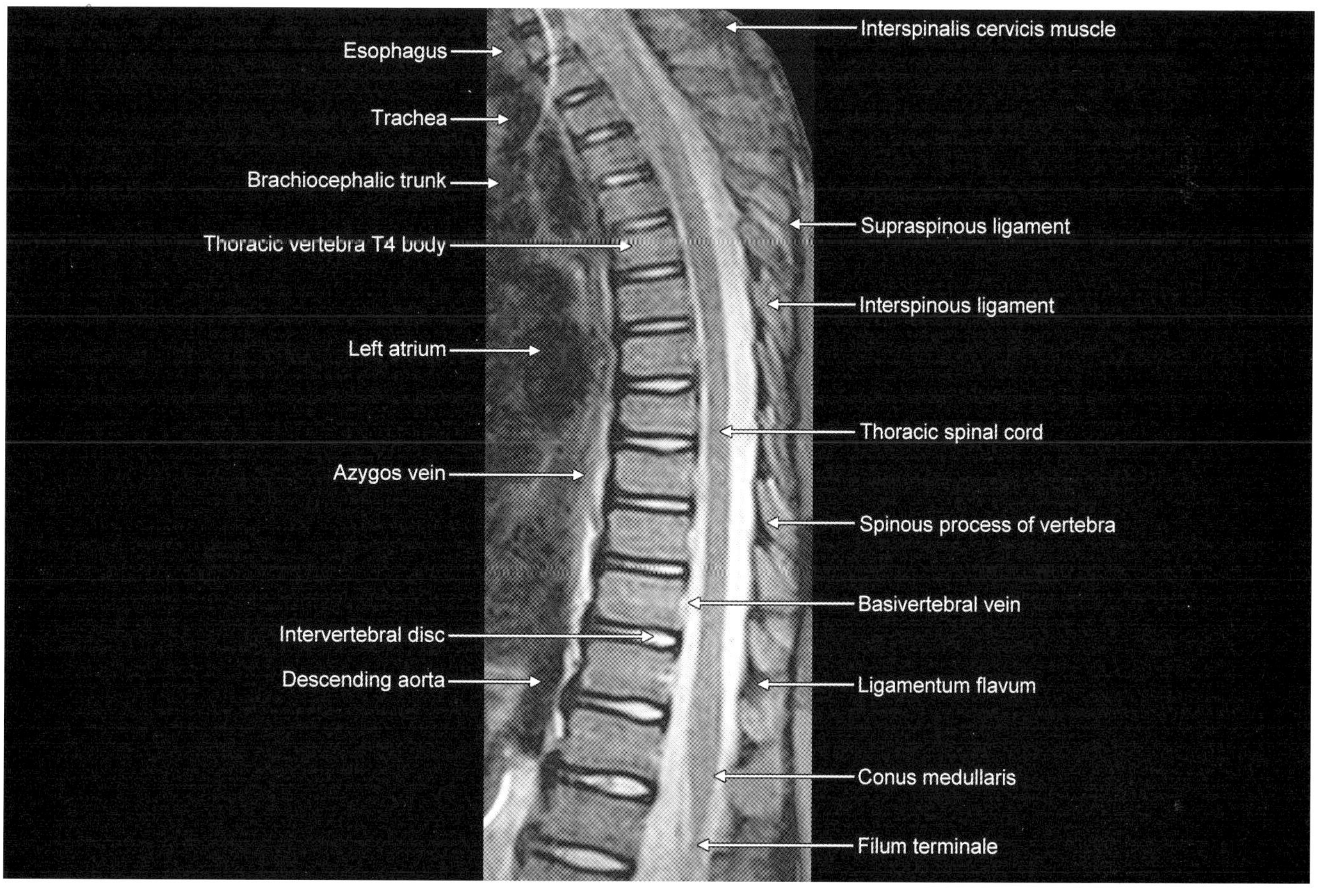

Fig. 25: Dorsal spine MRI: Sagittal T2WI (corresponds to level 1 in Fig. 24)

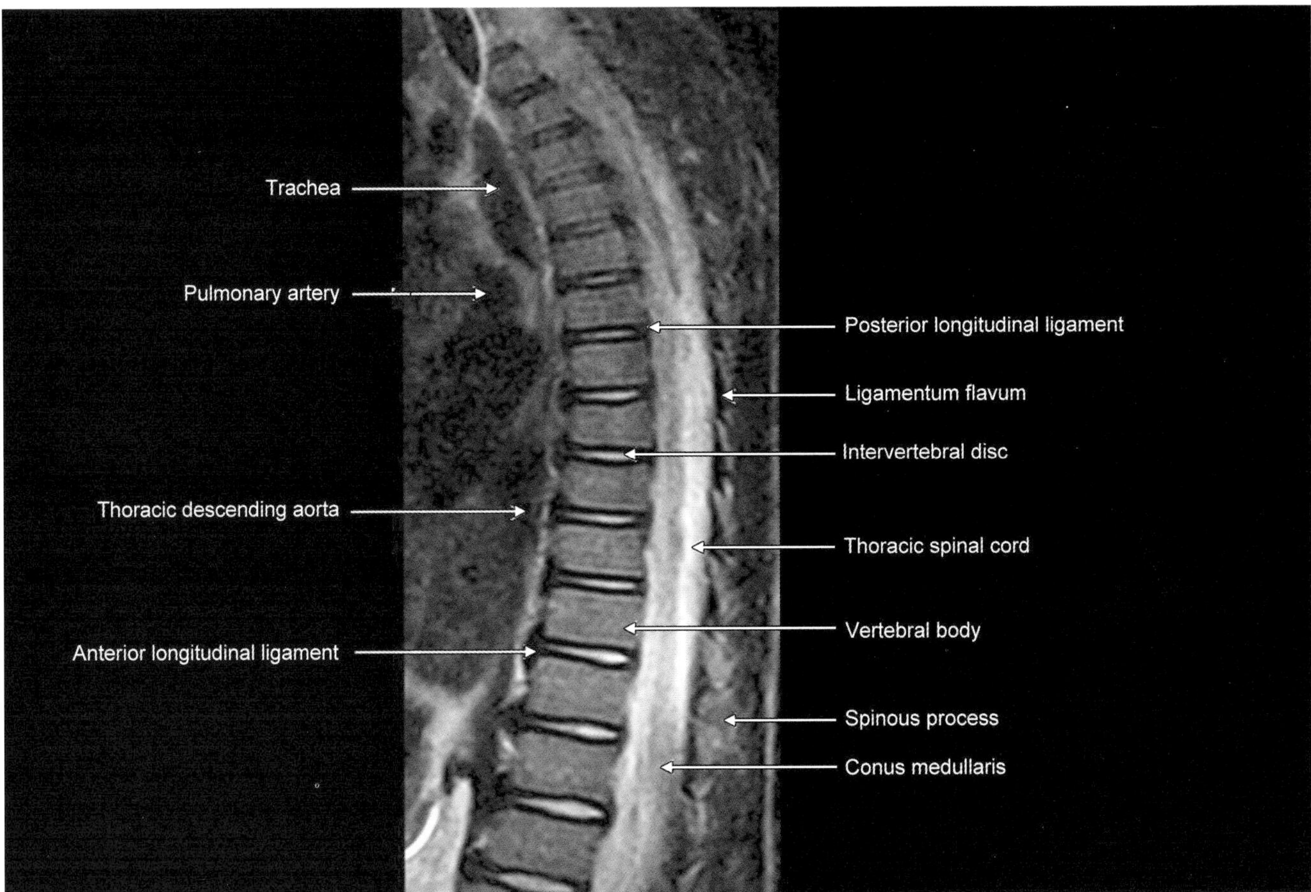

Fig. 26: Dorsal spine MRI: Sagittal T2WI (corresponds to level 2 in Fig. 24)

The lumbar vertebrae have neither a foramen in transverse process nor costal facets; they are also larger than the dorsal and cervical vertebrae in size.

Radiological importance of vertebral column in spinal injuries: The vertebral column can be subdivided as anterior column, middle column and the posterior column. Injuries involving the middle and posterior columns result in unstable injuries.

- Anterior column is formed by anterior longitudinal ligament, anterior annulus fibrosus and anterior part of vertebral body.
- Middle column is formed by posterior longitudinal ligament, posterior annulus fibrosus and posterior part of vertebral body.
- Posterior column includes posterior elements and ligaments.

Radiological importance of craniovertebral junction: Chamberlain line is the line between posterior part of hard palate and posterior margin of foramen magnum. Normally the tip of odontoid process lies at or below this line. Basilar line is the line along the clivus and it usually falls tangent to posterior aspect of tip of odontoid.

Craniovertebral angle (Clivus-Canal angle): It is angle between basilar line and a line along posterior aspect of odontoid process. If this angle is <150°, cord compression can occur on the ventral aspect.

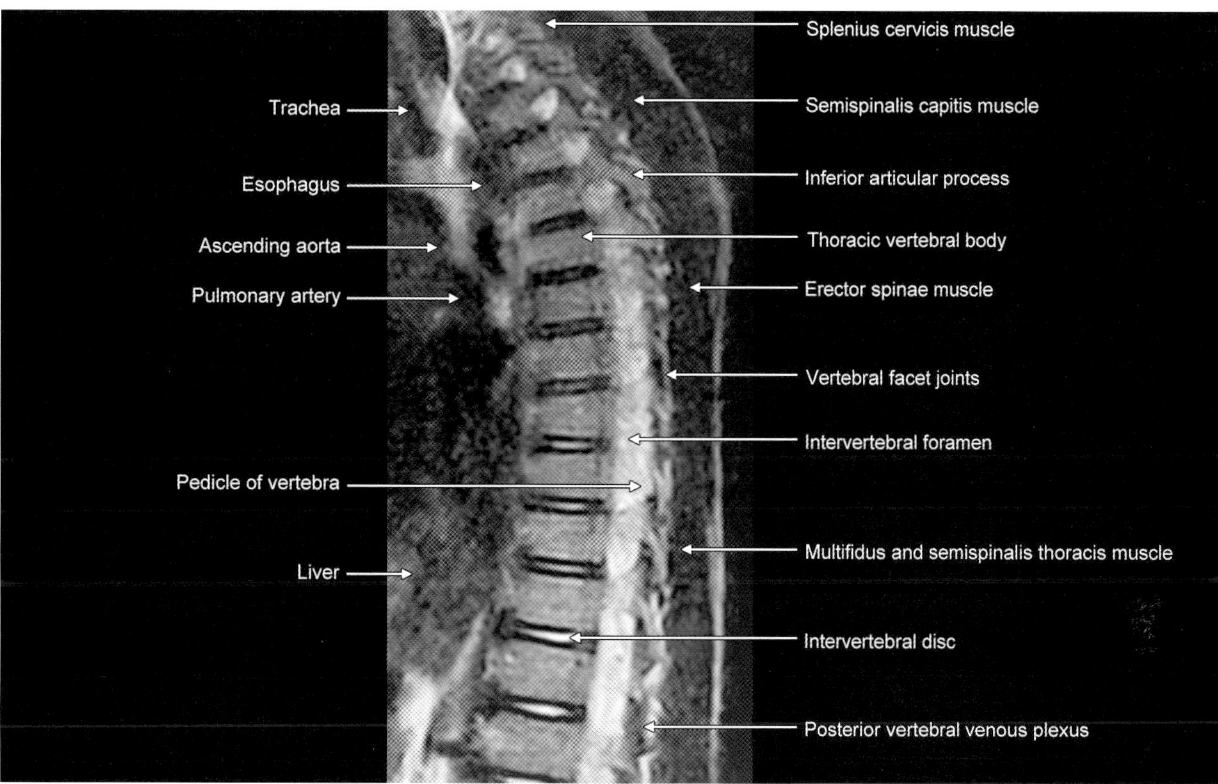

Fig. 27: Dorsal spine MRI: Sagittal T2WI (corresponds to level 3 in Fig. 24)

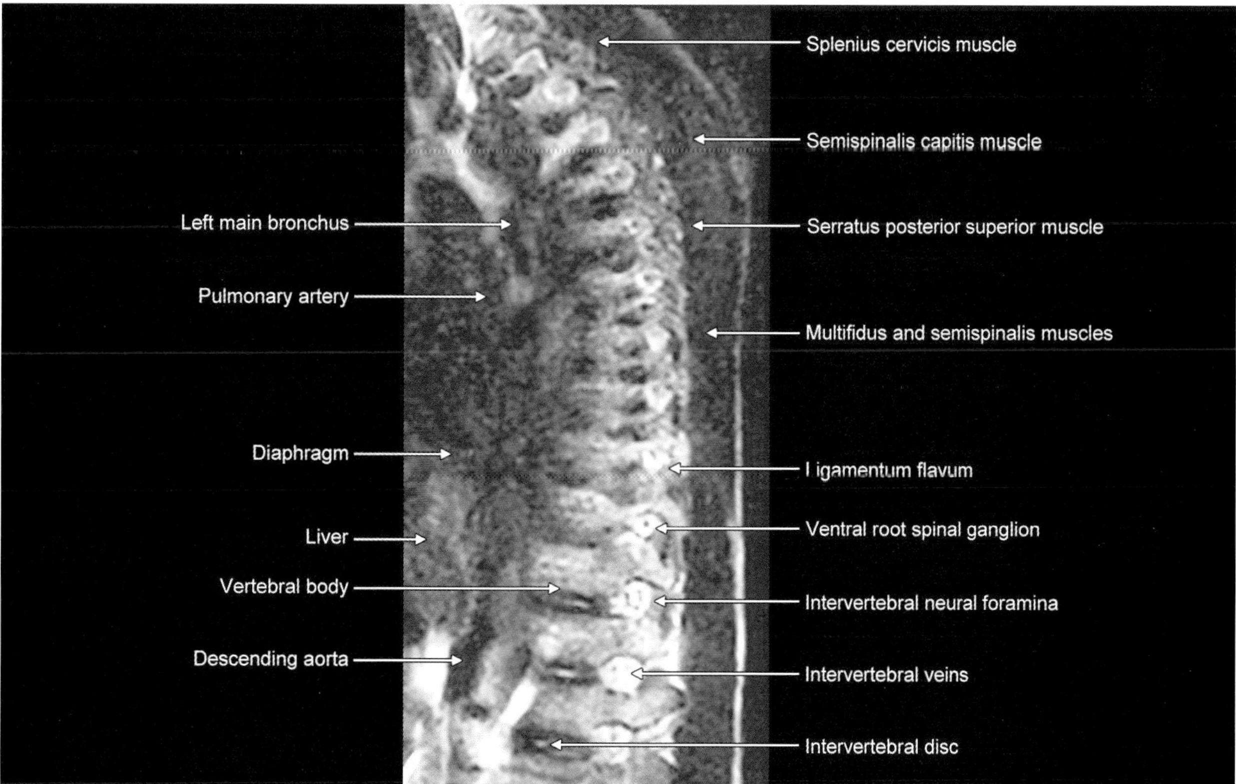

Fig. 28: Dorsal spine MRI: Sagittal T2WI (corresponds to level 4 in Fig. 24)

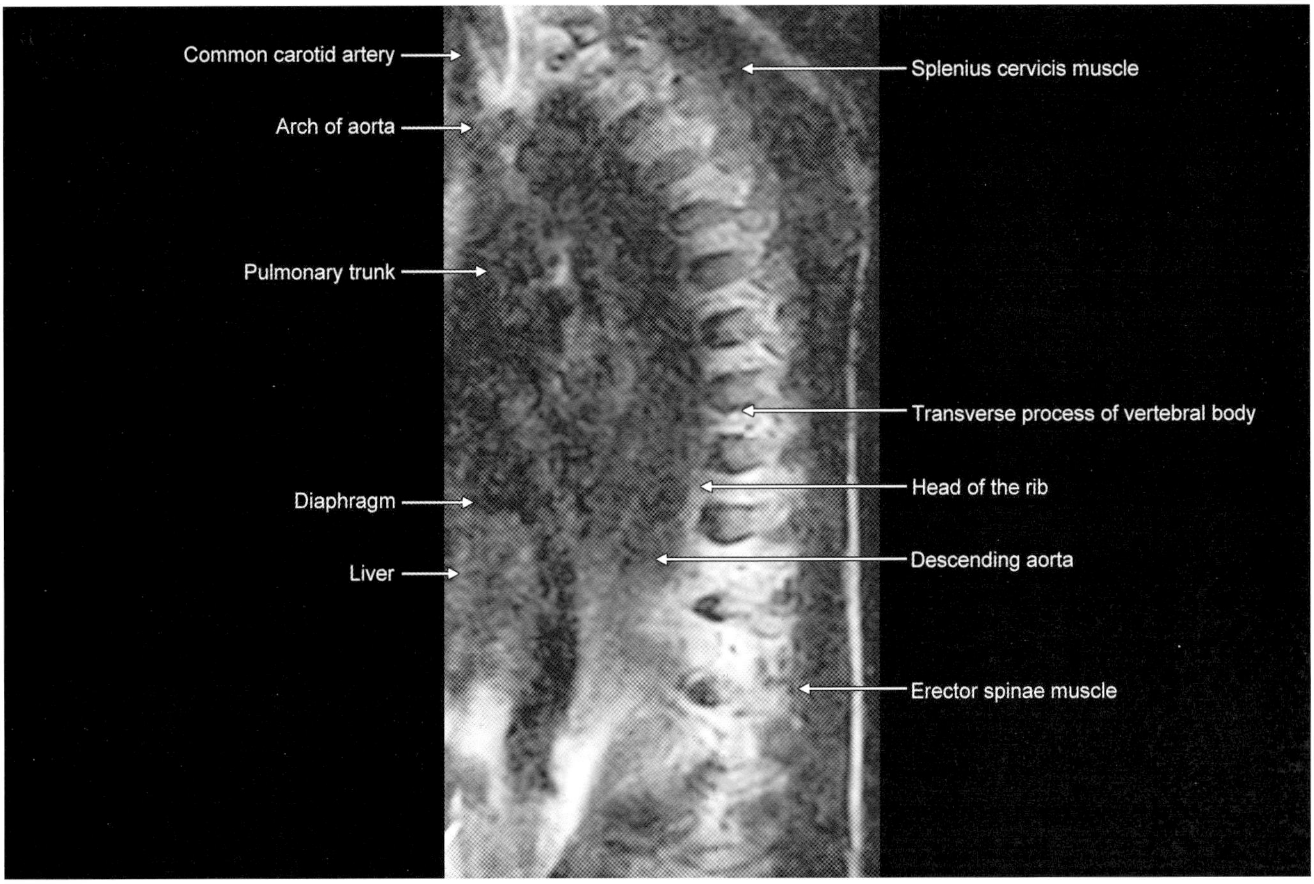

Fig. 29: Dorsal spine MRI: Sagittal T2WI (corresponds to level 5 in Fig. 24)

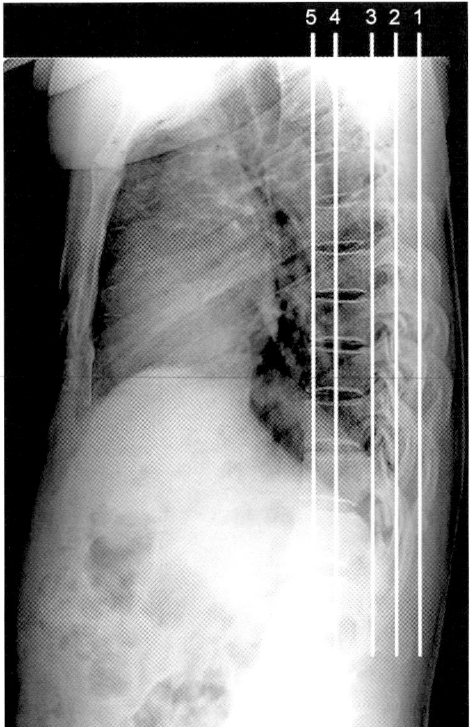

Fig. 30: Dorsal spine: Coronal section plan

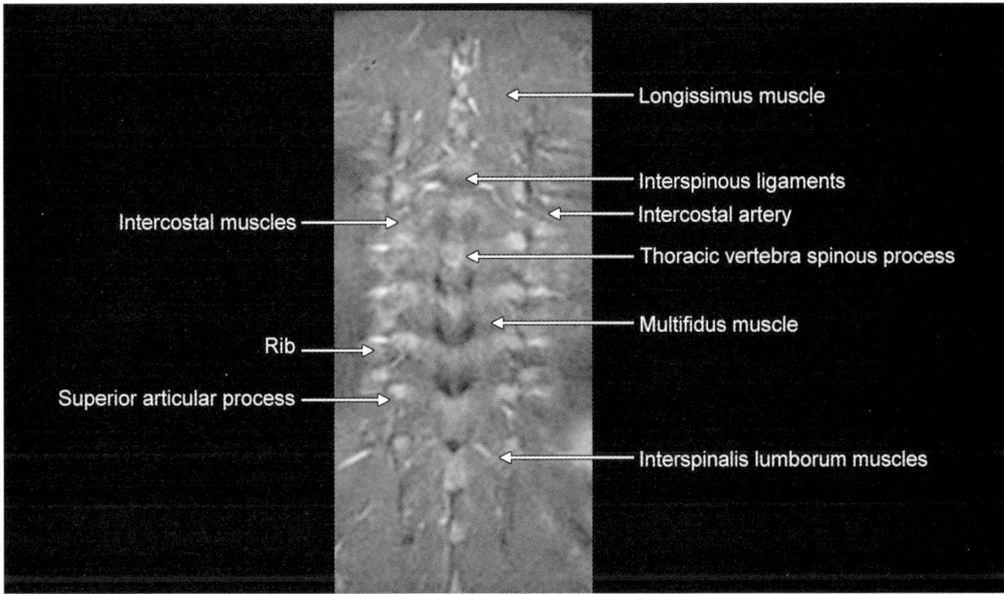

Fig. 31: Dorsal spine MRI: Coronal T2WI (corresponds to level 1 in Fig. 30)

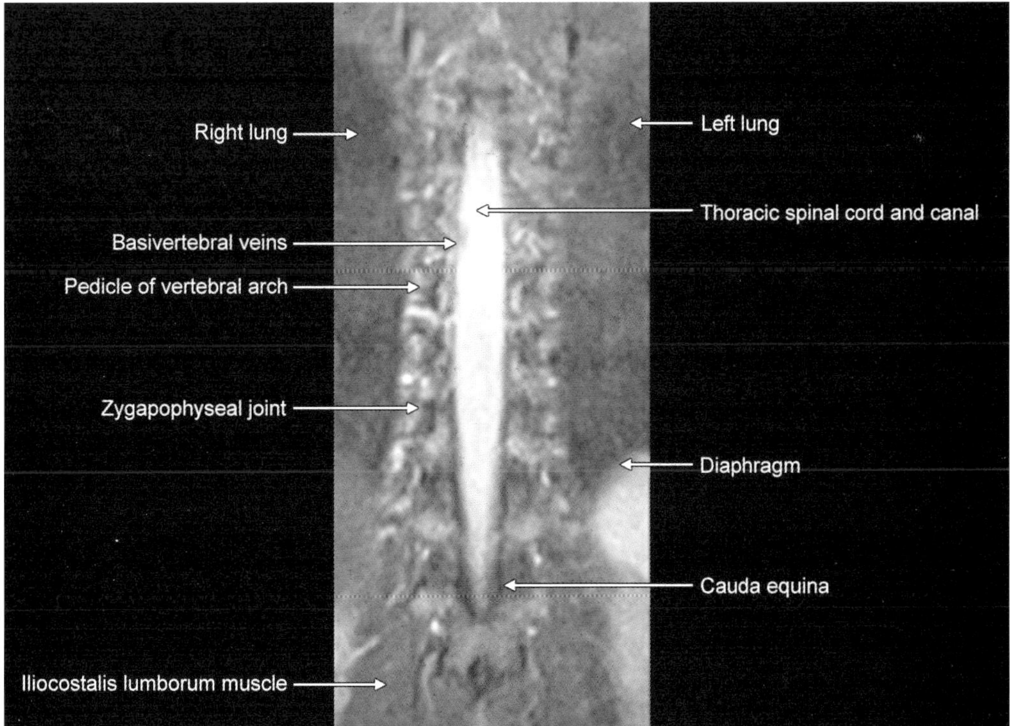

Fig. 32: Dorsal spine MRI: Coronal T2WI (corresponds to level 2 in Fig. 30)

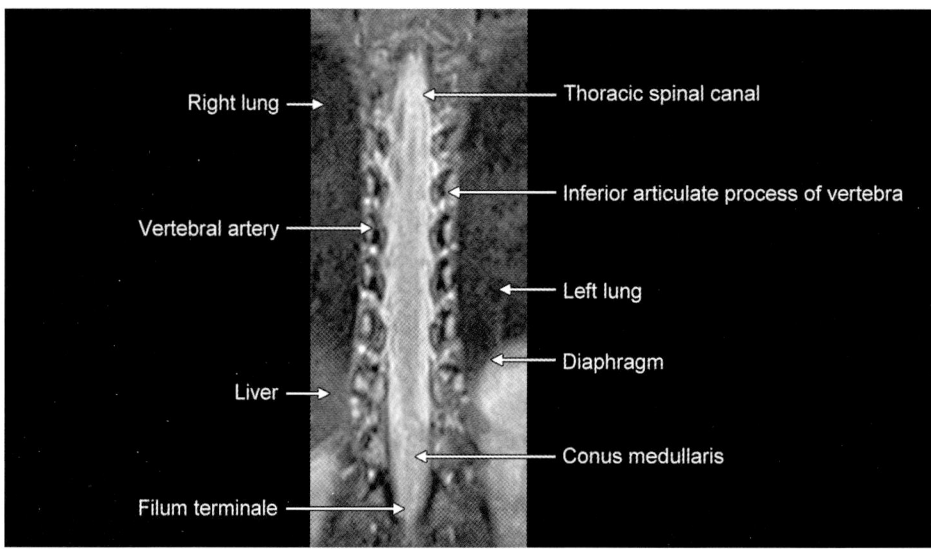

Fig. 33: Dorsal spine MRI: Coronal T2WI (corresponds to level 3 in Fig. 30)

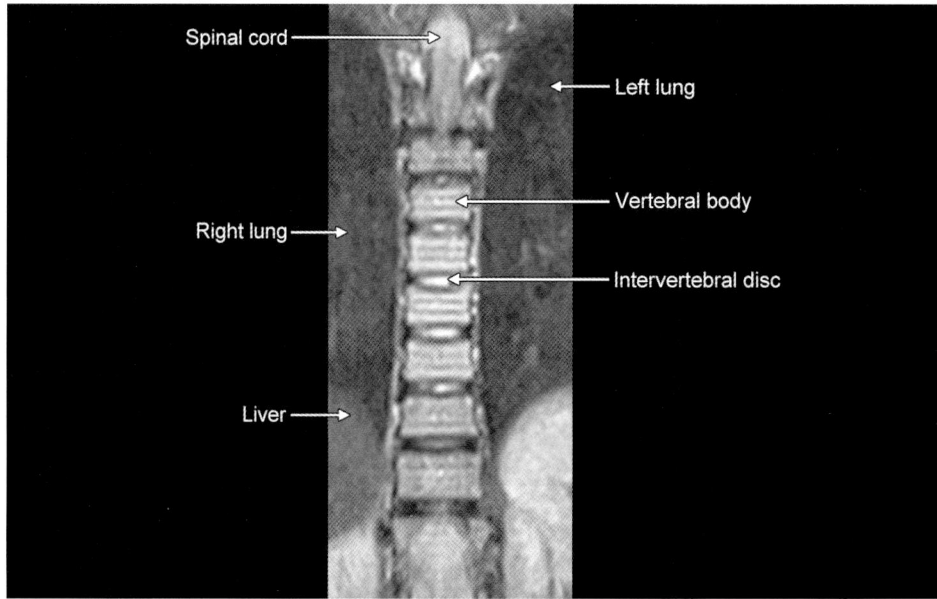

Fig. 34: Dorsal spine MRI: Coronal T2WI (corresponds to level 4 in Fig. 30)

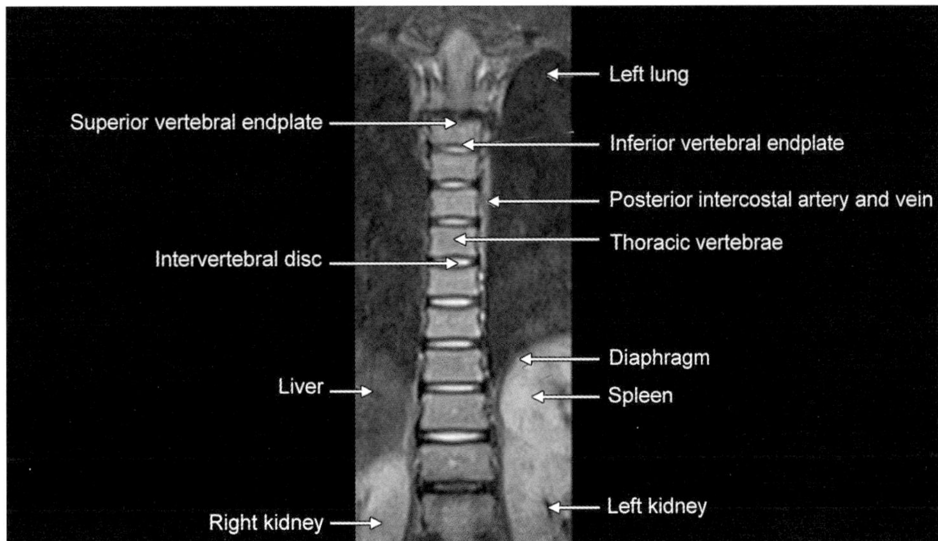

Fig. 35: Dorsal spine MRI: Coronal T2WI (corresponds to level 5 in Fig. 30)

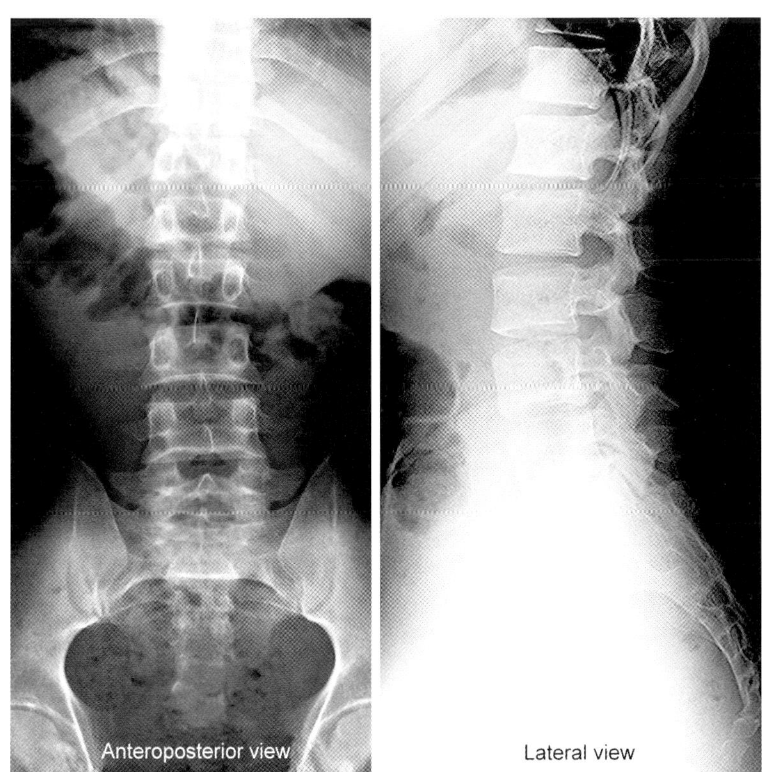

Fig. 36: Lumbosacral spine

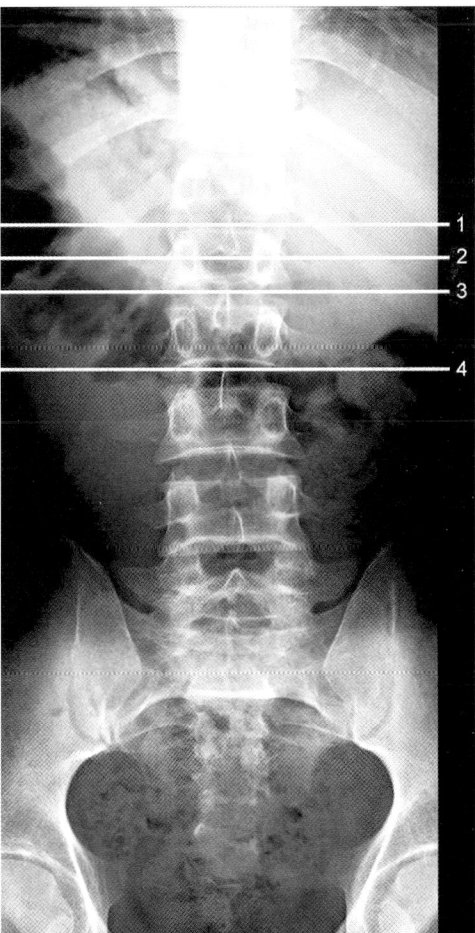

Fig. 37: Lumbosacral spine MRI: Axial section plan

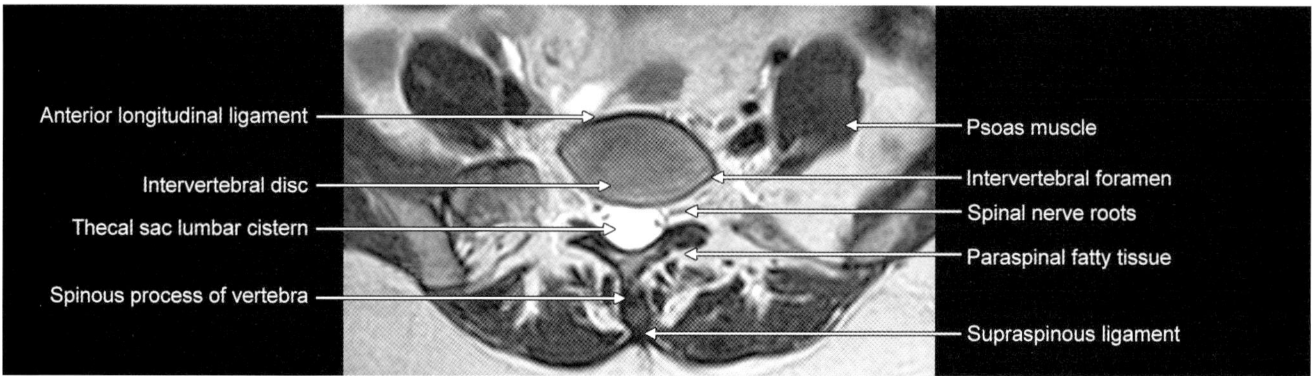

Fig. 38: Lumbosacral spine MRI: Axial T2WI D12-L1 disc level (corresponds to level 1 in Fig. 37)

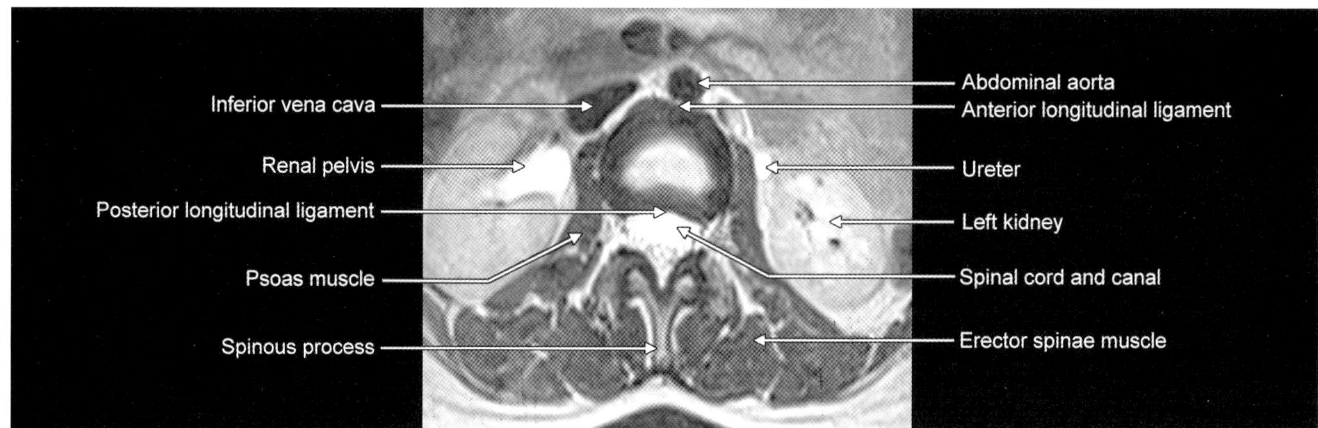

Fig. 39: Lumbosacral spine MRI: Axial T2WI L1 vertebral body level (corresponds to level 2 in Fig. 37)

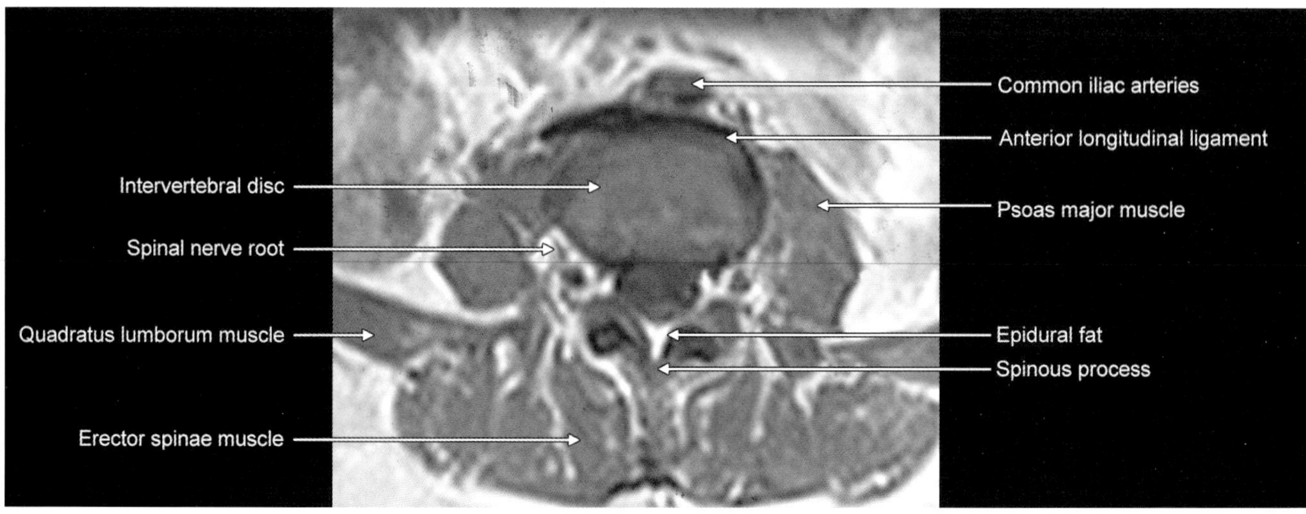

Fig. 40: Lumbosacral spine MRI: Axial T1WI L1-L2 disc level (corresponds to level 3 in Fig. 37)

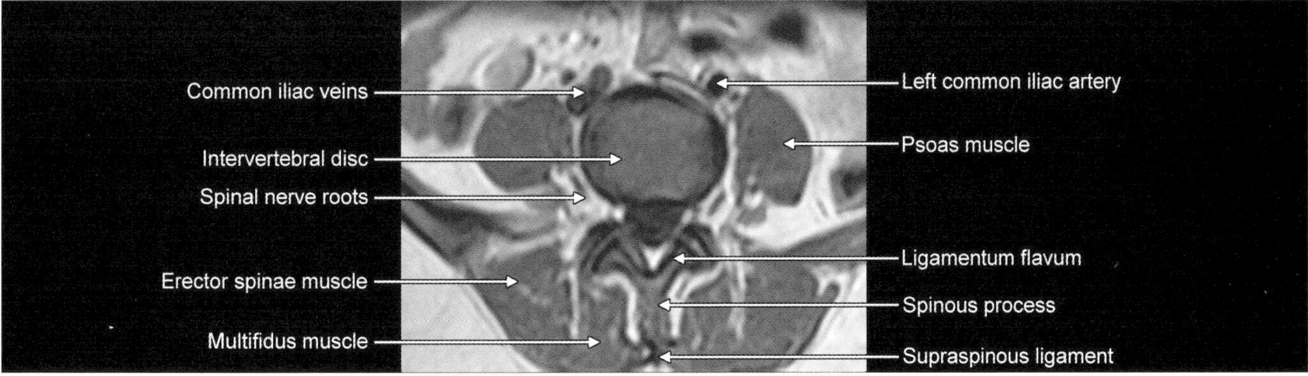

Fig. 41: Lumbosacral spine MRI: Axial T1WI L2-L3 disc level (corresponds to level 4 in Fig. 37)

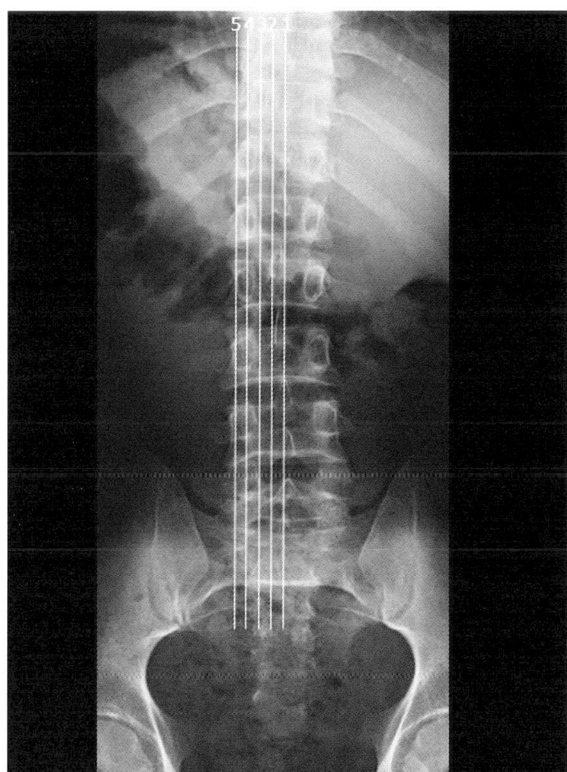

Fig. 42: Dorsolumbar spine MRI: Sagittal section plan

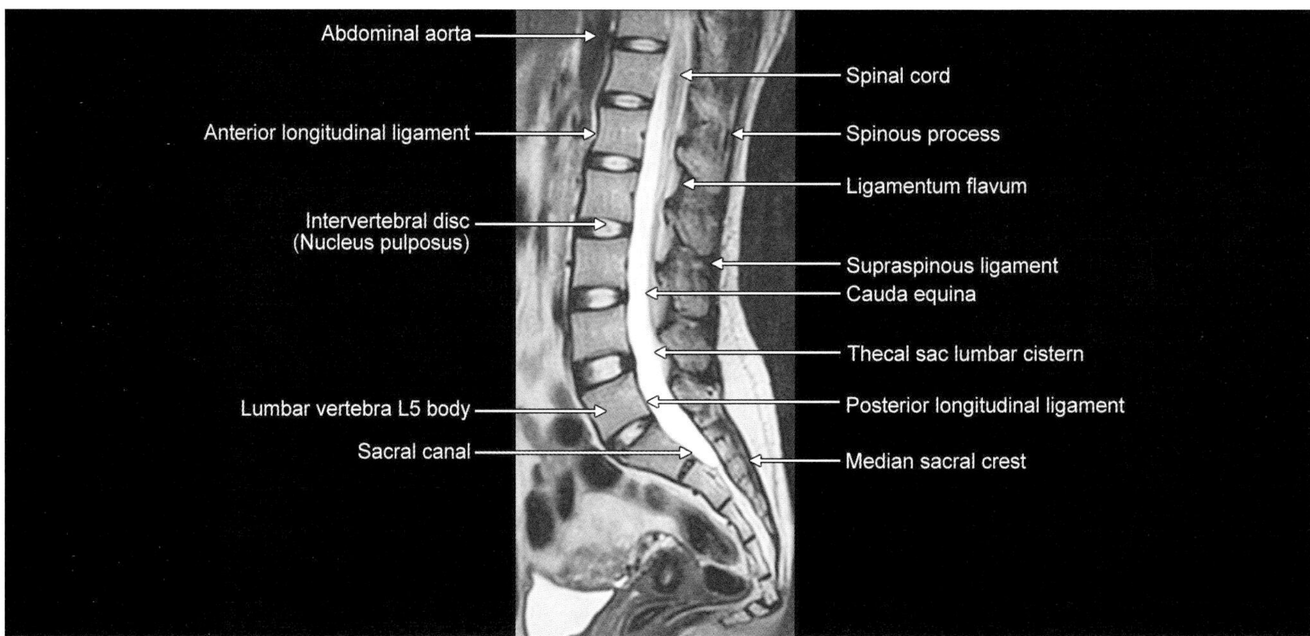

Fig. 43: Lumbosacral spine MRI: Sagittal T2WI (corresponds to level 1 in Fig. 42)

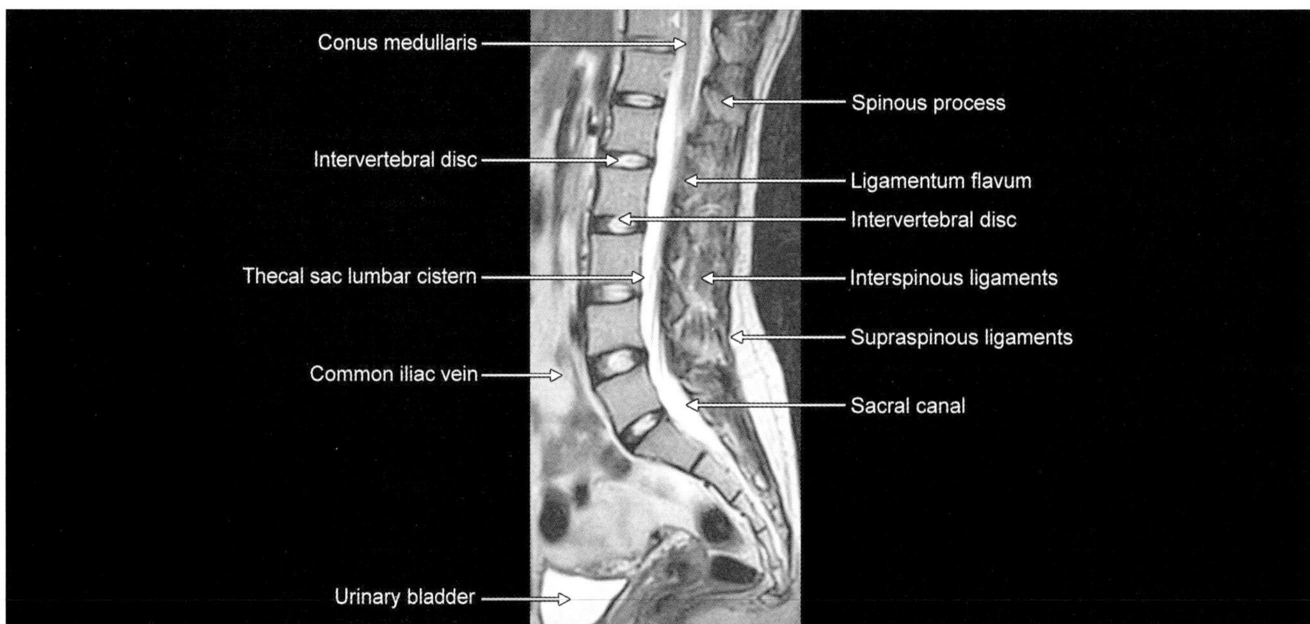

Fig. 44: Lumbosacral spine MRI: Sagittal T2WI (corresponds to level 2 in Fig. 42)

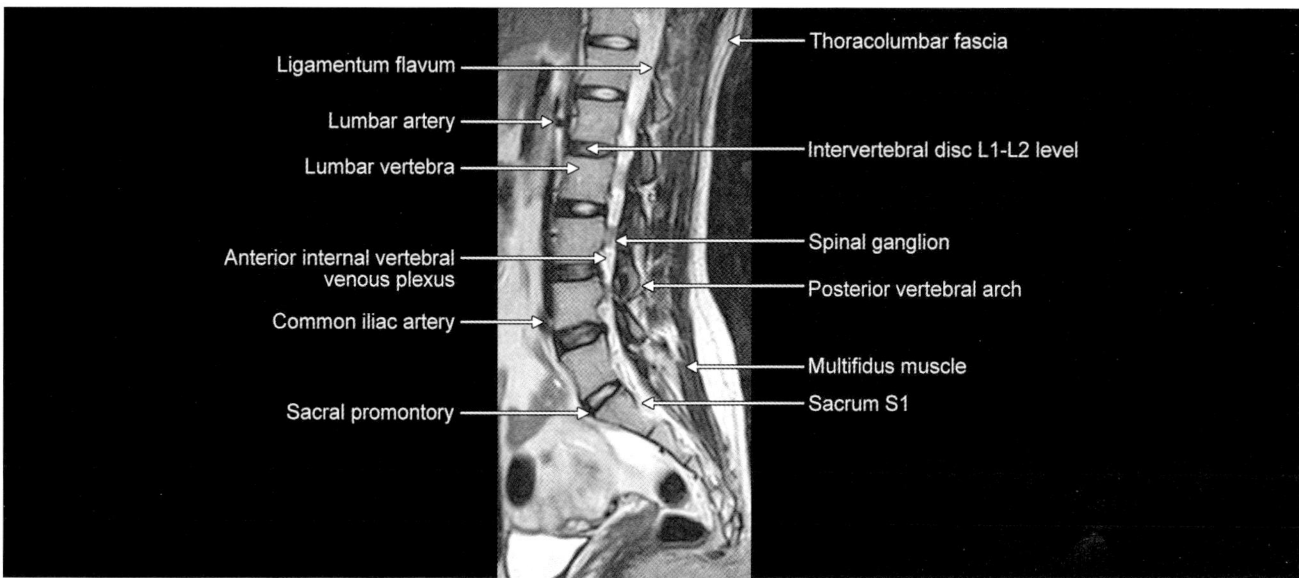

Fig. 45: Lumbosacral spine MRI: Sagittal T2WI (corresponds to level 3 in Fig. 42)

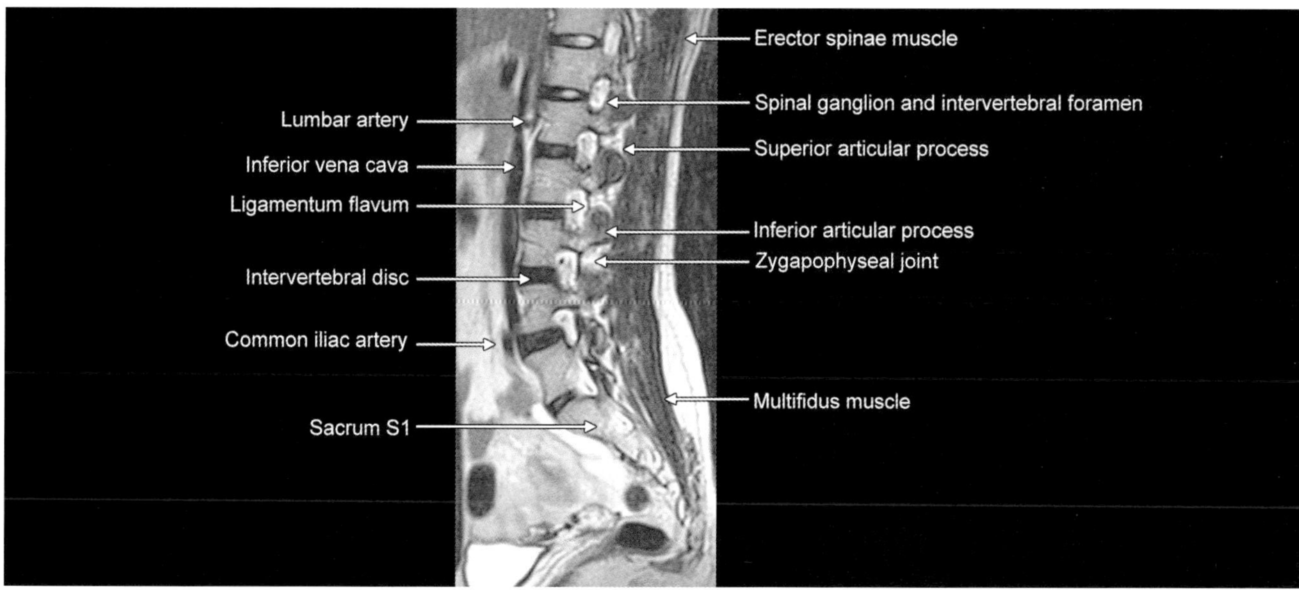

Fig. 46: Lumbosacral spine MRI: Sagittal T2WI (corresponds to level 4 in Fig. 42)

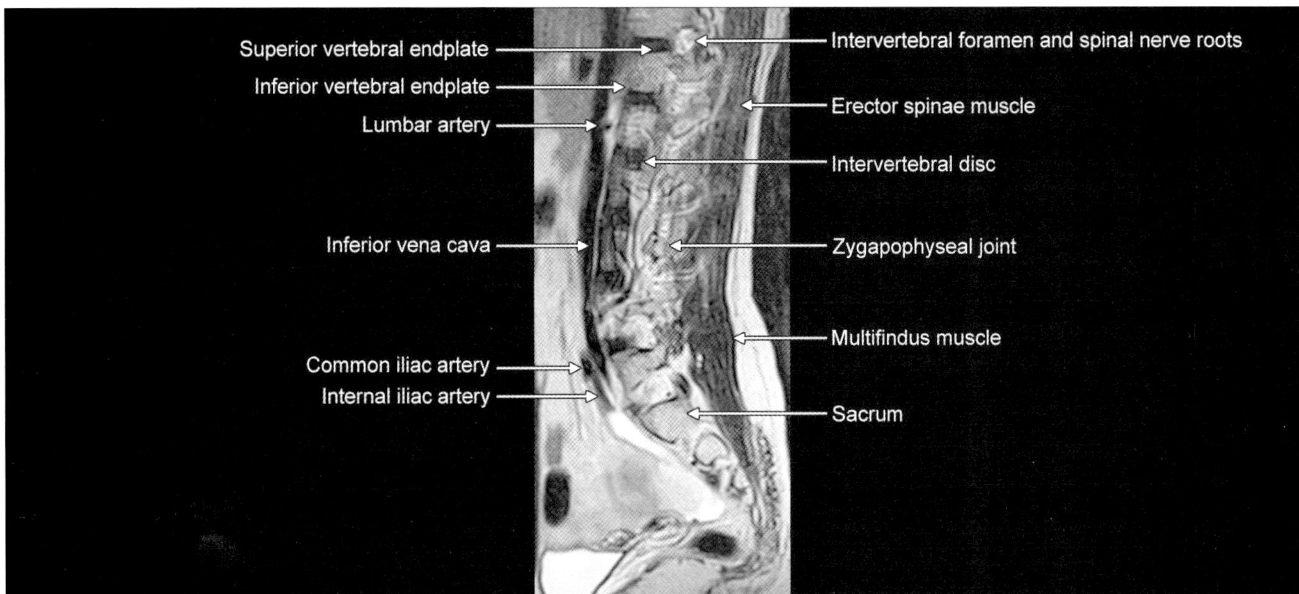

Fig. 47: Lumbosacral spine MRI: Sagittal T2WI (corresponds to level 5 in Fig. 42)

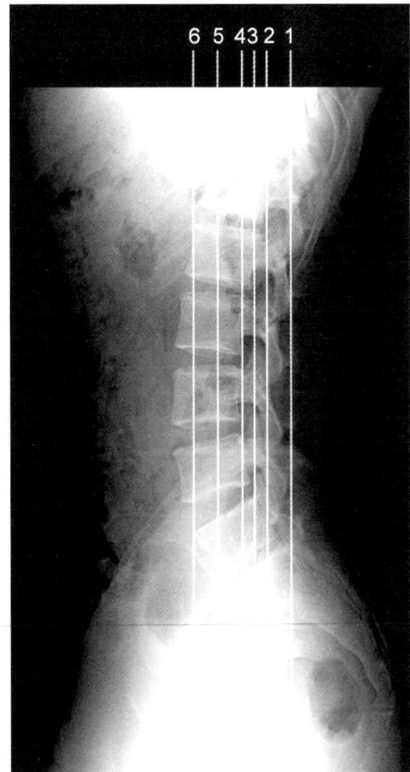

Fig. 48: Lumbosacral spine MRI: Coronal section plan

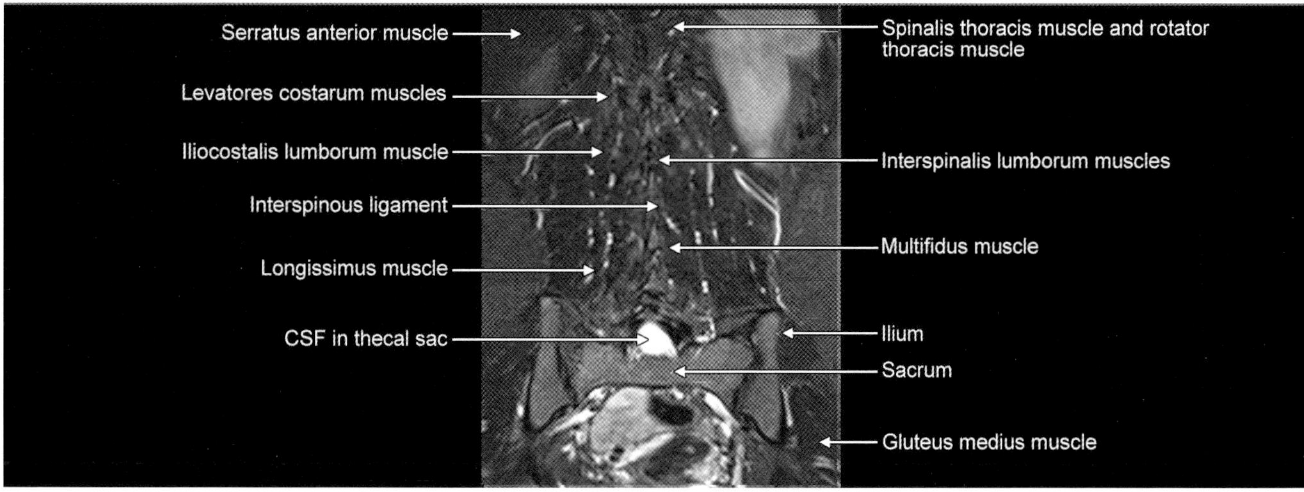

Fig. 49: Lumbosacral spine MRI: Coronal T2WI (corresponds to level 1 in Fig. 48)

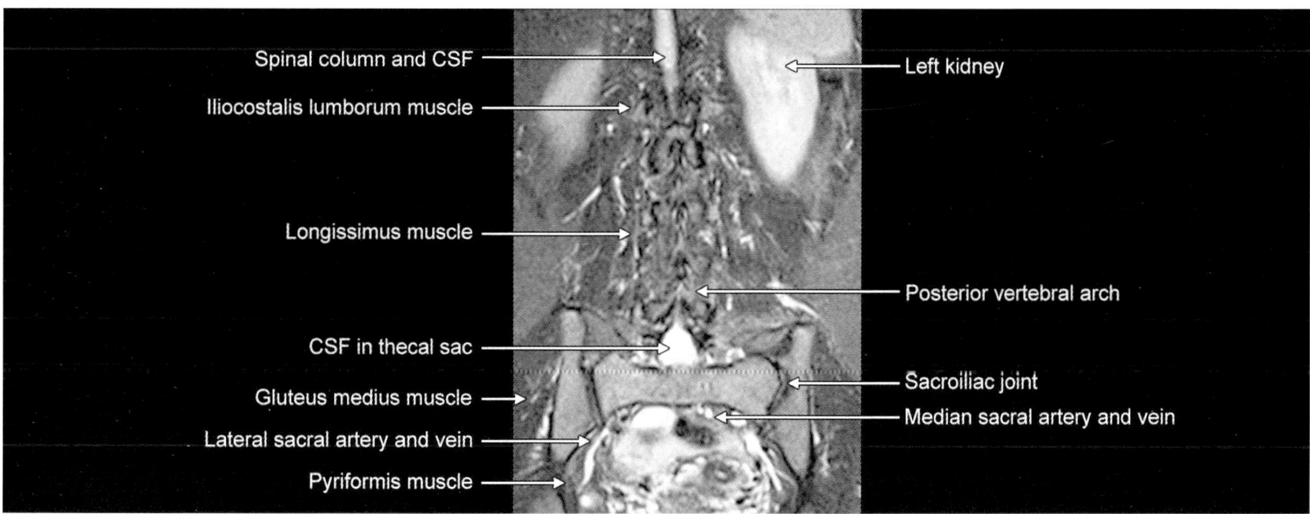

Fig. 50: Lumbosacral spine MRI: Coronal T2WI (corresponds to level 2 in Fig. 48)

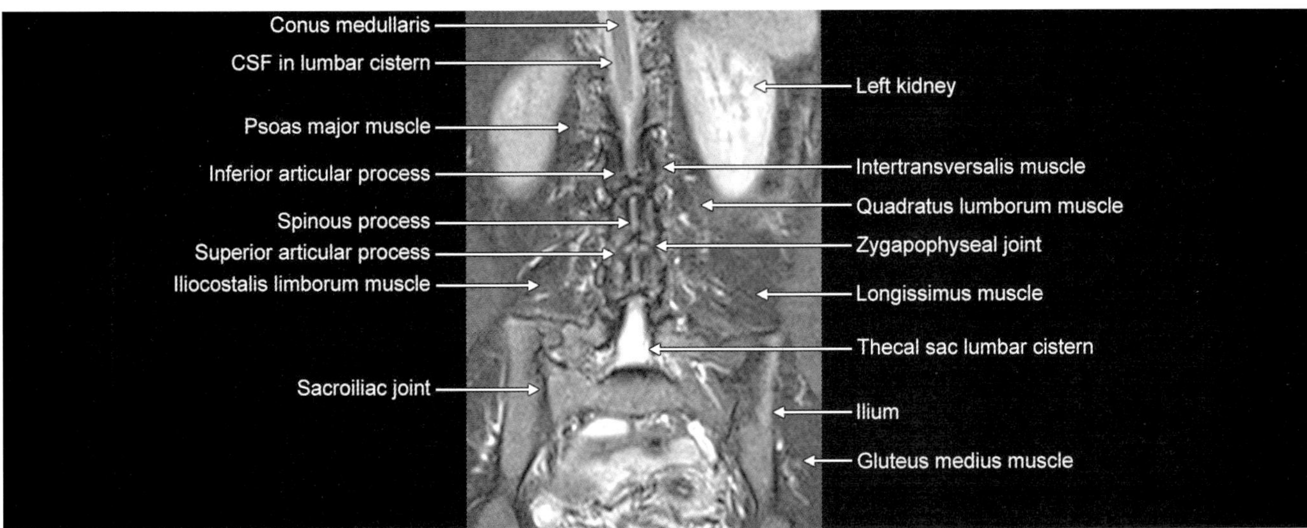

Fig. 51: Lumbosacral spine MRI: Coronal T2WI (corresponds to level 3 in Fig. 48)

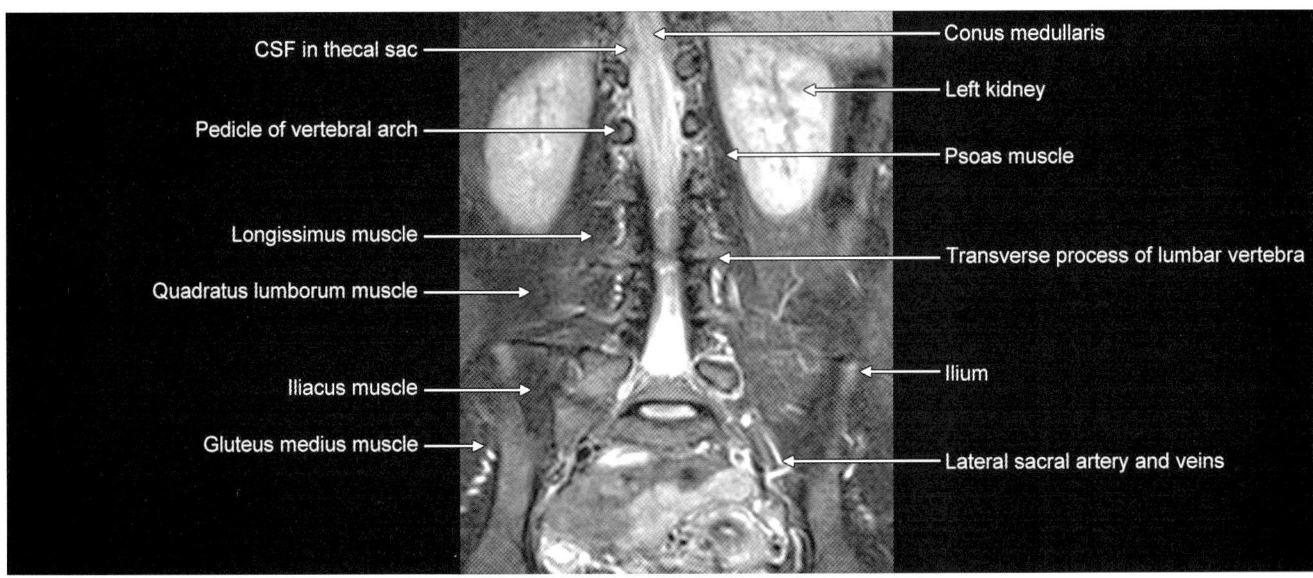

Fig. 52: Lumbosacral spine MRI: Coronal T2WI (corresponds to level 4 in Fig. 48)

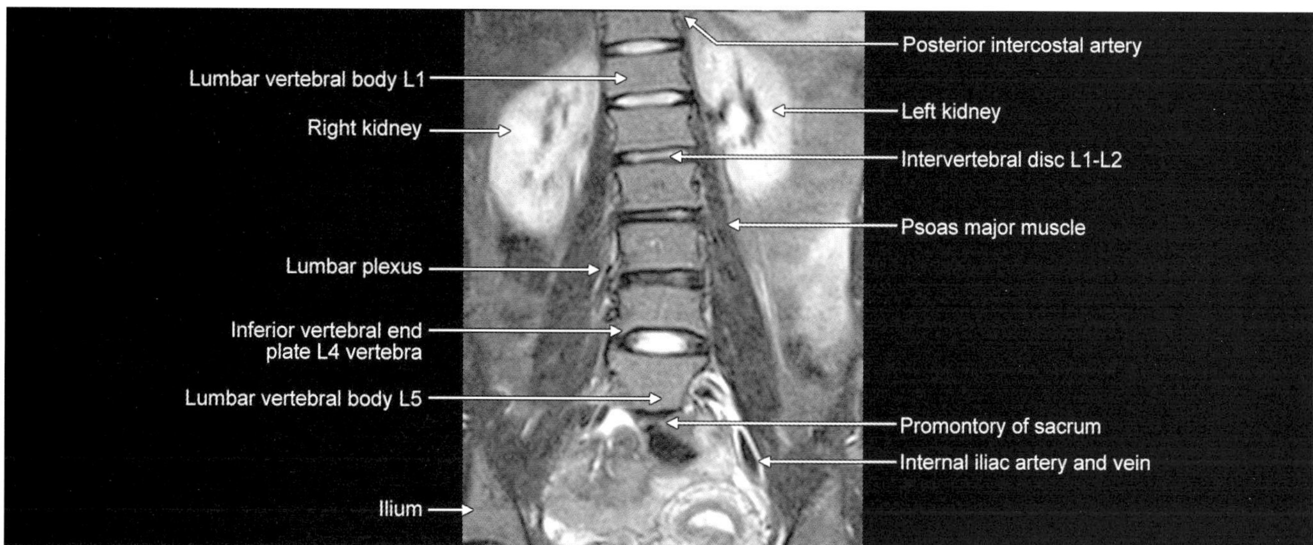

Fig. 53: Lumbosacral spine MRI: Coronal T2WI (corresponds to level 5 in Fig. 48)

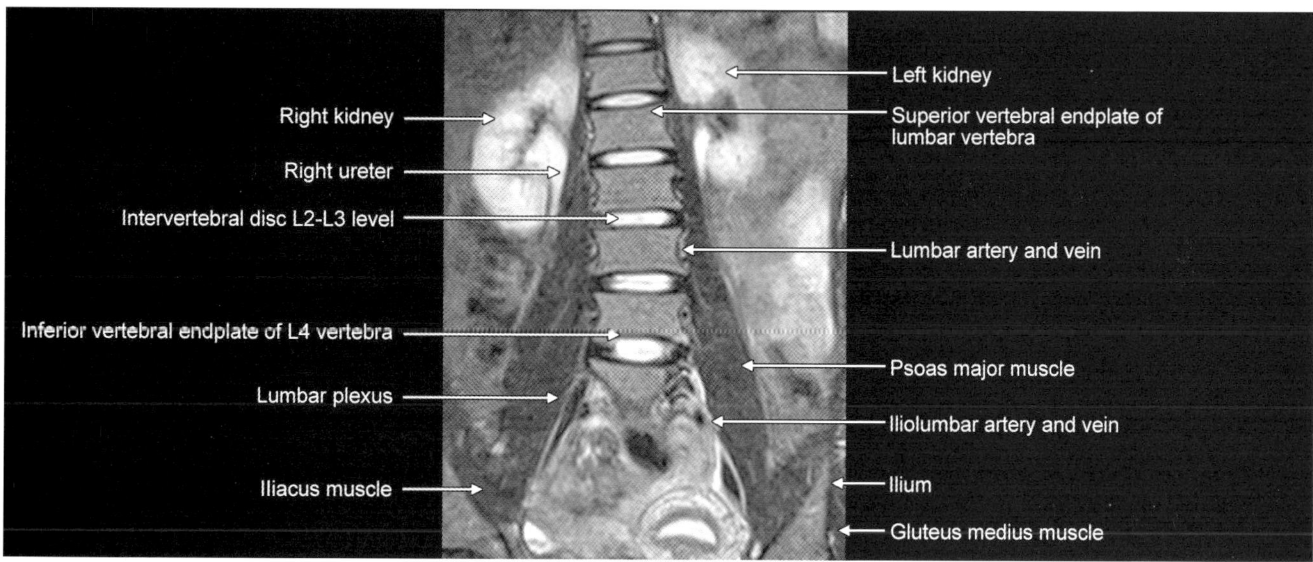

Fig. 54: Lumbosacral spine MRI: Coronal T2WI (corresponds to level 6 in Fig. 48)

CONGENITAL LESION

Spina Bifida

Spina bifida is a developmental congenital disorder caused by the incomplete closing of the embryonic neural tube.

Spina bifida malformations fall into four categories: spina bifida occulta, spina bifida cystica (myelomeningocele), meningocele and lipomeningocele. The most common location of the malformation is the lumbar and sacral areas. Myelomeningocele is the most significant form and it is this that leads to disability in most affected individuals. Spina bifida may be associated with vertebral defect, lipomeningocele, intraspinal dermoid, epidermoid cyst, myelocystocele, split notochord syndrome, meningocele, dorsal dermal sinus, tight filum terminale syndrome.

Plain X-ray demonstrate spina bifida well, however MR and CT provide additional information. USG can diagnose spina bifida in antenatal scan and in neonates.

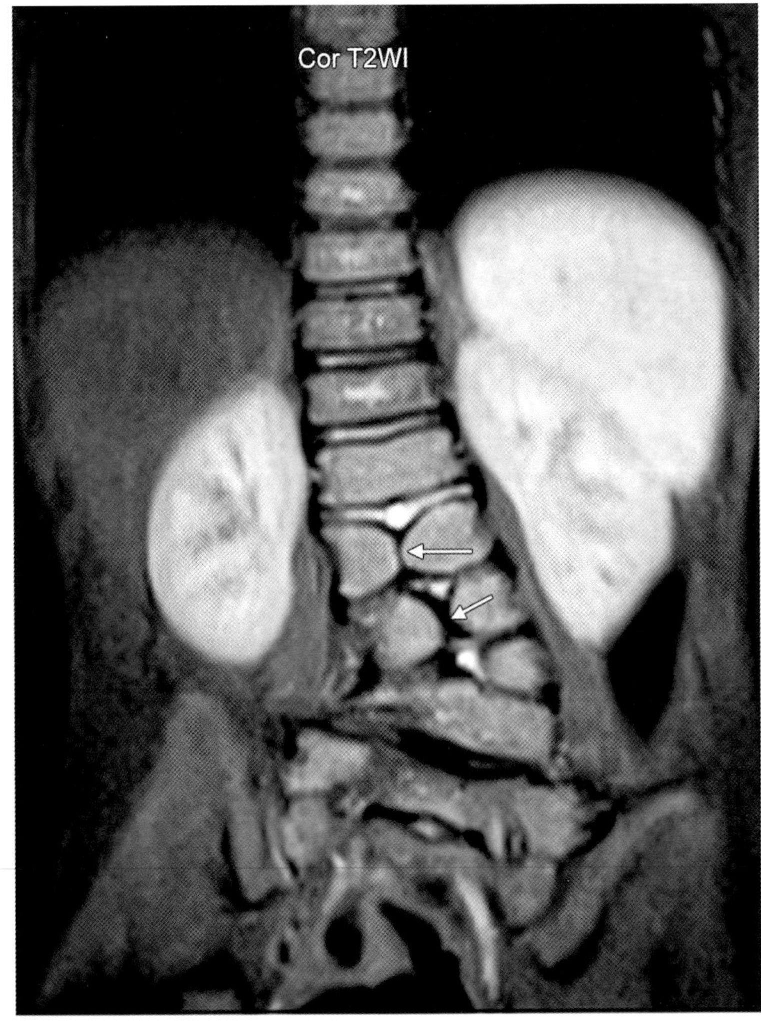

Fig. 55: Coronal T2WI shows fusion defect in the midline at L4 and L5 vertebra (arrows)

Scoliosis

Scoliosis (Figs 56A to C) is a deformity of the spine in which there is lateral curvature combined with anteroposterior deviation and axial rotation of the vertebra in the horizontal plane. Scoliosis is most commonly idiopathic but it may be due to a structural abnormality of the spine or due to central or peripheral neuromuscular diseases.

Idiopathic Scoliosis

This accounts for up to 80 percent of all cases of scoliosis. Idiopathic scoliosis is further subdivided into infantile, juvenile and adolescent forms. Infantile scoliosis appears before the age of 3, juvenile scoliosis occurs between the ages of 4 and 10 years and adolescent scoliosis develops after the age of 10.

Structural Scoliosis

Structural scoliosis may be congenital or acquired. Congenital scoliosis occurs secondary to congenital abnormalities of the spine such as wedge vertebra, hemivertebra, and failure of segmentation (Fig. 55). Asymmetry of bone growth may cause the scoliosis to progress. Acquired structural scoliosis may occur due to vertebral damage from neoplasm, infection, irradiation or trauma.

Neuromuscular Scoliosis

Scoliosis is a frequent complication of neuromuscular diseases such as cerebral palsy, poliomyelitis, traumatic paraplegia, neurofibromatosis and spinal muscular atrophy.

The role of imaging is to confirm the scoliosis, to detect any underlying cause and to monitor the progress of the scoliosis over time. Plain film frontal and lateral radiographs in the erect position are the initial investigation. If a structural spinal abnormality is identified, further detailed imaging of the spinal column may be undertaken using CT to evaluate the vertebral column and MRI if there is suspected spinal cord or nerve root abnormalities.

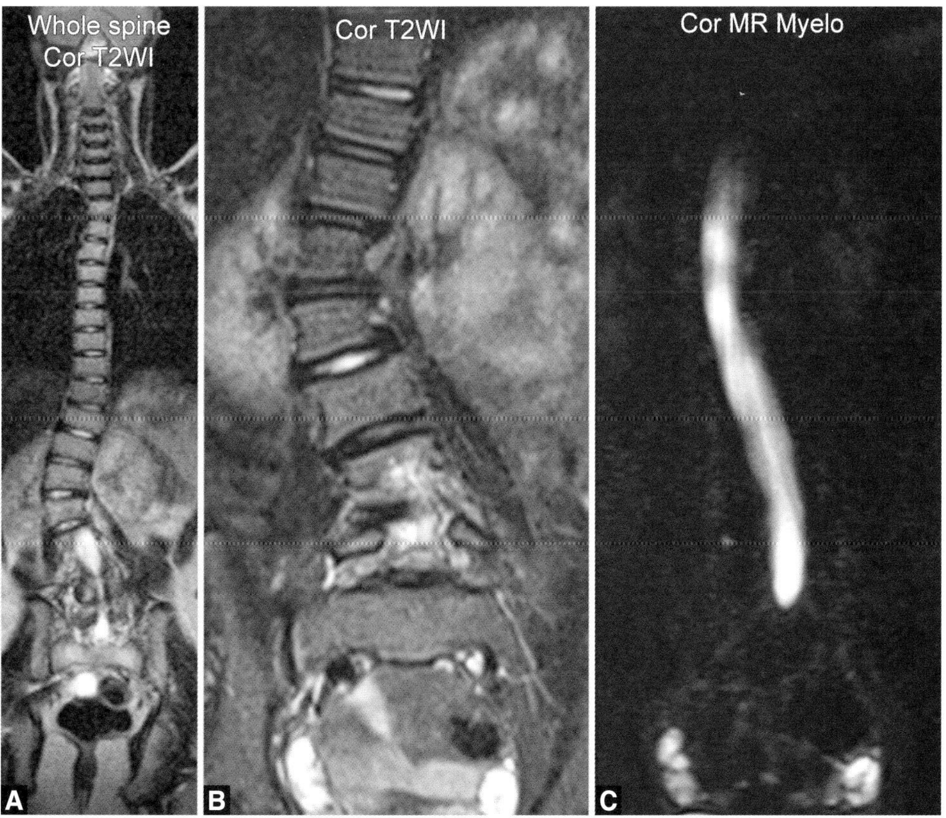

Figs 56A to C: (A and B) Coronal T2W whole spine image shows scoliosis of lumbar spine with convexity to right side; (C) Coronal MR myelogram shows scoliosis of lumbar canal with convexity to right side

Spinal Dysraphism

Spinal dysraphism (Figs 57 and 58), or neural tube defect (NTD), is a broad term encompassing a heterogeneous group of congenital spinal anomalies that result from defective closure of the neural tube early in fetal life and anomalous development of the caudal cell mass. The anatomic features common to the entire group is an anomaly in the midline structures of the back, especially the absence of some of the neural arches, and defects of the skin, filum terminale, nerves, and spinal cord. In cases of spinal dysraphism, MRI provides more information than myelography or CT in defining spinal cord anatomy.

Spinal dysraphism occurs in closed forms and open forms. Open forms include myelocele, meningocele, and myelomeningocele. These open forms are often associated with hydrocephalus and Arnold-Chiari malformation type II and may be classified as spina bifida aperta. Open NTD (ONTD) represents a serious congenital anomaly. If the neural tube fails to fuse at the skull, the result may be that of anencephalus or encephalocele. Meningomyelocele, occurs when the tube fails to fuse along the spine.

Spina bifida occulta is characterized by the variable absence of several neural arches and various cutaneous abnormalities, such as lipoma, hemangioma, cutis aplasia, dermal sinus, and hairy patch. It is often associated with a low-lying conus and other spinal cord anomalies. In infants, whenever the conus lies below the L2-L3 interspace, cord tethering should be considered. The term tethered cord implies that the cord may be attached to the vertebral column or subcutaneous tissues by a thickened filum terminale, fibrous band, dermal sinus tract, diastematomyelia or lipoma.

With spinal dysraphism, radiographs may show structural vertebral anomalies such as hemivertebra, butterfly vertebra, or incomplete fusion of posterior elements. Plain radiographs of patients with myelomeningocele demonstrate incomplete fusion of posterior elements and increased interpedicular distance.

CT myelography demonstrates splitting of the cord and, in some cases, splitting of the meningeal sheath in patients with diastematomyelia. In addition, other bony anomalies, such as an intervertebral septum, and aberrant fibroneural bands may be depicted.

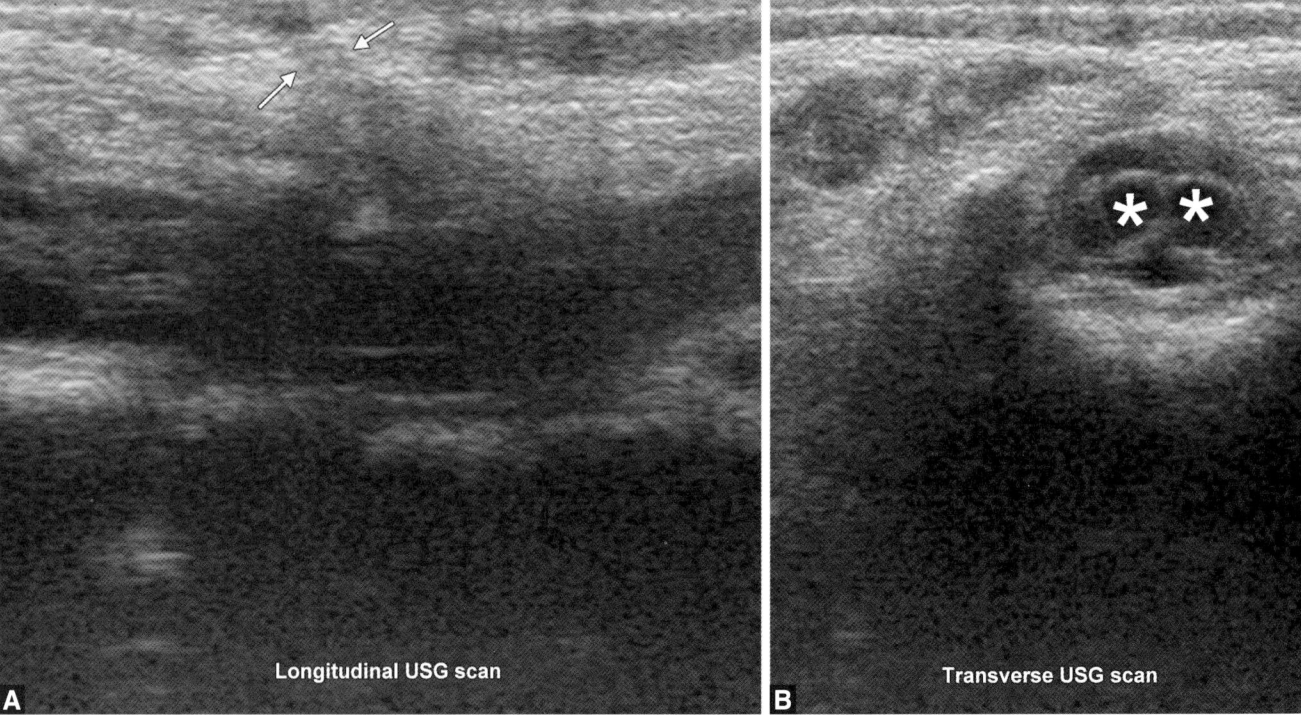

Figs 57A and B: Longitudinal (A) and transverse (B) USG scan with high frequency linear transducer reveals dorsal dermal sinus tract (arrow) extending from skin surface up to the spinal canal and split cord (*)

MRI findings include absent posterior bony elements at the site of the defect. The soft tissue sac containing CSF may be obvious, and the conus is invariably low, coursing dorsally within a capacious dural sac. Spinal lipomas, with their fatty tissue contents, are identifiable both on CT scans and on MRIs. On CT scans, fatty tissue has a strongly hypoattenuating appearance and on MRIs, fatty tissue is strongly hyperintense on images obtained with both short and long repetition times. Newer techniques of fat suppression, such as short-tau inversion recovery (STIR) imaging, may resolve any doubts. On the one hand, CT better shows osseous abnormalities associated with the lipomas; on the other, MRI is preferred because it allows better depiction of detail and contrast resolution of soft tissues. These two techniques are complementary to each other.

Arnold-Chiari II Malformations

Arnold-Chiari II malformations are noted in nearly all cases of myelomeningocele. These malformations are best assessed with MRI. The small posterior fossa, low insertion of the tentorium, and downward displacement of cerebellar tissue and medulla through a widened foramen magnum are seen.

Syringomyelia

Syringomyelia of the cervical cord or syringobulbia and progressive dilatation of the fourth ventricle may account for worsening neurologic deficit. Additional findings in Chiari II malformation include stenogyria, partial agenesis of corpus callosum, large massa intermedia, and a beaked tectum. Rarely, a Chiari I malformation is associated with myelomeningoceles in which only the cerebellar tonsils herniate below the foramen magnum.

Tethered Cord

A tethered cord manifests itself as a low conus with associated spinal lesions. By the age of 2 months, a conus below L2-L3 is considered abnormal (Figs 59A and B). Axial T1-weighted images are most accurate in determining the conus level. Other supporting evidence, such as dorsal displacement of the cord in

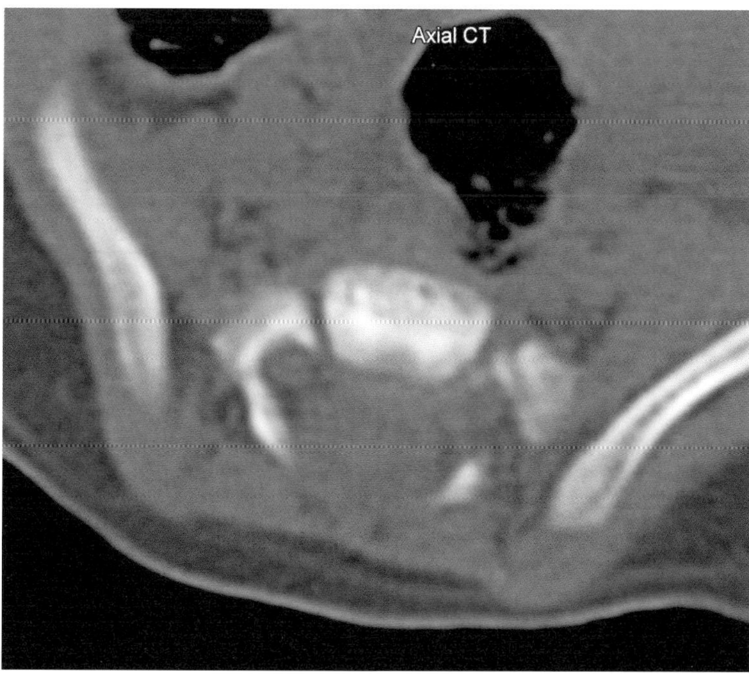

Fig. 58: Axial CT images reveals widening of spinal canal at L4-L5 level

association with obliteration of the surrounding CSF spaces, may support the clinical suspicion. A low cord invariably occurs with a myelomeningocele; retethering may occur after repair.

Neural Arch Defects

Posterior neural arch defects and an increased interpedicular distance are often associated with a lumbosacral lipoma. T1-weighted images have high sensitivity in the detection of lipomas because of the short relaxation time of fat, confirmed by using fat-saturation techniques.

Thickened Filum

The diagnosis of a thickened filum is made when the filum measures more than 2 mm at the L5-S1 disc space. In infants and young children, the filum is not discretely visualized on multiple axial images below the tip of the conus. Thus, visualization of the filum in this age group should be considered abnormal even if the thickness is less than 2 mm; in such cases, further investigation is warranted.

Diastematomyelia

In diastematomyelia, MRI is used to evaluate the extent of cord clefting; conus of low position (Figs 57 to 60); scoliosis; other bony anomalies; and syringohydromyelia, which is commonly associated with diastematomyelia. The bony spur is well seen on T1-weighted MRIs when fatty marrow is present. On T2-weighted images, less well-developed spurs are seen as areas of low signal intensity that split the thecal sac, which appears as an area of high signal intensity.

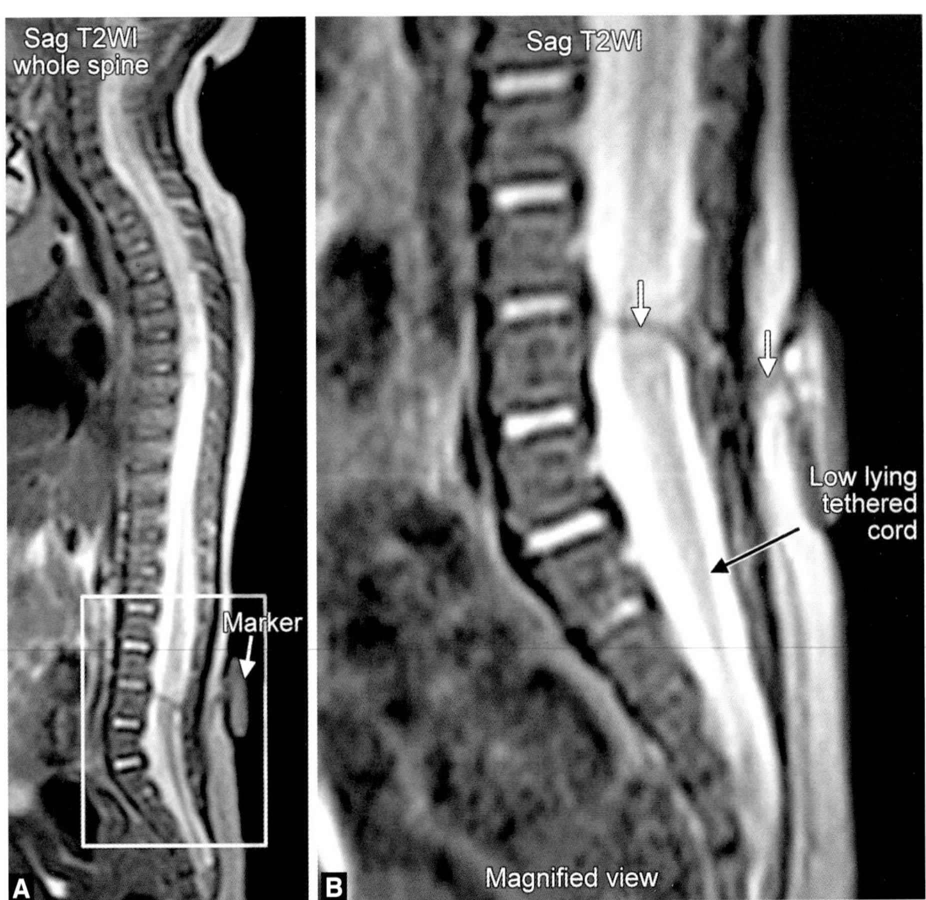

Figs 59A and B: Sagittal T2W images demonstrate focal hypointense tract at lumbar vertebrae level extending from skin surface up to the spinal canal splitting the spinal cord (white arrows). Low lying tethered cord is seen

Dermoids and Epidermoids

Dermoids and epidermoids may be associated with a dermal sinus or occur in isolation. When not associated with dermal sinuses, they may occur with progressive compressive myelopathy or with chemical meningitis of acute onset. The thoracic lumbar and sacral spine are affected. CT and MRI characteristics are similar to those seen in epidermoids at other sites.

Lipomas

Lipomas in the dura occur mainly in the caudal portion of the spine. Those in the region of the filum terminale are associated with congenital spinal anomalies. The lipoma is hyperintense on T1-weighted MRIs. Spinal lipomas are usually found in the extradural space in the thoracic region. The radiologic and MRI signal intensity characteristics are similar to those of intradural lipomas.

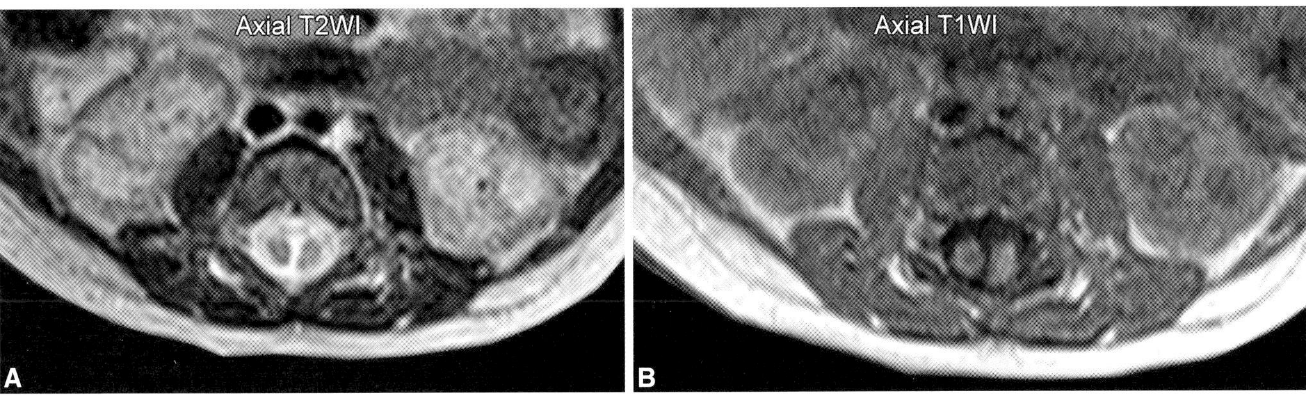

Figs 60A and B: Axial T2WI (A) and T1WI (B) images demonstrate splitting the spinal cord resulting in diastomatomyelia at lumbar spinal canal level

Spondylolisthesis

The word spondylolisthesis is derived from the Greek words *spondylo,* meaning spine, and *listhesis,* meaning to slip or slide. Spondylolisthesis is a descriptive term referring to slippage (usually forward) of a vertebra and the spine above it relative to the vertebra below it. It is the most common type and results from bilateral defects in the pars interarticularis. Posterior body remains fixed in position while the anterior part is free to slip forward.

Cause of spondylolysis appears to be a combination of a dysplastic pars at birth coupled with the long-term stresses of upright posture. Sports involvement (e.g. weight-lifting, wrestling, football, tennis) appear to increase these stresses.

Conventional radiography in the anteroposterior, lateral and both oblique projections are usually adequate to demonstrate both spondylolysis and spondylolisthesis. MRI reveals spondylolisthesis on sagittal view (Figs 61A and B).

Spondylolisthesis is graded as

Grade 1: Vertebral body above subtends 1/4 of the AP diameter of the vertebral body below.
Grade 2: Vertebral body above subtends 1/2 of the AP diameter of the vertebral body below.
Grade 3: Vertebral body above subtends 3/4 of the AP diameter of the vertebral body below.
Grade 4: Vertebral body above subtends the full AP diameter of the vertebral body below.

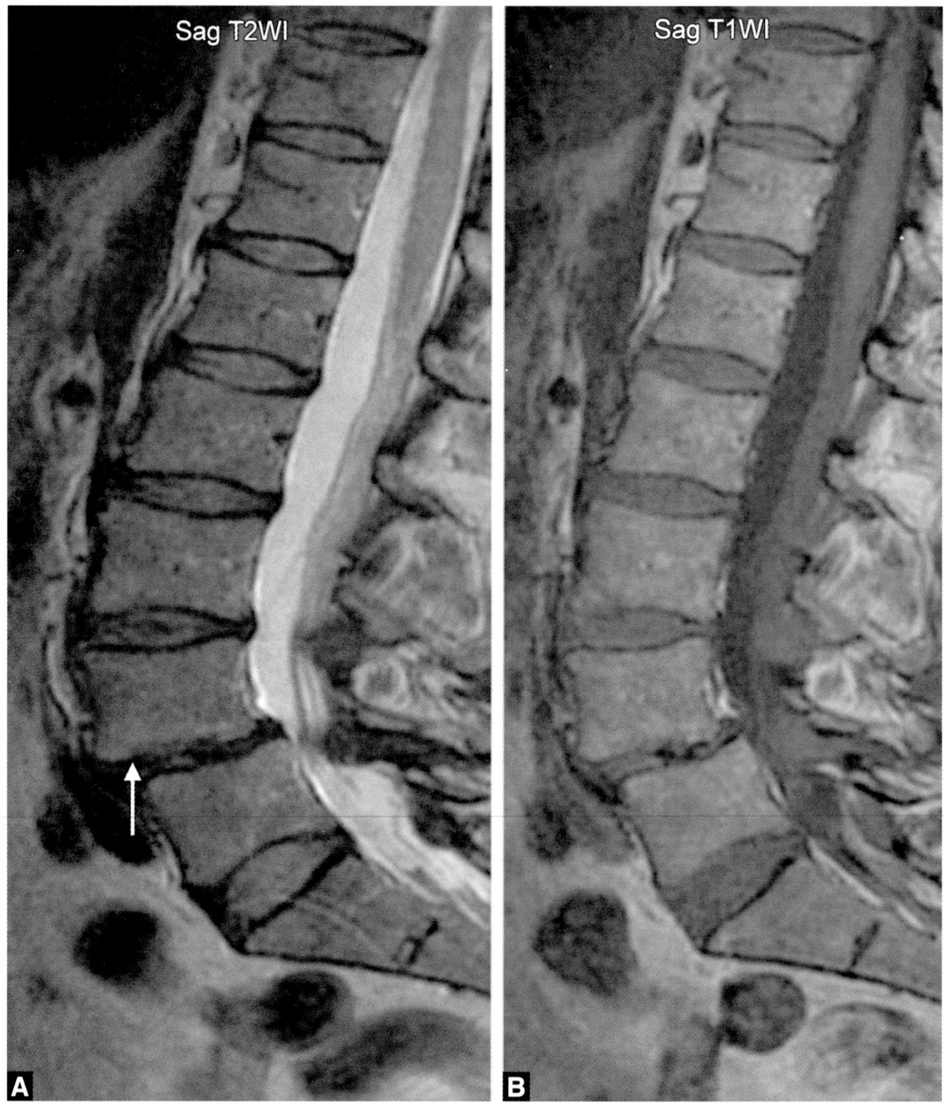

Figs 61A and B: Sagittal T2WI and T1WI shows anterior spondylolisthesis (arrow) of L4 vertebra over L5 vertebra

Myelomeningocele with Intraspinal Lipoma

Embryologically myelomeningocele derives from an incomplete dorsal fusion of the neural ectoderm during neurolation. This also prevents the separation of the neural and cutaneous ectoderm, the inward migration of the mesoderm and, as a consequence, the closure of the posterior elements of the spine and the formation of a cutaneous covering layer.

Myelomeningocele (Figs 62A to C) is evident at birth and requires immediate reparative surgery. Because the neural plate and meninges are anchored to the skin the spinal cord is tethered. There is an associated Chiari malformation. After repair the neurological deficit remains stable.

An intradural lipoma is a localized collection of fat and connective tissue contained wholly within the dura and separated from the subcutaneous fat. This is similar in embryological terms to a lipomyelomeningocele except that the neural tube closes after the mesenchyme has entered.

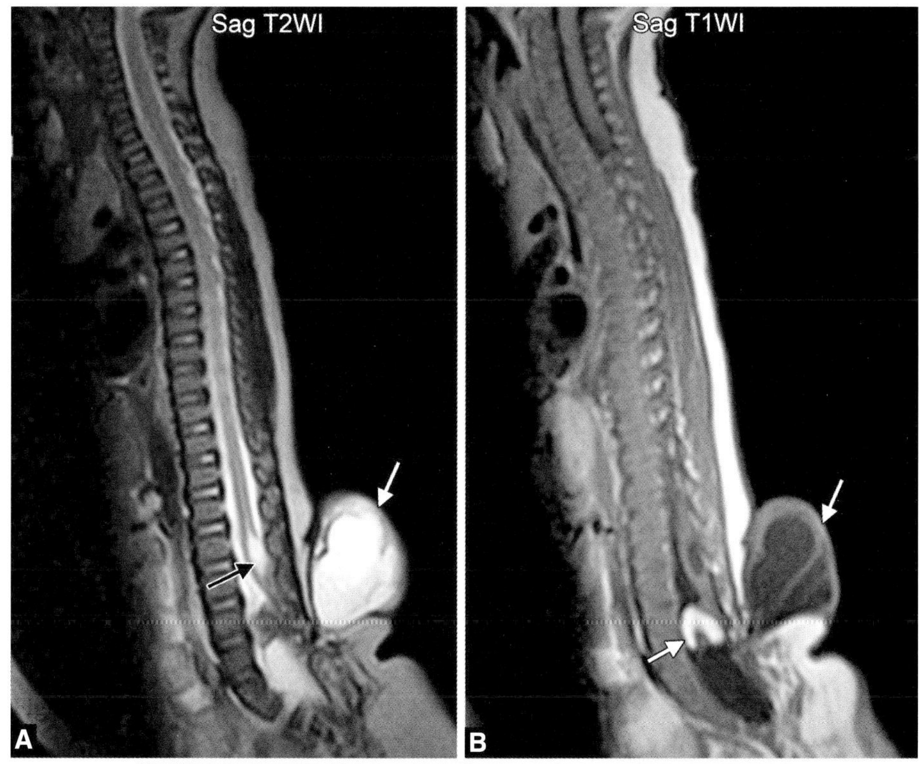

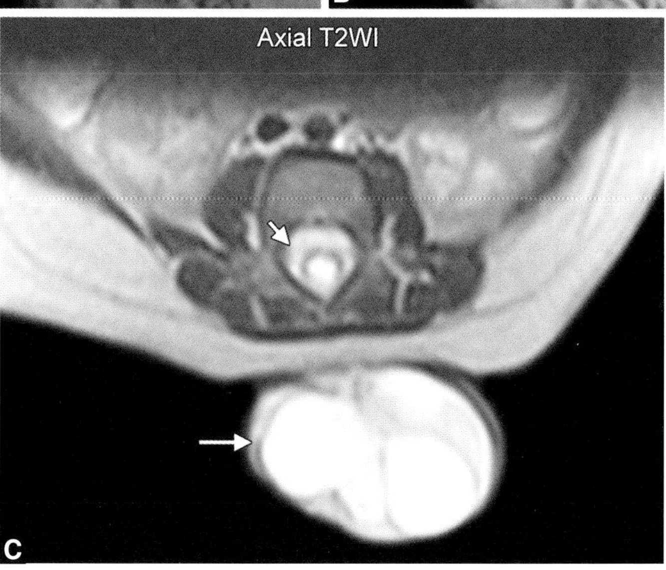

Figs 62A to C: Sagittal T1 and T2 WI (A and B) showing subcutaneous collection of CSF over lower back with cutaneous covering layer and communication with intraspinal CSF. Meninges are anchored to the skin the spinal cord is tethered. Intradural localized collection of fat noted at lower lumbar level which is hyperintense on both T1 and T2 WI. Axial T2WI (C) showing subcutaneous collection of CSF over lower back with cutaneous covering layer. Intradural localized collection of fat, which hyperintense on both T1 and T2 WI

CRANIOVERTEBRAL JUNCTION LESIONS

Os Odontoideum

Os odontoideum is an oval or round well corticated ossicle of variable size, found in the expected position of the odontoid process. Os odontoideum represents the result of prior unrecognized trauma. Fractures occur at the junction of the odontoid process with the body of the axis and disrupt the blood supply to the odontoid process. Nonunion leads to formation of an os odontoideum. Odontoid dysplasia is other cause, which results in failure of the normal development of the odontoid process of the axis.

Atlanto-axial instability occurs in cases of os odontoideum (Figs 63A to C). Therefore, when an os odontoideum is seen, flexion and extension MRI (Figs 63B and C) should be obtained to exclude instability.

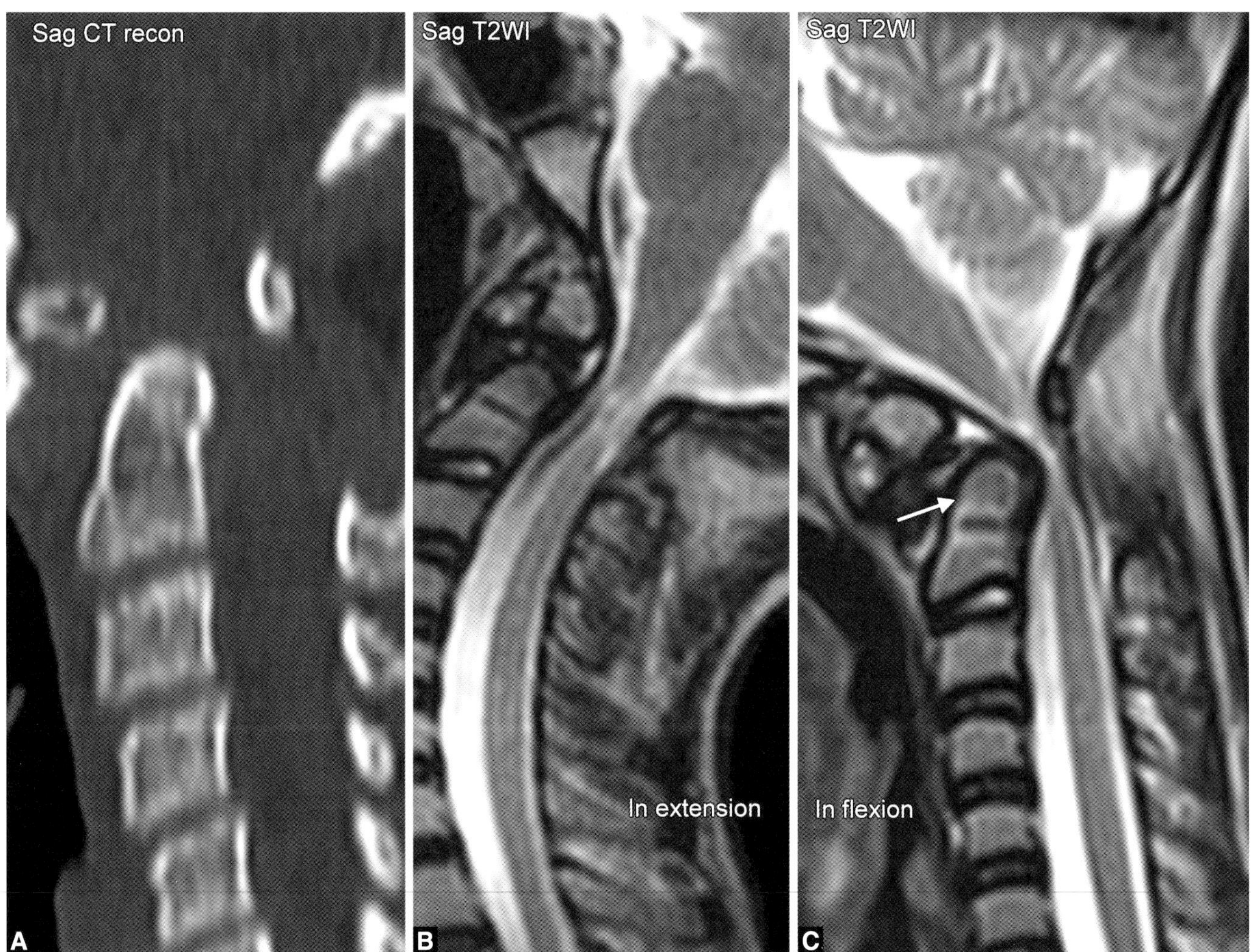

Figs 63A to C: In a 15-year-old male sagittal CT, T2W MR images in flexion-extension demonstrates high cervical cord compression with os odontoideum

Basilar Invagination

Basilar invagination is a mild form of craniovertebral junction anomaly characterized by an invagination of the margins of the foramen magnum upward into the skull (Figs 64 and 65). This may occur as a developmental anomaly or be associated with softening of the skull as in rickets. Causes of basilar invagination are osteogenesis imperfecta, Klippel Feil syndrome, Chiari malformation, cleido cranial dysplasias, condylus tertius, basi-occiput hypoplasia, Paget's disease, hyperparathyroidism, osteomalacia, rheumatoid arthritis, Marfan's syndrome and Ehlers-Danlos syndrome.

Occasionally it may also occur due to ligamentous laxity and vertical subluxation of C1 on C2. There may be resultant compression of the upper cervical cord or brainstem causing neurological symptoms.

Assessing the position of the dens relative to the foramen magnum has classically been determined using Chamberlin's line, McGregor's line, and McRae's line. Chamberlin's line is a line between the posterior aspect of the hard palate and the posterior margin of the foramen magnum. The tip of the dens should be below this line and not more than 5 mm above it. McGregor's line is a line from the posterior aspect of the hard palate to the lowest point of the

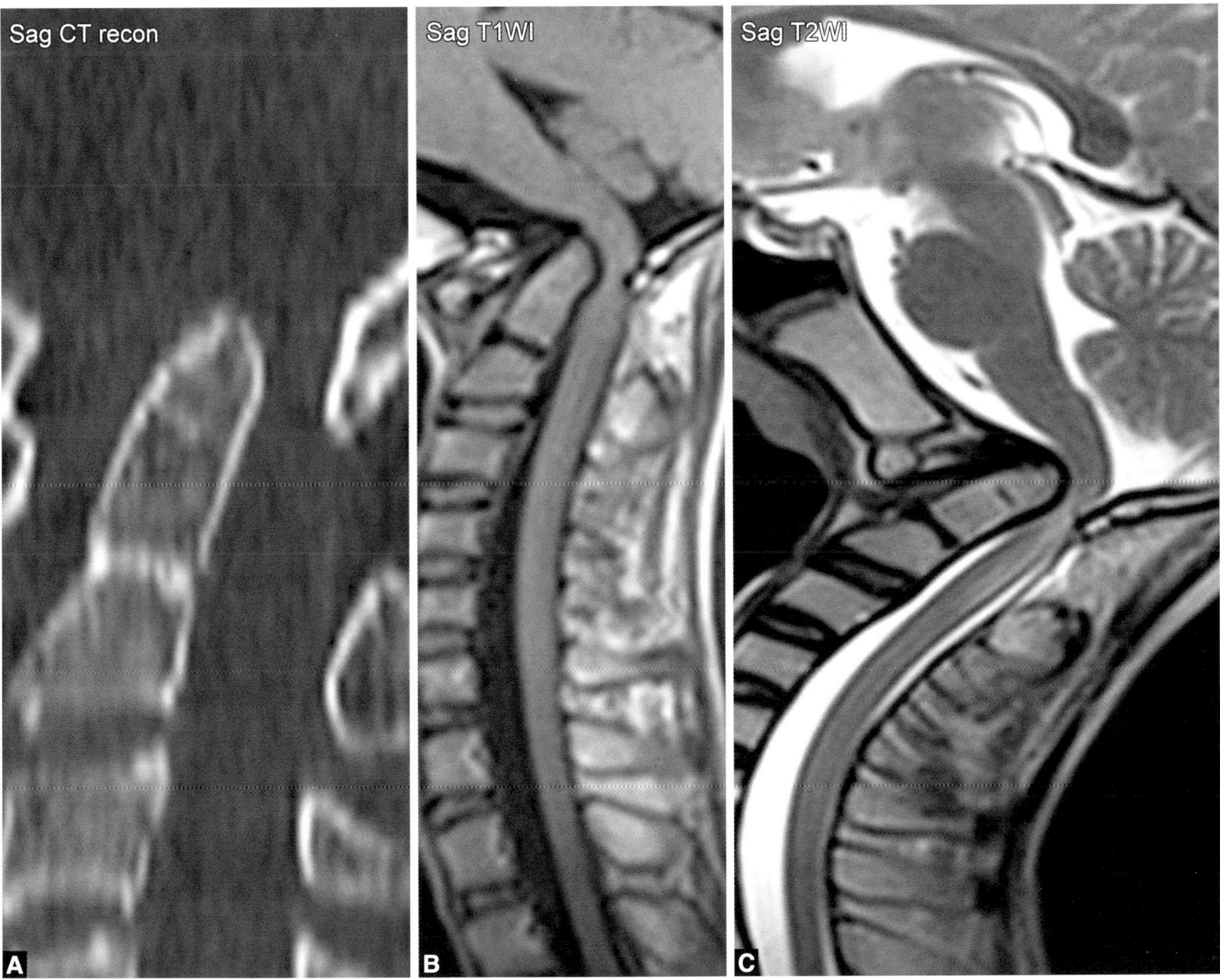

Figs 64A to C: Sagittal CT, sagittal T1WI and T2WI shows partial occipitalization of C1, the clivus is short and is more horizontally oriented, distance between anterior arch of C1 and dens has increased, dens is seen projecting into the posterior fossa and stretching of the apical ligament

occiput of the skull. The tip of the dens should be no more than 4.5 mm above this line. McRae's line is a line between the anterior and posterior aspects of the foramen magnum margin. The tip of the dens should always be below this line. Redlund-Johnell criterion refers to the distance between the McGregor line and the midpoint of the caudal margin of the second cervical vertebral body. A measurement less than 34 mm in males and less than 29 mm in females indicates basilar invagination.

Lastly, Runaway criterion refers to the distance between the center of the second cervical pedicle and the transverse axis of the atlas measured along the axis of the odontoid process. A measurement less than 15 mm in males and less than 13 mm in females indicates basilar invagination. Currently, the diagnosis ultimately is made by MRI or CT.

McGregor's line can be used for radiographic assessment on a lateral skull radiograph. Basilar invagination is suggested if the tip of the odontoid process is more than 4.5 mm above McGregor's line.

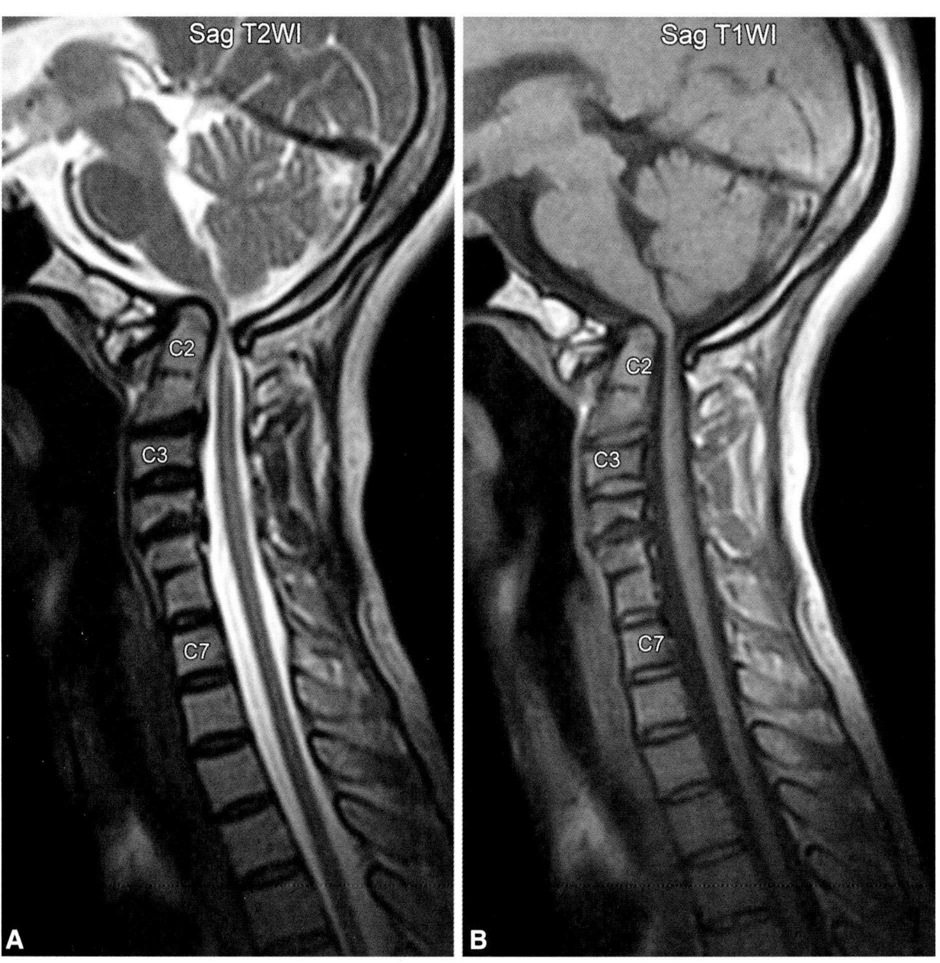

Figs 65A and B: Occipitalization of C1 with mild basilar invagination and protrusion of dens into the foramen magnum causing cord compression

DEGENERATIVE SPINE

Disc Lesions

Annular Tear

Lesion labeled annular tear or internal disruption is based on concept of leaking disc, one which permits the irritating liquid material normally restricted to the center of the disc to come into contact with the innervated tissue (Figs 66A to C).

The herniated disc has a significant capacity to be resolved with time; annular tear continues to produce symptoms indefinitely. Clinical picture is based on pain related to increased intradiscal pressure and irritability of neural structures. Annular tear is usually produced by injury that increases intradiscal pressure significantly. Predominant element in the history is back pain, either alone or in excess of leg pain. Pain is often worse when sitting than when standing; coughing and sneezing worsen the pain as do forward bending and lifting.

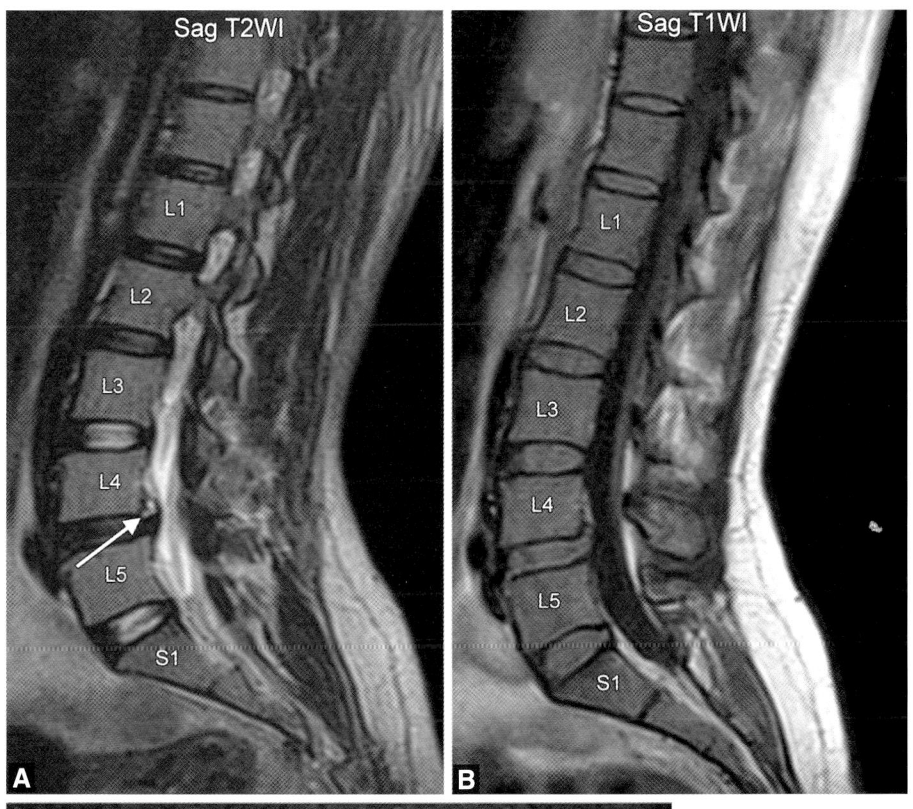

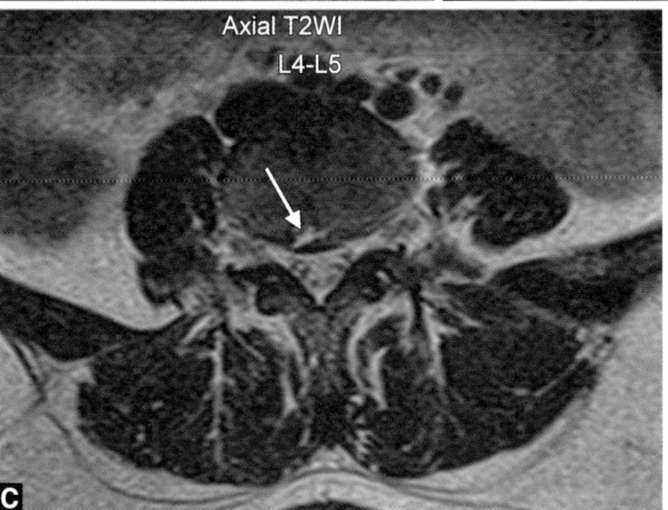

Figs 66A to C: (A and B) Sagittal T2W and sagittal T1WI images show desiccation of L4-L5 intervertebral disc with acute annular tear at L4-L5 level. Axial T2WI (C) shows acute annular tear as a hyperintense signal, and posterocentral protrusion compressing thecal sac and indenting bilateral traversing nerve root

Disc Bulge

Disc bulge refers to smooth symmetric circumferential extension of the disc (more than half of disc circumference) beyond the boundary of adjacent vertebral end plates. The cause of disc bulge is weakened end plates, weakened and lengthened but intact annulus fibrosus and posterior longitudinal ligament. Posterior disc bulge is common and anterior bulge is less frequent due to thicker annulus fibrosus anteriorly. Most commonly involved intervertebral discs are L4-5, L5-S1, C5-6 and C6-7. Associated disc degeneration is usually present and is seen as loss of intervertebral disc height, intradiscal gas and paradiscal osteophytes on plain radiograph.

Decreased disc height and loss of normal hyperintense signals are often seen in dessicated disc on T2 weighted MR scans. On axial MR images mildly bulging disc initially appears as loss of normal posterior disc concavity. Moderate disc bulge is seen as diffuse, non-focal, circumferential protrusion of disc material beyond the edges of ring apophyses on sagittal and axial MR scans (Figs 67A and B).

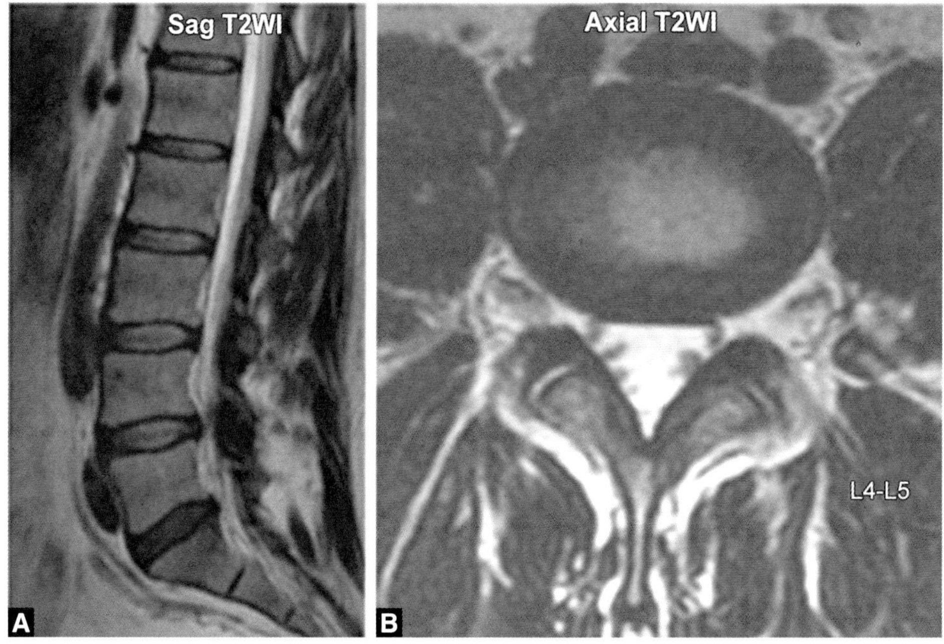

Figs 67A and B: Sagittal and axial T2WI shows posterior disc bulge indenting the thecal sac

Lumbar Disc Desiccation with Protrusion

The normal disc does not extend beyond the vertebral end plates and has intermediate signal intensity on T1W images and high signal intensity on T2W images. T2 weighted high signal is not uniform throughout the whole disc, central nucleus pulposus and inner annulus have high signal, while outer annulus and cortical band of vertebral end plates have low signal intensities. The signal returned from degenerated discs is usually lower than from healthy discs due to diminished water content and is best appreciated on T2WI. Sometimes due to calcium precipitation in healthy discs the signal may be paradoxically higher on T2WI. Presence of fluid filled clefts in the discs may also show high signals on T2WI. In infective discitis, there is high signal on T2WI with associated reactive changes in adjacent vertebrae. Tears in the external layers of the annulus fibrosus may be visible as high signal foci on T2WI. Signal from degenerative fibrocartilage within the spinal canal. It is quite variable on T2WI and is common for the migratory fragments to be conspicuously brighter than the nucleus of the disc of origin. Disc protrusions present as indentations on the anterior surface of thecal sac opposite the disc space and are better appreciated on T2WI (Figs 67 and 68).

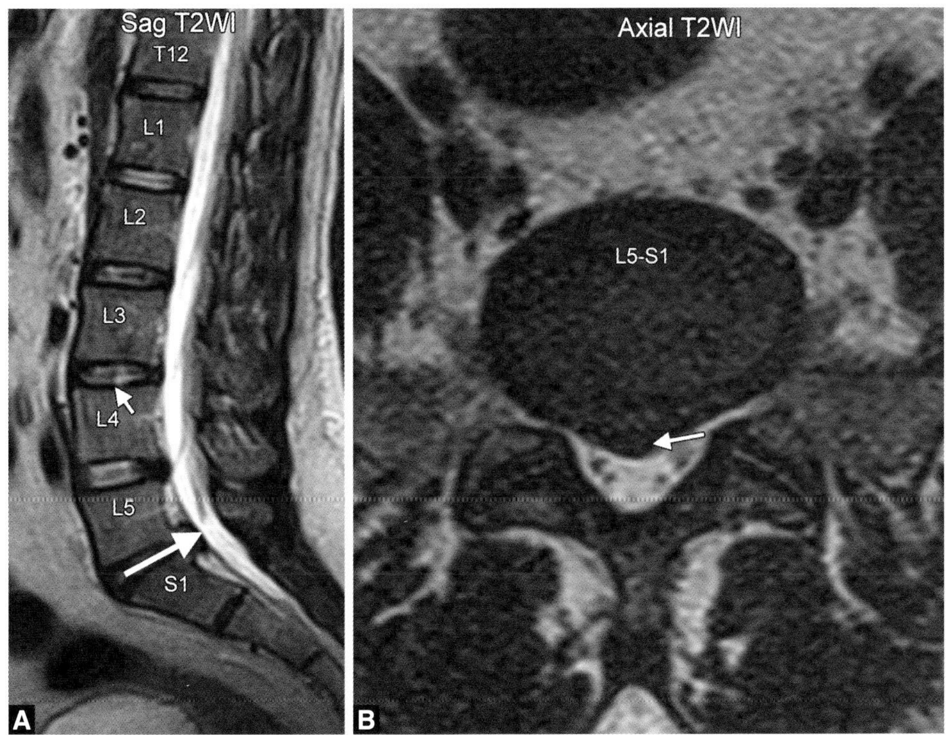

Figs 68A and B: T2W sagittal (A) and T2W axial (B) images of the lumbar spine reveal desiccation of L5-S1 disc with posterocentral disc protrusion (arrow)

Disc Herniation and Migration

Displacement of the disc material beyond the margins of the adjacent vertebral endplate, resulting in disc herniation which can be obtained (covered by annulus fibrosus) or uncontained. Trauma is the single most common cause of rupture of the nucleus pulposus through the annulus fibrosus. The result is protrusion or extrusion of the disc material into the vertebral canal. This outcome can be caused by a single event or by repeated trauma.

Herniation is defined as a localized displacement of disc material beyond the limits of the intervertebral disc. Localized displacement in the axial (horizontal) plane is classified as focal, in which less than 25 percent of the disc circumference is involved, or as broad-based, in which 25 to 50 percent of the disc circumference is involved. When 50 to 100 percent of the circumferential disc tissue extends beyond the edges of the ring apophyses, the disc is classified as bulging; such a condition is not considered a form of herniation.

A disc herniation is classified as an extrusion (Figs 69A to C) if any distance between the edges of the disc material beyond the disc space is greater than the distance between the edges of the base measured in the same plane (arrow). The disc is labeled as sequestrated disc when there is a lack of continuity of the disc material with the parent disc.

A radial tear of the annulus fibrosus is considered a sign of early disc degeneration. It is accompanied by other signs of disc degeneration, such as a bulging annulus, loss of disc height, herniation of the nucleus pulposus, and changes in the adjacent endplates. Although a radial tear of the annulus fibrosus can be detected as an area of increased signal intensity on T2 weighted images.

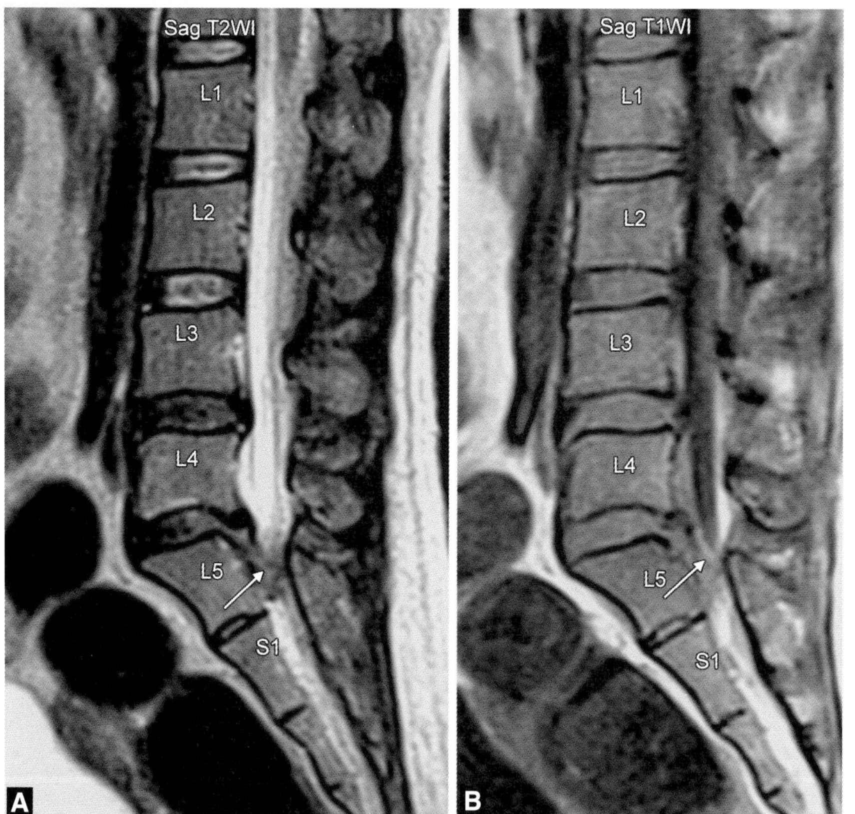

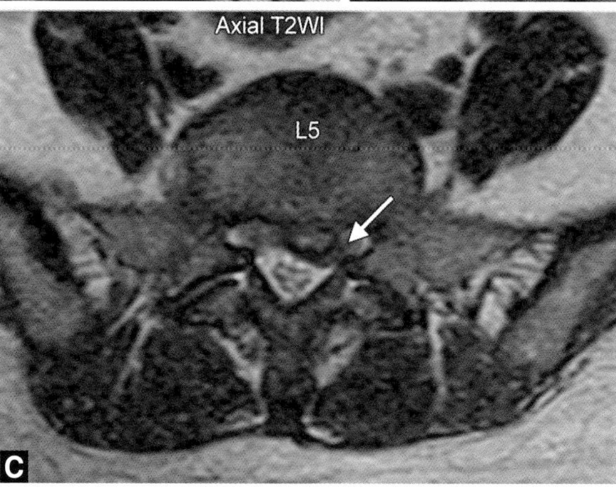

Figs 69A to C: (A and B) Large posterior herniation is seen in the L4-L5 disc with inferior migration; (C) Axial section shows a large posterior and left paracentral herniation. It has compressed the thecal sac and nerve roots on the left side

Schmorl's Node

Schmorl's node is a herniation of intervertebral disc in vertebral body. It is due to protrusion of disc material through the cartilaginous endplate. It may be associated with diseases that lead to weakening of the cartilaginous endplate or subchondral bone of the vertebral body such as intervertebral osteochondrosis, Scheuermann's disease, and trauma.

Radiographically Schmorl's nodes appear as a radiolucent lesion within the vertebral body surrounded by helmet-shaped sclerosis that borders on the intervertebral disc. CT scans and MR imaging also show characteristic features (Figs 70A and B).

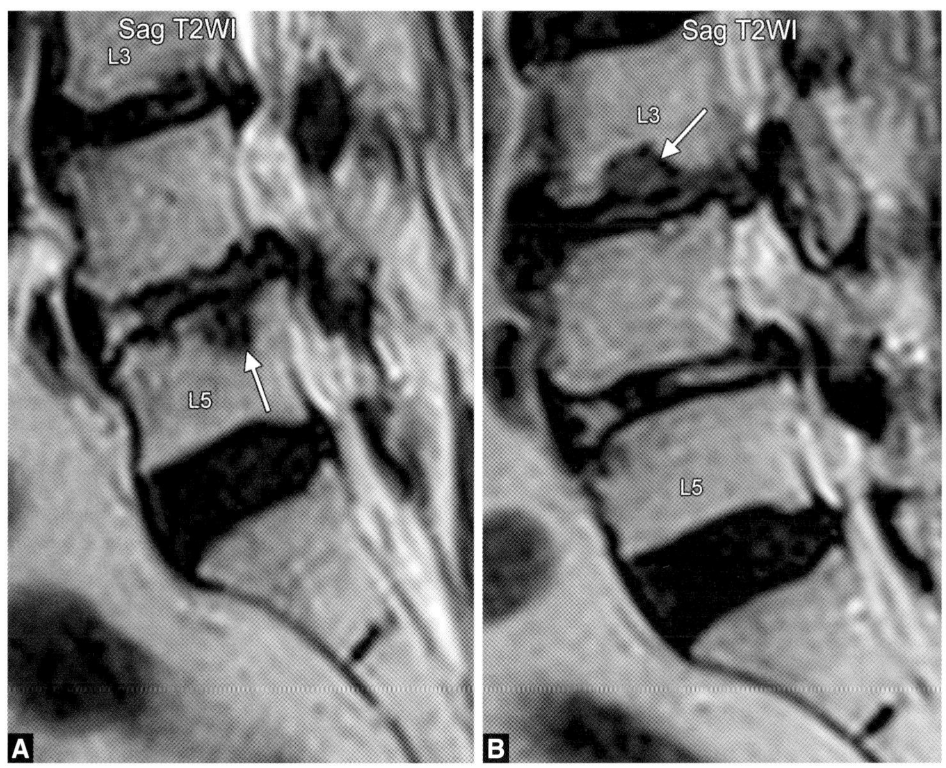

Figs 70A and B: Schmorl's node seen in superior endplate of L5 and inferior endplate of L3 vertebra

Vacuum Phenomenon

The presence of a linear hypointensity in the disc space (vacuum phenomenon) is a typical finding of degenerative disc disease. It is often associated to other findings of degenerative disc disease such as disc space narrowing and endplate sclerosis. This radiologic sign is related to the accumulation of gas in the fissures and clefts of the degenerated annulus fibrosus and nucleus pulposus at one or more spinal levels.

In the early stages of disc degeneration the nucleus pulposus begins to break down, resulting in fissuring of the fibrocartilage. These fissures can develop into spaces or clefts that fill with gas from the surrounding tissue because the vapor pressure in this space is lower than the vapor pressure of gas dissolved in the adjacent tissues.

The vacuum phenomenon is typically observed on routine positioning of the lumbar spine. Computed tomography and magnetic resonance imaging may also support this diagnosis. CT has a higher sensitivity for demonstrating vacuum phenomenon and disc calcification particularly on sagittal and frontal reformations. On T1WI linear streak of hypointensity is seen suggestive of presence of gas (Fig. 71).

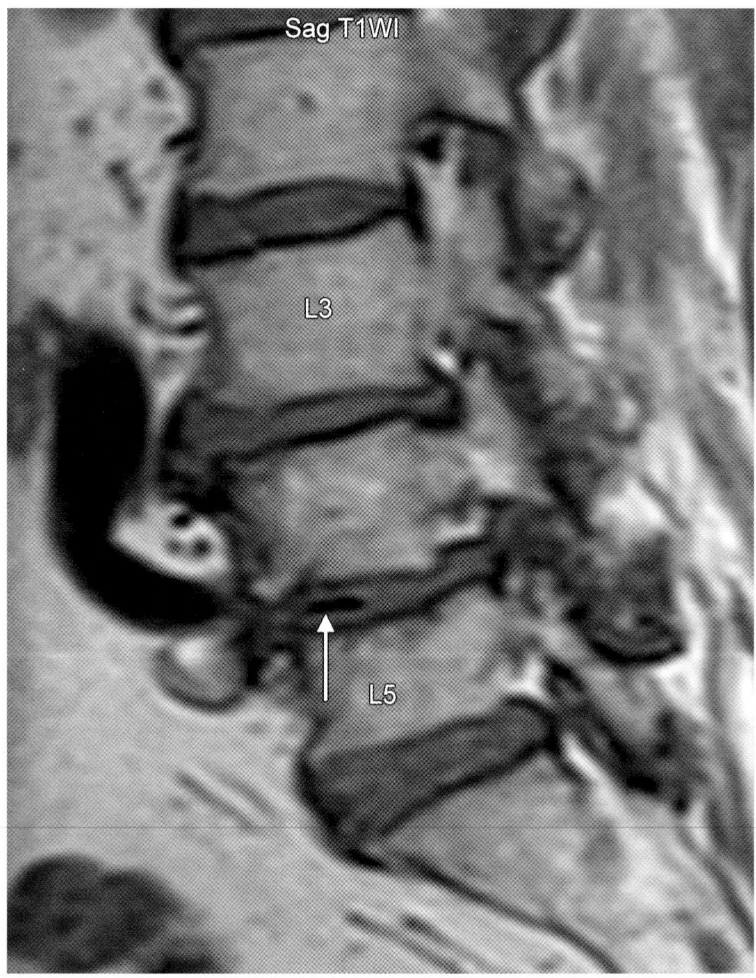

Fig. 71: Hypointense signal of air (arrow) on sagittal T1WI image in L4-L5 disc s/o vacuum phenomenon and disc degeneration

Modic Changes

Modic changes are dynamic markers of the normal age related degenerative process affecting the lumbar spine. The prevalence of modic changes among patients with degenerative disc disease of the lumbar spine varies between 19 and 59 percent, with type 1 and 2 changes being the most common and type 3 and mixed-type changes being relatively rare (Table 1). Modic changes appear in the vertebral bodies near the endplates of the disc. It confirms the diagnosis of degenerative disc disease.

Type 1 changes: Increased marrow signal intensity in T2-weighted MR images and decreased signal intensity in T1-weighted MR images due to fibrovascular tissue in endplates (Figs 72 and 73).

Type 2 changes: Increased signal intensity in T1- and T2-weighted MR images because of lipid deposits in endplates (Figs 73A and B).

Type 3 changes: Decreased signal intensity in T1 - and T2-weighted MR images due to endplate sclerosis.

Table 1: Modic classification for endplate degenerative changes

Modic type	*T1WI*	*T2WI*
I	Hypointense	Hyperintense
II	Hyperintense	Hyperintense
III	Hypointense	Hypointense

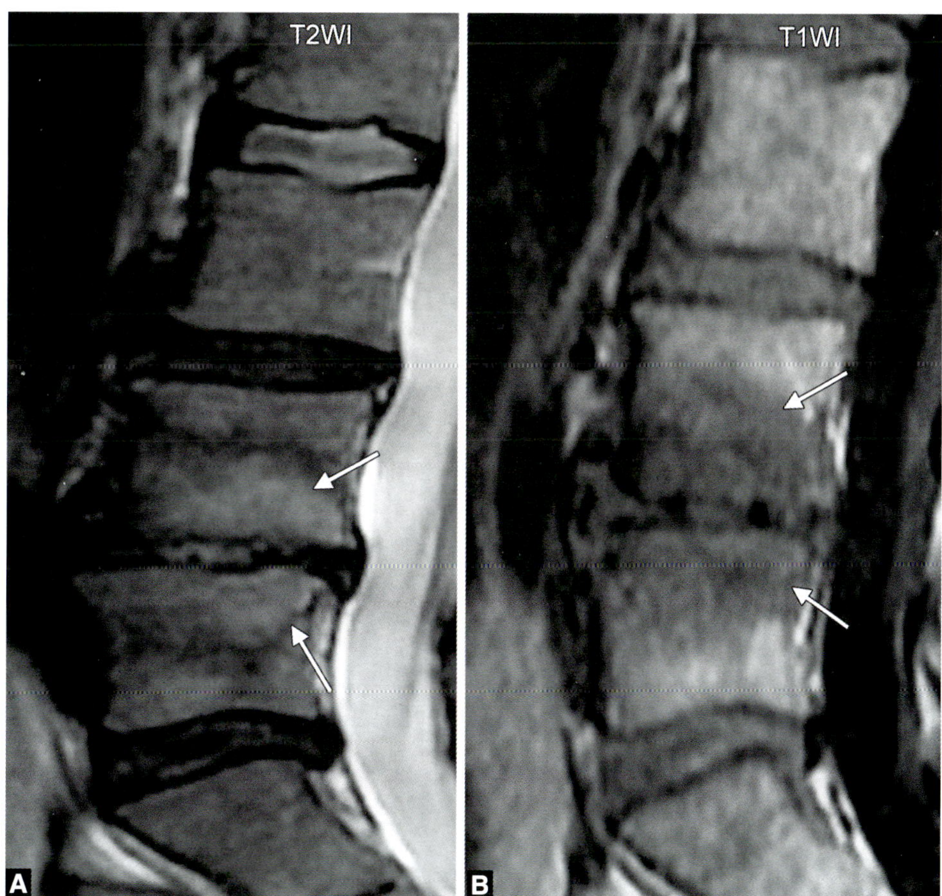

Figs 72A and B: Modic type 1 changes seen on sagittal T2WI (A) shows hyperintense signal change in lower endplate of L3 and upper endplate of L4 vertebra and sagittal T1WI (B), shows hypointense signal changes in lower endplate of L3 and upper endplate of L4 vertebrae

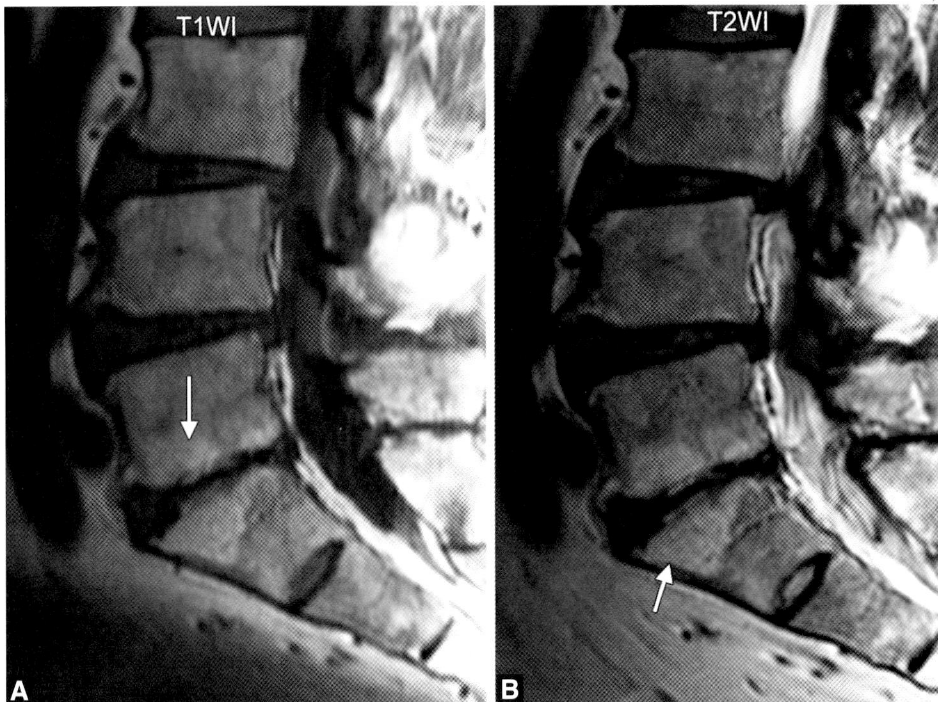

Figs 73A and B: Modic type 2 changes are seen as increased signal intensity in T1- and T2-weighted MR images due to lipid deposits in endplates

Osteoporotic Compression Fractures

MRI is particularly useful in distinguishing between benign compression fractures and those caused by underlying tumor or infection. The presence of a soft-tissue mass or signal change extending into the pedicle is strongly suggestive of tumor. In this setting, use of gadolinium contrast is typically not necessary to successfully differentiate osteoporotic from neoplastic fractures. Findings of decreased signal intensity on T1-weighted images and increased signal intensity on T2-weighted images is sensitive (Figs 74A and B), but not very specific for tumor as the same findings are common with acute osteoporotic compression fractures. Normal marrow intensity on T1 images, however, makes a diagnosis of tumor extremely unlikely. Diffusion-weighted magnetic resonance imaging is a relatively new technique that may allow for improved discrimination between osteoporotic and tumor-associated compression fractures.

Bone scintigraphy has been suggested as a means of confirming the presence of a symptomatic compression fracture in patients with osteoporosis. Technetium bone scintigraphy is sensitive for diagnosing compression fractures, but radionuclide uptake can persist for up to 2 years after injury, and the utility of bone scans in determining fracture acuity is limited. The relationship between persistent uptake on bone scan and pain is unclear. Single-photon emission computed tomography provides greater anatomic detail and allows localization of the radionuclide uptake observed on routine bone scan. Nuclear studies, in general, can suggest the presence of metastatic disease by revealing multiple foci of increased radionuclide uptake. Positron emission tomography with fluorine-18 deoxyglucose has been studied in patients with vertebral compression fractures in patients with osteoporosis and may be useful in distinguishing benign from pathological fractures. Increased uptake on positron emission tomography scan appears associated with malignant and inflammatory processes. However, this modality demonstrates relatively low specificity during the first 2 months after injury and in cases with moderate standard uptake values.

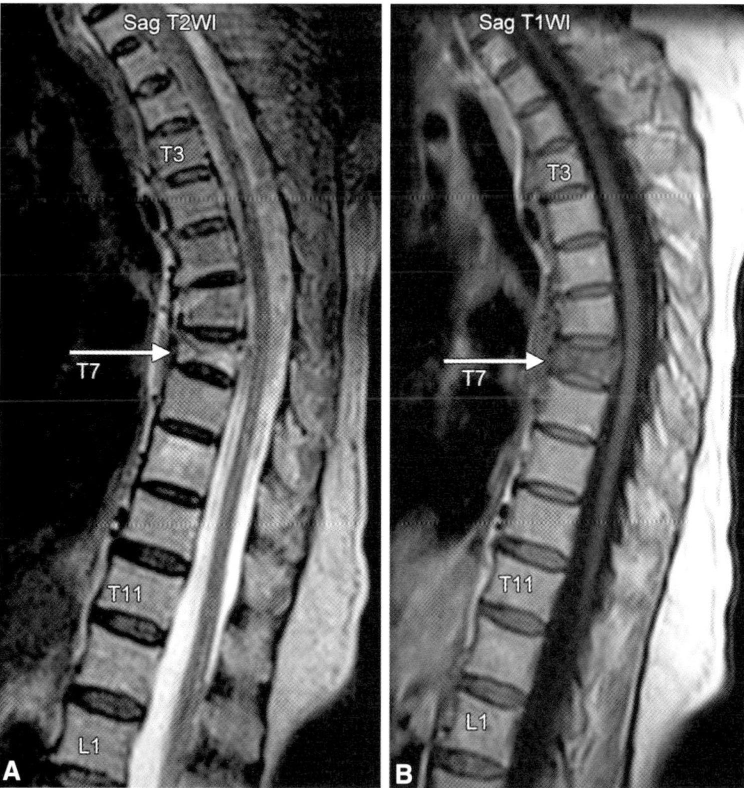

Figs 74A and B: Wedge compression collapse fracture with reduced height of D7 vertebral body on T2WI (A) with marrow edema appearing hypointense on T1WI (B) seen in a 65-year-old female

Ossification of Posterior Longitudinal Ligament

Ossification of posterior longitudinal ligament (OPLL) is seen as dense, ossified strip or plaque along the posterior margins of the vertebral bodies and intervertebral discs. It is most common in the midcervical (C3-5)and midthoracic (T4-7) spine. Ossification of the posterior longitudinal ligament (OPLL) begins with hypervascular fibrosis and hypertrophy of the posterior longitudinal ligament, followed by cartilaginous proliferation, lamellar bone formation, and Haversian canal production. OPLL mineralization progressively narrows the anteroposterior (AP) diameter of the cervical canal by 0.4 mm a year, while lengthening by 0.67 mm longitudinally. Once the average canal diameter is reduced by more than 30 to 50 percent (less than an average of 9.4 mm), myelopathy typically appears.

Direct demonstration of the calcification in OPLL by means of noncontrast computed tomography (CT), CT myelography, and 3D CT scans is the best way to define the full extent and type of OPLL. OPLL is classified into four types: segmental (39 percent of cases), continuous (27 percent), mixed (29 percent), and other (5 percent). Segmental OPLL is located behind the vertebral bodies and not at the disc spaces, whereas continuous OPLL extends from body to body. Mixed OPLL has both segmental and continuous components, and OPLL classified as other is confined to the disc spaces.

MRI is the gold standard as far as spinal imaging is concerned and shows the manifestations of the disease well. T1W and T2W MR images show marked thickening of posterior longitudinal ligament appearing hypointense on both sequences (Figs 75A to E).

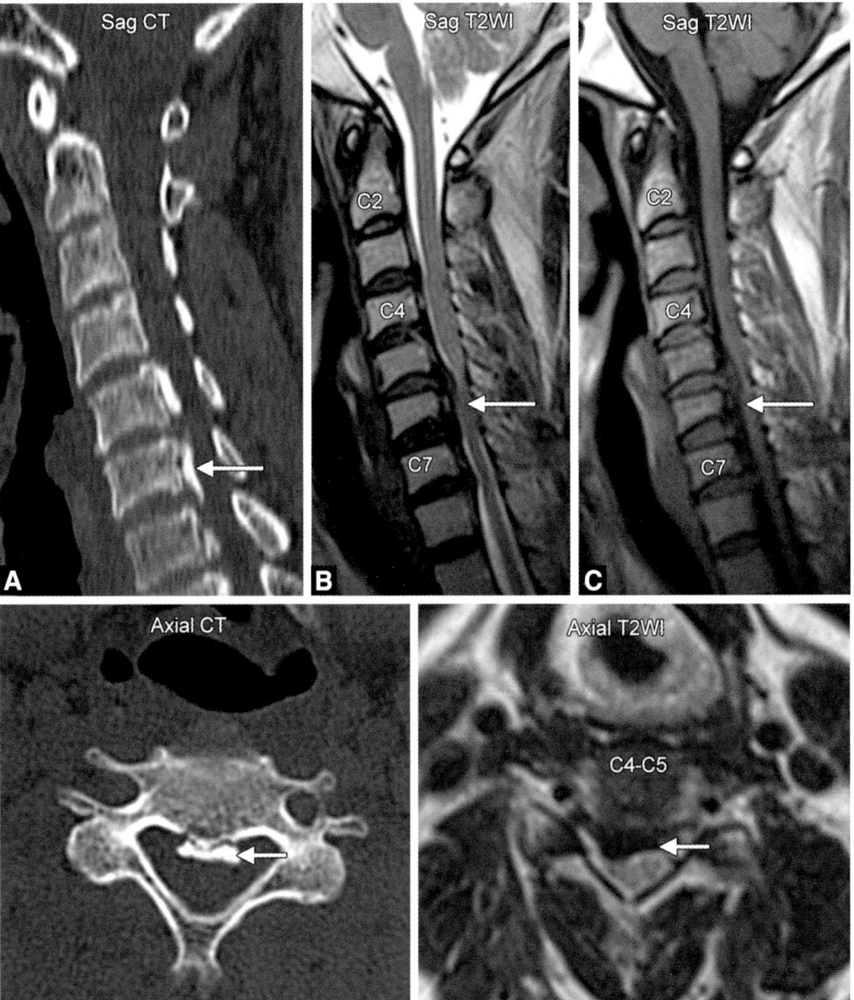

Figs 75A to E: Sagittal CT image (A) image demonstrates ossified posterior longitudinal ligament (arrow) posterior to C5, C6 and C7 vertebral bodies. Sagittal T2WI (B) and sagittal T1WI image (C) shows hypointense signal (arrow) posterior to C5, C6 and C7 vertebral bodies with narrowing of spinal canal suggesting segmental OPLL. Axial CT image (D) shows tongue like projection of ossified posterior longitudinal ligament (arrow) posterior to cervical vertebral body, it appears hypointense (arrow) on T2WI (E) with pronounced narrowing of the spinal canal

Ligamentum Flavum Hypertrophy

The ligamentum flavum are ligaments which connect the laminae of adjacent vertebrae from the axis to the first segment of the sacrum (C2 to S1). Each ligament consists of two lateral portions which commence one on either side of the roots of the articular processes, and extend backward to the point where the laminae meet to form the spinous process. In the cervical region the ligaments are thin, but broad and long. They are thicker in the thoracic region, and thickest in the lumbar region.

Hypertrophy of this ligament (Fig. 76) may cause spinal canal stenosis because it lies in the posterior portion of the vertebral canal. In some patients extensive calcification or ossification in hypertrophied ligamenta flava can occur in association with myelopathy or radiculopathy.

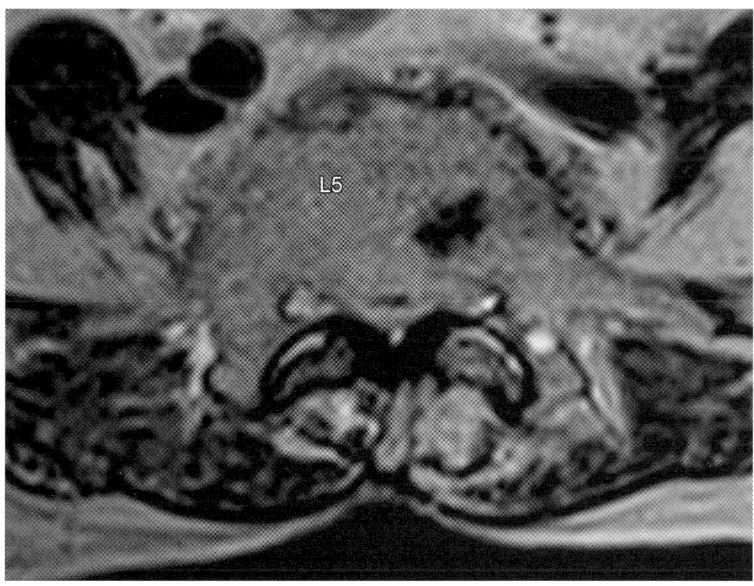

Fig. 76: Thickening of ligamentum flavum is seen at L5 disc level measuring 5 mm in thickness

Spinal Canal Stenosis

Spinal stenosis results from an overall decrease in the dimensions of the spinal canal, lateral recesses, or neural foramina. It occurs more commonly in the lumbar and cervical region.

Etiologically, stenosis can be divided into two main categories. The first is developmental or congenital, which is idiopathic and includes entities such as achondroplasia, Morquio disease, fluorosis, postoperative changes, and various bony dysplasias. Acquired stenosis that may be a result of degenerative disease, trauma, spondylolisthesis, or postoperative and various miscellaneous conditions such as ankylosing spondylosis, ossification of the posterior longitudinal ligament, degenerative disease. The common denominator of spinal stenosis is narrowing of the canal, which may be central, lateral, or both. In the lumbar spine, central stenosis tends to occur at multiple levels but is most common at L4–L5. Degenerative diseases is most severe at L4–L5. Neural foraminal stenosis can result from bony overgrowth, spondylolisthesis, or degenerative disc bulge or herniation of the intervertebral disc. Symptomatic spinal stenosis of the thoracic spine is much less common than of the cervical and lumbar spine. This is to a large degree caused by the relatively large size of the thoracic canal relative to the cord. On MR imaging (Figs 77 to 79), the following features are important for analysis: facet joint size and contour, osteophyte formation of the facet joints or the vertebral bodies, hypertrophy or calcification of the ligamentous structures, and transverse and sagittal dimensions of the canal, lateral recess, and the neural foramina. Lumbar canal stenosis is characterized by circumferential narrowing of the central canal to an area less than 1.5 cm^2 or anteroposterior diameter of less than 1.15 cm.

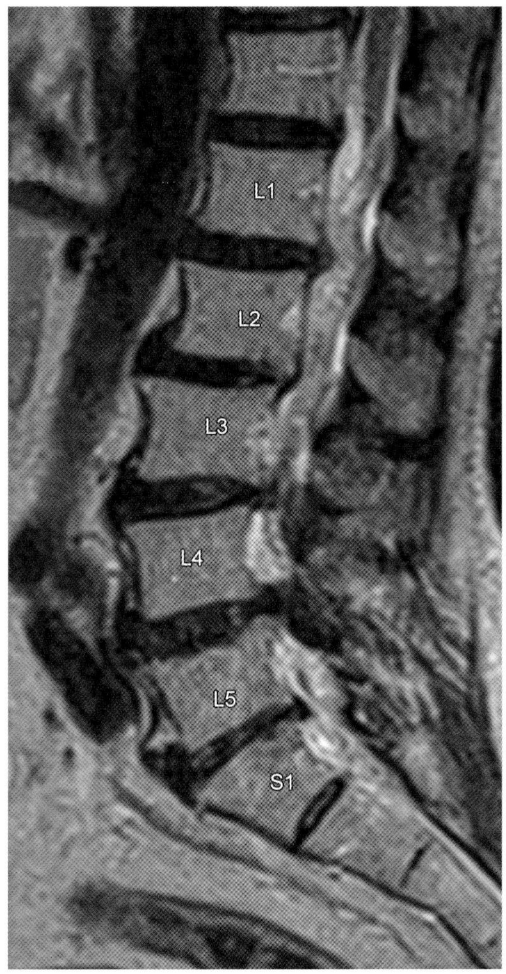

Fig. 77: Sagittal T2W image shows multilevel lumbar disc protrusions compressing the thecal sac and the nerve roots with resultant secondary lumbar canal stenosis

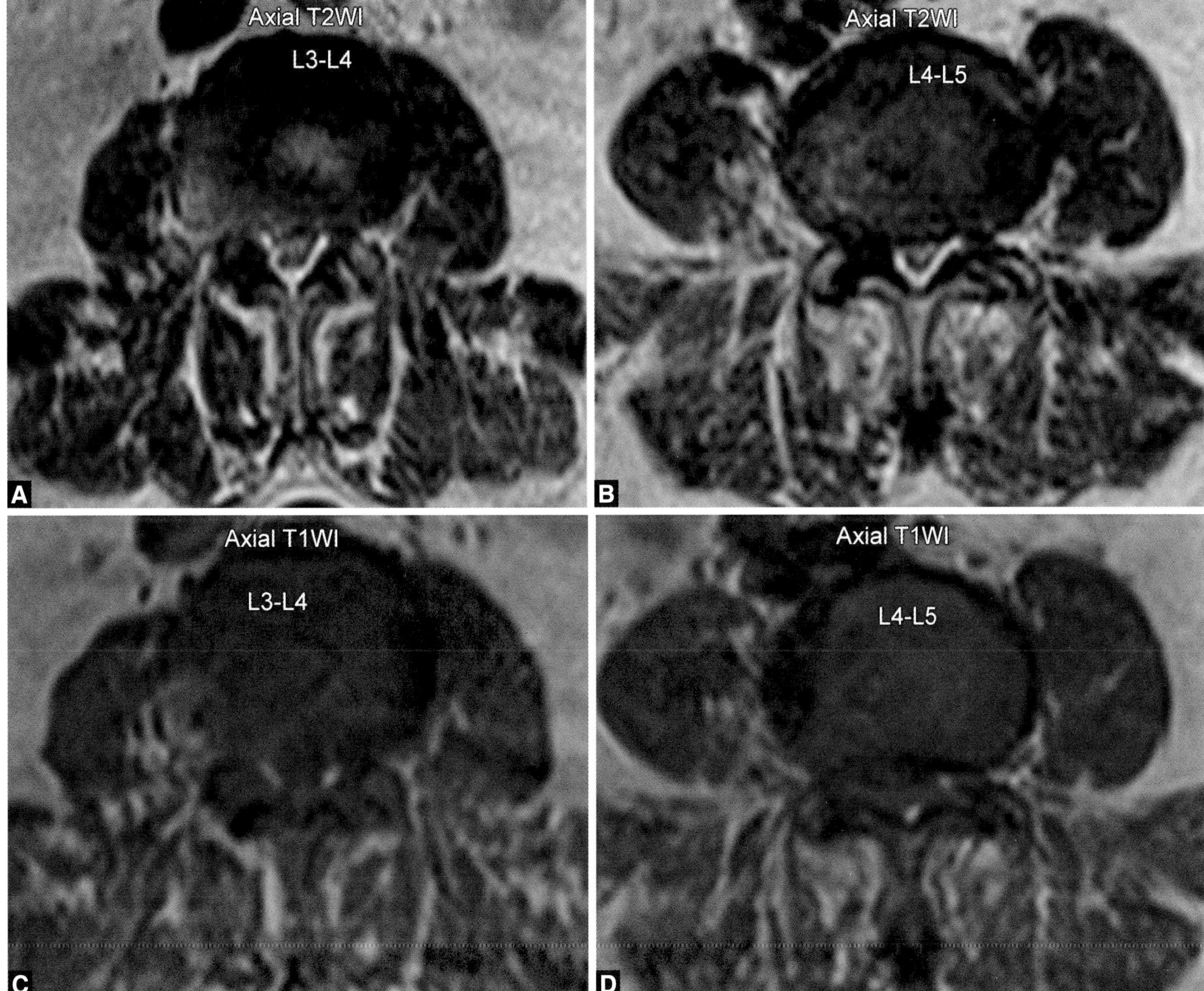

Figs 78A to D: Axial T2WI (A and B) and axial T1WI (C and D) show disc protrusion compressing the thecal sac, and the presence of ligamentum flavum hypertrophy and facetal arthropathy adds to the canal stenosis

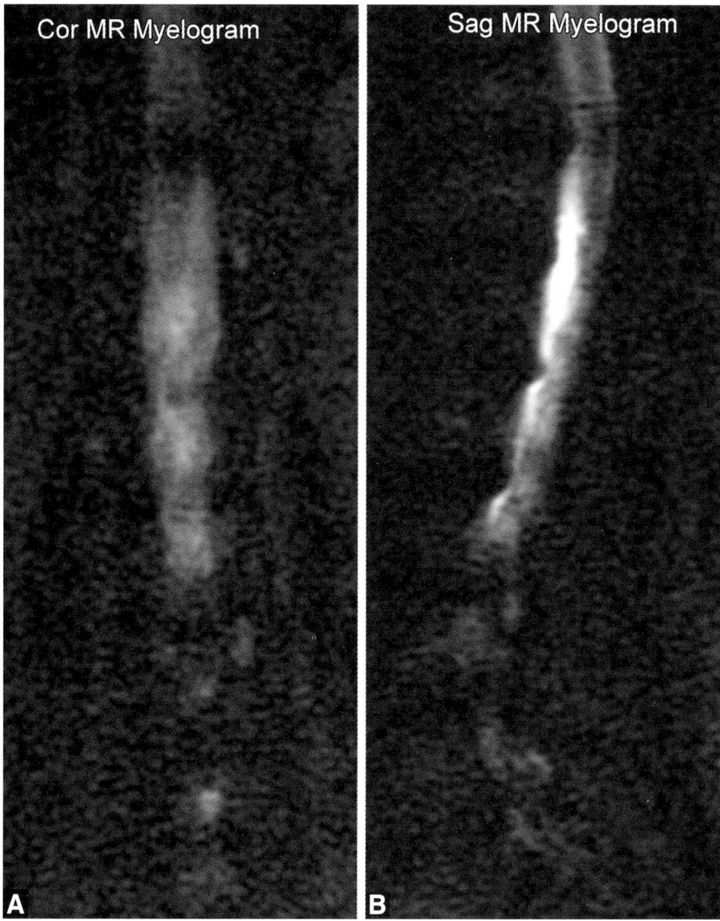

Figs 79A and B: Coronal and sagittal MR myelogram show indentation over the thecal sac at multiple levels with secondary canal stenosis

SPINAL TRAUMA

Spinous Process Fracture

Isolated fractures of the spinous process are usually benign injuries and are considered stable injuries. However spinous process fractures can also present with lamina fractures, facet dislocations, and various other injuries to the cervical spine including extension of avulsion into the laminae.

Clay Shoveler's fracture is type of hyperflexion avulsion injury that causes fractures of spinous process at base. Most commonly occurs at C7 level followed by C6 and T1. It is due to abrupt flexion against the tense posterior ligaments of the neck. This is a stable fracture.

Plain radiographs are often good enough for diagnosis if there are no neurological symptoms. However if there is an associated injury and neurological deficit, MRI should be done (Figs 80A to E).

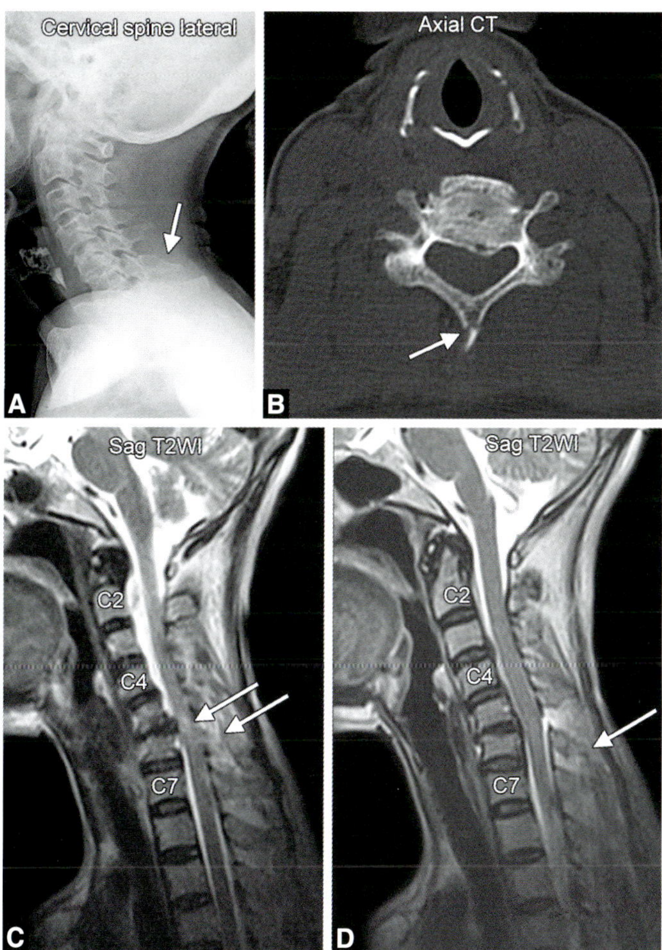

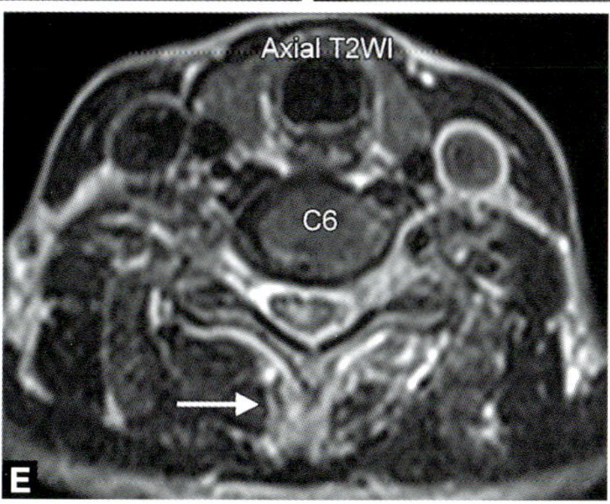

Figs 80A to E: (A) X-ray cervical spine lateral view of a 50-year-old female with history of trauma with weakness in upper limbs shows fracture of C6 spinous process; (B) Axial CT image showing fracture of C6 spinous process; (C and D) Sagittal T2WI showing fracture of C6 spinous process and mild cord edema at C5-C6 level; (E) Axial T2WI showing fracture of C6 spinous process and mild cord edema at this level

Compression Fracture

A compression fracture occurs when the normal vertebral body of the spine is squished, or compressed, to a smaller height. This injury tends to happen first, in patients involved in traumatic accidents commonly seen after a fall. Secondly when the spine takes a load which for a vertebrae exceeds its stability, it may collapse, which is much more common specially in patients with osteoporosis. Compression fracture is usually diagnosed by the history, physical examination and X-rays. In any patient over the age of 60 years with the acute onset of sudden low back pain, a compression fracture should be suspected. Physical exam will usually show tenderness directly over the area of pain as well as mild kyphotic deformity. Plain X-rays will demonstrate the wedge shape of the vertebral body on a lateral view. If osteoporosis is suspected, a bone mineral density test and thyroid function test may be requisitioned. They help determine the severity of the bone thinning. CT scan is occasionally needed to help differentiate a compression fracture from a burst fracture. MRI scans rule out disc herniation or any other pathology along with a compression fracture. It provides accurate status of spinal cord (Figs 81 and 82). MRI scan may also help differentiate pathologic compression fractures and osteoporotic compression fracture. In any patient with a known history of cancer, a compression fracture should tip off the physician to look for evidence of a metastatic lesion and pathologic fracture.

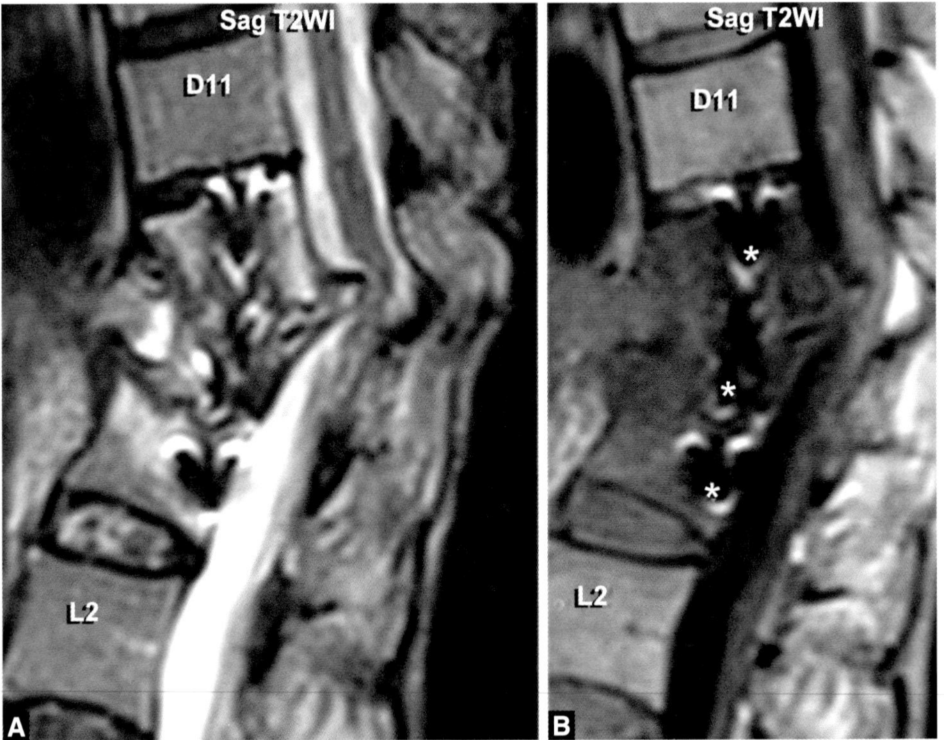

Figs 81A and B: Postoperative sagittal T2W (A) and T1W (B) images show wedge compression collapse fracture of the D12 and L1 vertebral bodies and break in the superior endplate of L2 vertebral body with retropulsion and compression of the lower end of cord at same level. Postoperative susceptibility artifact seen in D12 to L2 vertebral bodies (*)

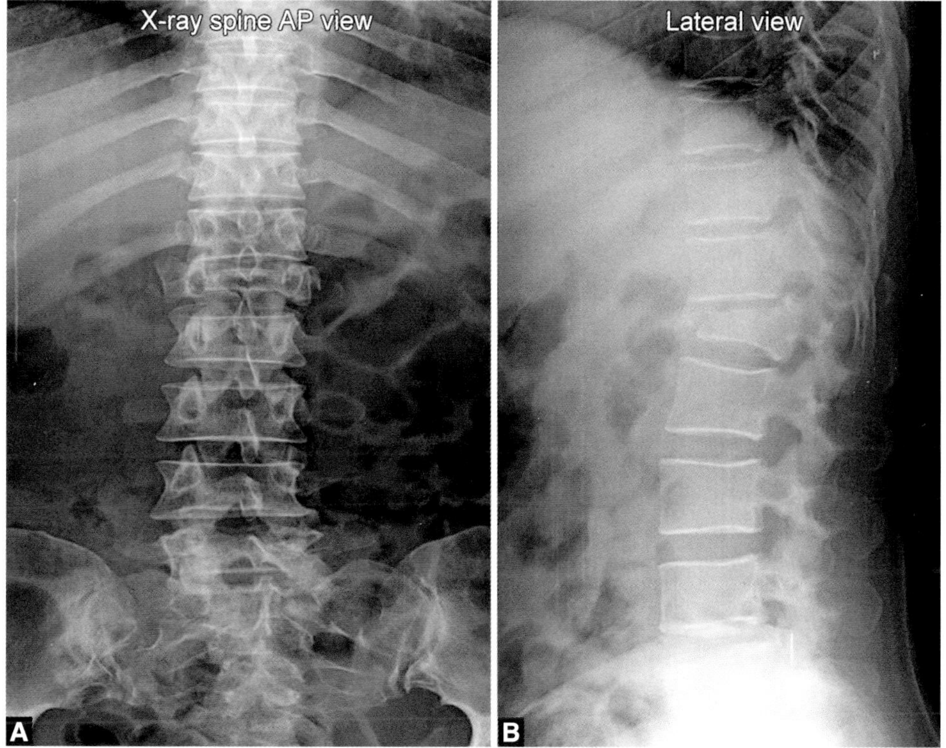

Figs 82A and B: AP (A) and lateral (B) X-rays show wedge compression collapse fracture of L1 vertebral body with retropulsion of bone fragment with mild reduction in height of L5 vertebral body

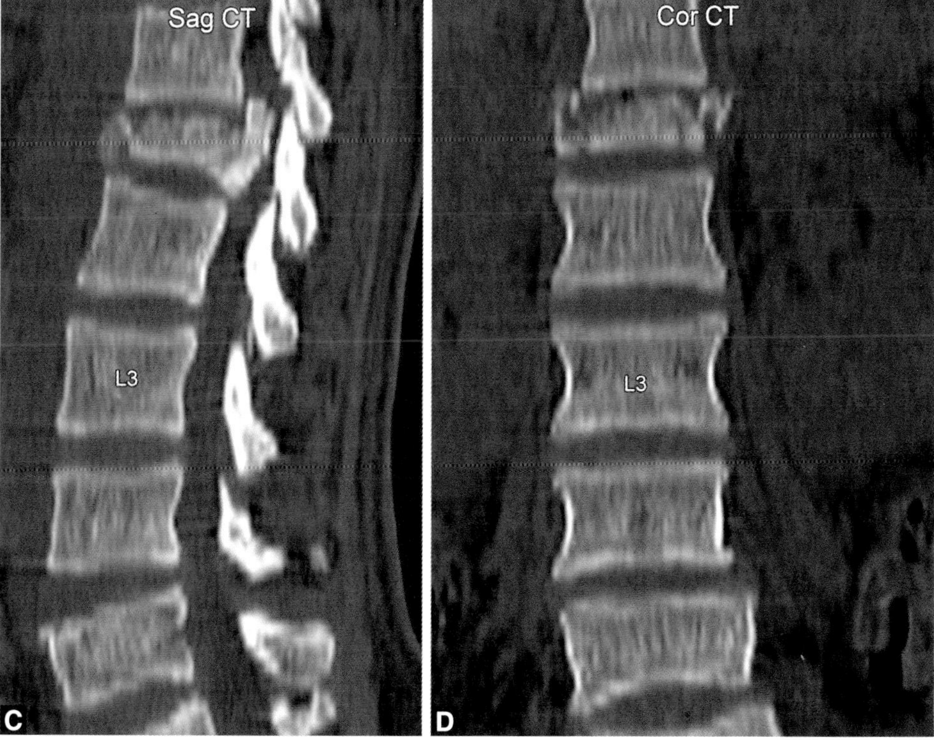

Figs 82C and D: Reformatted sagittal and coronal CT image show wedge compression collapse fracture of L1 vertebral body with retropulsion of bone fragment with mild reduction in height of L5 vertebral body

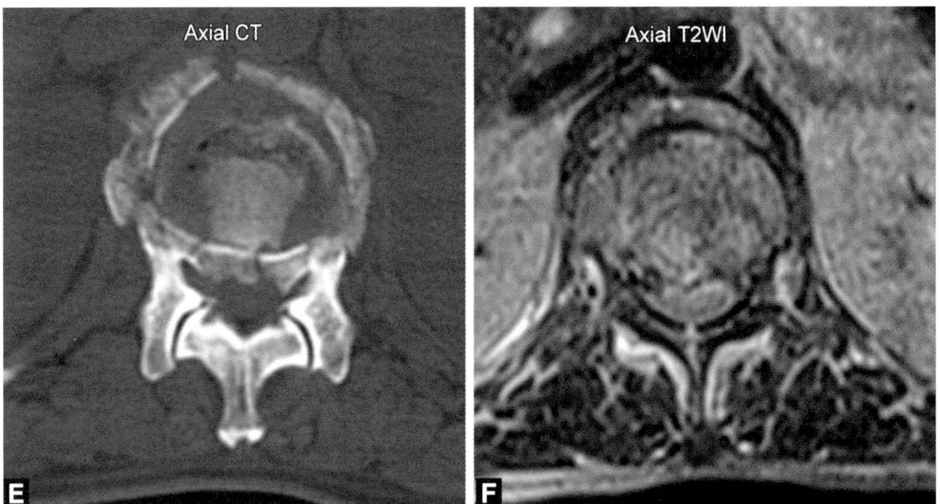

Figs 82E and F: Axial CT (A) and MRI (B) show fracture of the L1 vertebral body with retropulsion of the bone fragment in spinal canal

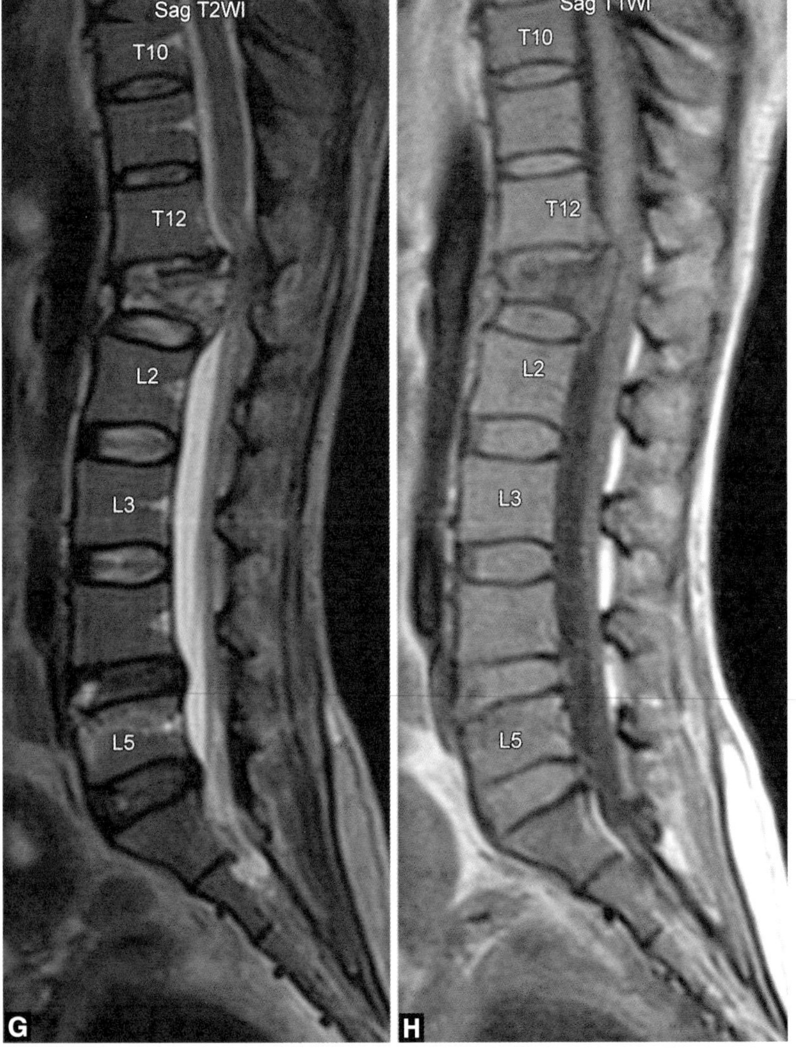

Figs 82G and H: Sagittal T2WI (A) and sagittal T1WI (B) show wedge compression collapse fracture of L1 vertebral body with retropulsion of bone fragment with marrow edema and mild reduction in height of L5 vertebral body with marrow edema

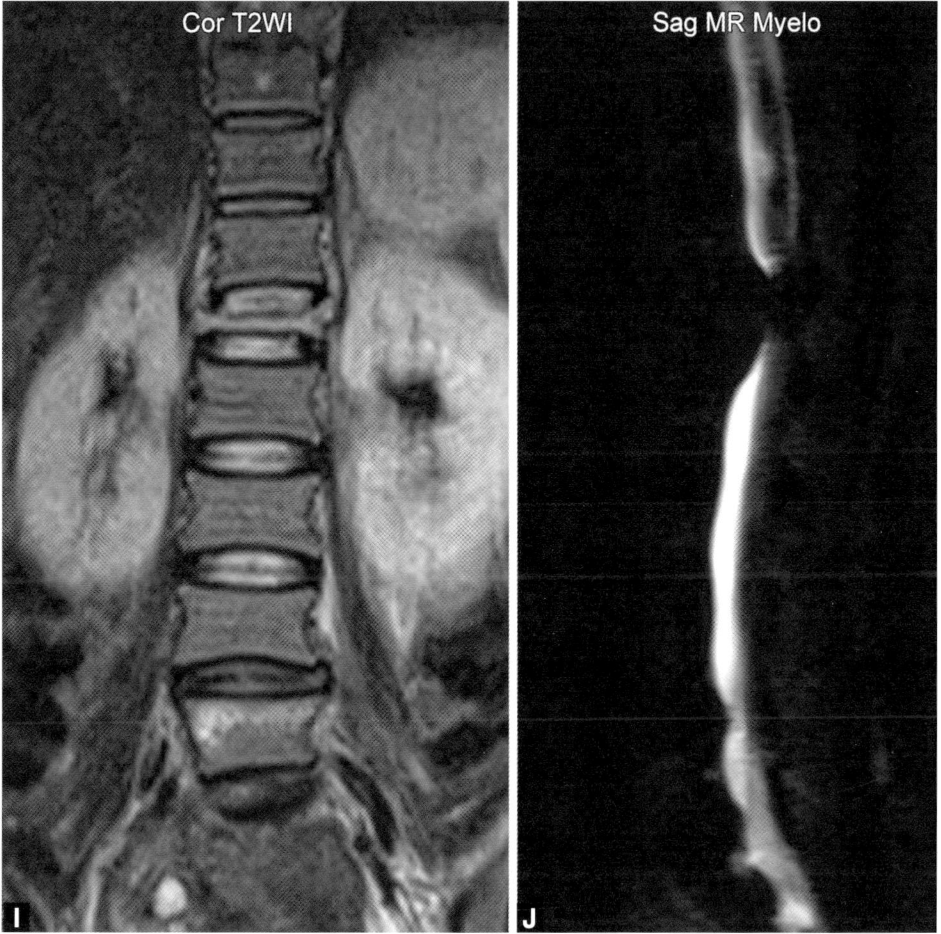

Figs 82I and J: Coronal T2WI (A) show wedge compression collapse fracture of L1 vertebral body with retropulsion of bone fragment with marrow edema and mild reduction in height of L5 vertebral body with marrow edema; (B) Sagittal MR myelogram show severe cord compression with myelographic block at L1 level

Spinal Cord Contusion

MR imaging can help detect spinal cord contusion (Figs 83A to C), compression, and transection and provide additional prognostic information. The presence of edema alone indicates a more favorable prognosis with potential for reversibility. MRI is the modality of choice for evaluation of cord injury, syrinx and atrophy of cord. In case of cord injury MRI scan should be performed in flexion and extension to evaluate spinal stability facetal locking and cord compression. CT can demonstrate fractures of spine accurately.

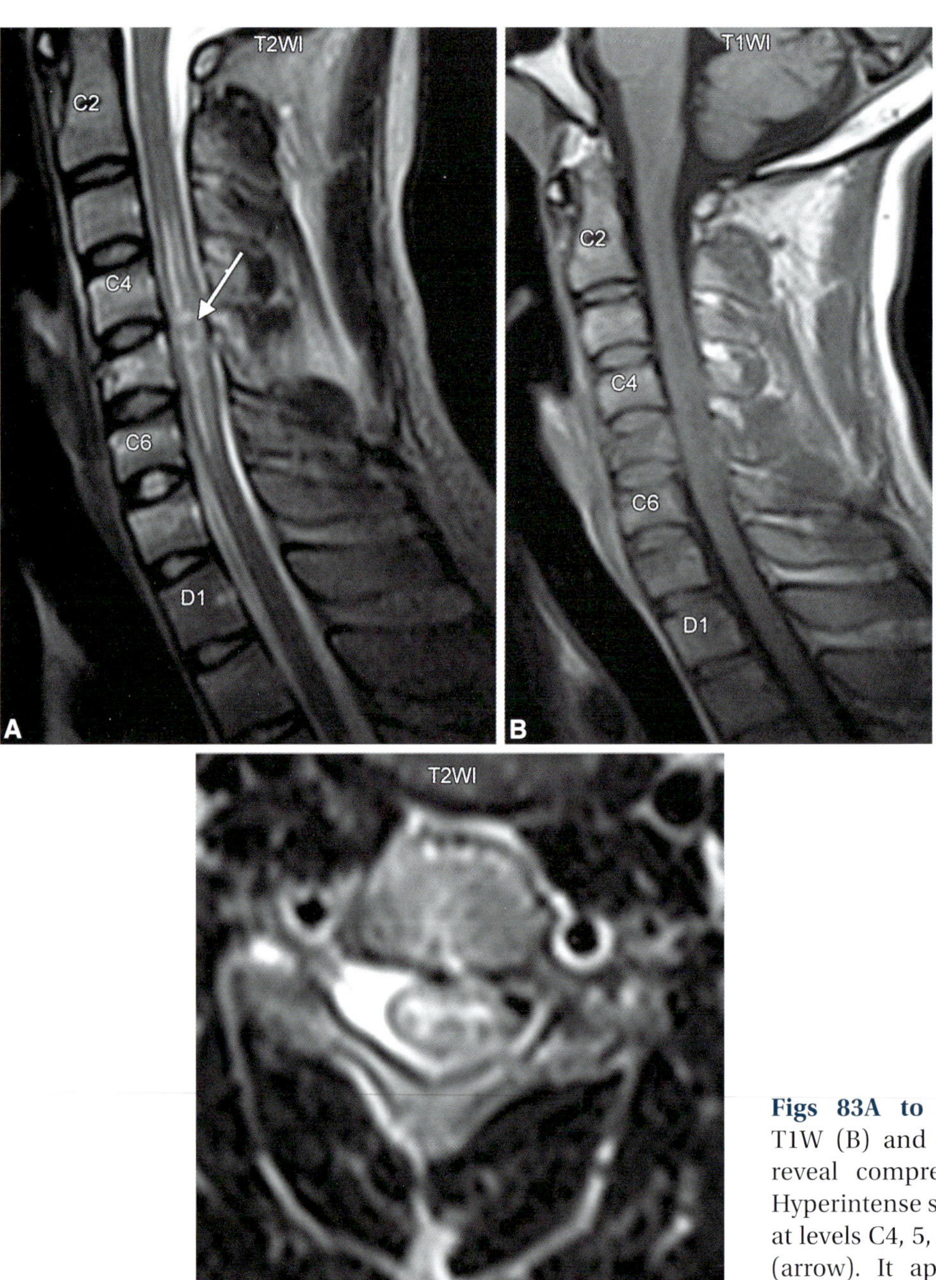

Figs 83A to C: Sagittal STIR (A) T1W (B) and axial T2W (C) images reveal compression fracture of C5. Hyperintense signal is seen in the cord at levels C4, 5, 6, and 7 on T2W image (arrow). It appears hypointense on T1W image and represents edema. Focal cord contusion is seen at C4-5 level with surrounding edema (A)

Pott's Spine

Spinal tuberculosis, the most common form of skeletal tuberculosis, it is increasing in prevalence because of the resurgence of tuberculosis during the past decade in patients with AIDS, the spread of tuberculosis among the homeless, and low socio-economic strata. Spinal infection is usually the result of hematogeneous seeding of the vertebral body, and the diagnosis often remains elusive because of the indolent nature of tuberculous infection. As a result, the radiographic findings and the signs and symptoms are typically far advanced when the diagnosis is finally established. Radiographic manifestations of tuberculous spondylitis include intraosseous and paraspinal abscess formation, subligamentous spread of infection, vertebral body destruction and collapse, and extension into the spinal epidural space. Significant instability and deformity of the spine can result, mandating prompt diagnosis and treatment to prevent permanent neurologic damage.

Imaging of Pott's disease on plain radiographs more commonly shows involvement of the thoracic spine and the lumbar spine. The infection usually begins in the anterior aspect of the vertebral body, either inferiorly or superiorly, adjacent to the vertebral endplate. Focal areas of erosion and osseous destruction in the anterior corners of the vertebral body are typical plain film findings for tuberculous spondylitis. Involvement of the adjacent intervertebral disc or vertebral body results from penetration through the disc itself or spread of infection beneath the anterior longitudinal or posterior longitudinal ligament. Contiguous vertebra body involvement, destruction of the intervertebral disc and progressive vertebral body collapse result in the characteristic gibbus deformity of the spine commonly associated with tuberculosis. Multiple vertebral levels may be involved in a noncontiguous fashion, manifested on plain radiographs as skip lesions of vertebral body destruction and collapse. The posterior elements of the spine are usually secondarily involved by spread of infection from the vertebral body.

Paraspinal abscess formation may be detected clinically if large enough. On plain radiographs it is seen as areas of fusiform soft-tissue swelling around the spine and is refered as a cold abscess which is a specific type of abscess that forms without the heat or inflammation characteristically associated with standard abscesses. It usually forms gradually over time, which results in less irritation or inflammation. Pain only occurs when pressure is applied. These swellings can be chronic, persisting after initial growth with no sign of either healing or worsening. Cold abscesses are usually of tuberculosis etiology. One common site of cold abscesses is the *psoas muscles*, in which case the abscess is known as a psoas abscess.

Features of Pott's spine on CT include anterior vertebral body destruction, vertebral body collapse, disc space narrowing, and large paraspinal soft tissue masses representing abscess formation. During the course of the infection, a cloaca may be visualized and may result from spontaneous decompression and drainage of the vertebral body abscess. Paraspinal abscesses form as a result of this drainage, which can then travel through fascial planes and lead to the development of mediastinal abscesses, pleural effusions, or psoas and flank abscesses, depending on the level and direction of spread. The multiplanar imaging capability of MR imaging greatly improves the detection of vertebral intraosseous abscesses, skip lesions, subligamentous spread of infection (Figs 84 to 88) and epidural extension commonly associated with tuberculous spondylitis. T1W images of the spine typically show decreased signal within the affected vertebral bodies, loss of disc height, and paraspinal soft-tissue (Figs 84A to E). Contrast-enhanced sequences are helpful in distinguishing between tuberculous spondylitis (Figs 85 and 86) and other granulomatous spinal infections. There is presence of a thick rim of enhancement around paraspinal and intraosseous abscesses. Involvement of the paraspinal soft tissues and subligamentous spread of infection often are best evaluated with coronal contrast-enhanced images. Because of its multiplanar capability and sensitivity in detecting osseous and soft-tissue changes associated with osteomyelitis, MR imaging should be considered the method of choice for imaging spinal tuberculosis. The lack of ionizing radiation and the multiplanar capability of MR imaging make it advantageous for postoperative assessment of the spine and follow-up studies for monitoring the response.

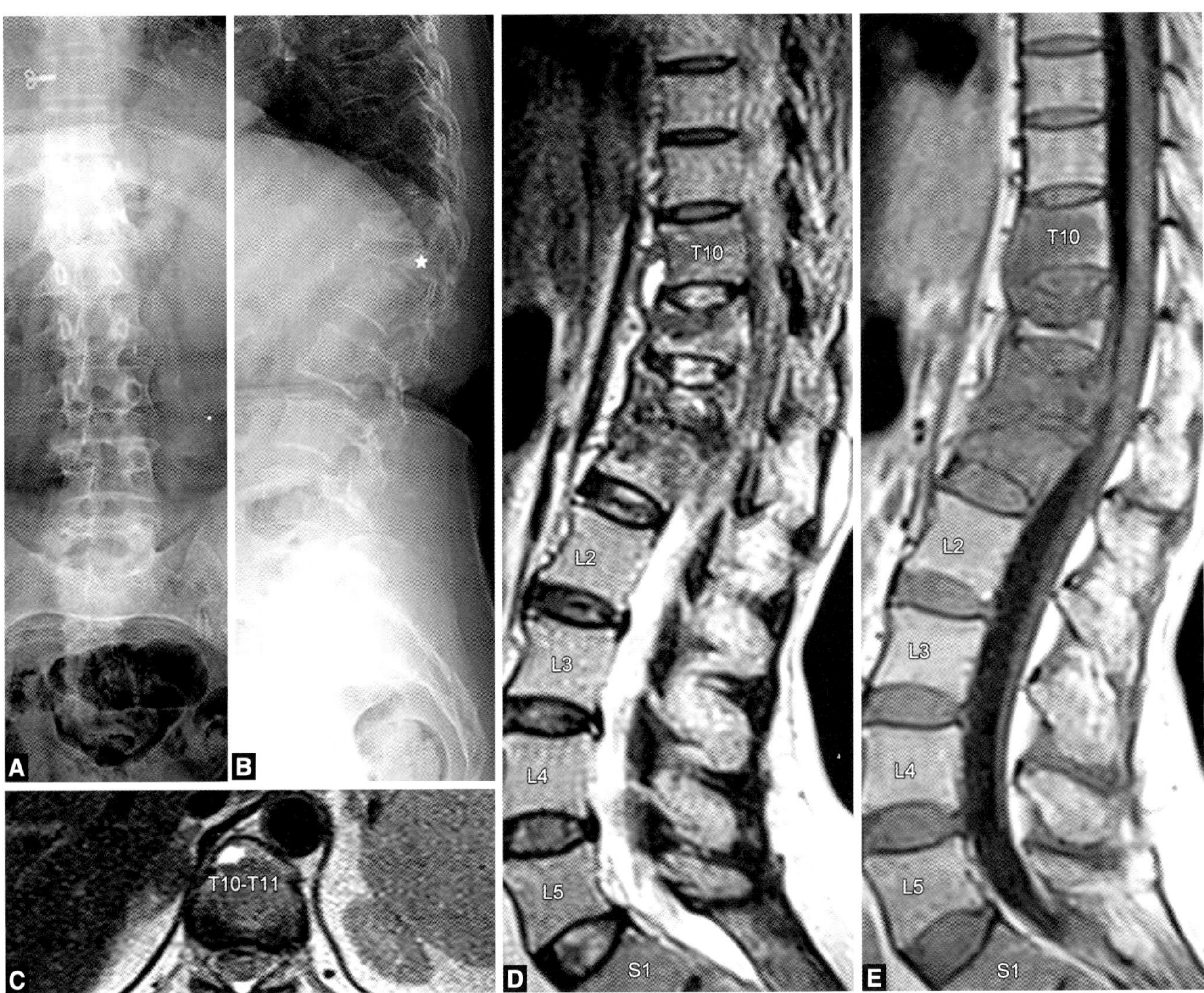

Figs 84A to E: (A and B) AP and lateral views of dorsolumbar spine show wedge-shaped collapse of D11 vertebral body (*) with questionable paravertebral abscess; (C to E) MRI confirms the finding of X-ray and show destruction of D11 to L1 vertebral bodies and discs with anterior prevertebral abscess

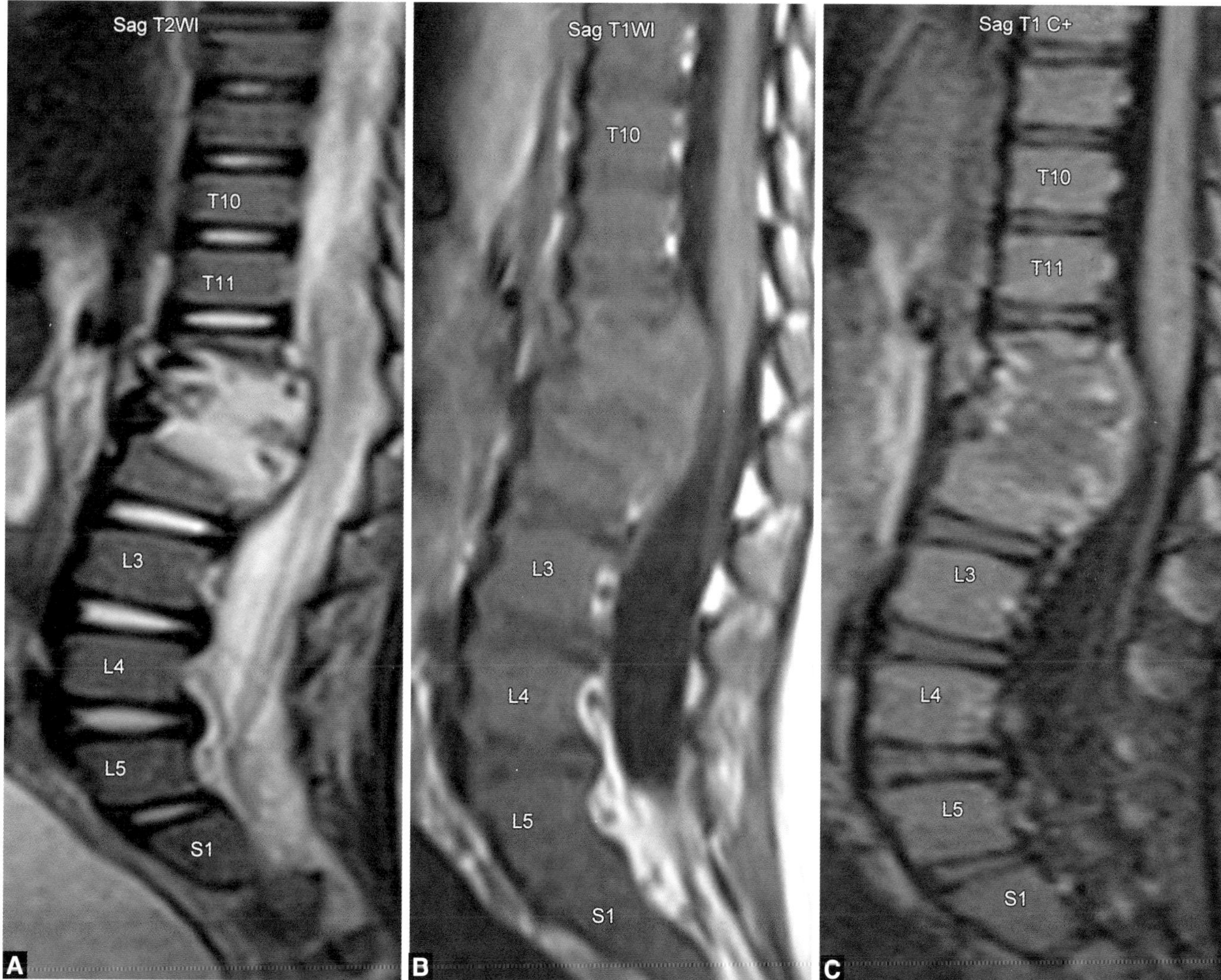

Figs 85A to C: Sagittal T2WI and T1WI shows abnormal signal in T12, L1 and L2 vertebra with involvement of intervening discs and abnormal prevertebral and epidural soft tissue component, causing indentation over thecal sac (A and B). T1W contrast image (C) shows irregular peripheral enhancing lesion involving T12, L1 and L2 vertebra suggestive of vertebral abscess formation

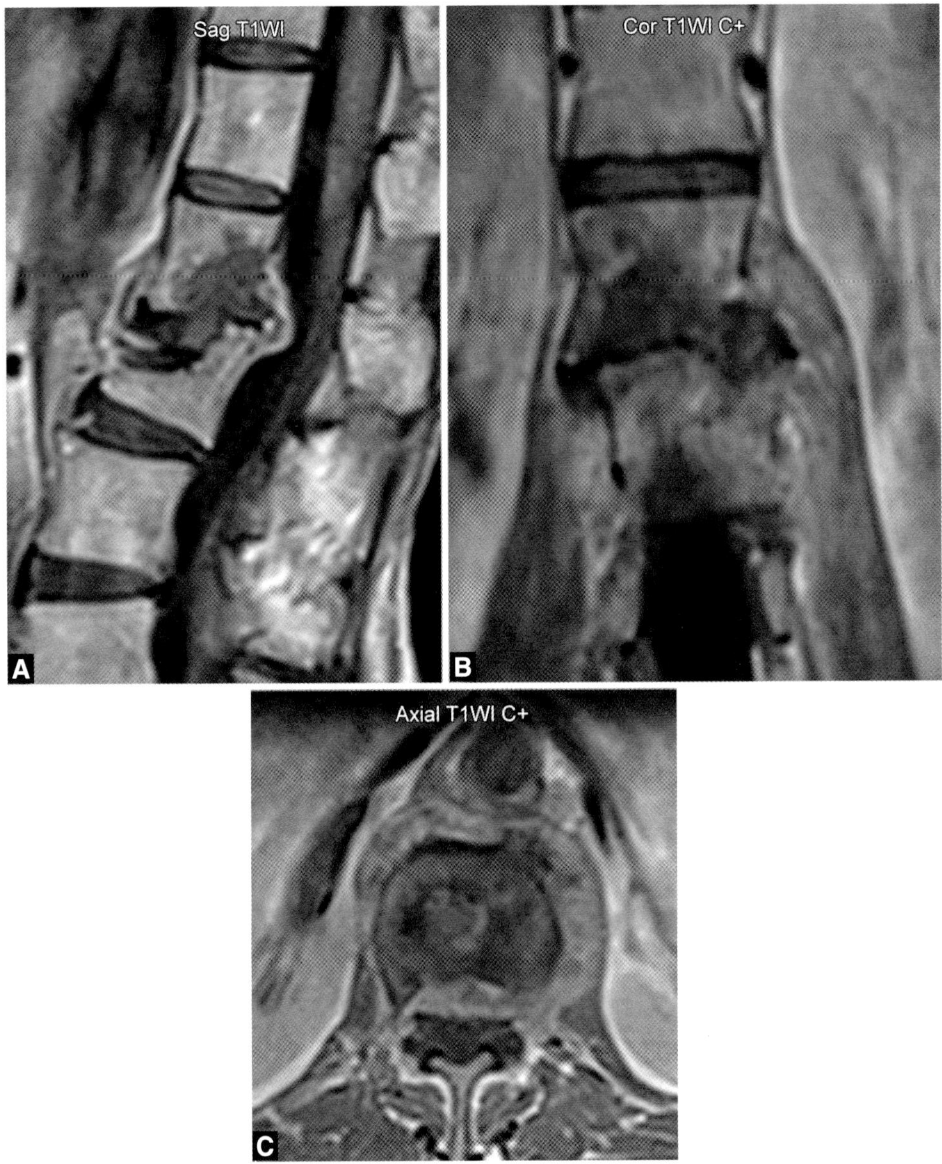

Figs 86A to C: Sagittal T1WI shows altered signal intensity lesion involving L1 and L2 vertebrae with the intervening disc, with soft tissue component and wedge collapse of both vertebrae (A). Coronal postcontrast T1W image (B) show enhancement within the altered signal area involving L1 and L2 vertebrae with involvement of bilateral psoas muscle

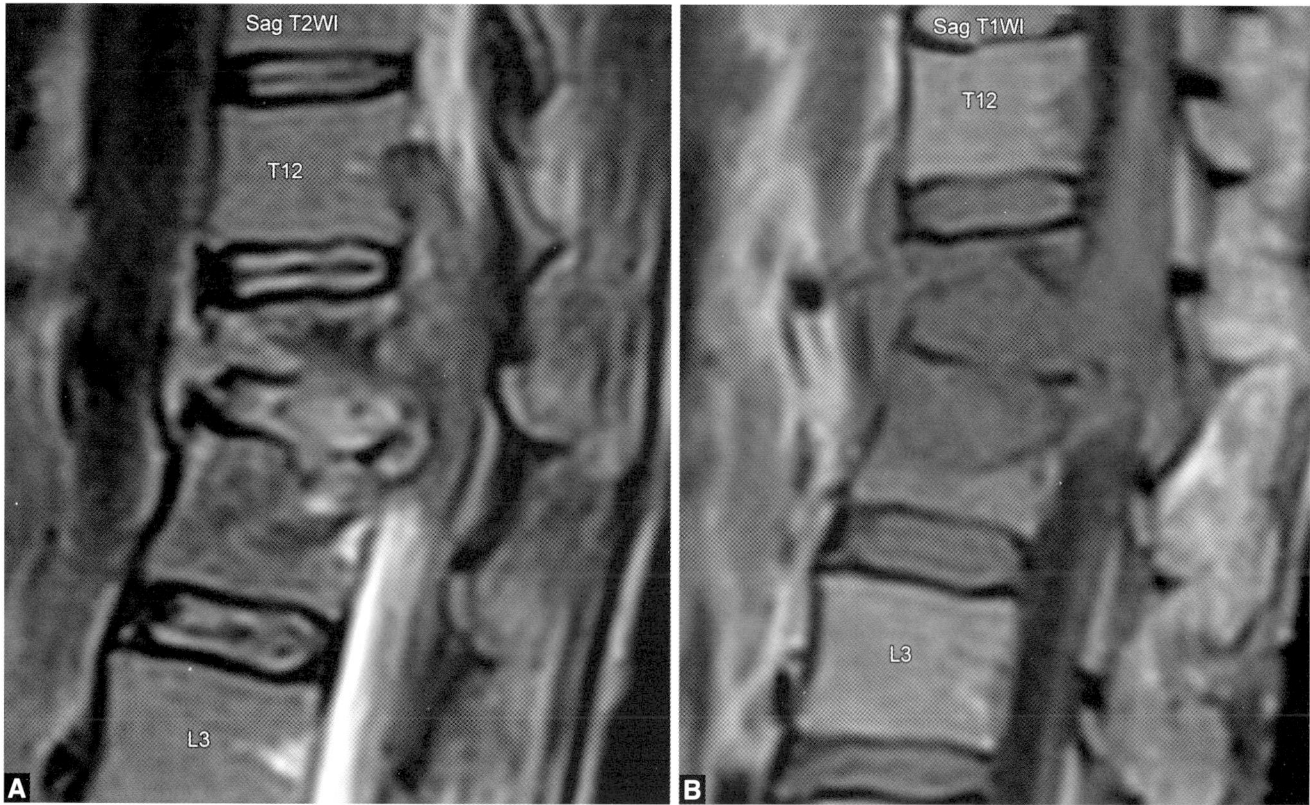

Figs 87A and B: In a case of Pott's spine sag T2WI (A) and T1WI (B) shows altered marrow signal with destruction of the body of L1, superior half of L2 vertebral body and the intervening L1-L2 intervertebral disc

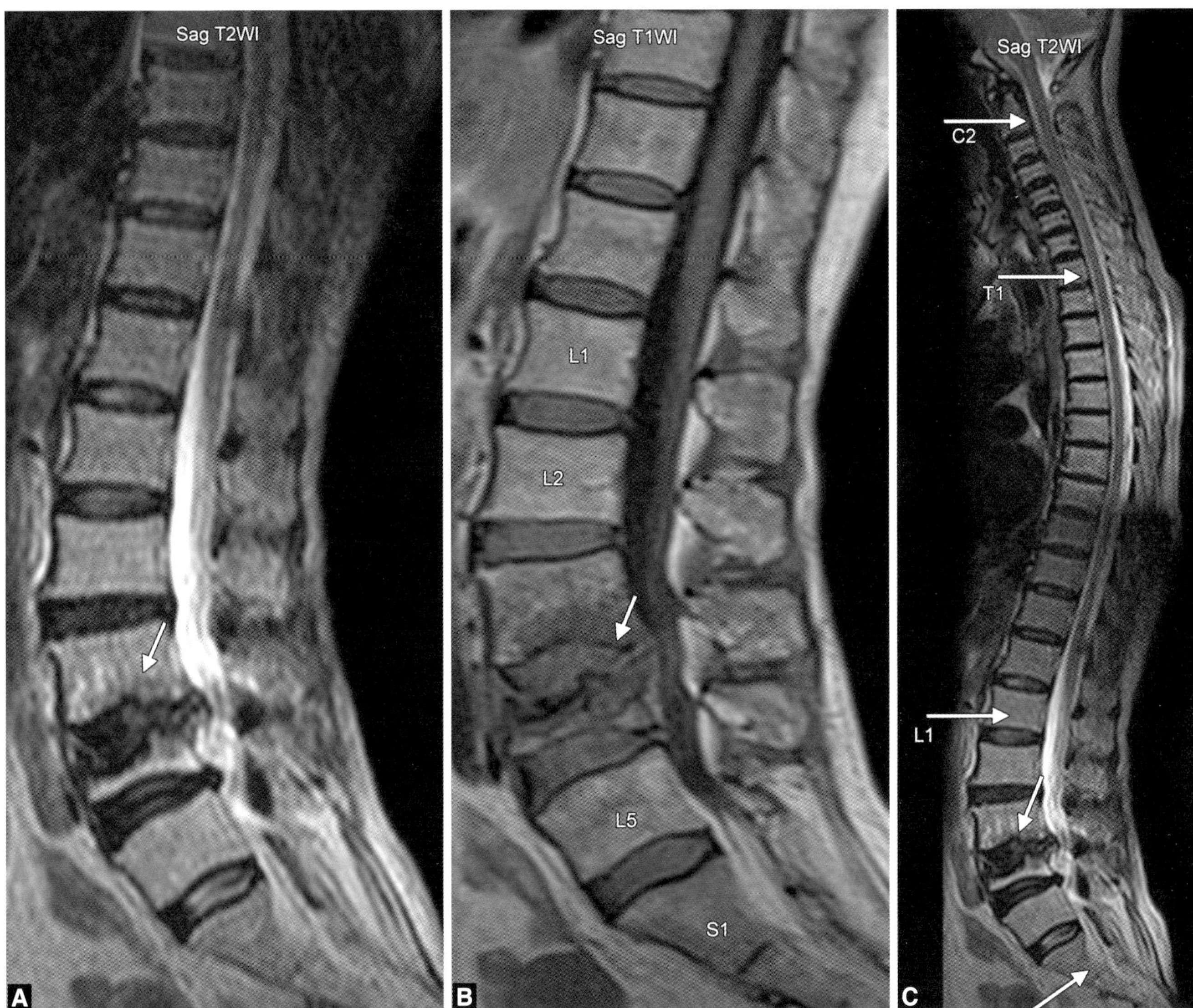

Figs 88A to C: Sagittal T2W image (A and C) and T1WI (B) reveal abnormal signal with destruction of the L3-L4 disc with destruction of the inferior half of the L3 and superior half of the L4 vertebral body with abnormal soft tissue causing secondary canal narrowing

Pott's Spine in Pediatric Group

Tuberculosis is a necrotizing bacterial infection with protean manifestations. Skeletal tuberculosis accounts for 5 to 20 percent of all extra pulmonary cases and Pott's spine is the most common form of skeletal involvement.

In Pott's spine up to the age of 10 years, the involvement is florid and associated with large abscesses formation without neurological involvement. After the age of 10 the lesions are more like adult, and are associated more often with neurological deficits. Commonly thoracic and thoracolumbar areas are involved. The lumbar spine is next to get involved.

On MR imaging T1 and T2 weighted images give good soft tissue differentiation and even the earliest inflammation can be picked up. The soft tissue extension is well demonstrated. The effect of the disease on soft tissues like disc is pin pointed (Figs 89A to D). Involvement of the cord and nerve roots can be diagnosed and the cause of neural compression can be established.

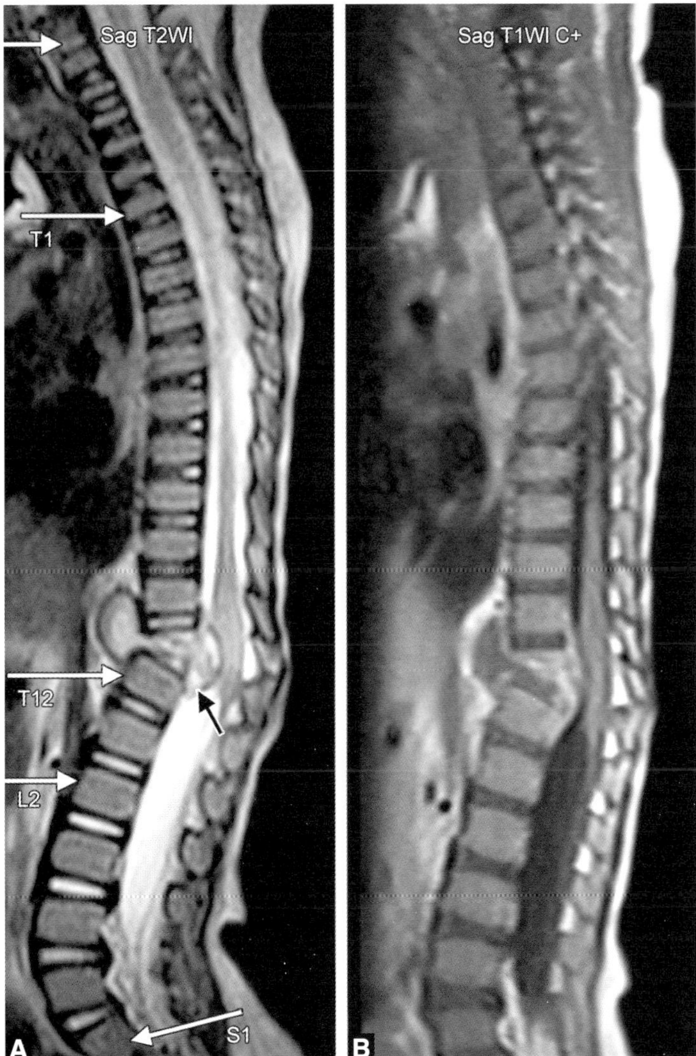

Figs 89A and B: In an 18-month-old child sagittal T2W (A) and TW postcontrast (B) images show destruction of D11 vertebral body with involvement of D11-12 disc and superior endplate of D12 vertebra with abnormal signal and enhancement. Prevertebral and anterior epidural abscess (arrow) is seen

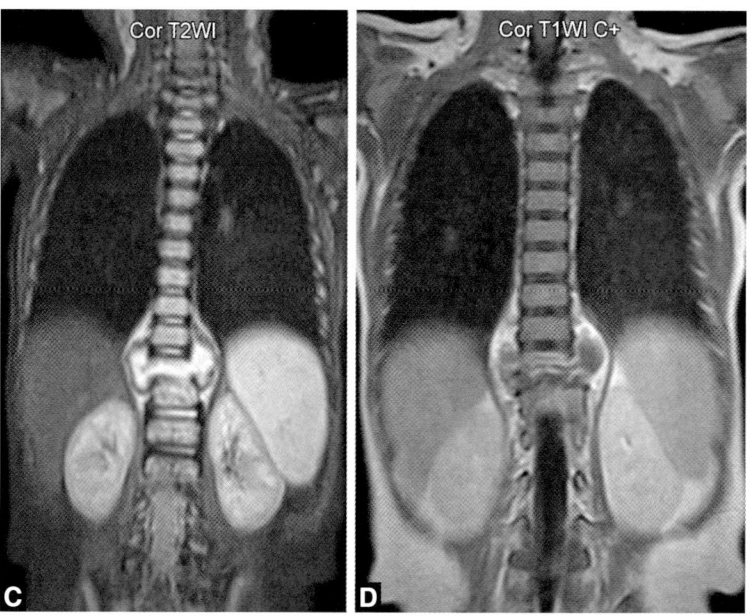

Figs 89C and D: Coronal T2 and T1 postcontrast weighted images show destruction of D11 vertebral body with involvement of D11-12 disc and superior endplate of D12 vertebra with bilateral paravertebral abscess

Transverse Myelitis

Transverse myelitis is a neurological disorder caused by an inflammatory process of the spinal cord, and can cause axonal demyelination. The disease commonly begins with back or radicular pain followed by the abrupt onset of bilateral paresthesias of the legs, an ascending sensory level, and a paraparesis that often progresses to paraplegia. Young adults are commonly affected, and the thoracic spinal cord is the most frequent site of involvement.

There are many etiologic associations such as with viral diseases, vaccinations, demyelinating processes such as multiple sclerosis, collagen-vascular diseases like as systemic lupus erythematosus, vascular disorders, and paraneoplastic syndromes. Polio virus, herpes zoster, and human immunodeficiency viruses are known to involve the spinal cord directly.

Transverse myelitis are divided into acute, sub-acute, or chronic varieties. MRI demonstrate abnormal intramedullary signal, that is, low signal on T1WI and high signal on T2WI (Figs 90A and B), with segmental and peripheral pattern of involvement. The disease may affect cervical, thoracic, or both segments of the cord. The abnormal signal may be extend above the level of clinical deficit. After gadolinium administration, the abnormal areas may show enhancement.

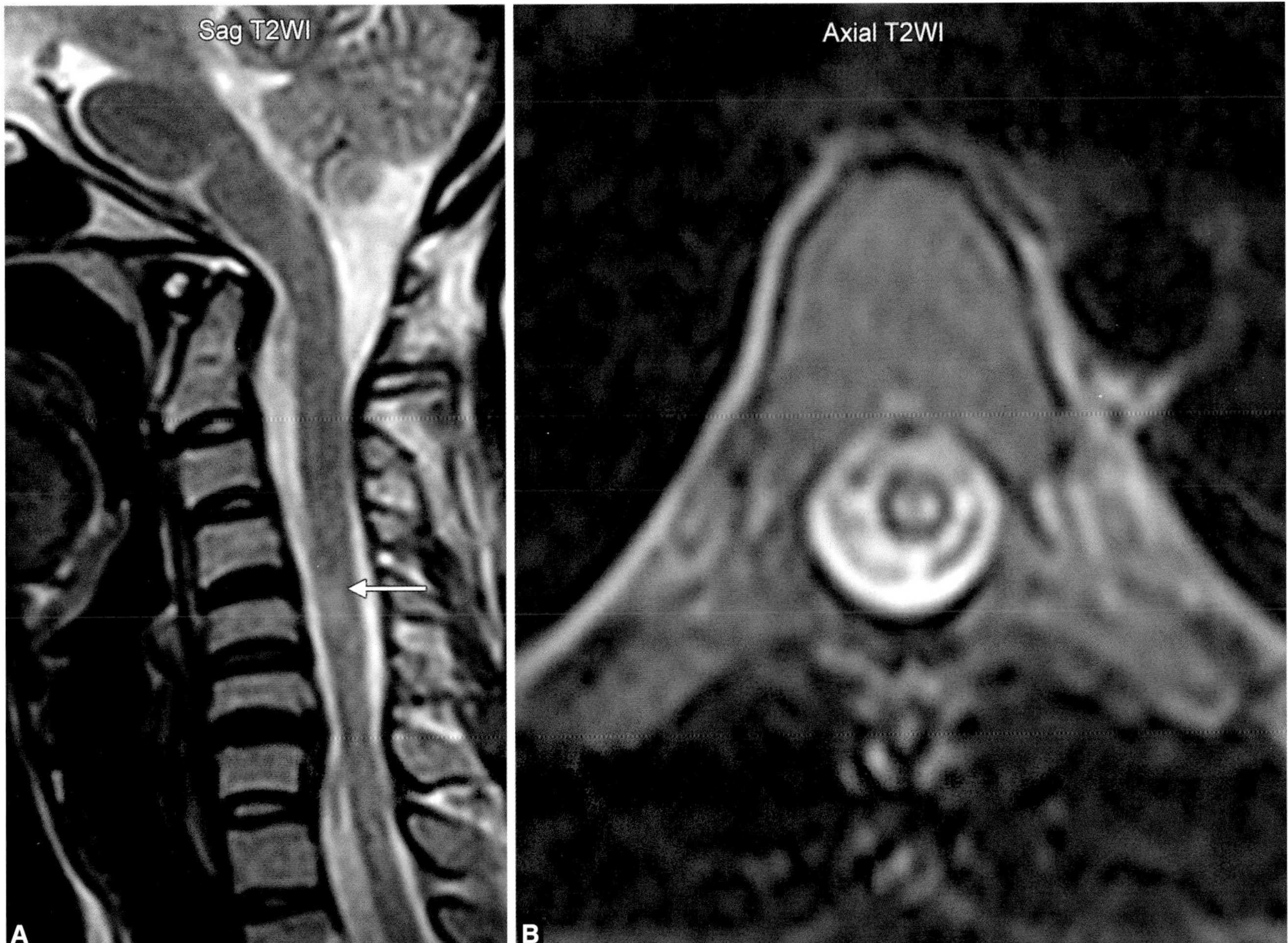

Figs 90A and B: Sagittal and axial T2WI shows high signal intensity within the cord and mild expansion of cord

NEOPLASM

Vertebral Hemangioma

Vertebral hemangiomas are slow-growing benign primary neoplasms of capillary, cavernous or venous origin. The most common histologic type is cavernous hemangioma. These lesions are composed of mature thin-walled vessels and large blood-filled endothelium-lined spaces. They are usually asymptomatic, but may very occasionally be associated with spinal cord compression requiring surgery. Most vertebral hemangiomas are located in the vertebral body; some lesions involve only part of the vertebral body.

On MR, T1W and T2W images, fatty matrix is seen as hyperintense (Figs 91A to C) in the vertebral body. The matrix shows hypointense foci due to bony trabeculation or vascular channels. Vertebral hemangiomas always have a relation to the course of the basivertebral vessels and their anastomosis with intraspinal and paraspinal vessels. Hemangiomas may be discrete and well-defined or diffuse and ill-defined. They may be single or multiple.

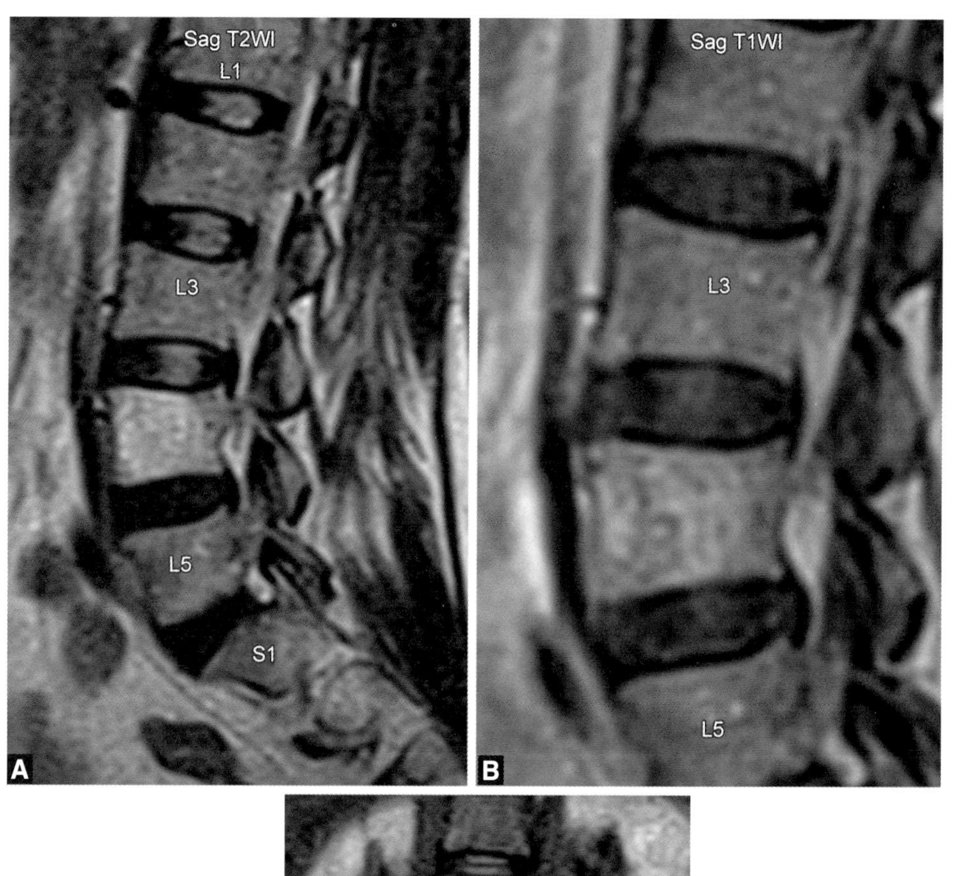

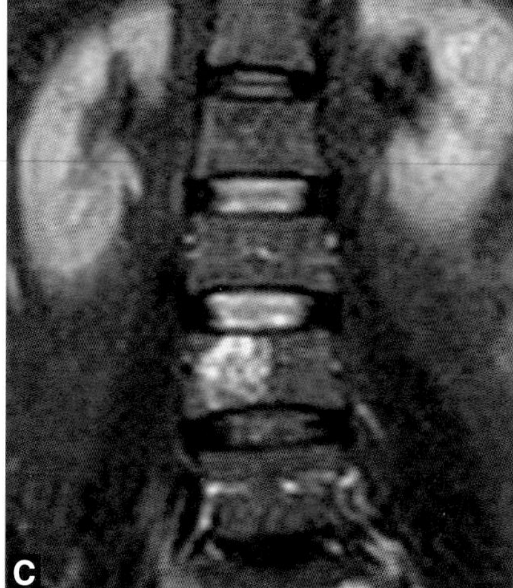

Figs 91A to C: Sagittal T2WI (A and B) and coronal T1WI (C) shows hyperintense lesion seen in the body of L4 vertebra suggestive of hemangioma

Spinal Dermoid

Spinal dermoid is rare developmental benign, slow growing tumor arising from more than one of the three primitive germ cell layers. It is commonly intramural in location, most often seen in lumbosacral region and cauda equina but rarely in cervical and thoracic spine. Dermoid tumors have variable imaging appearance depending upon presence of fluid, soft tissue, calcium and lipid contents in the lesion and typically demonstrate heterogeneous signal intensity on MR imaging.

MR is helpful in detecting intraspinal dermoid tumors and delineating their extent. Most lesions are hyperintense on T1W and T2W sequences due to presence of fat in the lesion which is confirmed on fat-suppression sequences. The soft tissue component usually enhances after administration of intravenous contrast medium. Non-enhanced CT scan help in diagnosis of dermoid tumor by confirming the presence of fat and calcification within the lesion (Figs 92A to F).

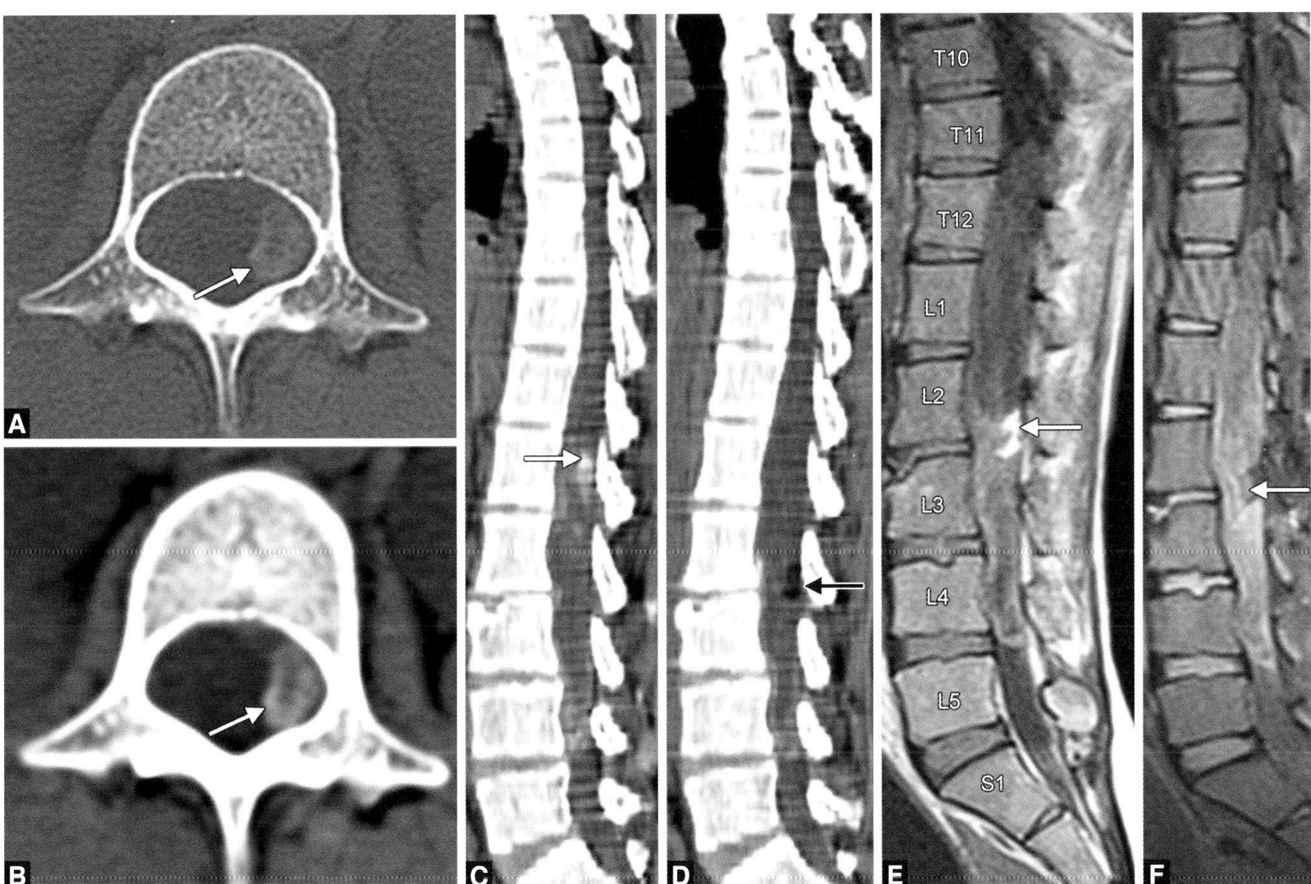

Figs 92A to F: CT scan of spine in bone window (A) and soft tissue window (B) show intradural mass lesion. Sagittal reformation (C and D) shows the presence of calcification (white arrow) and fat (black arrow) within the lesion with widening of spinal canal. Sagittal T1 (E) MRI images reveal heterogeneous intraspinal mass lesion extends from D11-12 to L4-L5 level with suppression of hyperintense signal (arrow) on fat suppression image (F)

Spinal Cord Lipoma

Lipomas are rare spinal cord tumors, representing 6 percent of intramedullary tumors. It is important to differentiate true intramedullary lipoma from cauda equina lipomas or lipomas associated with dysraphism. Often no cleavage plane from the surrounding spinal cord is found at surgery. Therefore, the tumor usually cannot be completely resected without causing neurological damage.

The tumor shows hyperintensity on T1WI and T2WI (Figs 93A and B) and is suppressed on fat sat images (Fig. 93C). These tumors consist of fully differentiated adipose tissue with or without a minor component of fibrous or vascular tissue.

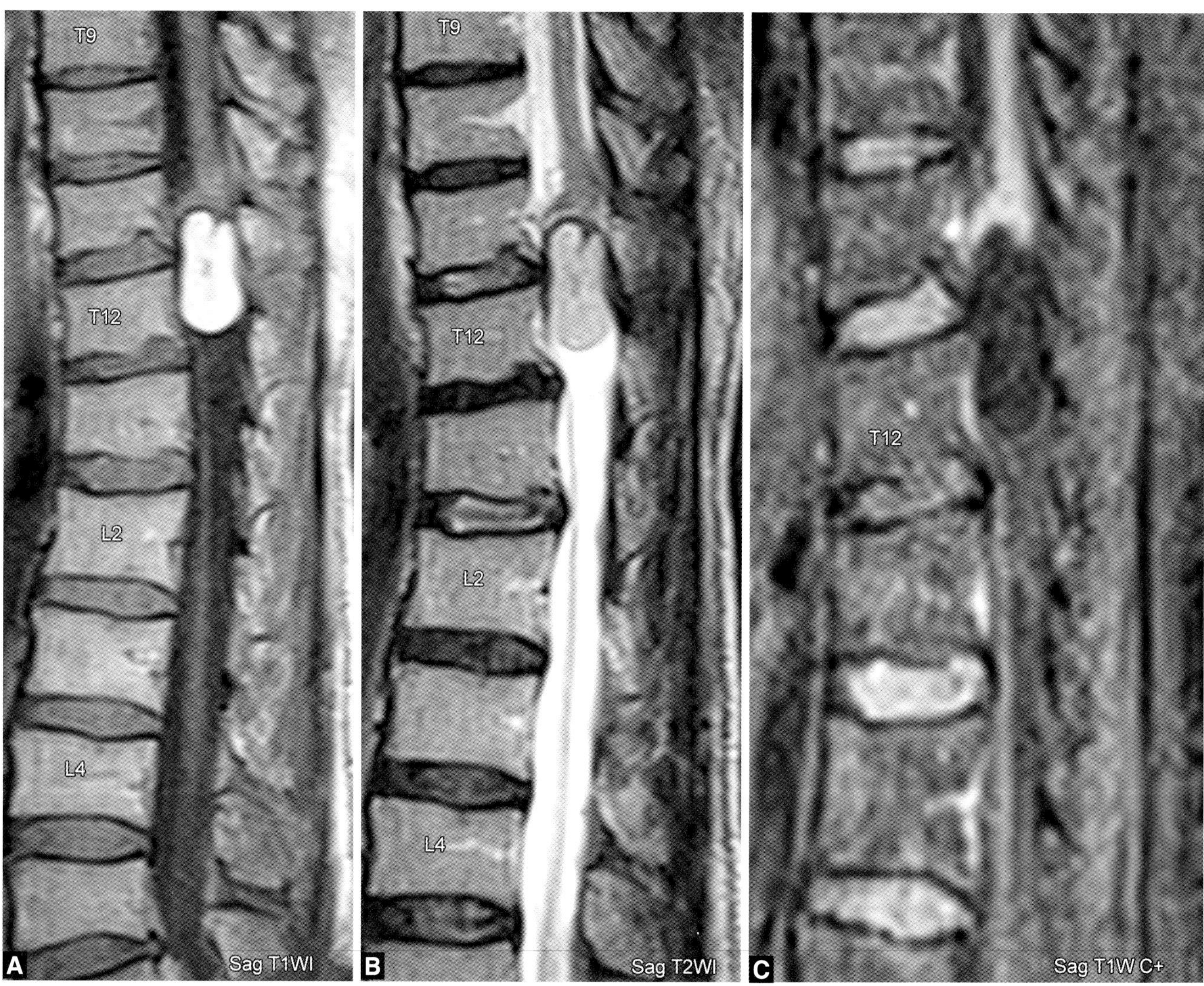

Figs 93A to C: Sagittal T1WI (A) and T2WI (B) shows hyperintense mass lesion extending from lower half of D11 vertebral body upto D12 level. The mass appear hypointense on postcontrast fat sat image (C) confirming the diagnosis to be spinal lipoma

Spinal Meningioma

Spinal meningiomas are benign tumors. The ratio of spinal to intracranial meningiomas is about 1:8. The peak incidence is in the fifth and sixth decade, more commonly seen in women. Ninety percent of spinal meningiomas are intradural, most occour lateral to spinal cord. The thoracic spine is the most common site, followed by the cervical spine.

Motor and sensory deficits are presenting symptoms in 90 and 60 percent of patients respectively. Sphincter dysfunction and pain occour in about 50 percent of cases. Spinal meningiomas are slow growing neoplasms, and complete tumor removal is achieved in the vast majority of patients.

Plain films are usually normal. MR myelography demonstrares a mass localized to the intradural, extramedullary compartment (Fig. 94C). The subarachnoid space on the side of the lesion are displaced away from the mass and sharp meniscus is generally seen.

MR scans demonstrate most intradural meningiomas, clearly delineating their extension and relationship to the spinal cord. Most meningiomas are isointense with the spinal cord on both T1 (Fig. 94A) and T2WI. Moderate, relatively homogeneous enhancement (Fig. 94B) is seen following contrast administration. Most spinal meningiomas have a broad base dural attachment and a dural tail sign is seen in some cases.

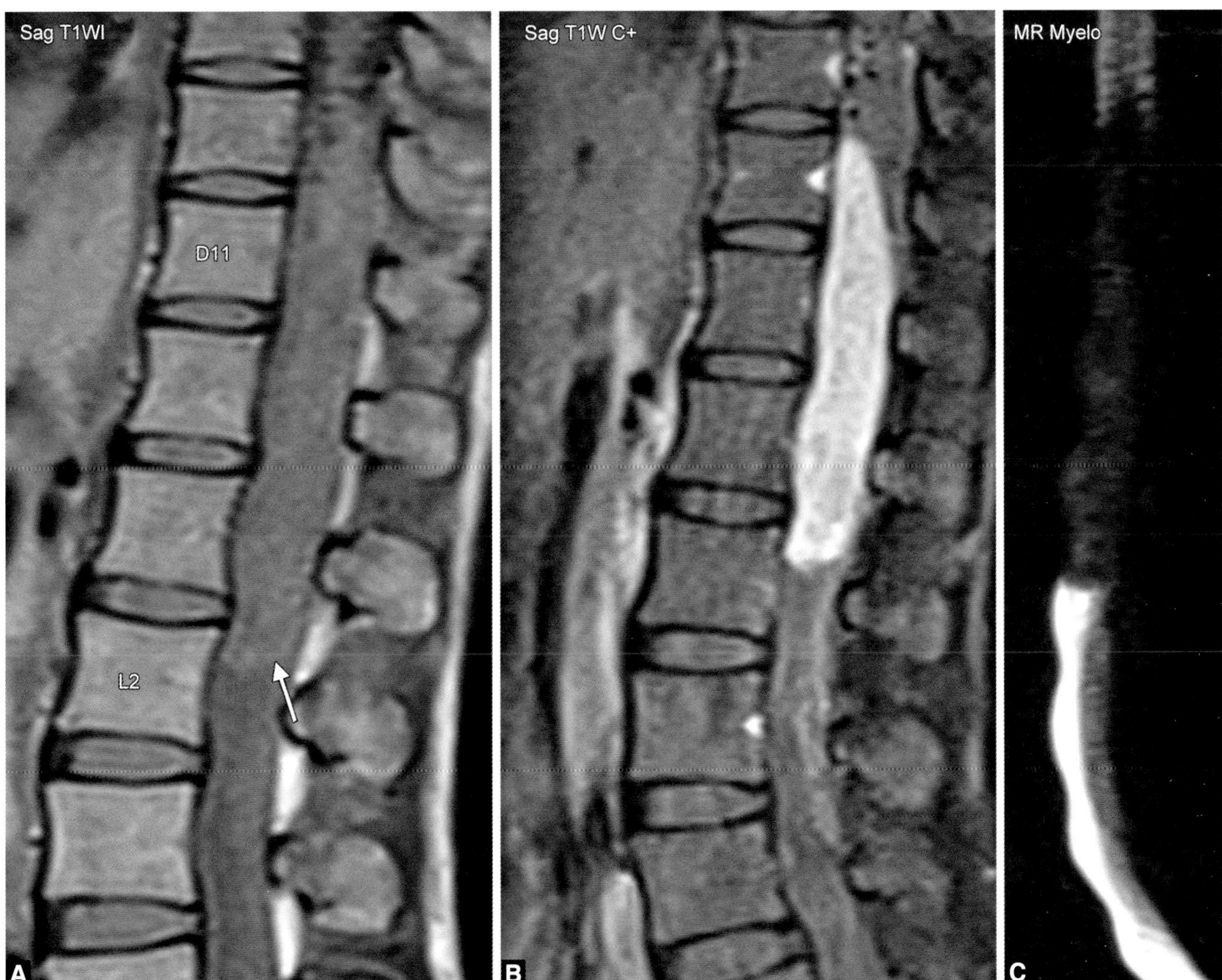

Figs 94A to C: In a 52-year-old female sagittal T1WI (A) shows isointense intradural mass extending from D11 to L2 vertebra (arrow), postcontrast sagittal T1WI (B) shows moderately homogeneous enhancing intradural mass. MR myelography (C) shows a mass localized to the intradural, extramedullary compartment

Spinal Cord Ependymomas

Ependymomas originate from the ependymal or subependymal cells that line the ventricular walls and the central canal of the spinal cord. The typical ependymoma is located in the cervical region. An ependymoma is a well-delineated tumor of neuroepithelial tissue, composed of neoplastic ependymal cells developing perivascular pseudorosettes. Most ependymomas are slow growing and correspond to WHO grade II. Some ependymomas show histological anaplasia and vascular proliferation. This type of tumor corresponds to WHO grade III.

On noncontrast CT ependymomas are isodense with calcification in 50 percent. Enhancement is mild to moderate. On MR ependymomas are hyperintense on T2WI (Figs 95A and B) and iso-to hypointense on T1WI. The lesions are well circumscribed and show post contrast enhancement. Calcification is less conspicuous than on CT, whereas cysts and small hemorrhagic foci are frequently better and are better demonstrated on MRI.

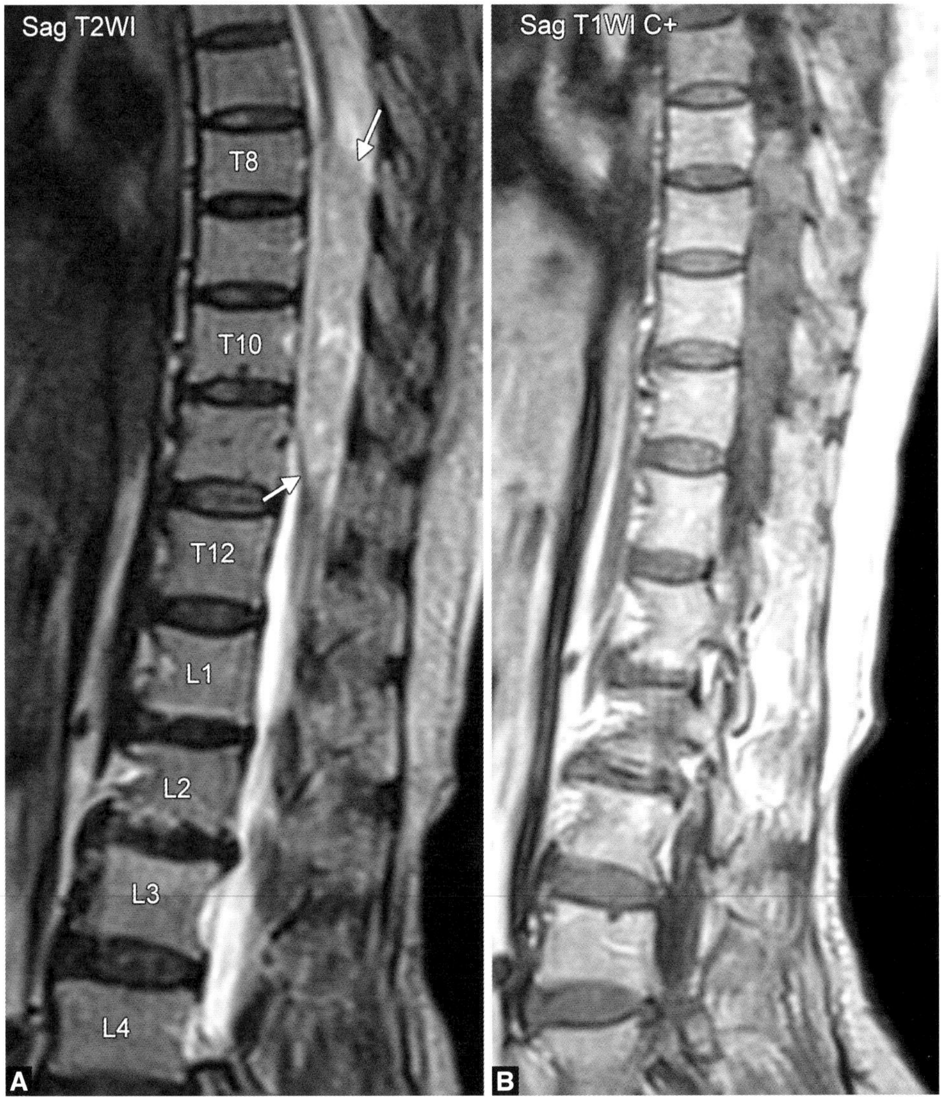

Figs 95A and B: Sagittal T2WI shows isointense to hyperintense intramedullary mass extending from D8 to D11 (arrow). Postcontrast sagittal T1WI shows mild to moderate enhancement within the mass

Neurogenic Tumors

Neurogenic tumors account for 16 percent of mediastinal tumors; about 10 percent of neurogenic tumors invade the spinal canal, and are called dumb-bell tumors because of their shape. Surgery is the first-choice of treatment, in these cases surgical resection is difficult because it expands outside and inside the spinal canal via the intervertebral foramen.

Nerve sheath tumors are one of the most common intraspinal tumors and together with meningiomas, constitute 90 percent of all intradural-extramedullary tumors. Schwannoma, neurilemmoma, neuroma and neurofibroma are all grouped under nerve sheath tumors. MR imaging differentiation between these tumors is difficult and is preferably referred as "neurogenic tumors".

Neurofibroma arises from nonspecific cells in the nerve sheath. It is a benign expansile lesion through which the nerve passes. When it grows in size it enlarges the foramina through which it passes giving it a dumb-bell appearance (Figs 96A and B) or contiguous bones undergo pressure erosion leading to bony defect. On MRI, neurofibromas have intermediate signal intensity on T1-weighted images, very high signal intensity on T2-weighted images and following gadolinium enhancement (Figs 96A to D).

The clinical symptoms and presentation of nerve sheath tumors are usually indistinguishable from those associated with disc herniation. Back pain,

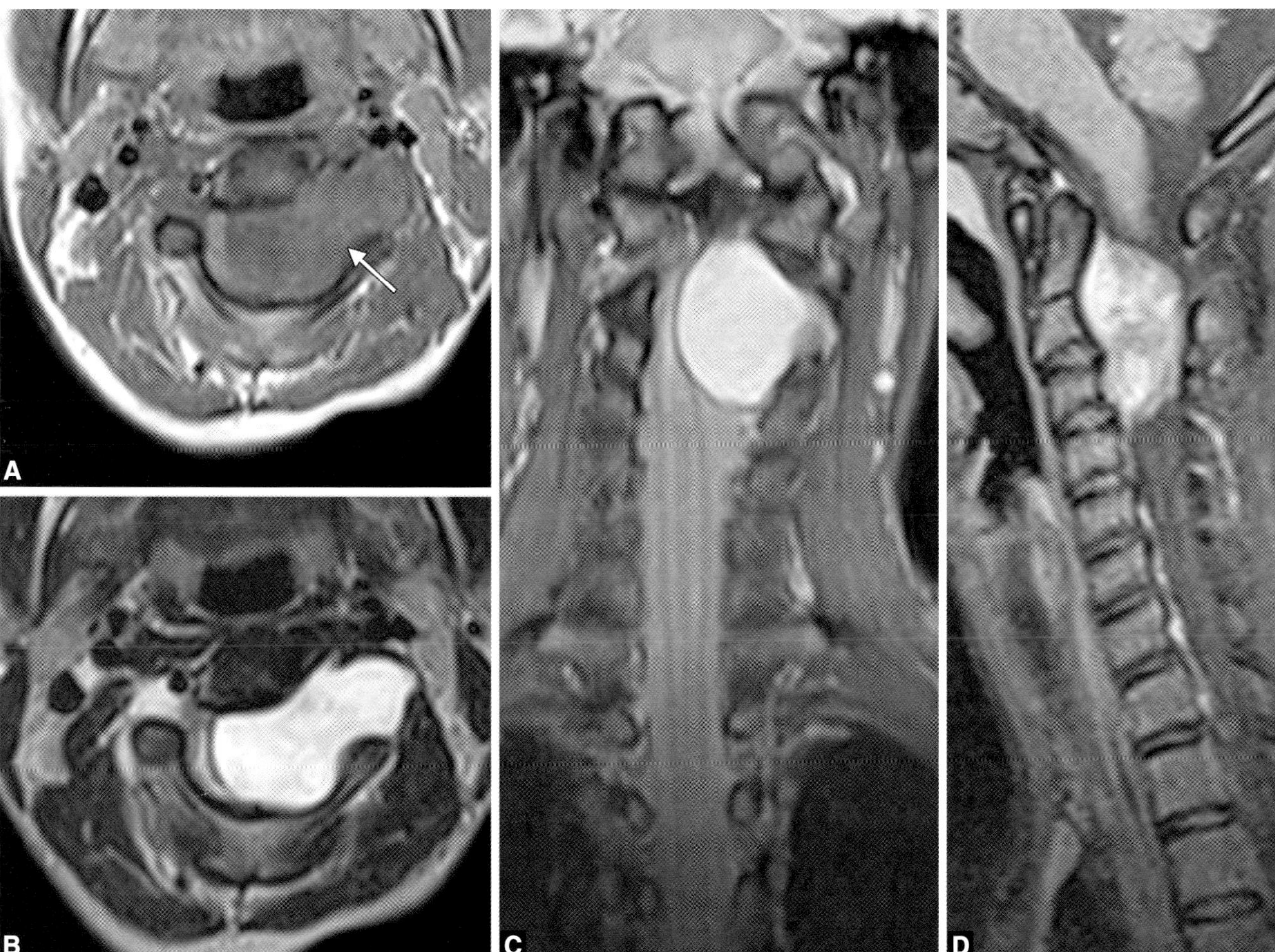

Figs 96A to D: A well-defined dumb-bell shaped lesion is seen in the spinal canal, left neural foramen and left paraspinal region. The left neural foramen is widened. It is hypointense on T1 (A), hyperintense on T2 (B) and shows moderate homogeneous enhancement on postcontrast T1W images (D). Coronal T2W (C) image reveals compression and displacement of the cord to right

radiculopathy, paraesthesia and limb weakness are the most common presenting symptoms. Myelopathic symptoms may occur if the tumor compresses the spinal cord.

The radiographic findings if present are characteristic (Figs 97A and B) with scalloped bony erosion of the posterior vertebral bodies, erosion of the pedicles and widening of neural foramina are the most common radiographic findings. In the presence of a dumb-bell tumor, a paraspinal soft tissue mass may be detected radiographically.

On CT, the lesions appear either as an intraspinal mass or intraspinal lesion with an extradural and or paraspinal component. Bony erosion of the vertebral bodies is well seen on CT (Figs 98A to F).

MR imaging is presently the imaging modality of choice for all forms of spinal tumors. The majority of neurogenic tumors are isointense relative to the spinal cord on T1-weighted images, while 25 percent are hypointense (Figs 99A to D). These tumors appear hyperintense relative to spinal cord on T2-weighted images (Figs 100 and 101). Homogeneous intense contrast enhancement is commonly seen as seen in (Figs 102 and 103). Bony erosion of the vertebral bodies and widening of intervertebral foramina are also well seen on MR imaging.

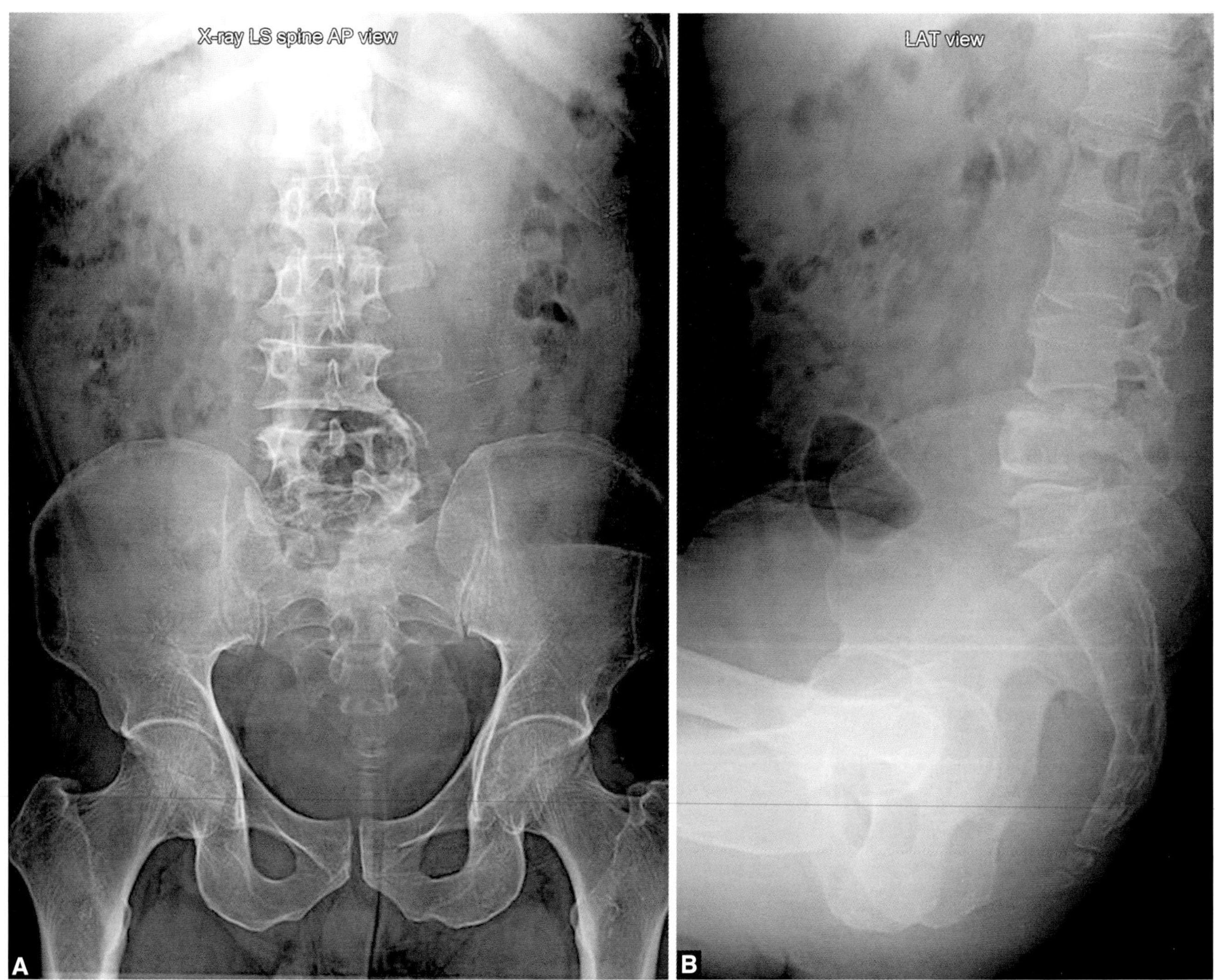

Figs 97A and B: X-ray LS spine AP and lateral views reveals lytic lesion involving L4 and L5 vertebral bodies with erosion of left pedicle and widened neural foramen

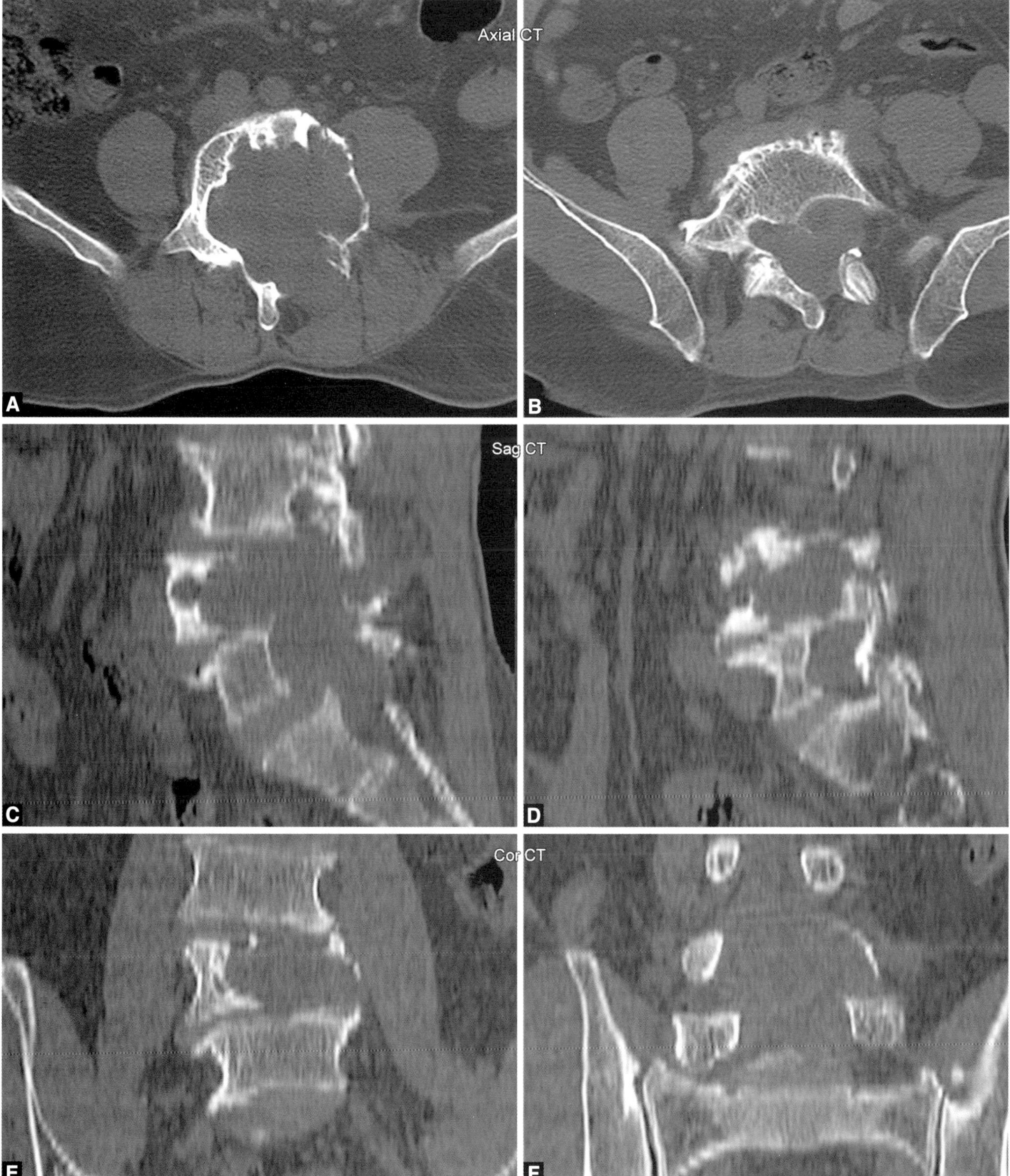

Figs 98A to F: CT axial (A and B), reformatted sagittal (C and D) and coronal (E and F) images demonstrates severe scalloping of L4 and L5 vertebrae with widened spinal canal and left neural foramen with thinning of pedicles

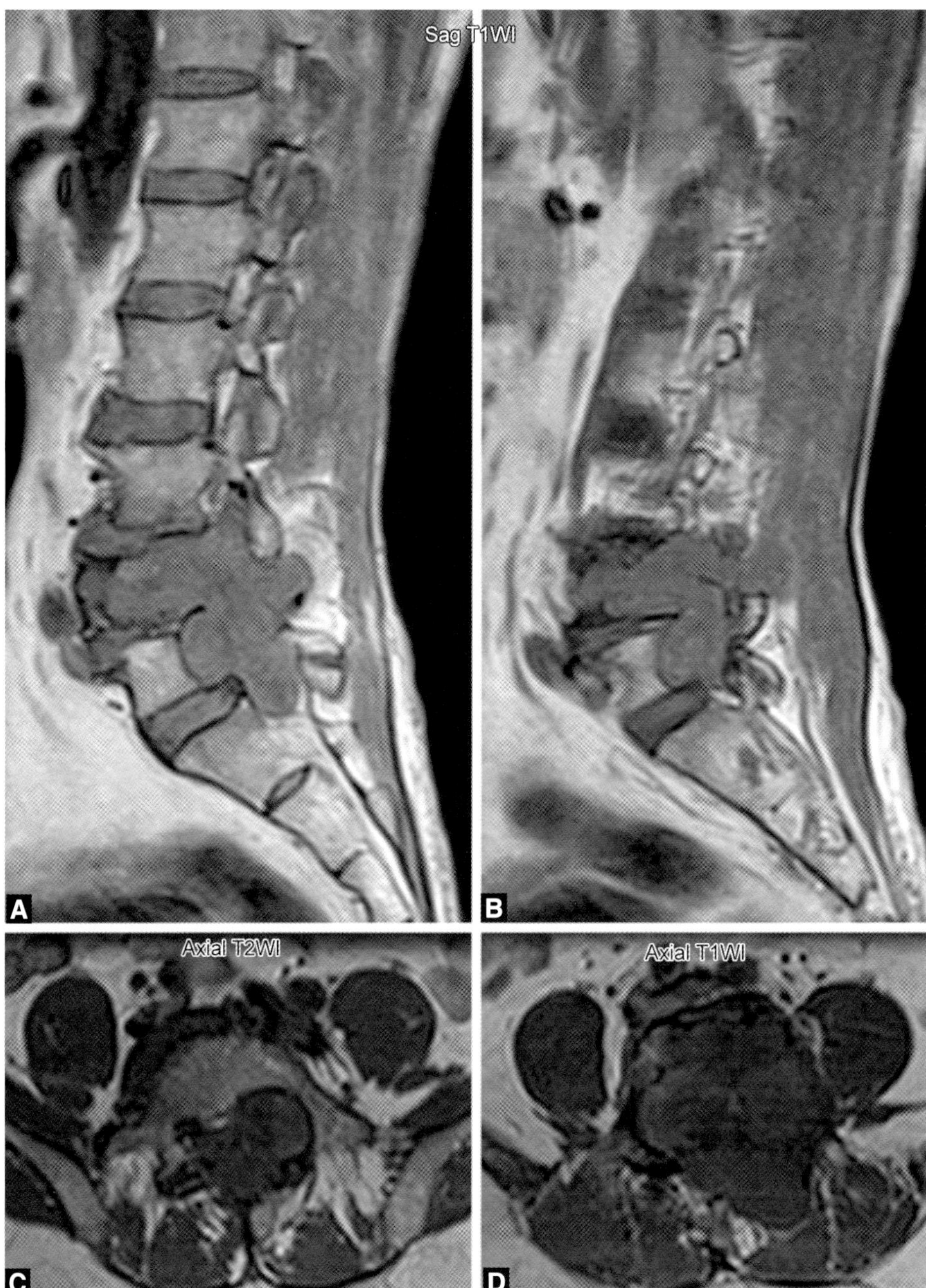

Figs 99A to D: Sagittal T1 (A and B) and axial T1WI (C and D) weighted images reveals hypointense lesion involving the spinal canal with its widening and scalloping of the surrounding bones

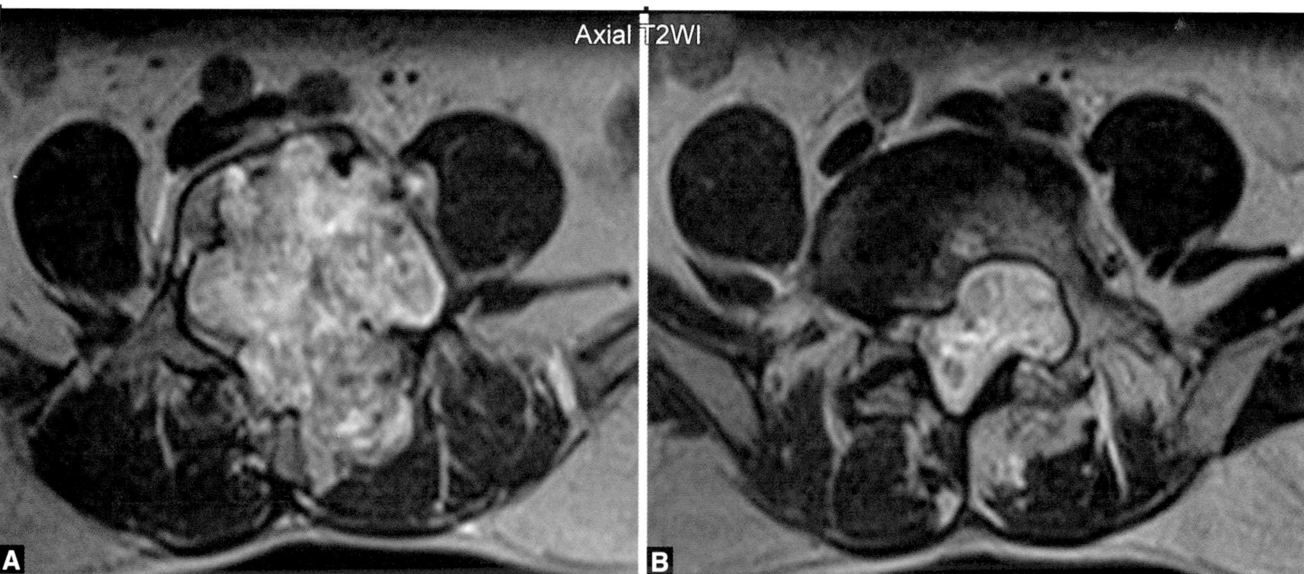

Figs 100A and B: Axial T2WI reveals large hyperintense lesion involving the spinal canal with its widening and scalloping of the surrounding bones including vertebral body

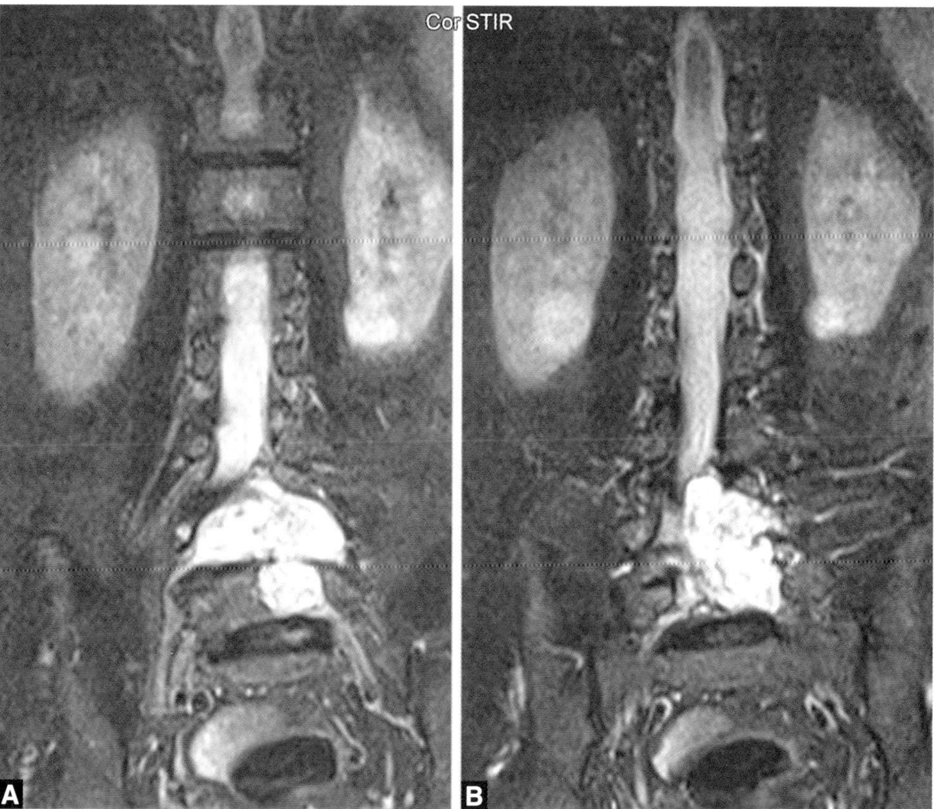

Figs 101A and B: The lesion is hyperintense on coronal STIR images

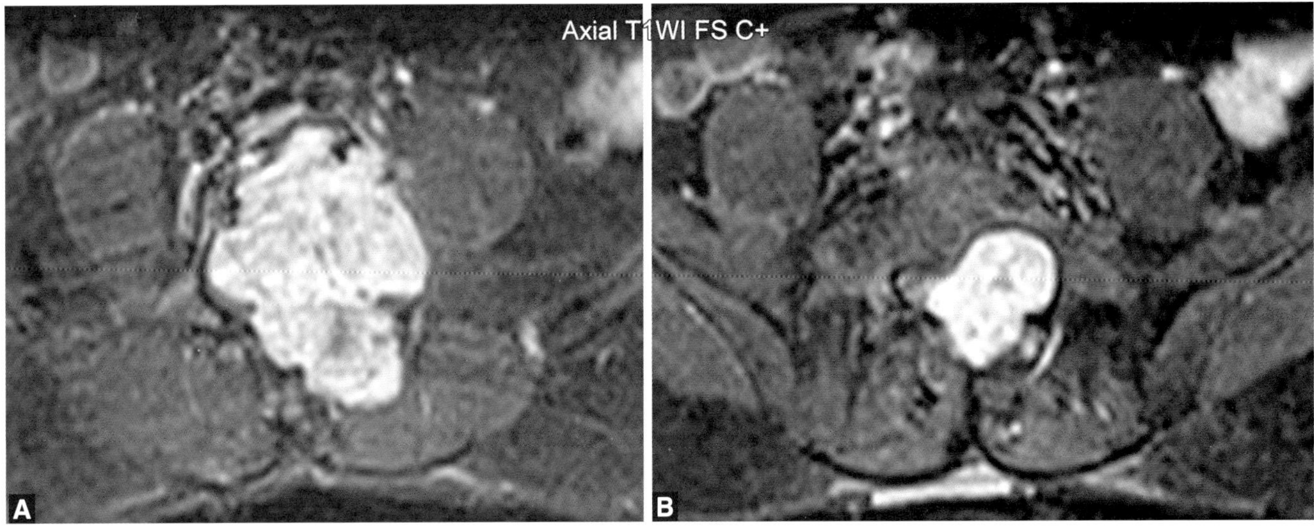

Figs 102A and B: Intense postcontrast enhancement of the lesion is seen in the post Gadolinium contrast T1 FS axial images

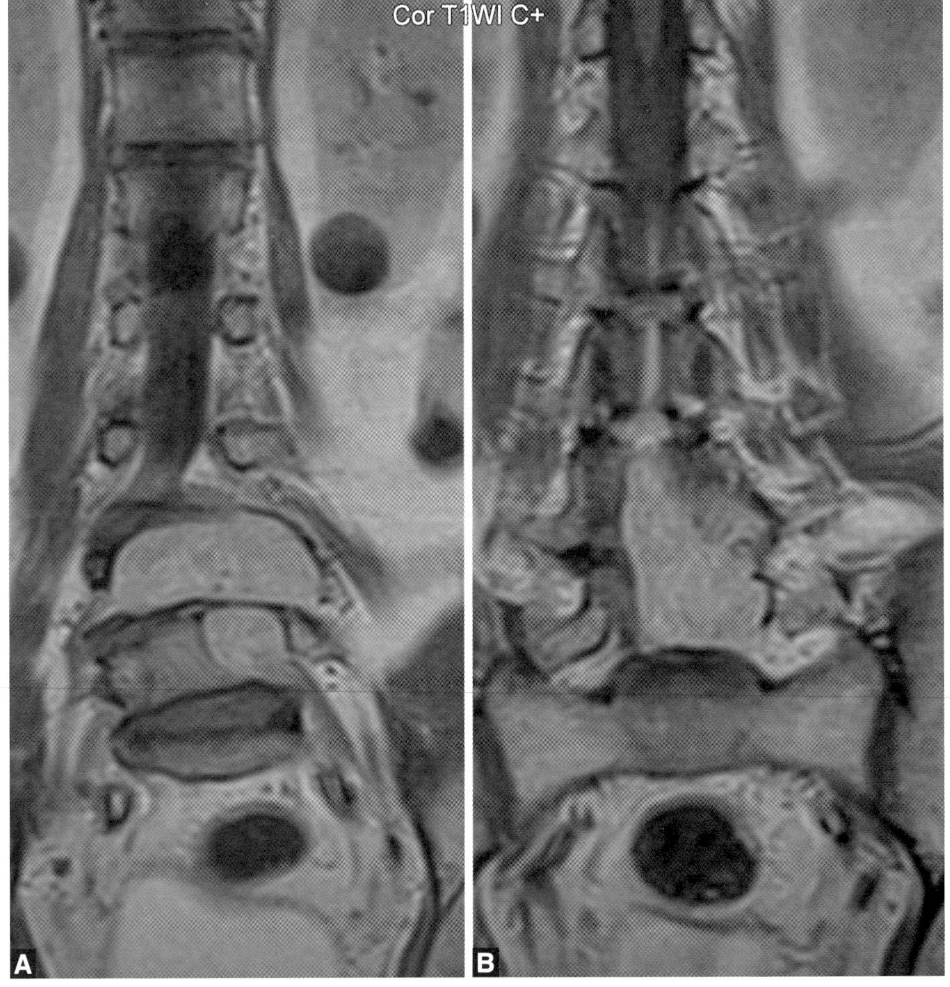

Figs 103A and B: Intense postcontrast enhancement of the lesion is seen in the post Gadolinium contrast T1 coronal images

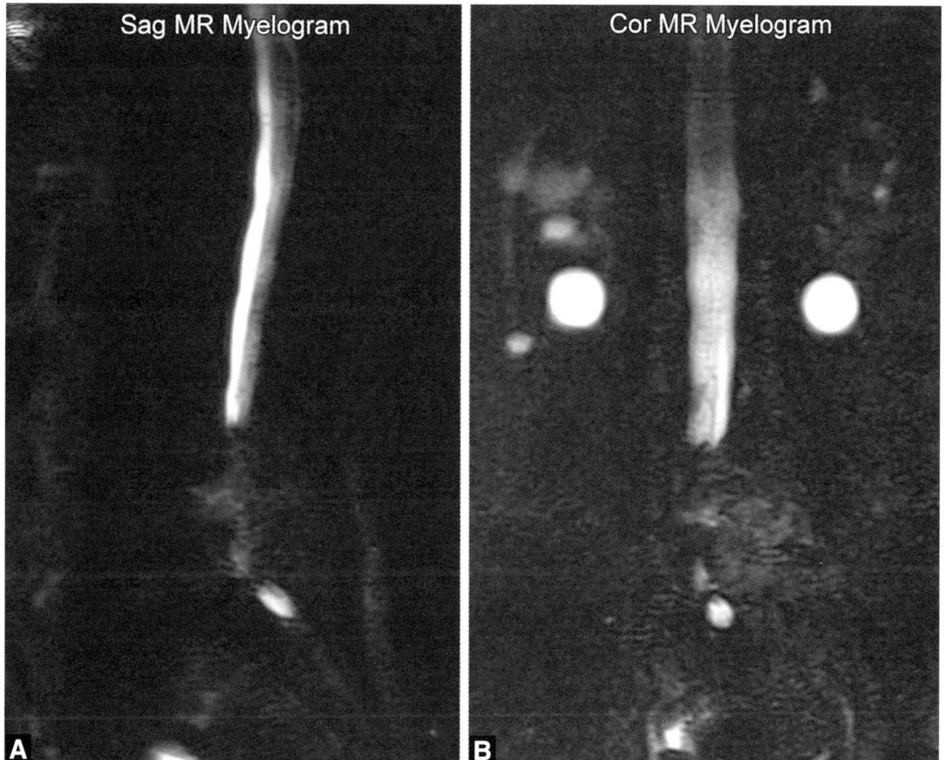

Figs 104A and B: MR myelography images reveal complete myelographic block at L4 and L5 vertebral levels

On MR myelogram these appear as an intradural extramedullary lesion with displacement of the spinal cord. The subarachnoid space is widened above and below the tumor ipsilaterally, and there is a sharp interface between the contrast and undersurface of the tumor (Figs 104A and B).

Other tumors such as paraganglioma and ganglioglioma are rarer. Paragangliomas may present as intraspinal tumors that are most commonly located in the cauda equine and filum terminale. These lesions are isointense on T1-weighted and hyperintense on T2-weighted MR images. Intense enhancement is usually present after the administration of contrast agent. Ganglioneuromas are tumors composed of mature ganglion cells and frequently arise from the paraspinal region, mimicking dumb-bell tumors. Scalloped bony erosion of the vertebral bodies and extension into the intervertebral foramina are frequently present. However, the age of the patient may help suggest the correct diagnosis, as these tumors are most typically found in children and young adults.

The major differential diagnoses of intraspinal extramedullary tumors include meningioma and drop metastases. Meningiomas are slightly less common than nerve sheath tumors, and account for 25 percent of all spinal tumors. Meningiomas tend to occur in the thoracic region in women over 40 years of age. The location is somewhat different from that of nerve sheath tumors. Metastasis is another differential diagnosis of an intradural-extramedullary lesion. Intradural metastatic lesions may arise from primary tumors of the central nervous system (CNS) or from outside the CNS. The most common primary CNS tumor is germinoma, pineal tumor, ependymoma and medulloblastoma. Carcinomas of the breast, lung, melanoma, lymphoma and leukemia are the most frequent non-CNS sources of intradural metastases.

Sacrococcygeal Teratoma

A teratoma is a germ cell tumor, 40 percent of which are found in the sacrococcygeal region. A mature teratoma is benign, but on imaging it is impossible to exclude malignant components. In the neonate histological malignancy is present in up to 30 perent. The malignant component is usually due to embryonal carcinoma, yolk sac carcinoma or choriocarcinoma. Though histologically malignant, if the tumor is completely excised the prognosis is good. If elements are left behind, or the diagnosis is delayed, the incidence of malignancy increases. Elevated alpha fetoprotein levels can indicate malignancy but unfortunately in the neonatal period this is normally high and does not fall to normal levels until 9 months of age.

A sacrococcygeal tumor in the neonate usually presents as an external mass and where there is a presacral component the infant may also have urinary frequency or retention, or constipation. These are the symptoms in children who present later. Any intra-abdominal extent of disease renders the lesion more likely to be malignant.

The plain film will usually show a rounded mass extending externally in the buttock region. Calcification may be present and there are sometimes formed structures such as bone or occasionally teeth in solid lesions. The spectrum varies from being completely solid through mixed solid and cystic lesions to an almost completely cystic mass.

Full evaluation is best performed by MRI (Figs 105A and B). If there is invasion of the soft tissues or bone it implies malignancy, but the majority of the teratomas do not show this feature and the diagnosis has to be made by histology.

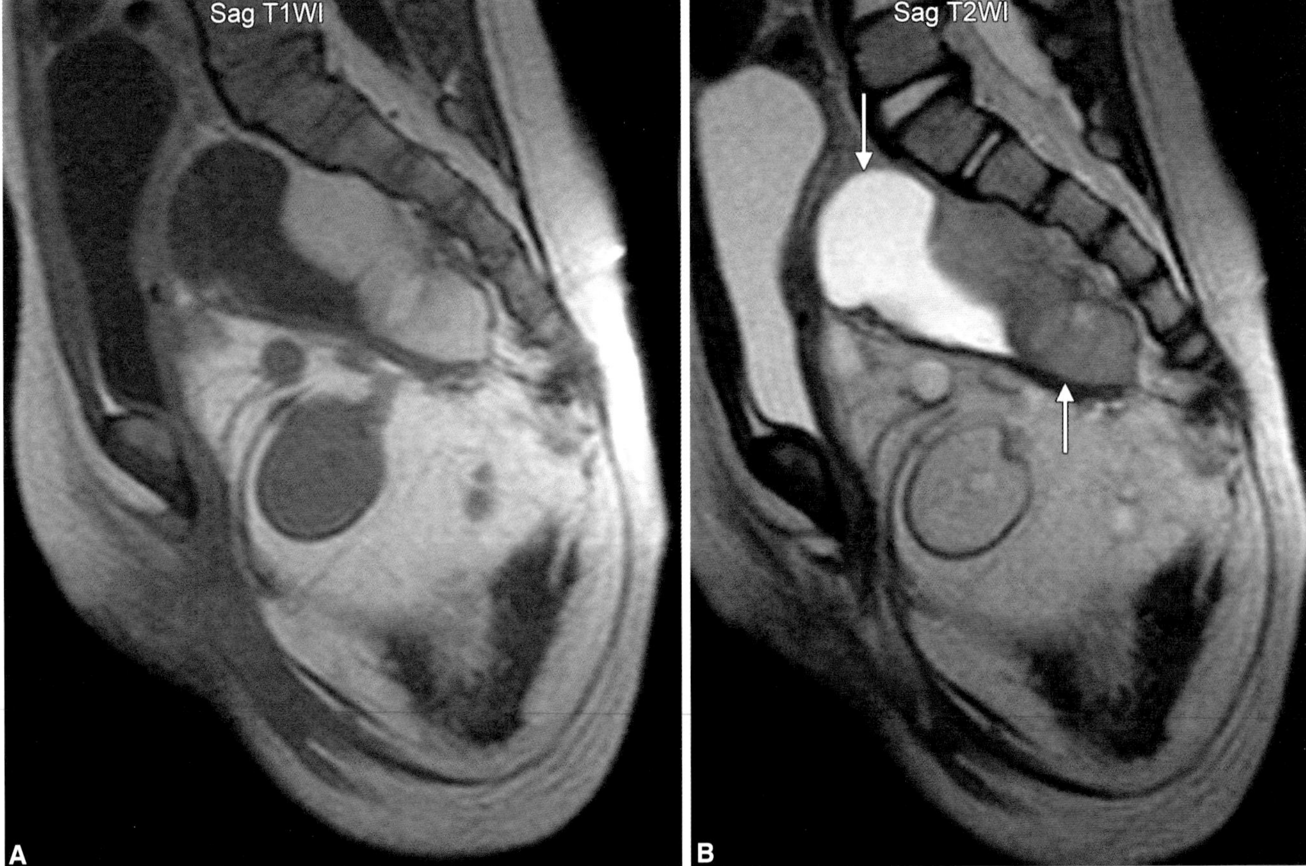

Figs 105A and B: A 1-year-old female child with swelling over the buttock since birth and inability in walking on MR shows a large well-defined heterogeneous lesion in the pelvis posterior to the bladder. It is predominantly fatty with cystic soft tissue component. Superiorly it extends upto the pelvic inlet, inferiorly into the right ischiorectal fossa and laterally upto the lateral pelvic wall (image not displayed). The coccygeal vertebrae reveal altered marrow signal. There is no intraspinal extension (A and B). This lesion measures 11.9 × 5.8 cm. On STIR sequence (not in the figure) the fat component was suppressed with bright cystic component

Pelvis 5

Abhijit Pawar

BICORNUATE UTERUS

Bicornuate uterus is an anomaly resulting from partial failure of Müllerian duct fusion. The resultant septum, composed of myometrium, may extend to the external os (bicornuate bicollis uterus) or to the internal os (bicornuate unicollis uterus). Surgery is required to correct the anomaly.

The diagnosis of bicornuate uterus can be suggested by hysterosalpingography (HSG) or ultrasound but the most definitive and most accurate diagnosis is obtained by magnetic resonance imaging. On MR scans, in bicornuate uterus the intercornual distance is increased; there is an outward fundal concavity compared with the normal convexity; endometrial and myometrial width and ratio are normal; two uterine cornua (Figs 1A and B) and two endometrial cavities are easily identified, and the myometrial characteristics of the septum are accurately diagnosed.

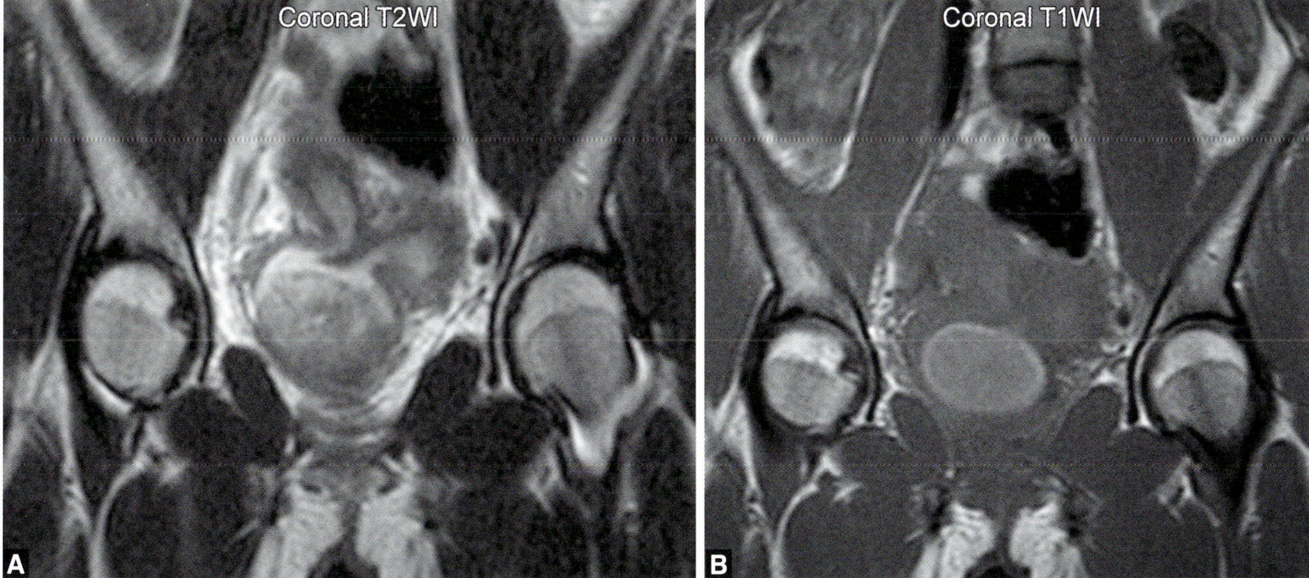

Figs 1A and B: Coronal T2 and T1WI shows two uterine cornua suggestive of bicornuate uterus

UTERINE FIBROIDS

Leiomyomas of the uterus (or uterine fibroids) are benign tumors that arise from the overgrowth of smooth muscle and connective tissue in the uterus. The preferred imaging modality for the evaluation of uterine fibroids is ultrasonography, specifically, transabdominal and transvaginal US.

There are four primary types of uterine fibroids, classified primarily according to location in the uterus:

1. *Subserosal uterine fibroids:* These fibroids develop in the outer portion of the uterus and continue to grow outward.
2. *Intramural uterine fibroids:* The most common type of fibroid. These develop within the uterine wall and expand making the uterus feel larger than normal (which may cause "bulk symptoms").
3. *Submucosal uterine fibroids:* These fibroids develop just under the lining of the uterine cavity. These are the fibroids that have the most effect on heavy menstrual bleeding and the ones that can cause problems with infertility and miscarriage.
4. *Pedunculated fibroids:* Those grow on a small stalk that connects them to the inner or outer wall of the uterus.

Calcified fibroids are often depicted on conventional radiographs of the pelvis. In some patients, Magnetic resonance imaging (MRI) provides additional information.

Fibroids appear as sharply marginated areas of low to intermediate signal intensity on T1 and T2 weighted MRI scans (Figs 2A to E). One third of fibroids have a hyperintense rim on T2-weighted images, as a result of dilated veins, lymphatics, or edema. An inhomogeneous area of high signal intensity may be depicted on T2-weighted images; this results from hemorrhage, hyaline degeneration, edema, or highly cellular fibroids. Intravenous administration of gadolinium-based

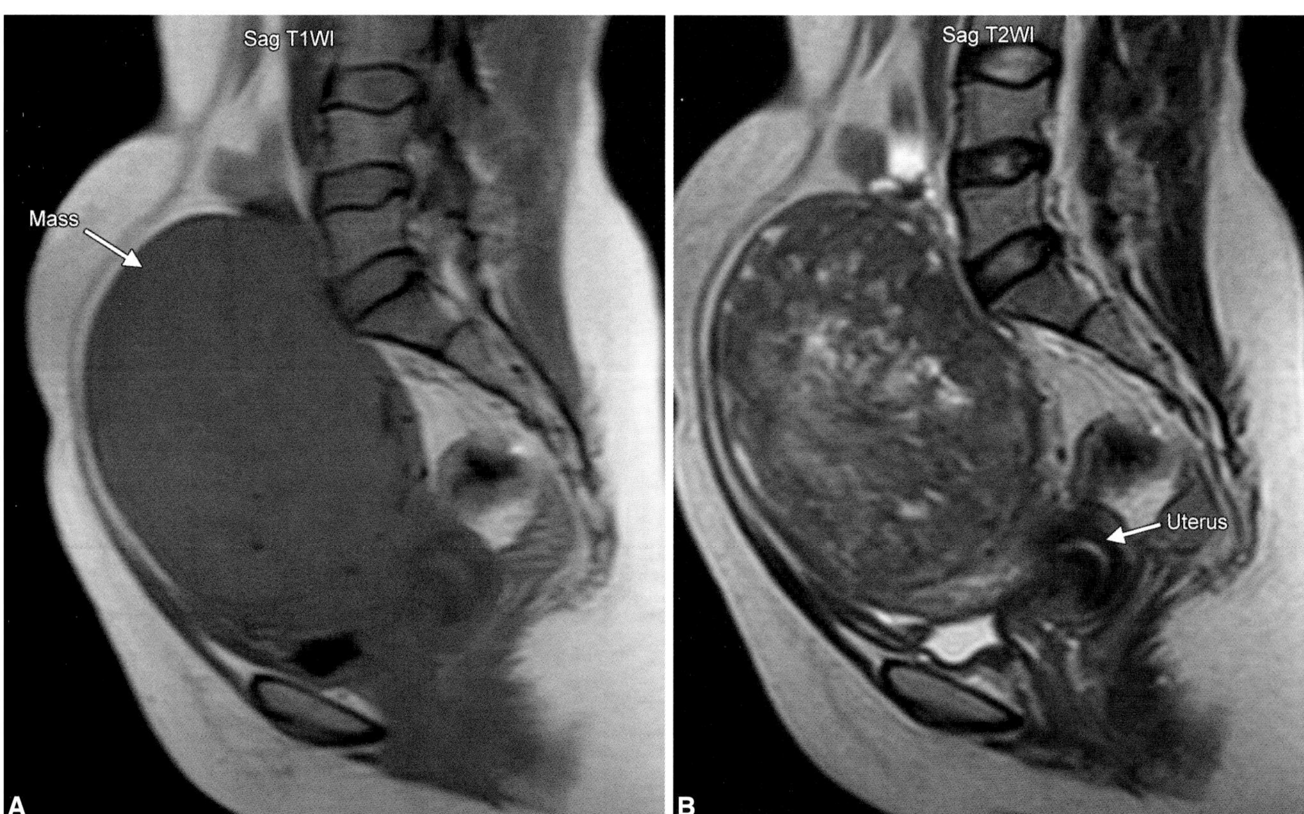

Figs 2A and B

contrast material usually is not required; however, if it is administered, fibroids usually enhance later than does the healthy myometrium. Fibroid enhancement can be hypointense (65%), isointense (23%), or hyperintense (12%) in relation to that of the myometrium.

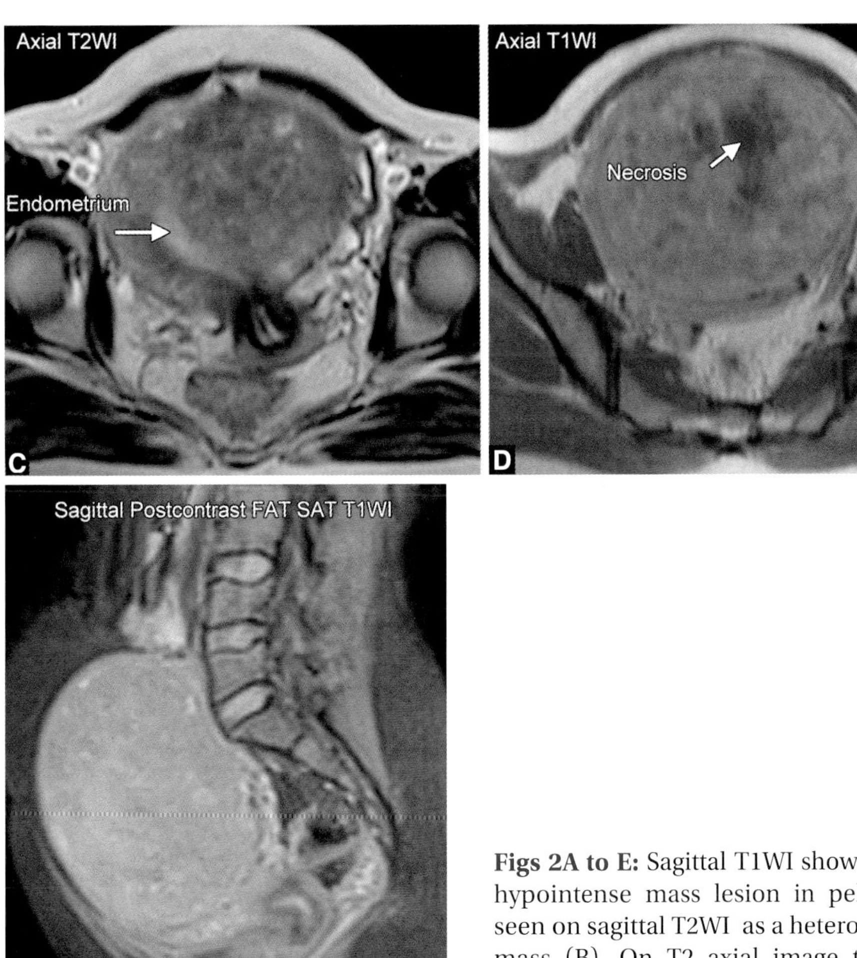

Figs 2C to E

Figs 2A to E: Sagittal T1WI shows a large rounded hypointense mass lesion in pelvis (A) which is seen on sagittal T2WI as a heterogeneous intensity mass (B). On T2 axial image the mass is seen arising from the anterior wall of uterus (C). T1 axial shows hypointense areas within the lesion (D). Postcontrast sagittal fat saturated T1WI shows patchy enhancement within the lesion (E)

BROAD LIGAMENT FIBROID

Tumors of the broad ligaments are rare. The most common solid tumor of the broad ligament is the fibroid. Fibroid can arise from any tissue that contains smooth muscle cells, but most commonly from the uterus. Broad ligament leiomyoma (fibroid) can originate from the uterus and invade the broad ligament or it can originate from the broad ligament itself. These benign tumors are usually asymptomatic. However, if the leiomyoma reaches significant size, it can distort the anatomy of the pelvis, pushing the uterus to the contralateral side (Figs 3A and B), and it can potentially compress the ureter, which leads to hydronephrosis. This tumor is extremely difficult to remove without interfering with important organs or the blood supply to the uterus.

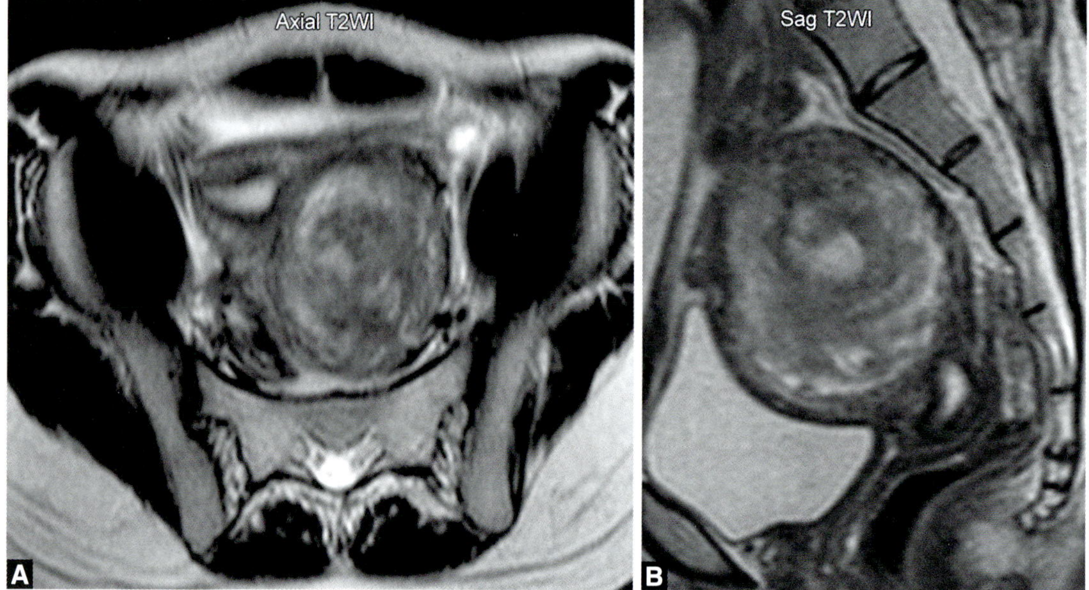

Figs 3A and B: Axial and sagittal T2W images reveal broad ligament fibroid on left side appearing hypointense on T2W image, displacing uterus to right side

OVARIAN DERMOID CYST

Ovarian dermoid is a cyst lined by an epidermis-like epithelium and containing variable mesodermal, endodermal and ectodermal derivatives such as sebaceous secretions, hair, teeth, bone or fat. Dermoid cysts are common, accounting for 20 to 25 percent of all ovarian neoplasms. They can occur at any age, but are commoner in the reproductive years. Unilateral it may be associated with pregnancy (Figs 4A and B). They are the most common ovarian tumor under the age of 30. The tumor is bilateral in 10 to 15 percent of cases. The tumors are slow growing, and many are discovered incidentally. The tumors may cause pain, dysmenorrhea and pelvic pressure.

Complications include torsion, rupture, infection and hemorrhage. Torsion occurs in up to 10 percent of dermoids, and is common in dermoids when compared to other ovarian tumors. This may be because the tumor is often pedunculated. Perforation is rare, and may be acute, presenting as an acute abdomen, or chronic. In the latter case, slow leakage of sebaceous material from the cyst may cause a granulomatous peritonitis and result in a gross appearance resembling ovarian cancer, both on imaging and at surgery. Rupture may be triggered by pregnancy. Three very rare medical complications may develop; thyrotoxicosis (due to thyroid tissue), carcinoid syndrome (due to carcinoid tissue), or autoimmune hemolytic anemia.

Malignant transformation is rare, occurring in 1 to 2 percent of cases. The risk is greater in postmenopausal women.

Plain radiographs show pelvic calcifications, resembling teeth or bone, in 50 percent of cases, ultrasound (US) may show a solid cystic, or mixed solid and cystic adnexal mass. Sonographic features that suggest the specific diagnosis of dermoid cyst are the presence of hair, teeth, or Rokitansky protuberances (rounded polypoid soft tissue masses projecting into the lumen). CT and MRI show contents of the cyst and are diagnostic modalities.

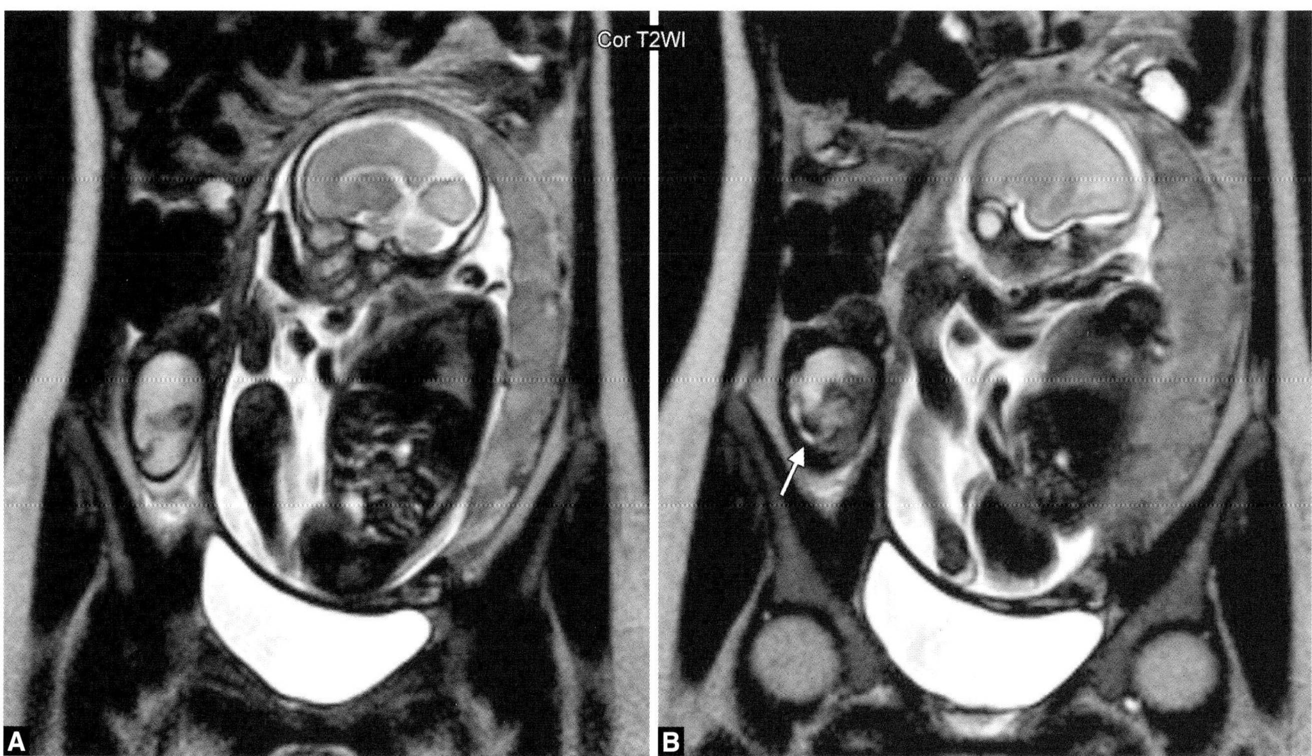

Figs 4A and B: MR of a 25-year-old pregnant female on coronal T2W images show intrauterine fetus and a heterogeneous lesion in right ovary, predominantly hyperintense with few hypointense areas within the lesion, suggestive of calcification or hemorrhage

OVARIAN MASSES

Functional cysts and benign neoplasms are the most common ovarian masses. Ovarian cancer is the most common genital tract malignancy.

Ovarian cysts: The most commonly encountered benign ovarian condition is physiologic cysts. Ultrasonography is the primary imaging tool. Simple cysts are unilocular and have a uniformly thin wall surrounding a single cavity that contains no internal echoes (Figs 5A to D), most commonly represent functional follicular or luteal cysts and less commonly, serous cystadenomas (Figs 6A to E) or inclusion cysts. Ovarian torsion occurs as a result

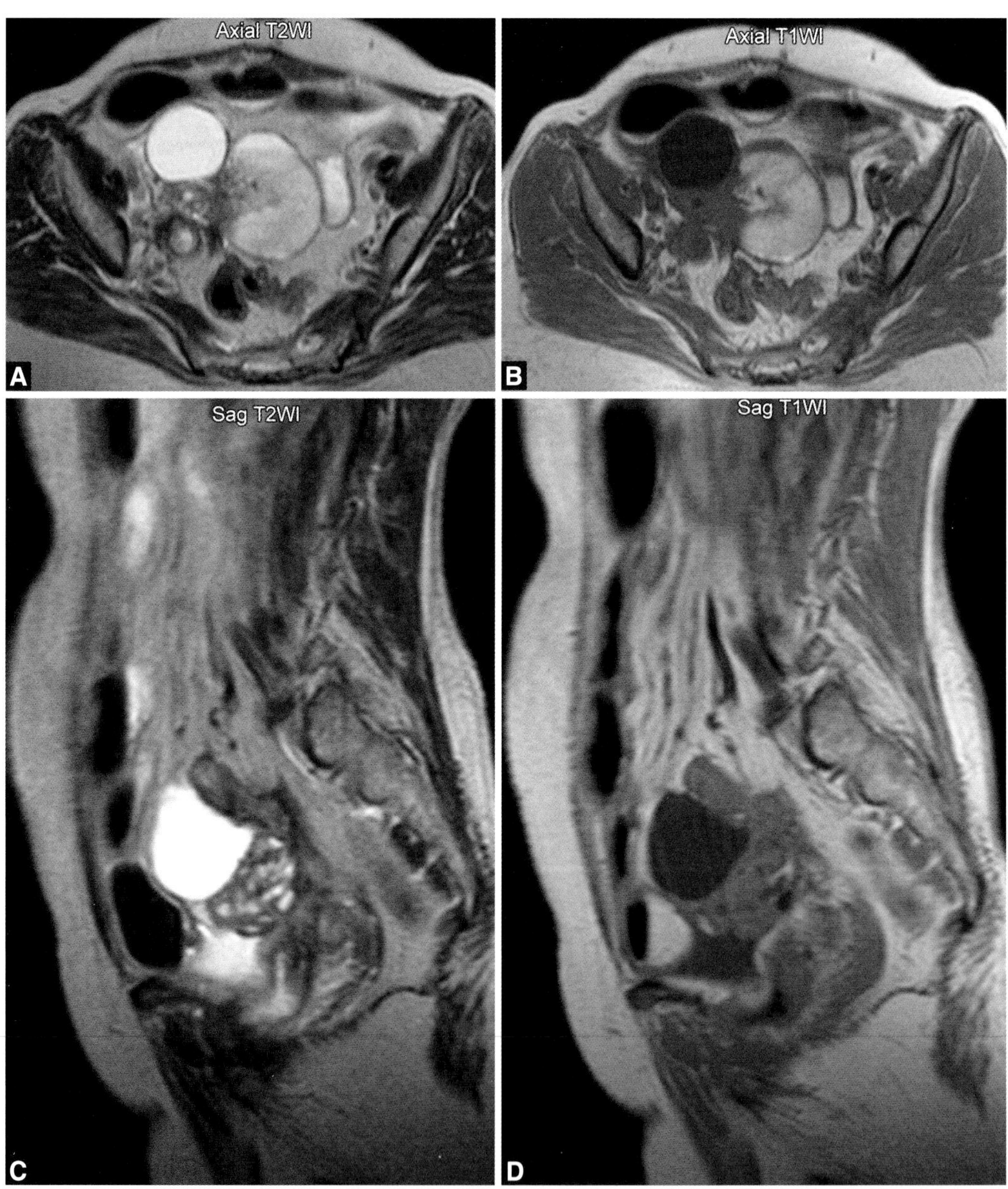

Figs 5A to D: An approximately 4 cm in diameter, well-defined cystic lesion is seen in the right adnexa, it is hyperintense on T2WI and hypointense on T1W image suggestive of simple ovarian cyst

of twisting of the ovary around its vascular pedicle, leading to ischemia, most commonly associated with ovarian or paraovarian cysts. Complex cysts have more than one compartment (multilocular) with thickening of the wall, projections sticking into the lumen or on the surface and abnormalities within the cyst contents (Figs 6A to E). Malignant cysts usually fall within this category, as do many benign neoplastic cysts. Hemorrhagic cysts, endometriomas and dermoids tend to have characteristic features on sonograms that may help to differentiate them from malignant complex cysts. CT scanning is inferior to ultrasonography and MRI for helping define ovarian cysts and pelvic masses. MRI images have better soft tissue contrast particularly for identifying fat and blood and give better idea of the organ of origin.

Ovarian carcinoma: Ovarian cancers are typically large heterogeneous masses with both cystic and solid components, however may be just cystic. Rather than predicting the exact histology of an ovarian cancer, the real strength of the imaging is in suggesting whether or not a lesion is malignant.

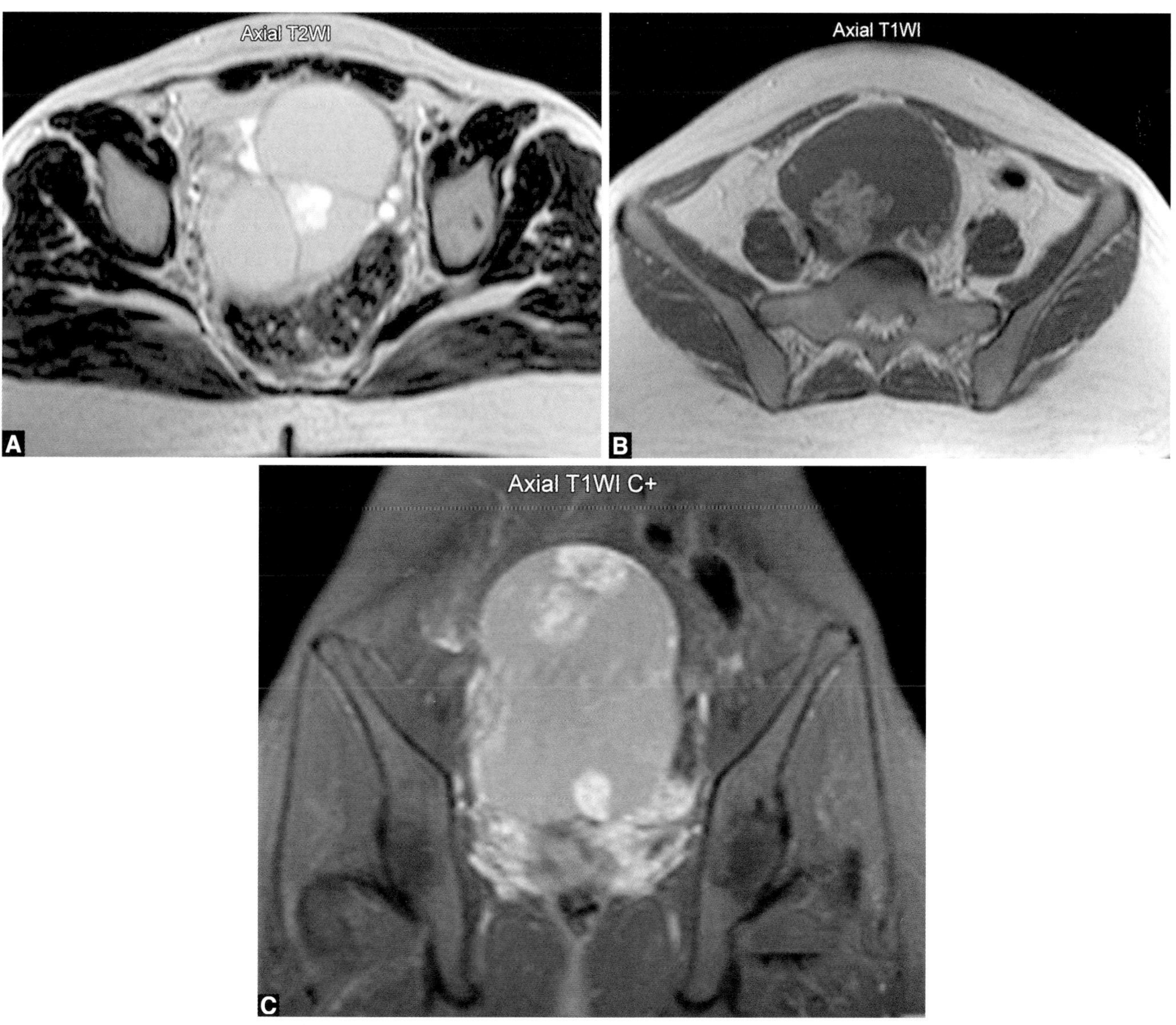

Figs 6A to C

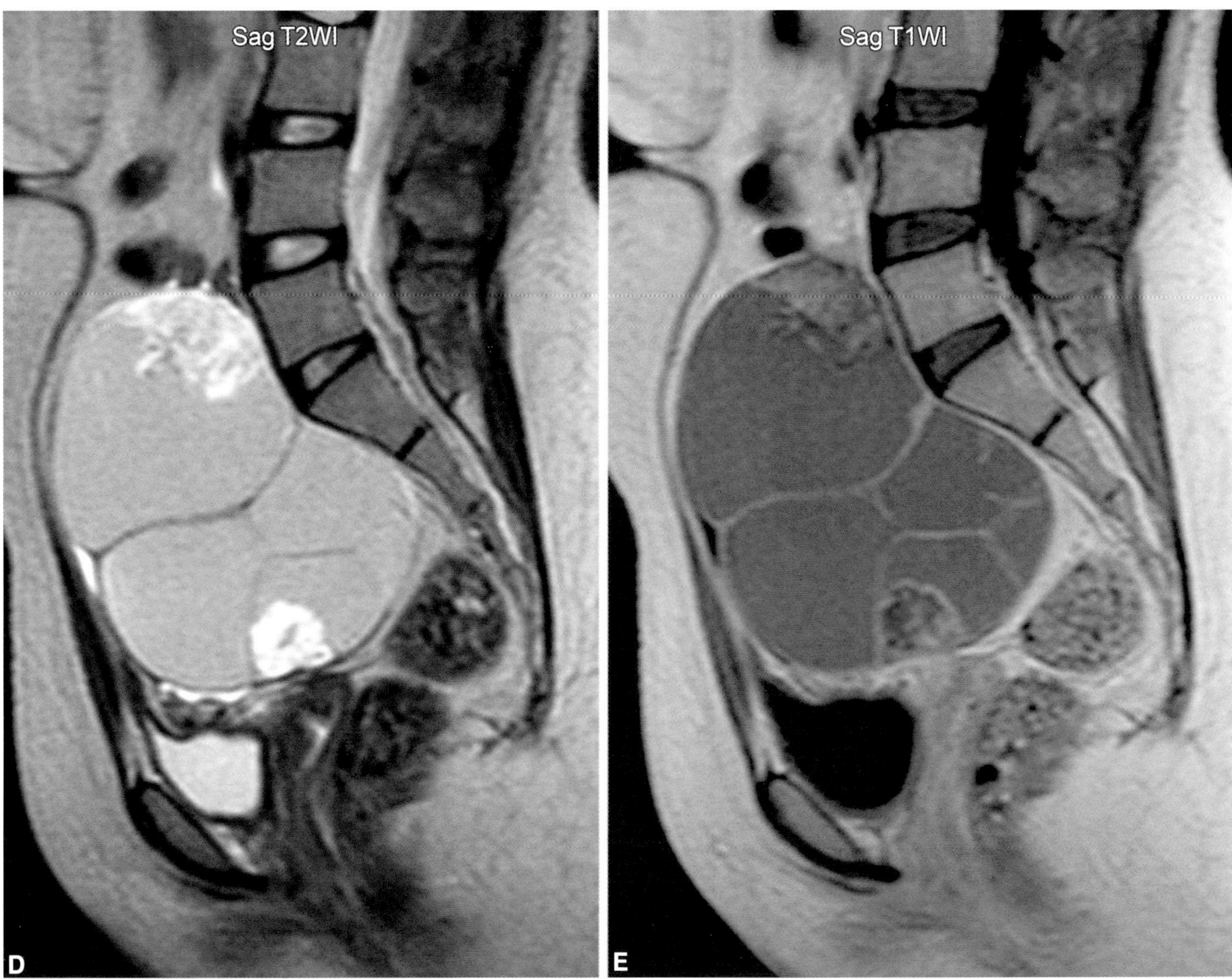

Figs 6D and E

Figs 6A to E: A large multicystic lesion with few enhancing solid components appearing hyperintense on T2 WI (A) and hypointense on T1WI (B) show postcontrast enhancement; (C) The lesion is posterior to the uterus and is suggestive of ovarian neoplastic mass lesion (cystadenocarcinoma). The large multicystic lesion with few solid components appear hyperintense on sagittal T2WI (D) and hypointense on sagittal T1WI (E)

Primary criteria for malignancy include size greater than 4 cm, solid or predominantly solid lesion, wall thickness greater than 3 mm, septae with thickness greater than 3 mm, nodularity, and presence of necrosis. Ancillary criteria include involvement of pelvic organs or sidewall, peritoneal, mesenteric or omental disease, ascites and lymphadenopathy. Necrosis within a solid lesion, vegetations within a cystic lesion, ascites and peritoneal metastases are the features most predictive of malignancy.

OVARIAN TORSION

Ovarian torsion is the twisting of an ovary with vascular pedicle on its axis which leads to lymphatic, venous and arterial obstruction. It is most commonly seen in women during their reproductive years, whereas increased rate of ovarian masses are seen at extremes of age. Clinical features are often nonspecific and include left or right quadrant pain and pelvic tenderness, hence in most cases it is difficult to differentiate the torsion from the other causes of lower quadrant pain. Since US is noninvasive, cost-effective and has high accuracy, it is the primary modality to evaluate ovarian torsion. The color doppler flow has limited specificity to demonstrate absence of arterial flow in torsion of the adnexa, because the dual blood supply of the ovaries and the symptoms of the ovarian torsion result from venous obstruction which occurs before arterial obstruction. The identification of twisted pedicle, the whirlpool sign, is very definitive for the torsion, but it is not commonly seen. The most common finding in the gray-scale US is the enlargement of the ovary with multiple homogeneous peripheral cysts. CT and MRI are useful when sonographic findings are ambigous. MRI helps to characterize the ovarian mass further and evaluate preoperative viability of the ovary (Figs 7A and B).

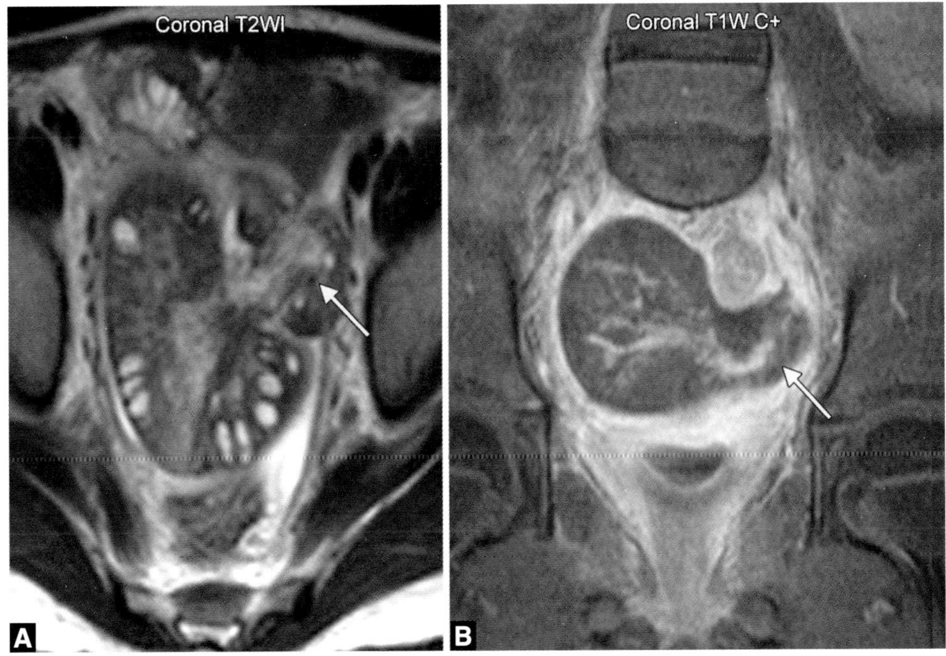

Figs 7A and B: T2W, T1W postcontrast images reveal enlarged ovary twisted around the vascular pedicle with multiple small follicles

ENDOMETRIAL CARCINOMA

Carcinoma of the endometrium is among the most common female pelvic malignancies and may develop in normal, atrophic, or hyperplastic endometrium. Most of the cancers are detected at an early stage, with the tumor confined to the uterine corpus in 75 percent of patients. The prognosis is generally favorable.

Magnetic resonance imaging (MRI) is preferred modality for imaging as advantages of MRI include superior spatial and tissue contrast resolution, multiplanar capabilities, lack of exposure to ionizing radiation, and availability of noniodinated, non-nephrotoxic IV contrast material. MRI findings include thickened endometrium (Figs 8A and B) with postcontrast enhancement.

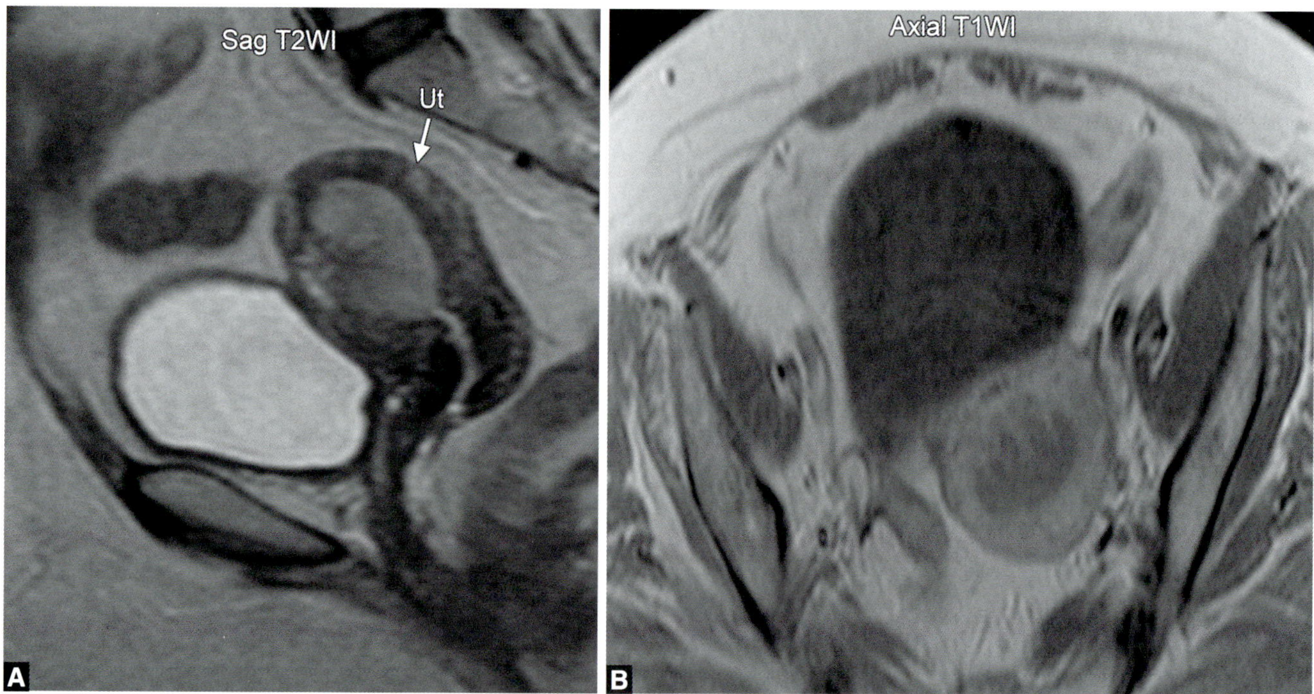

Figs 8A and B: Sagittal T2W axial T1W images show thickened endometrium

CARCINOMA CERVIX

After breast cancer, carcinoma of the uterine cervix is the second most common malignancy in women and accounts for two-thirds of malignant tumors found in the female genital tract. Most cases of cervical carcinoma occur between the late thirties and the mid-fifties. Early detection of cervical carcinoma due to gynecologic examination and the PAP smear has led to a significant reduction in mortality. Imaging is used for staging of cytologically proven disease.

Transvaginal ultrasound is usually the first imaging modality employed. Additional cross-sectional imaging is especially useful if the tumor size is large. MRI (Figs 9 and 10) is superior to CT in the local staging of cervical carcinoma. T2-weighted MR sequences are most helpful for local staging of cervical disease. The tumor presents with high signal intensity compared with the low intensity cervical stroma. Stage-IB International Federation of Gynecology and Obstetrics (FIGO) carcinoma is restricted to the cervix and presents on T2-weighted images with a fully preserved hypointense rim of normal cervical stroma surrounding the tumor. In patients with parametrial invasion (stage FIGO IIB), the normal stroma is disrupted. Contrast-enhanced sequences may be useful in selected cases with suspected invasion of the bladder or rectum (Table1).

Absence of a defining capsule to the cervix and a rich lymphatic network contribute to the spread of the tumor to parametrial tissues and pelvic lymph nodes. Loss of the fat planes between the cervix with the rectum or bladder or ureters indicate stage 3. Extension to the vagina, and then to the bladder, may cause vesicovaginal fistula. Direct spread from the supravaginal portion of the cervix may also reach the

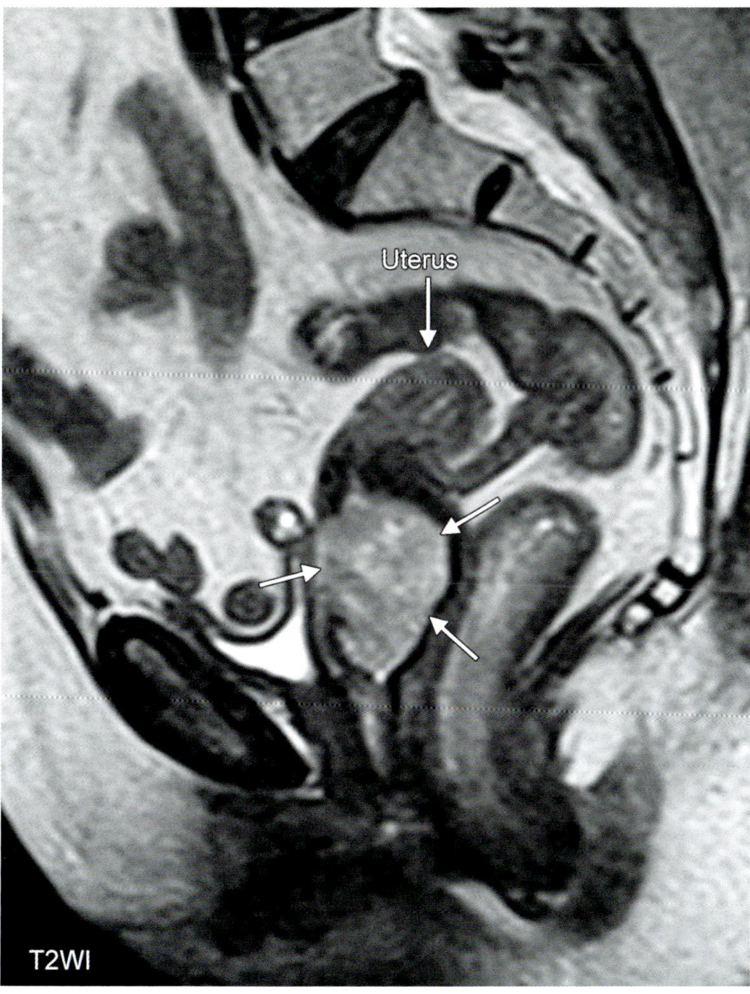

Fig. 9: Carcinoma cervix on MRI present as a soft tissue mass lesion in the cervix (arrows), it appears hyperintense on T2W image

bladder. The ureters often become obstructed when there is parametrial spread. The rectum is not often directly involved, because of its separation from the cervix by the Pouch of Douglas. Extension to the pelvic sidewall is seen as soft tissue strands extending to the obturator internus muscle and/or pyriformis muscle. Distant metastases may occur in the para-aortic lymph nodes, lungs or skeleton. The treatment and prognosis of cervical carcinoma depends on volume, extent, vascular, lymphatic spread and histology.

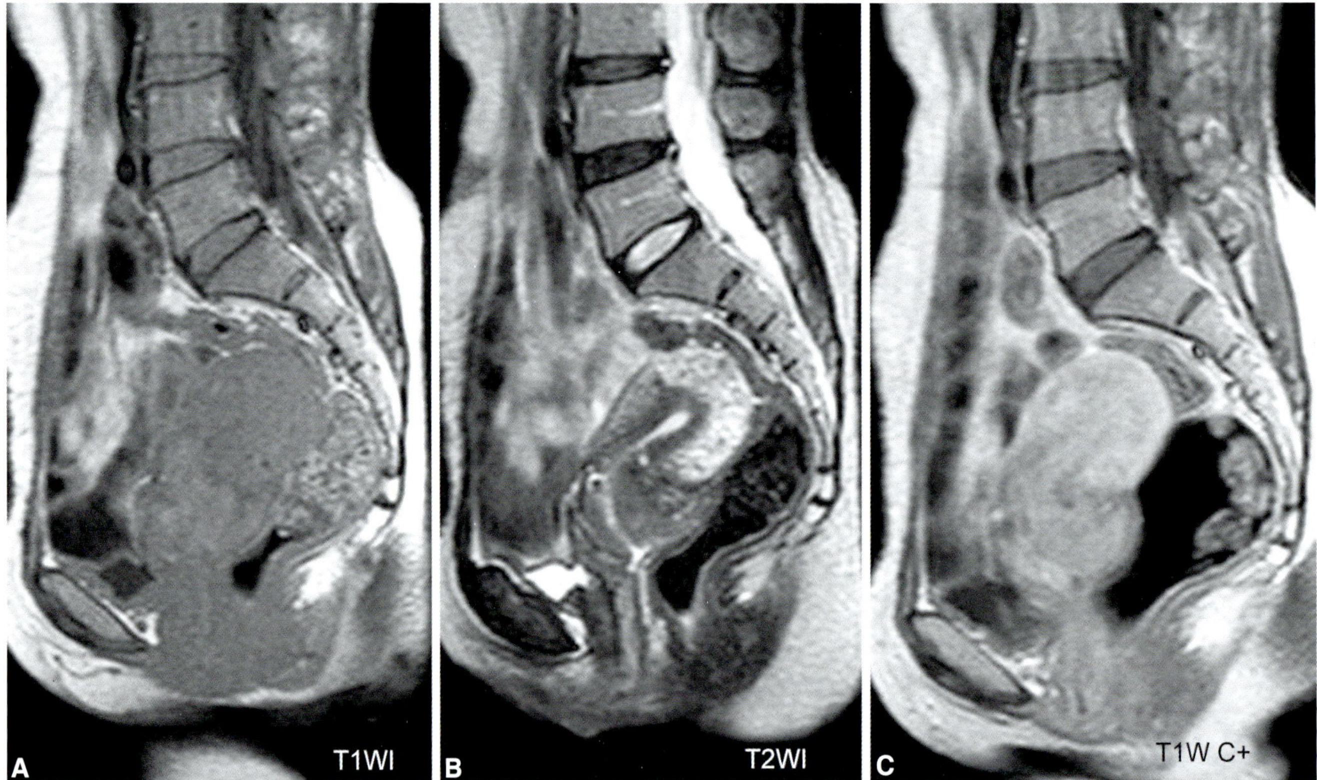

Figs 10A to C: Carcinoma cervix in a 40-year-old female who presented with history of PV bleeding of 12 days duration. Cervix is bulky and reveals altered heterogeneous signal. It is iso-to-mildly hyperintense on T1W image (A) and iso-to-hypointense on T2W image (B). It shows heterogeneous enhancement (C). The posterior wall is predominantly involved. The lower uterine segment is also involved. The fibrous stroma appears to be intact. Biopsy confirmed as adenocarcinoma

Table 1: Correlation between FIGO staging of cancer uterine cervix with MRI findings

Stage		*MRI T2WI features*
Ia	Microinvasion	No tumor evidence
Ib	Invasive, confined to the cervix	Hyperintense tumor on T2WI in contrast with hypointense signal from cervical stroma
IIa	Tumor invades the upper-vaginal-third, but does not affect the lower-vaginal-third	Segmental interruption of hypointense signal on the upper-third of the vaginal wall
IIb	Tumor invades the parametrium, but not the pelvic wall neither the lower-vaginal-third	Hyperintense tumor interrupting hypointense halo of the interface between cervical stroma and parametrium
IIIa	Involvement of the lower-vaginal-third, without affecting the pelvic wall	Segmental interruption of the hypointense signal of the lower-vaginal-third
IIIb	Pelvic wall involvement or hydronephrosis	Tumor extending to the musculature or causing hydroureter
IVa	Tumor invades the bladder or rectum mucosa	Loss of hypointense signal of the mucosa of the bladder or rectum
IVb	Distant metastasis	Distant metastasis

Müllerian Duct Cyst

Müllerian duct cyst (Fig. 11A) is an uncommon congenital anomaly. It is usually small, asymptomatic, midline, cystic lesion, located behind the superior half of the prostatic urethra and connected to the verumontanum by a thin stalk. Rarely a Müllerian duct cyst may be associated with renal agenesis (Figs 11B to F) and hypospadias. MRI accurately defines anatomic relationship when one is planning to excise a Müllerian duct cyst, due to multiplanar imaging capacity, superior soft tissue contrast, and absence of ionizing radiation.

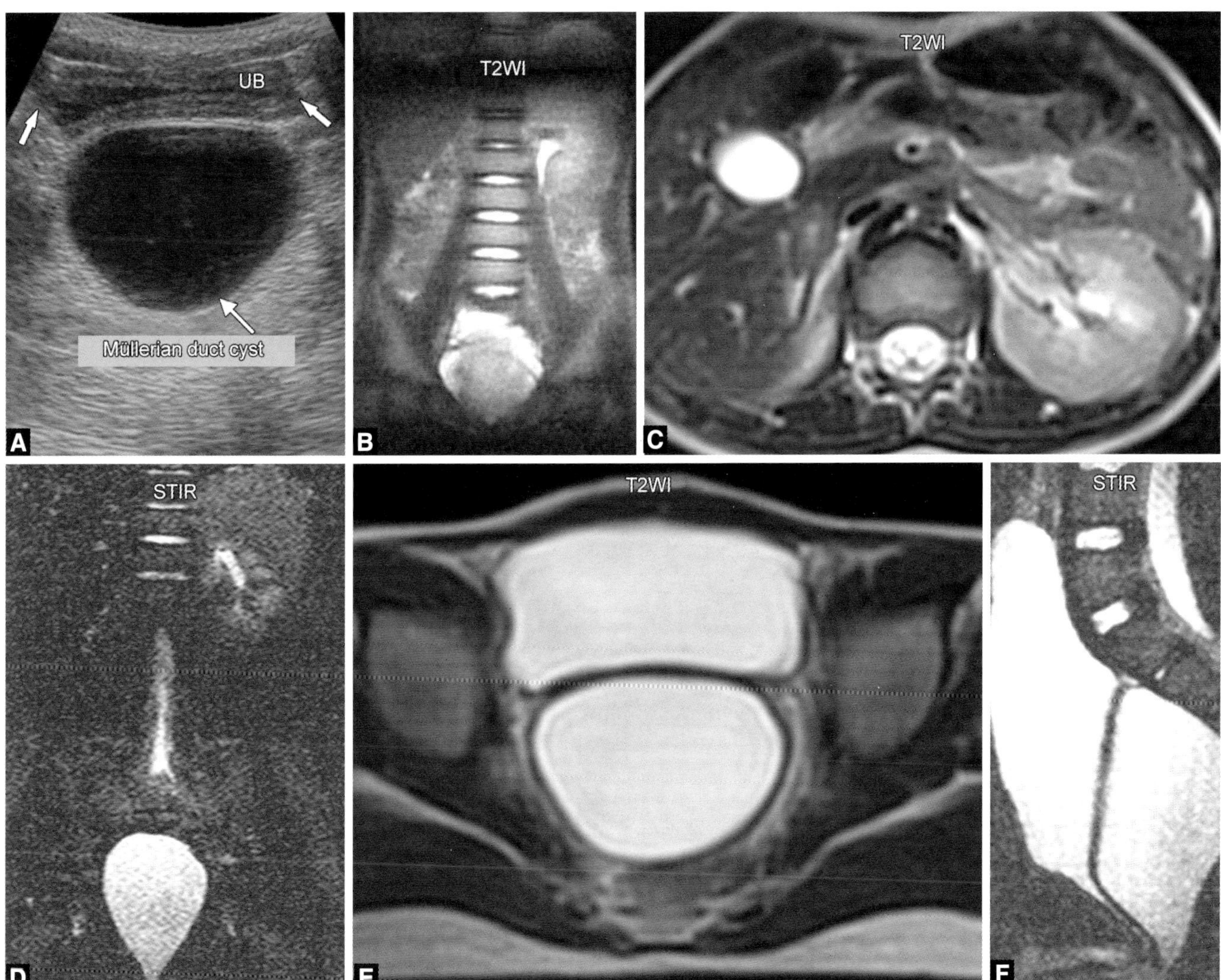

Figs 11A to F: In a 5-year-old male child, transabdominal USG (A) shows cystic nature lesion posterior to bladder (arrows). Agenesis of right kidney with normal left kidney is seen in coronal and axial T2-weighted images (B and C). Pear shaped cystic nature mass lesion is seen hyperintense on STIR and T2-weighted images (D and E). Sagittal STIR MR image (F) shows that there is no communication between cystic lesion and urinary bladder

CARCINOMA URINARY BLADDER

MR urography is useful in patients where use of ionizing radiation is to be avoided. The procedure is performed using heavily T2-weighted images such as RARE sequence (rapid acquisition with relaxation enhancement) and HASTE (Half fourier Acquisition Single Shot Turbo Spin Echo) sequence (Fig. 12). The sequence is performed in a single breath hold. The urine gives a bright signal, this aspect is used to create the urographic images while the fat signals from the background are suppressed. While using RARE and HASTE sequences no information about the renal function is obtained, and may not visualize a nondilated system. A T1WI gadolinium enhanced 3D image FLASH sequence is used, thin sections obtained and processed with maximum intensity projection, the images obtained provide information on renal anatomy and function similar to conventional urography, low doses of a diuretic agent can be administered before this examination to demonstrate filling of the pelvicalyceal system.

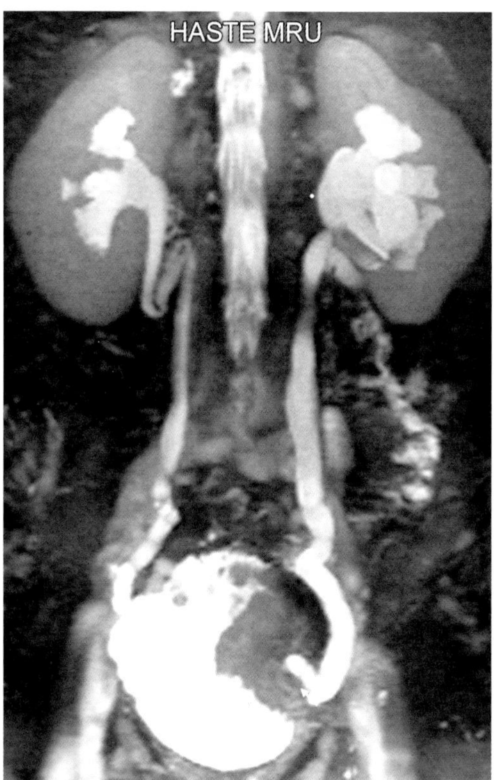

Fig. 12: In a case of carcinoma urinary bladder, HASTE coronal MR urography image reveals a large mass with irregular margins seen as a filling defect in the anterior and left part of the urinary bladder involving the left uretero-vesical junction with resultant moderate hydronephrosis and hydroureter on left side. The bladder wall is irregular. Mild hydronephrosis and hydroureter is also present on right side

CARCINOMA PROSTATE

Carcinoma prostate (PCa), it is the most common malignancy in men (excluding skin cancer) and the second leading cause of male cancer deaths (after lung cancer). The lifetime risk of developing PCa is 18 to 19 percent. Twenty-five to thirty-three percent of men who develop PCa will die of the disease. A significant part of the increase in incidence is probably due to an increase in PCa screening using serum prostate-specific antigen (PSA) and transrectal prostate ultrasound with biopsy.

Ninety percent of prostatic cancers are adenocarcinomas or anaplastic tumors. Other histological types are transitional cell carcinoma (2%), squamous cell carcinoma and mucinous and endometrioid carcinoma. Primary prostatic sarcoma is very rare. In lymphoma, primary as well as secondary manifestations in the prostate are possible. In leukemia prostate involvement is seen in 10 percent. Metastasis in the prostate has been reported, the most common primary being malignant melanoma.

On MR images the signal intensity and the detection of PCa depends on the type of imaging sequence used. On T1-weighted images, the prostate is of homogeneous medium signal intensity. On T2-weighted MR images, prostatic carcinoma is most commonly shown as decreased signal intensity within the high-signal-intensity of normal peripheral zone (Figs 13A and B).

While axial planes of section are essential in the evaluation of extracapsular invasion (Fig. 13C), visualization of the invasion of the seminal vesicles is facilitated by the evaluation of transaxial and coronal plane of section. In the evaluation of lymph node metastases, efficacy data for MRI and CT are similar. The recent developments of MR spectroscopic imaging expand the diagnostic assessment beyond anatomical information. MR spectroscopic imaging provides metabolic information specific to the prostate through the detection of the cellular metabolites citrate, creatine and choline. The information obtained from this new technology may allow an expanded assessment of tumor aggressiveness and the attendant risk of disease progression.

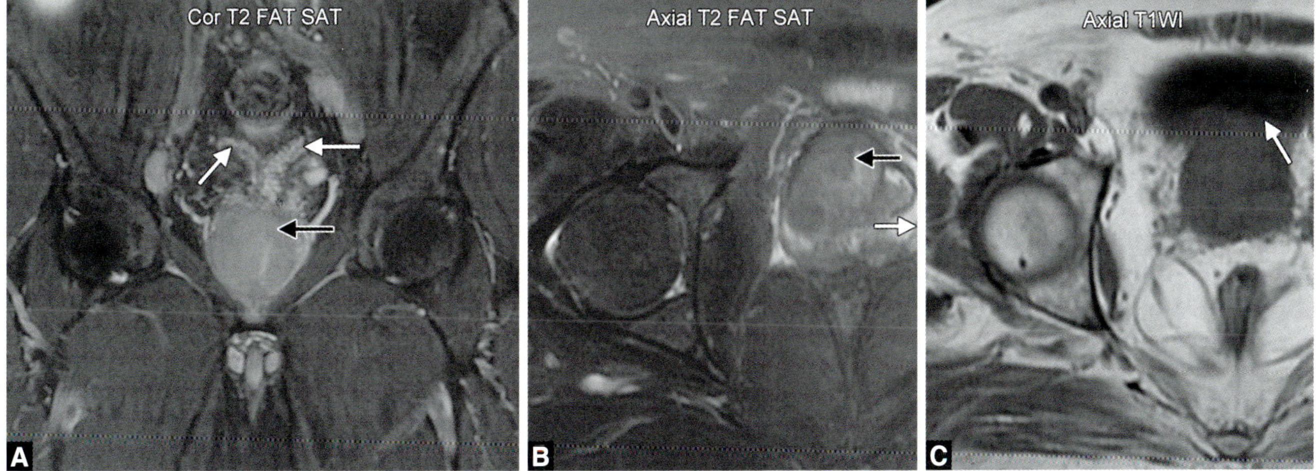

Figs 13A to C: Coronal T2 fat saturated image of prostate (A and B) shows enlarged soft tissue intensity heterogeneous lesion in prostate (black arrow). Normal hyperintense prostate parenchyma is compressed. Normal seminal vesicles are seen (white arrows). Axial T1WI of prostate (C) shows soft tissue intensity hypointense lesion of enlarged prostate indenting the urinary bladder

EJACULATORY DUCT CYST

Ejaculatory duct cyst is usually congenital and unilateral. There is frequently co-existent ipsilateral renal agenesis. The cysts may partially or completely replace the seminal vesicle, and may be unilocular or multilocular. These cysts are sometimes acquired, usually secondary to partial or complete obstruction of the ejaculatory duct. Cysts are usually incidental asymptomatic findings, although larger cysts may cause dysuria, frequency, perineal pain and painful ejaculation. Bladder outlet obstruction has also been reported. Seminal vesicle cysts can be recognized on ultrasound, CT and MRI. In contrast to Müllerian duct cysts, seminal vesicle cysts are lateral in location and often cause obstruction of the ipsilateral seminal vesicle. Medial seminal vesicle cysts can occur, but unlike Müllerian duct cysts, they do not communicate with the prostate. Since hemorrhage is relatively frequent, seminal vesicle cysts may be relatively hyperdense on CT, echogenic on ultrasound, and hyperintense on T1-weighted MRI sequences. High T2 signal intensity and lack of enhancement after gadolinium confirms the cystic nature of the structures on MRI (Figs 14A and B).

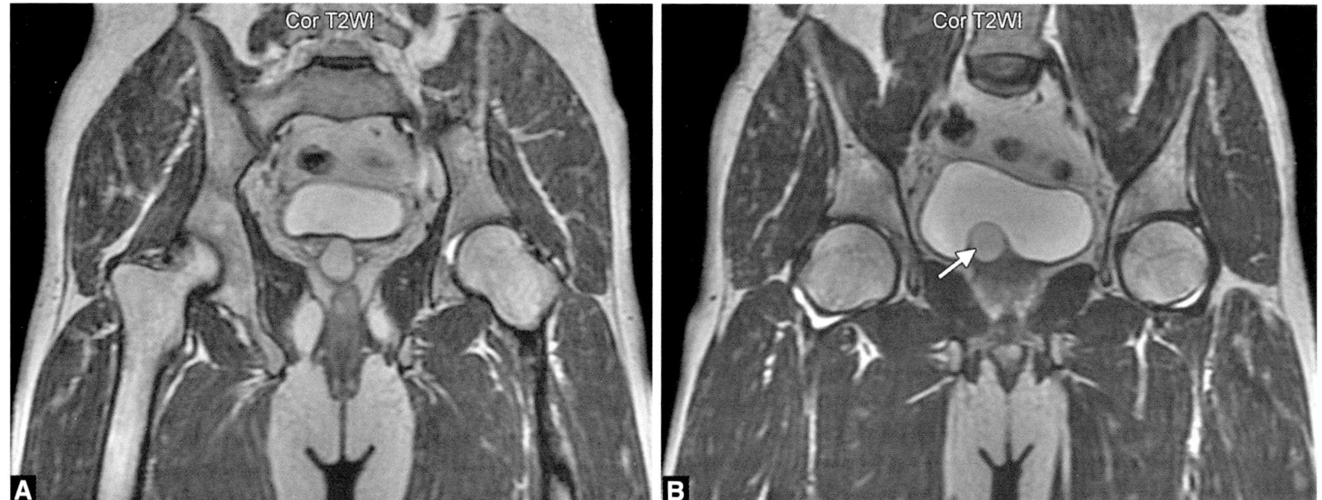

Figs 14A and B: MR in 25-years with dysuria and painful ejaculation on coronal T2WI shows hyperintense cystic structure, inferolateral to bladder base on right side, extending into midline and indenting the bladder base

TESTICULAR AGENESIS AND UNDESCENDED TESTIS

Failure of testicular development can occur all along the developmental time line. Early failure results in absence of the testis and the Wolfian structures on that same side. Testosterone must be produced locally to induce development of the vas, epididymis and seminal vesicles. Failure in the later stage may result in absence of the testis with presence of a vas.

When the testis fails to develop, it cannot be palpated on examination. However, the converse is not true; a boy with nonpalpable testes does not always have failure of testicular development. A testis that does not descend into the patent processus vaginalis in the inguinal canal is not palpable. Most cases of nonpalpable testes are a result of failure of descent of testis.

MR is the modality of choice for investigating undescended or absent testis as it does not involve ionizing radiation and has superior soft tissue resolution. The testis typically shows low signal intensity on T1-weighted images and high signal intensity on T2-weighted images (Figs 15A to C). MR imaging is highly accurate in localizing the testis in abdominal or canalicular region (Figs 16A to C).

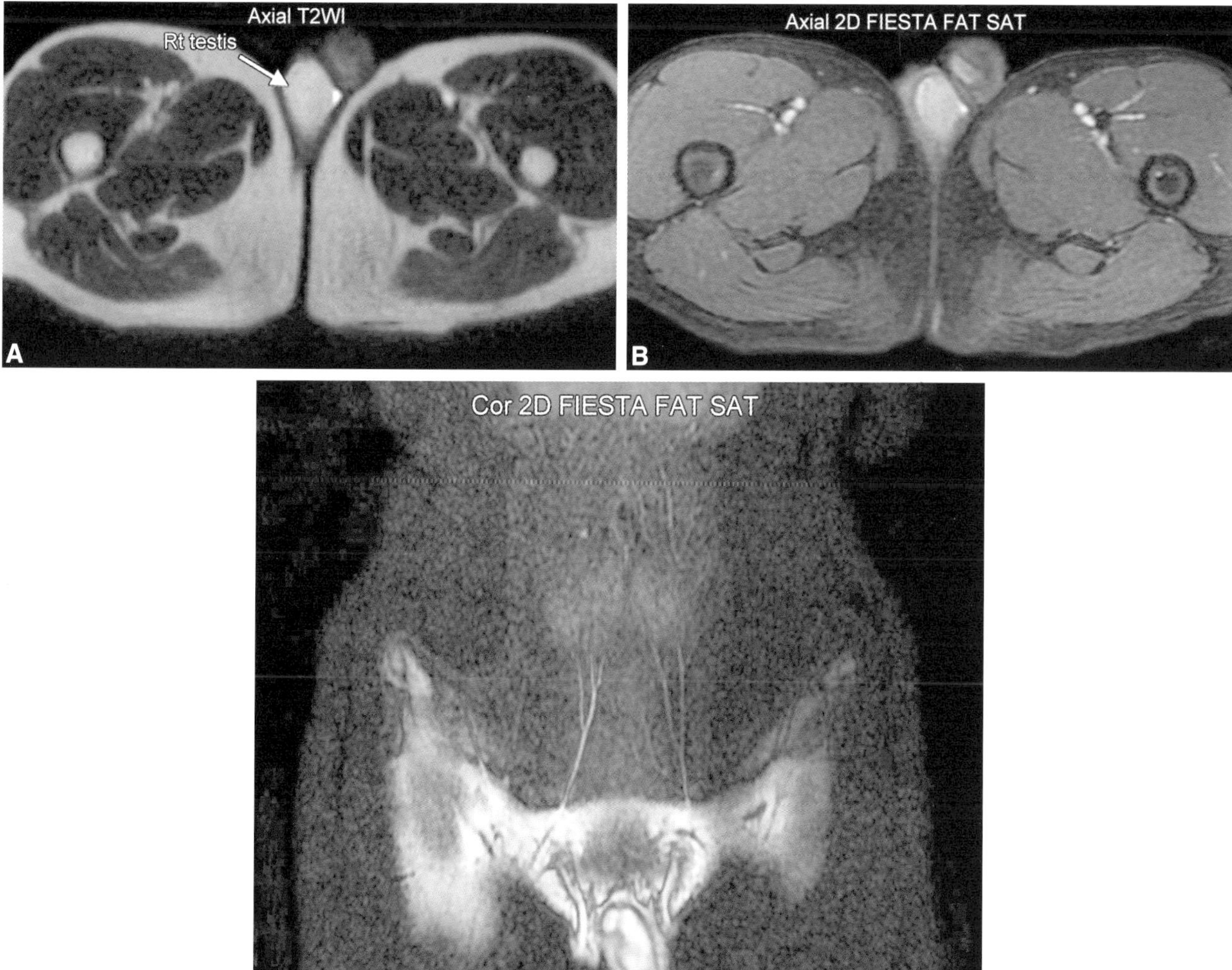

Figs 15A to C: 21-year-old male axial T2WI (A), 2D fiesta fat saturated (B) and coronal 2D fiesta fat saturated (C) sequence only right testis is seen, which is hyperintense. Left testis not seen in left scrotal sac or along the course of descent

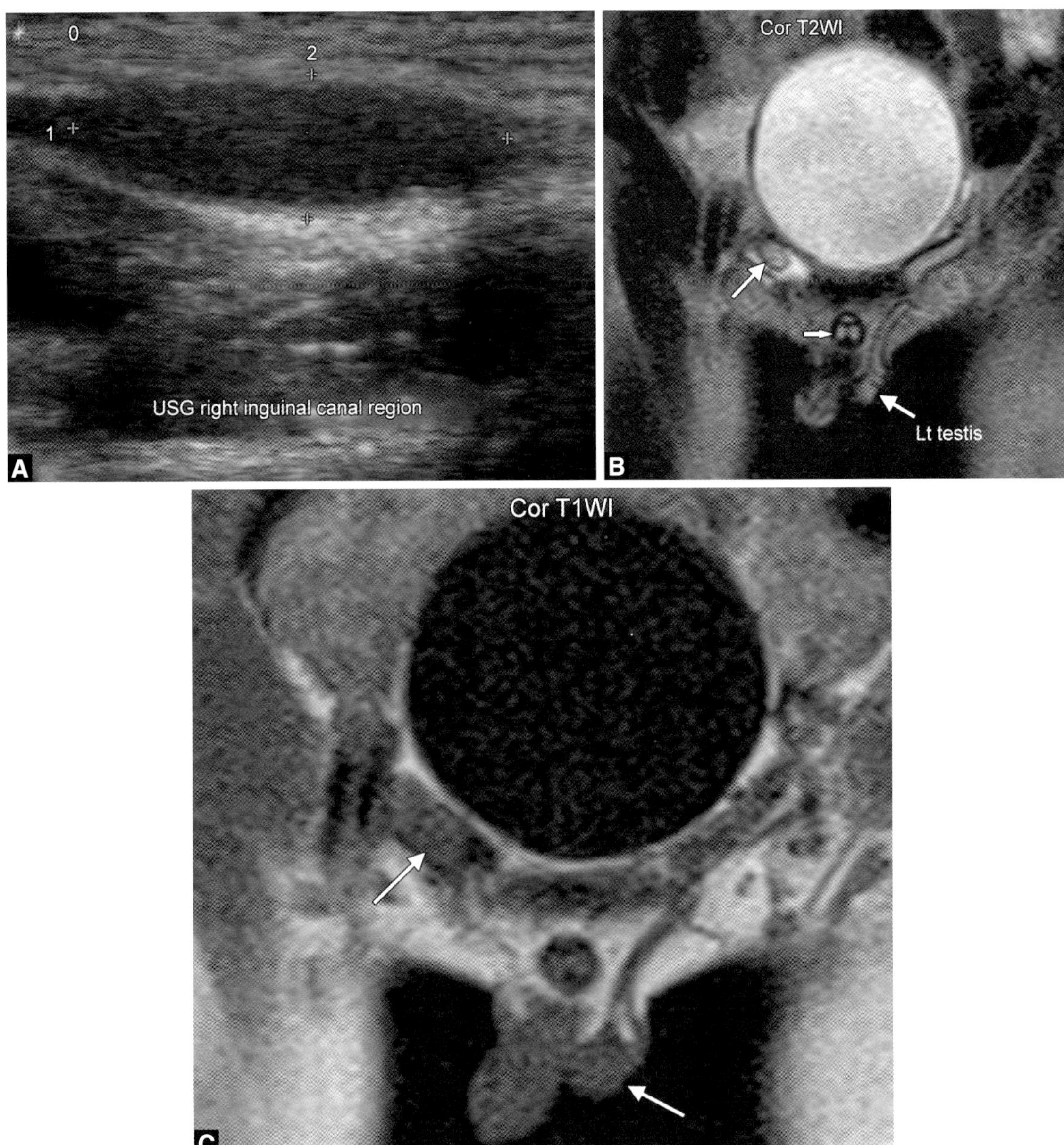

Figs 16A to C: In another patient 8-year of age right inguinal canal region USG (A) shows hypoechoic oval structure, similar in echogenicity as left scrotal testis. (B) Coronal T2WI shows hyperintense right undescended testis in right inguinal canal, it is similar in intensity to left scrotal testis (black arrow). The penis in cross section is well-demonstrated. (C) Coronal T1WI shows hypointense right undescended testis in right inguinal canal, it shows same hypointensity as the normally place left testis

Musculoskeletal System

6

Santosh Konde, Hariqbal Singh

SHOULDER JOINT

Anatomy Shoulder Joint

The shoulder or glenohumeral joint is the most flexible joint in the body. It consists of bones, ligaments, muscles and their tendons, and connects the arm to the chest (Figs 1 and 2). It is a ball and socket joint. The glenoid cavity forms a shallow socket and is inherently unstable. The added stability to the joint is made available by the capsule, ligaments, glenoid labrum and the rotator cuff.

The articular capsule completely encircles the joint; it is attached to the circumference of the glenoid cavity beyond the labrum. Inferiorly, it is attached to the anatomical neck of the humerus.

The ligaments of the glenohumeral joint are coracohumeral ligament and glenohumeral ligaments. Glenohumeral ligament has superior middle and inferior divisions. They are designed to stabilize the shoulder in the abducted or functional position.

The labrum is a fibrocartilaginous rim attached around the margin of the glenoid cavity. It cushions

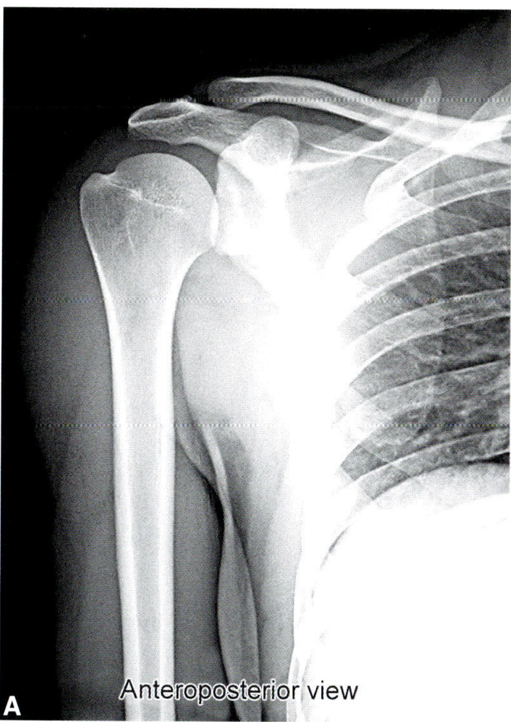

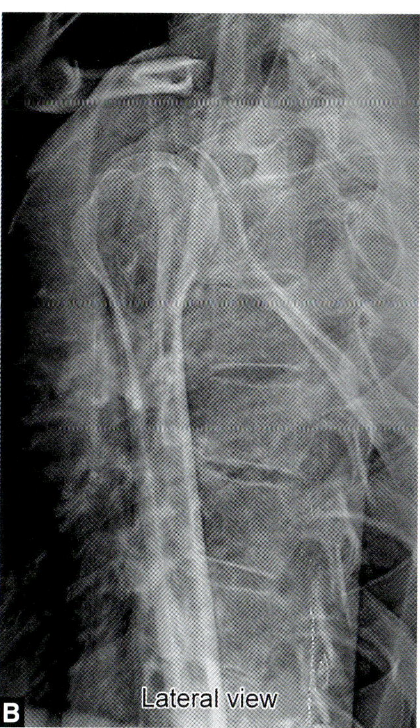

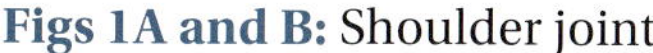
Figs 1A and B: Shoulder joint

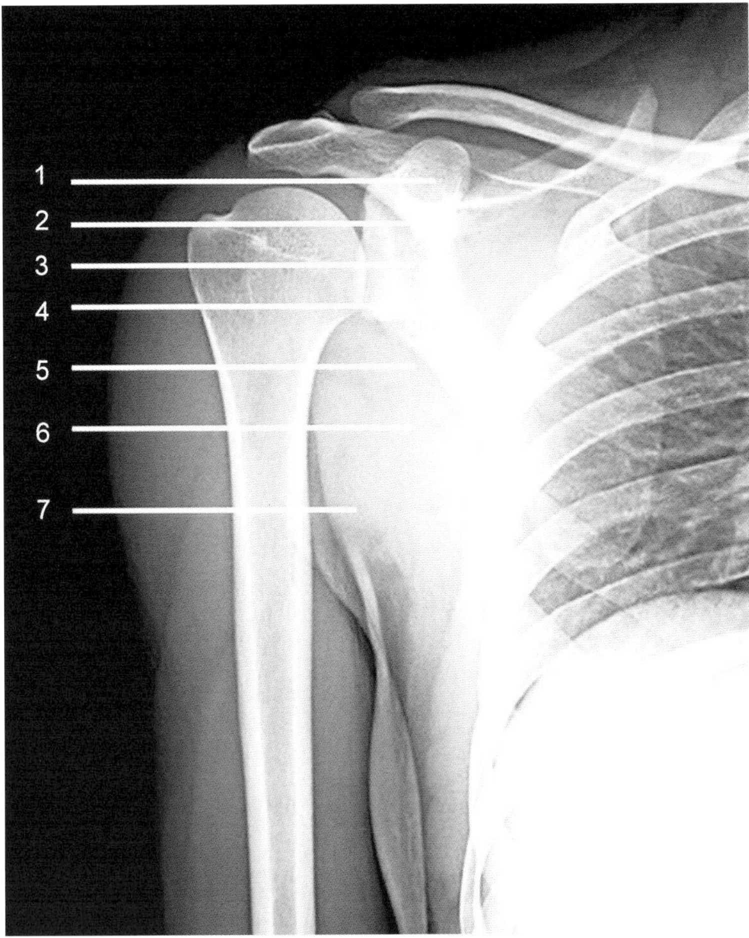

Fig. 2: Shoulder joint: Axial sections plan—superior to inferior sections

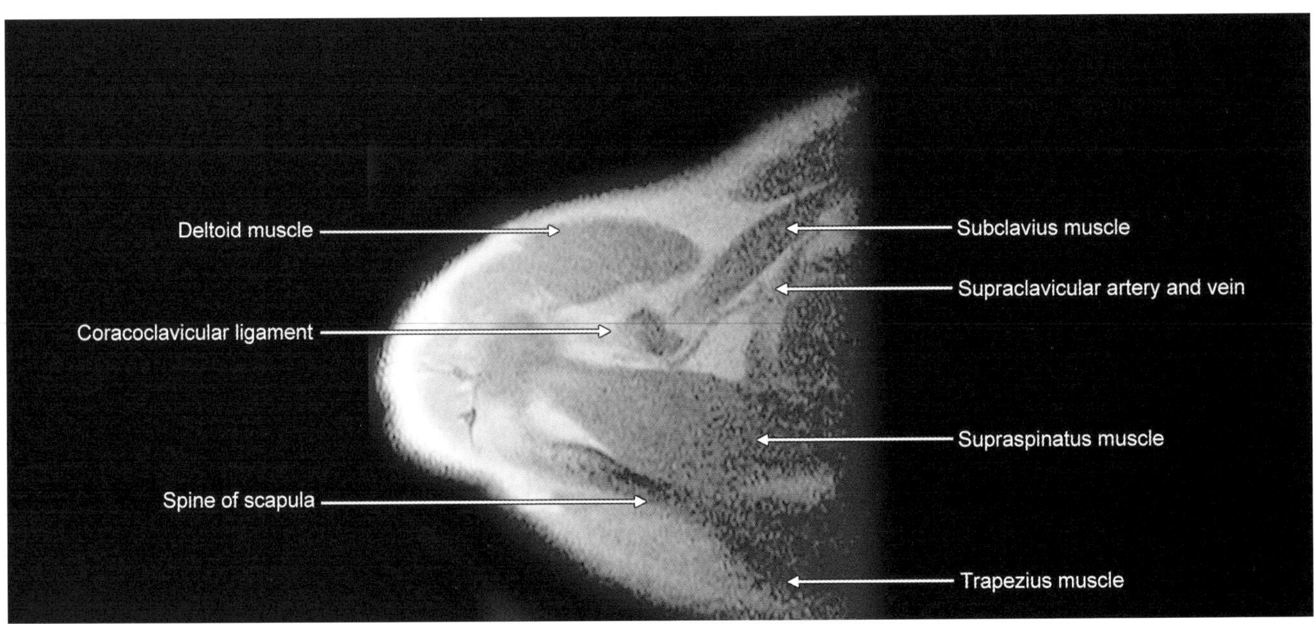

Fig. 3: Shoulder joint MRI: Axial T1WI (corresponds to level 1 in Fig. 2)

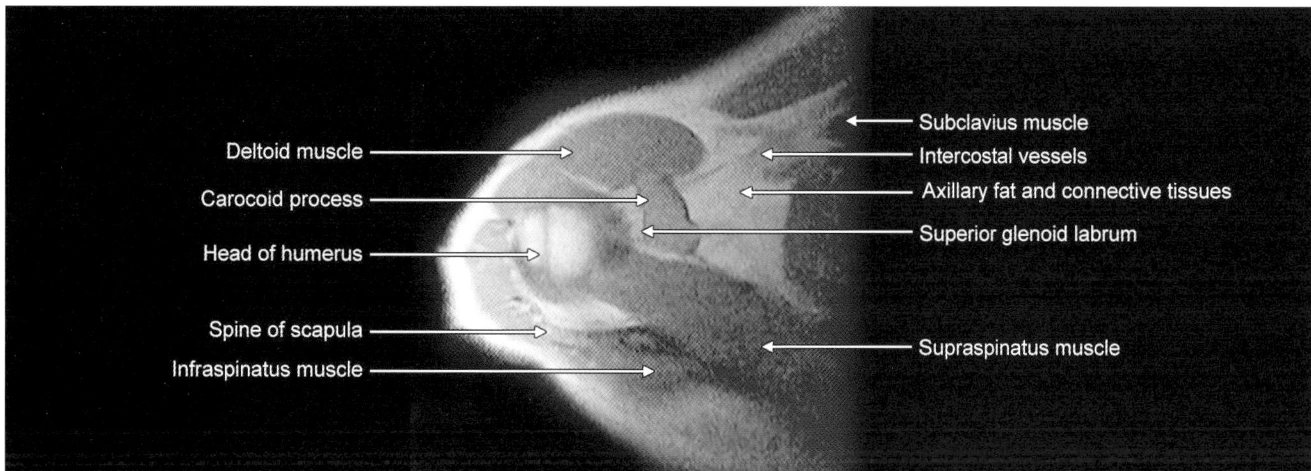

Fig. 4: Shoulder joint MRI: Axial T1WI (corresponds to level 2 in Fig. 2)

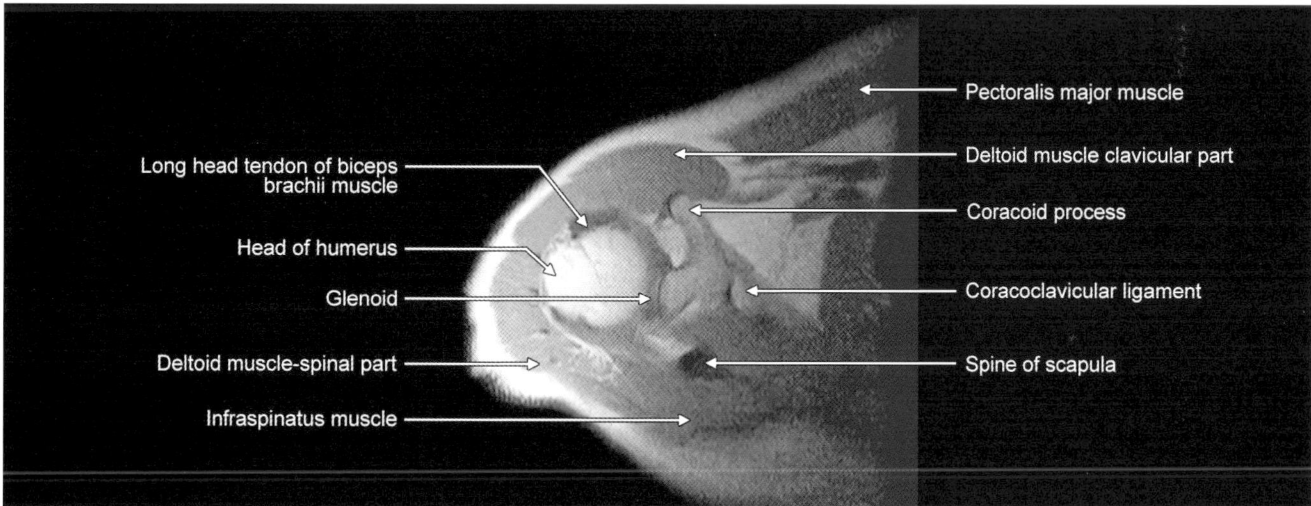

Fig. 5: Shoulder joint MRI: Axial T1WI (corresponds to level 3 in Fig. 2)

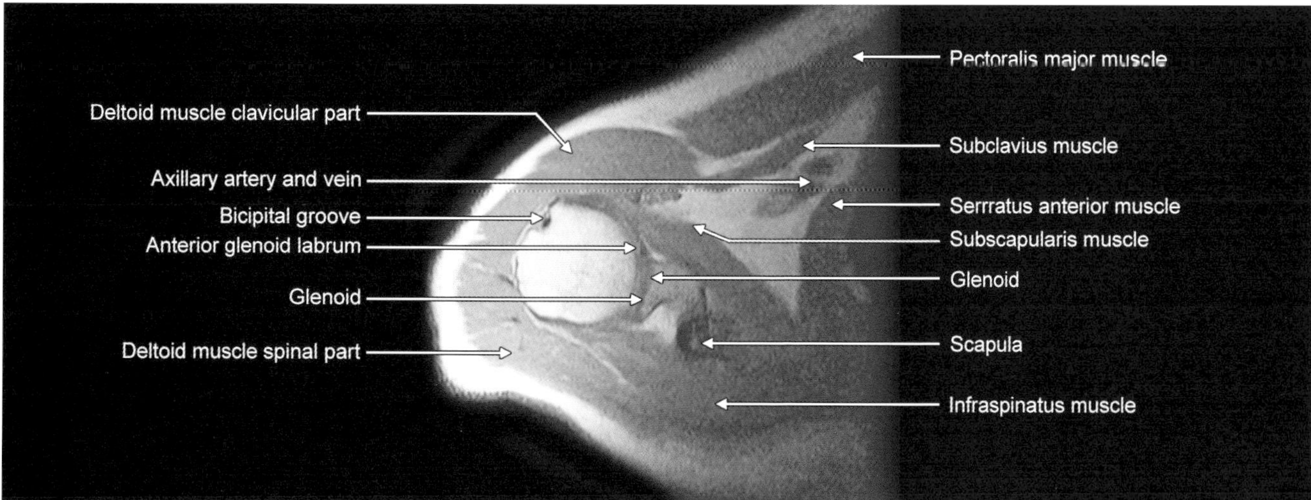

Fig. 6: Shoulder joint MRI: Axial T1WI (corresponds to level 4 in Fig. 2)

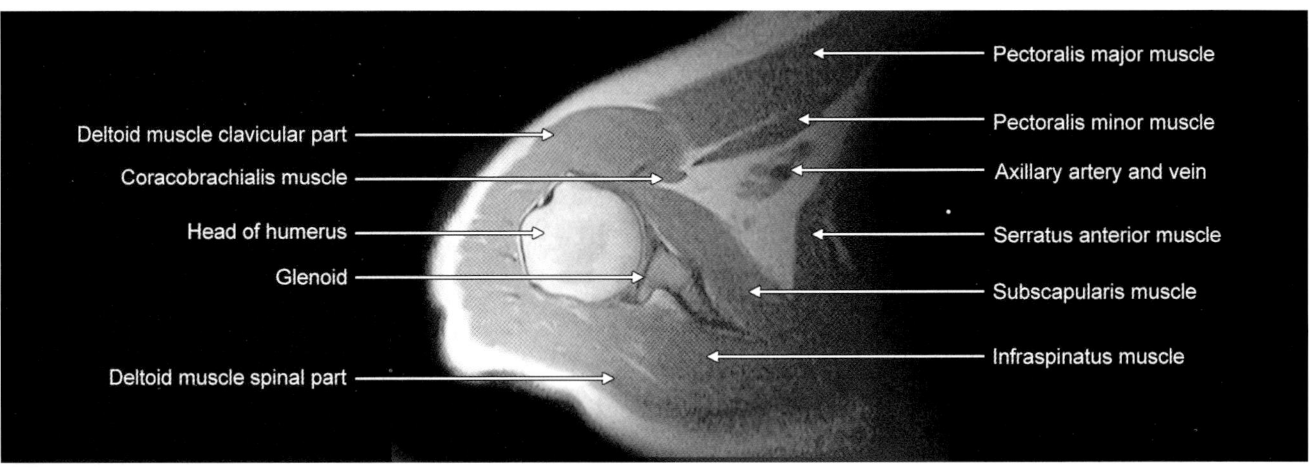

Fig. 7: Shoulder joint MRI: Axial T1WI (corresponds to level 5 in Fig. 2)

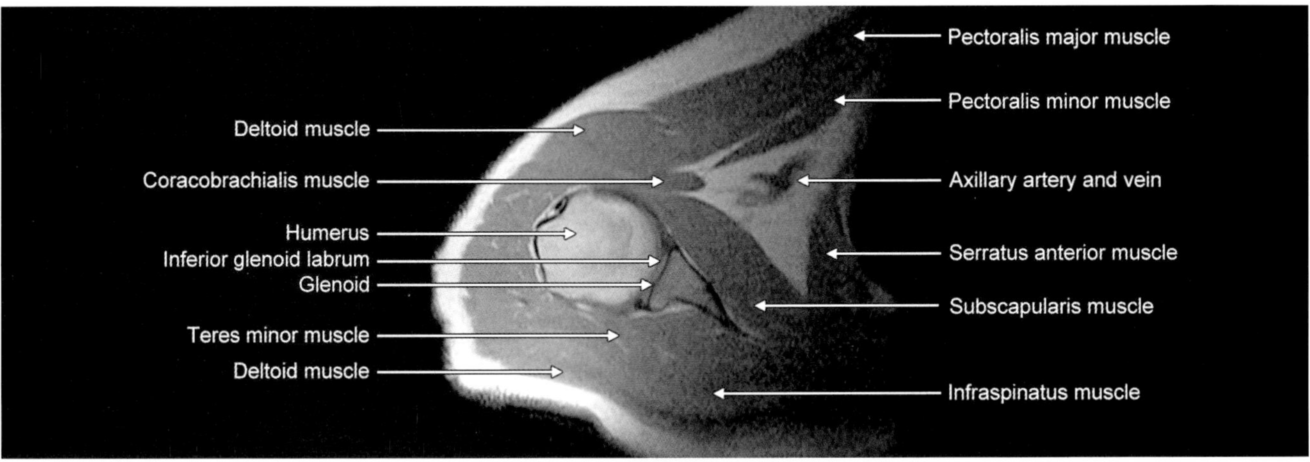

Fig. 8: Shoulder joint MRI: Axial T1WI (corresponds to level 6 in Fig. 2)

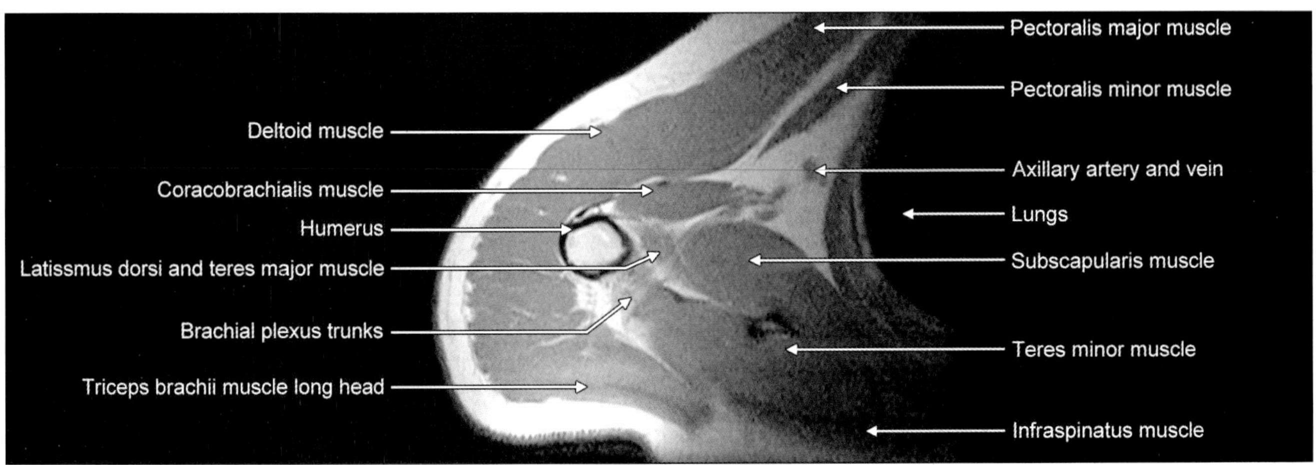

Fig. 9: Shoulder joint MRI: Axial T1WI (corresponds to level 7 in Fig. 2)

and stabilizes the humerus head. It increases the superoinferior diameter of the glenoid by 75 percent and the anteroposterior diameter by 50 percent. The base of the glenoid labrum is fixed to the circumference of the cavity. It is continuous above with the tendon of the long head of the biceps, which blends with the fibrous tissue of the labrum. It deepens the articular cavity.

The tendon of the long head of biceps forms biceps-labral complex with superior glenohumeral ligament and inserts on the supraglenoid tubercle. The tendon traverses laterally in the rotator cuff interval to lie in the bicipital groove. Glenohumeral joint is in connection with the sheath of biceps tendon.

The rotator interval is the portion of the joint capsule which lies between the supraspinatus and subscapularis tendons.

This lies between the superior and middle glenohumeral ligaments. The interval is reinforced by the coracohumeral ligament and underlying joint capsule. It is designed to limit flexion and external rotation.

Rotator cuff is formed by supraspinatus, infraspinatus, teres minor and subscapularis muscles and mostly by their flat tendons (Figs 3 to 23). The tendons fuse together and surround the shoulder joint. When the muscles contract, resulting in the rotator cuff tendon to rotate upward, inward, or outward. Supraspinatus tendon lies over the summit of humeral head and is an abductor. Infraspinatus and teres minor tendon cover the backside of humeral head and are external rotators. Subscapularis tendon crosses the front of the shoulder joint and is an abductor of shoulder joint.

There are two pouch-like bursae located in the shoulder which produce a lubricating fluid (Fig. 13), which helps reduce friction between the moving parts of the joint.

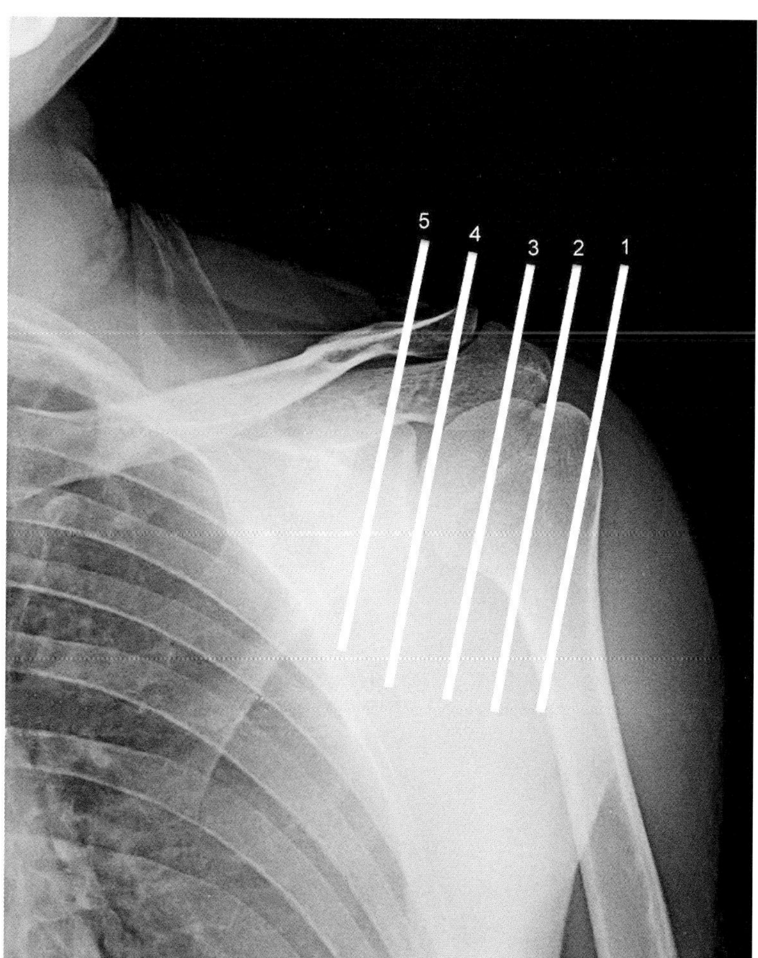

Fig. 10: Shoulder joint: Sagittal sections plan—lateral to medial sections

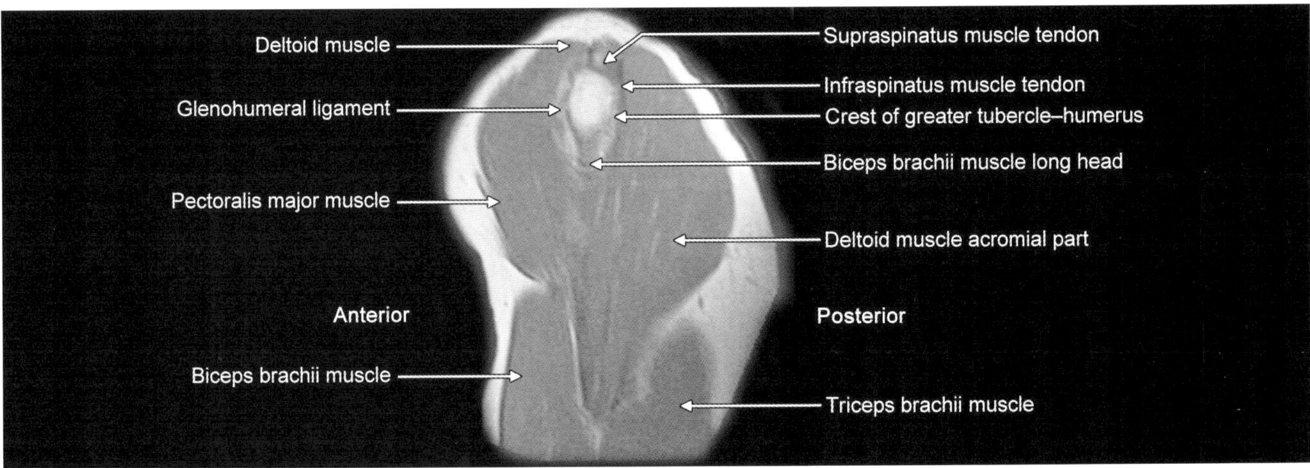

Fig. 11: Shoulder joint MRI: Sagittal T1WI (corresponds to level 1 in Fig. 10)

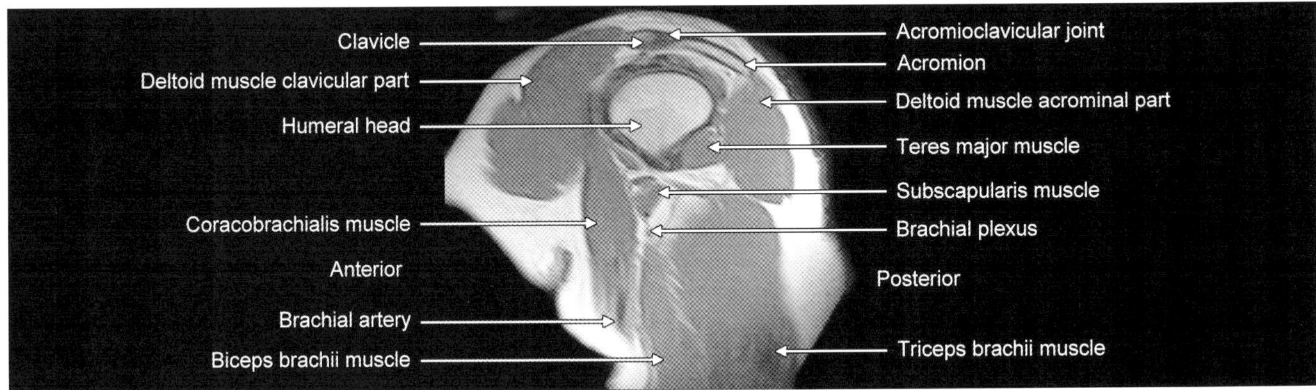

Fig. 12: Shoulder joint MRI: Sagittal T1WI (corresponds to level 2 in Fig. 10)

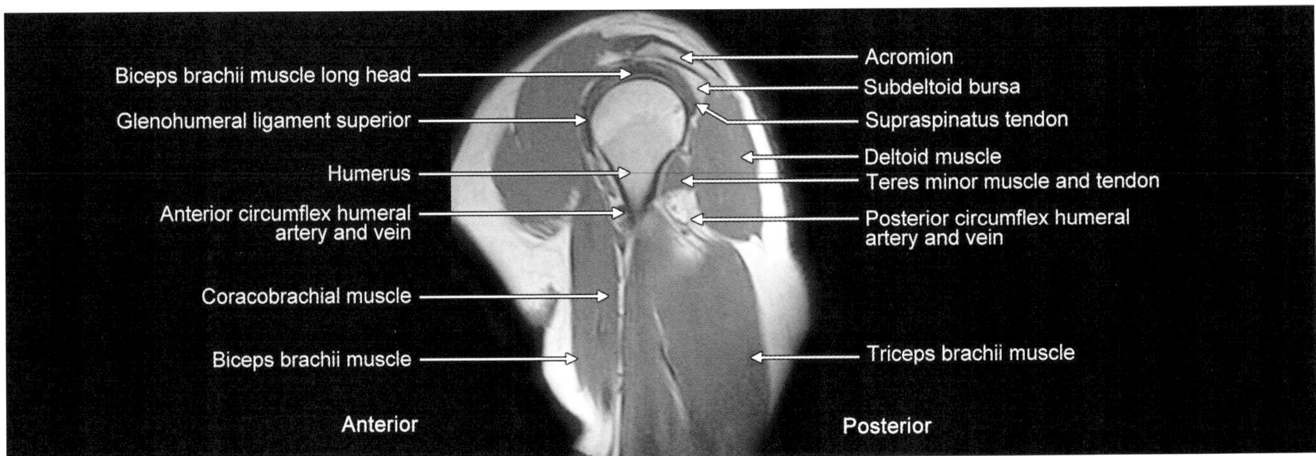

Fig. 13: Shoulder joint MRI: Sagittal T1WI (corresponds to level 3 in Fig. 10)

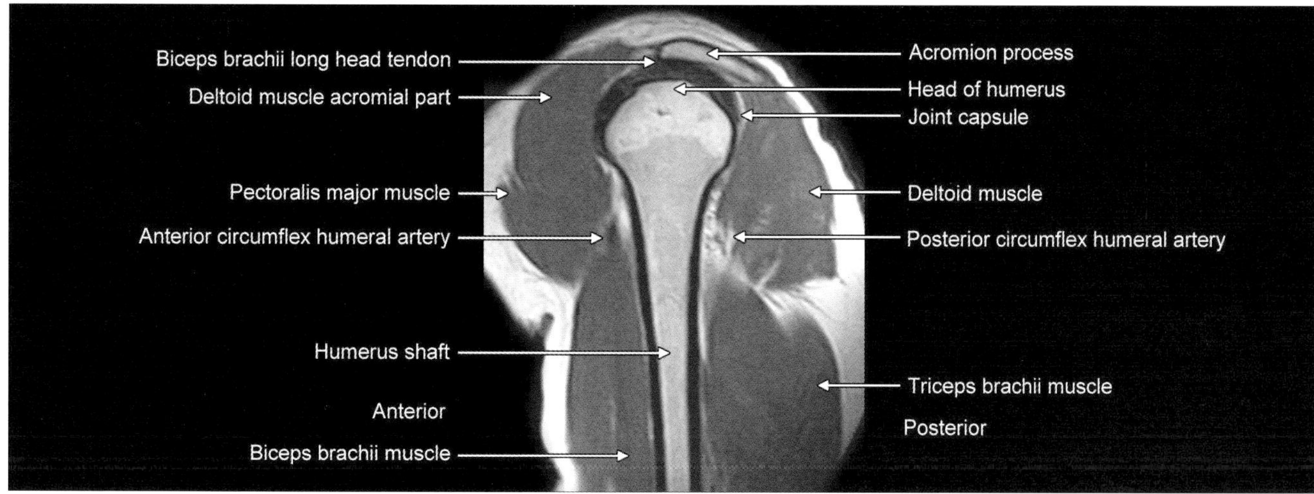

Fig. 14: Shoulder joint MRI: Sagittal T1WI (corresponds to level 4 in Fig. 10)

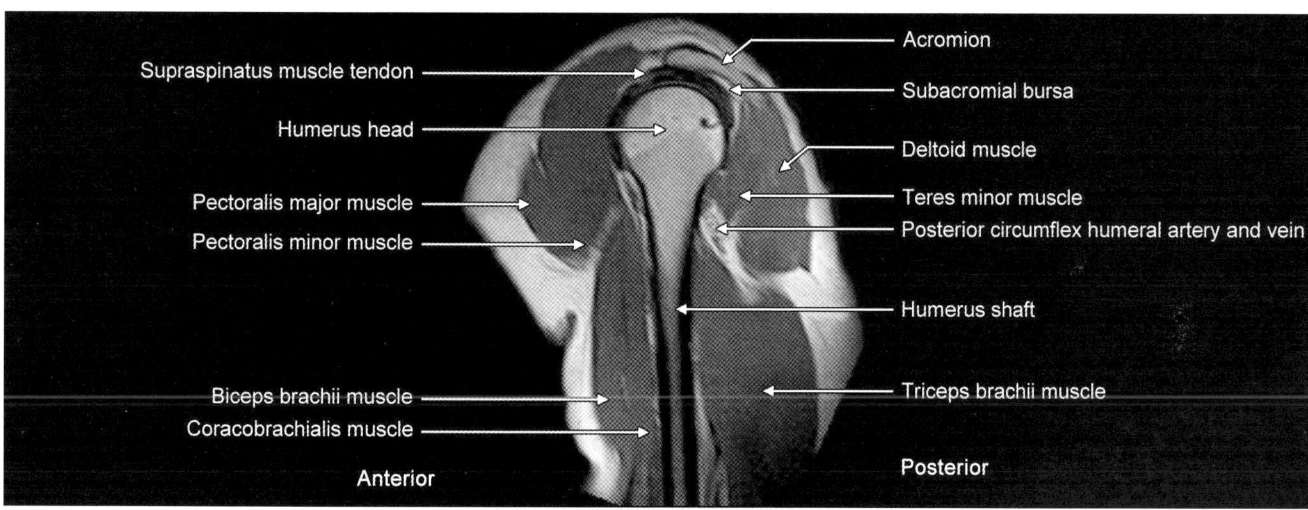

Fig. 15: Shoulder joint MRI: Sagittal T1WI (corresponds to level 5 in Fig. 10)

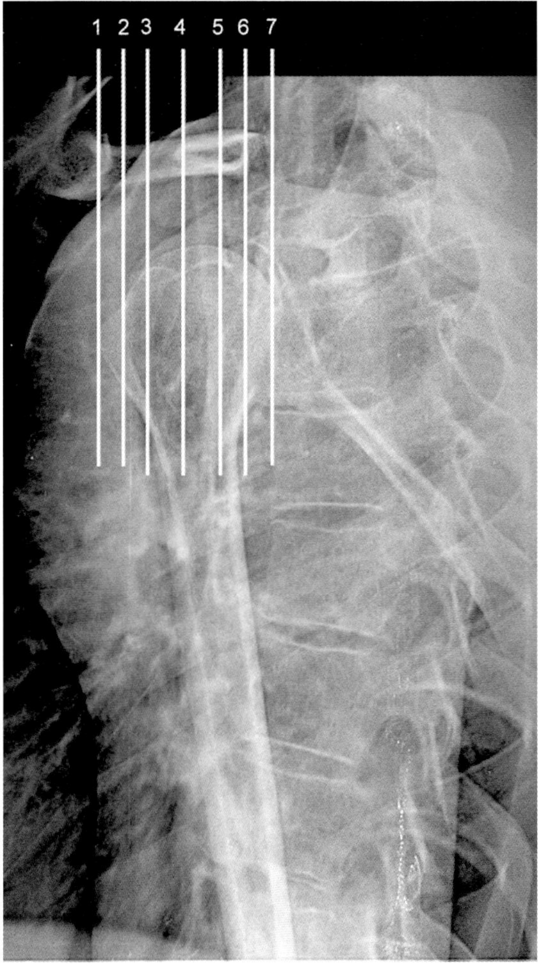

Fig. 16: Shoulder joint coronal sections plan

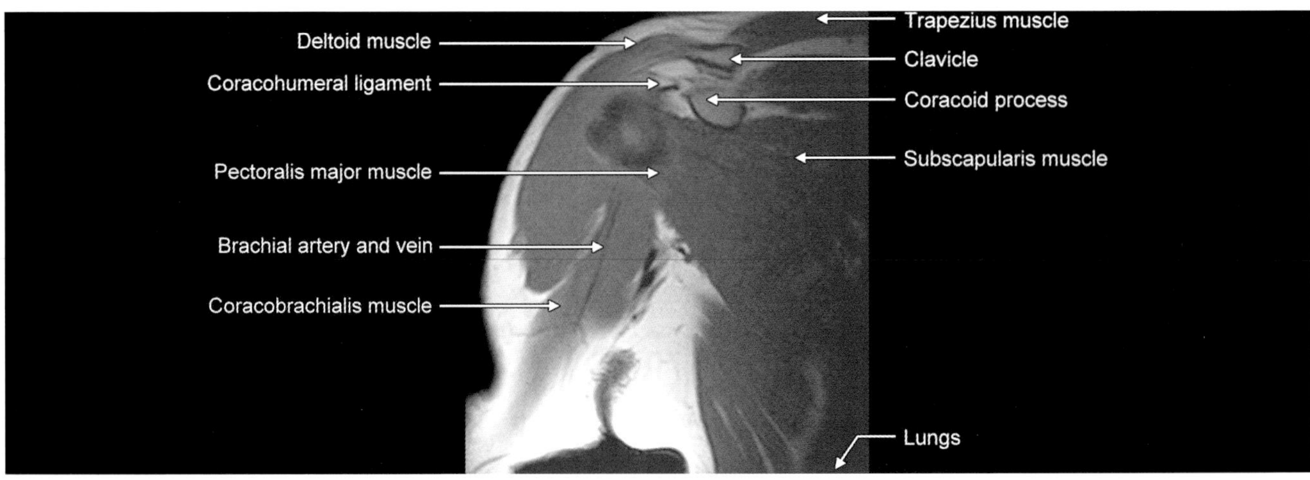

Fig. 17: Shoulder joint MRI: Coronal T1WI (corresponds to level 1 in Fig. 16)

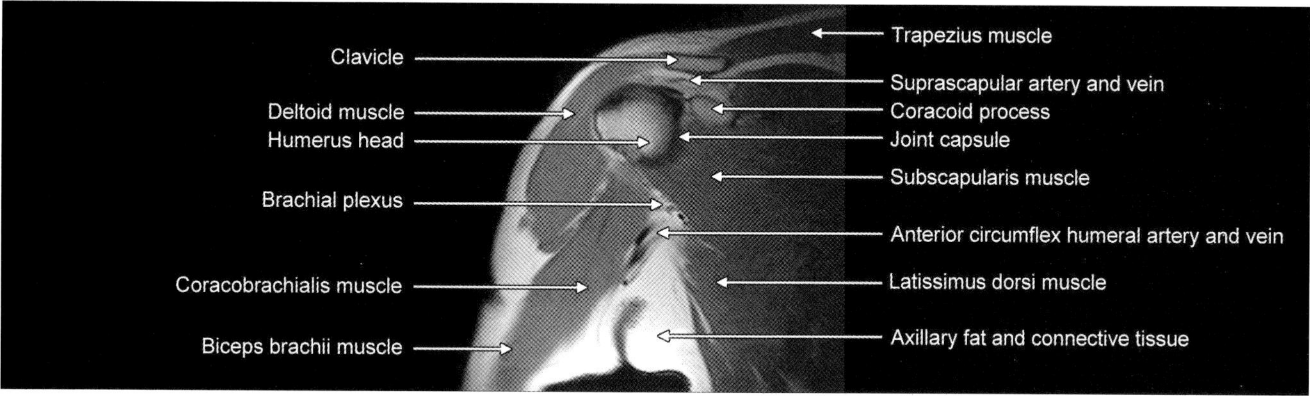

Fig. 18: Shoulder joint MRI: Coronal T1WI (corresponds to level 2 in Fig. 16)

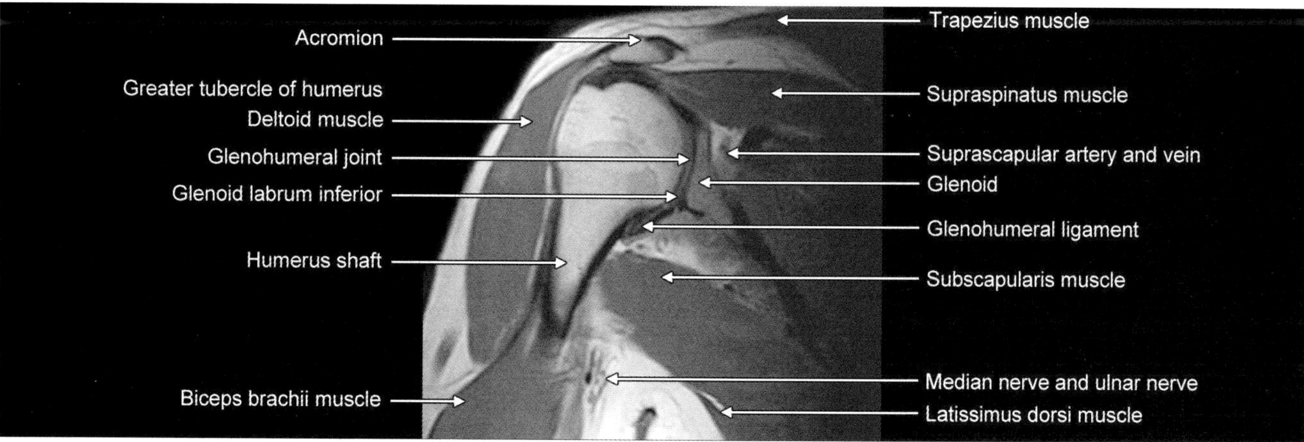

Fig. 19: Shoulder joint MRI: Coronal T1WI (corresponds to level 3 in Fig. 16)

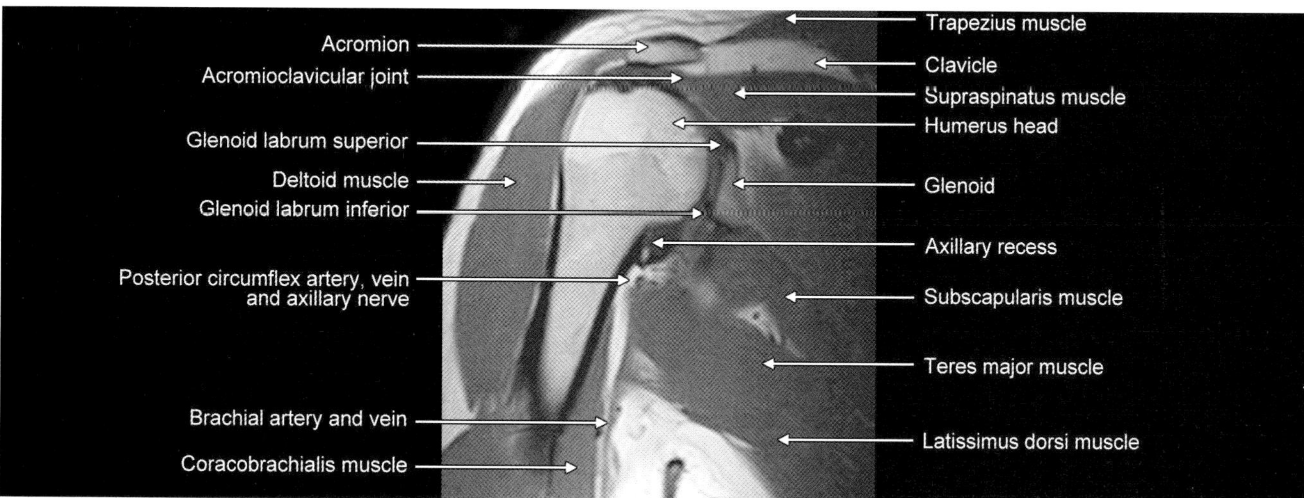

Fig. 20: Shoulder joint MRI: Coronal T1WI (corresponds to level 4 in Fig. 16)

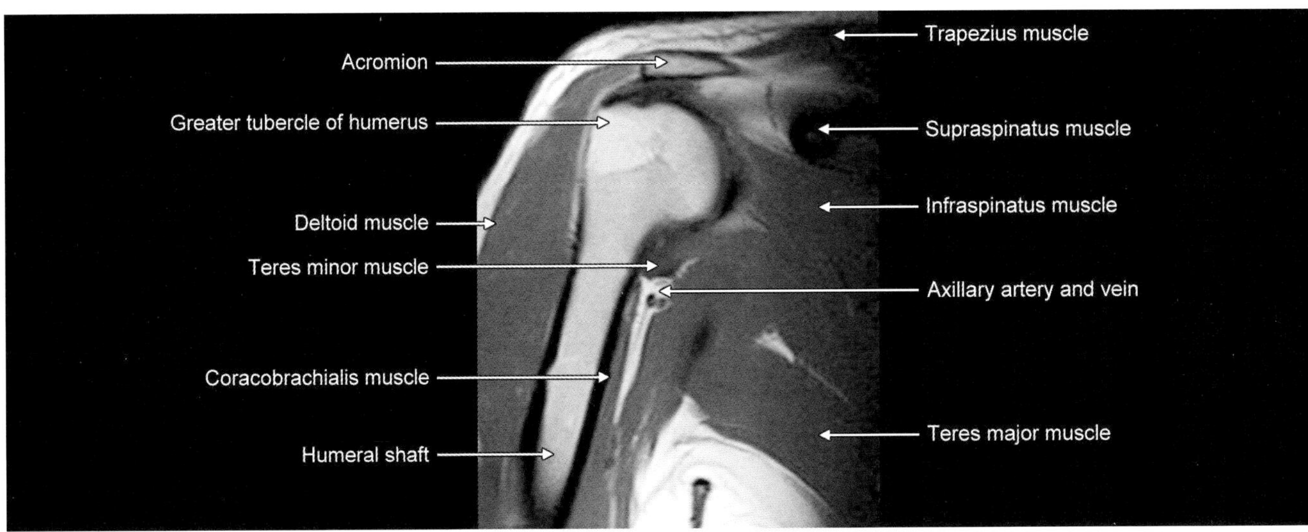

Fig. 21: Shoulder joint MRI: Coronal T1WI (corresponds to level 5 in Fig. 16)

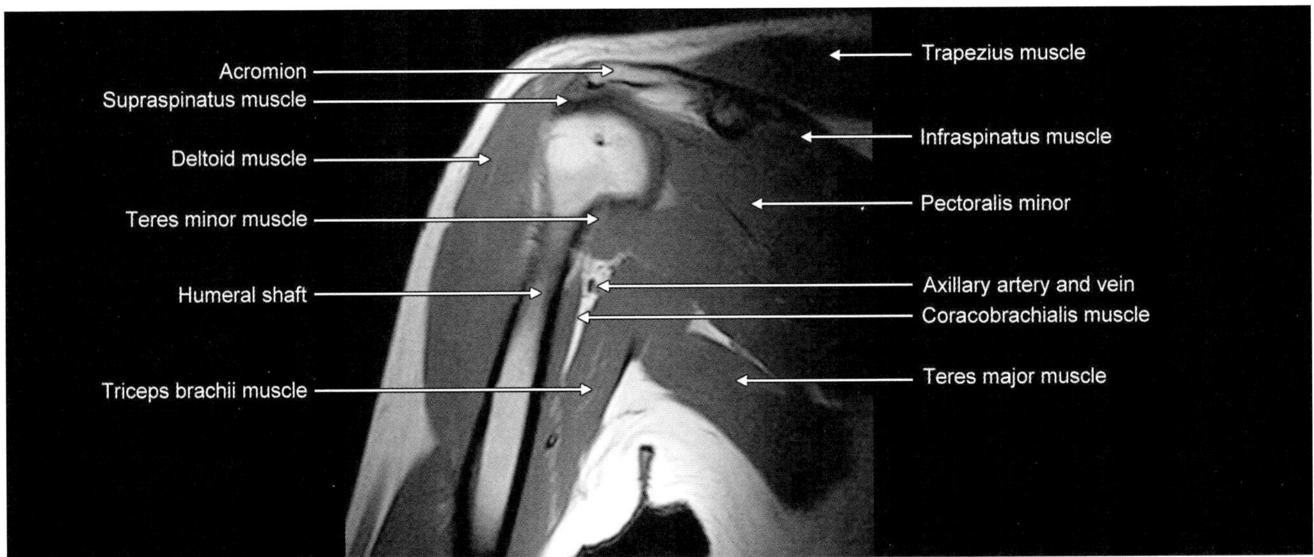

Fig. 22: Shoulder joint MRI: Coronal T1WI (corresponds to level 6 in Fig. 16)

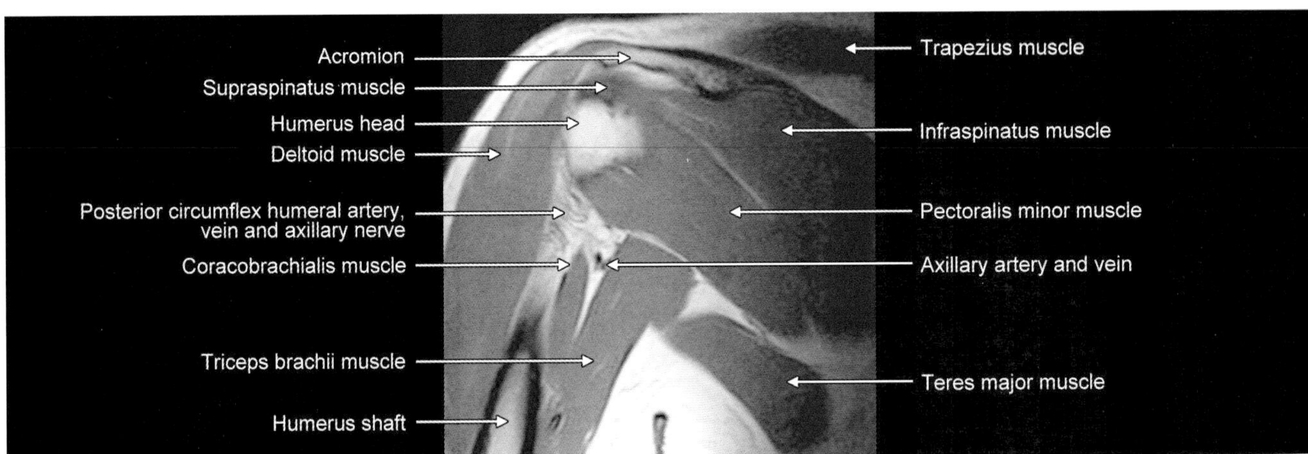

Fig. 23: Shoulder joint MRI: Coronal T1WI (corresponds to level 7 in Fig. 16)

Avulsion of Greater Tuberosity

Avulsion fracture is a pull-off fracture at a musculotendinous or ligamentous insertion site caused by sudden forceful muscle contraction or ligament traction. Such fractures are relatively common in athletic adolescents. The child characteristically describes acute onset of pain during muscle contraction. There is usually focal tenderness.

At most of these sites the fracture plane is through the physis of an apophysis as an apophysis acts as the insertion site for muscle and the physis represents a weak link in the immature skeleton.

Conventional radiographs generally confirm the diagnosis by demonstrating a bony fragment displaced at variable distance from the parent bone. Ultrasound can show displacement of the apophysis and dynamic examination allows confirmation that this corresponds with the site of tenderness. Ultrasound may also demonstrate associated hematoma within the adjacent muscle. Magnetic resonance imaging (MRI) will demonstrate reduced signal on T1 and increased signal on T2-weighted or STIR sequences, particularly within the fatty marrow of the secondary ossification center (Figs 24A and B). It is important to recognize the fracture by its characteristic site and radiographic appearance so as to avoid misdiagnosis.

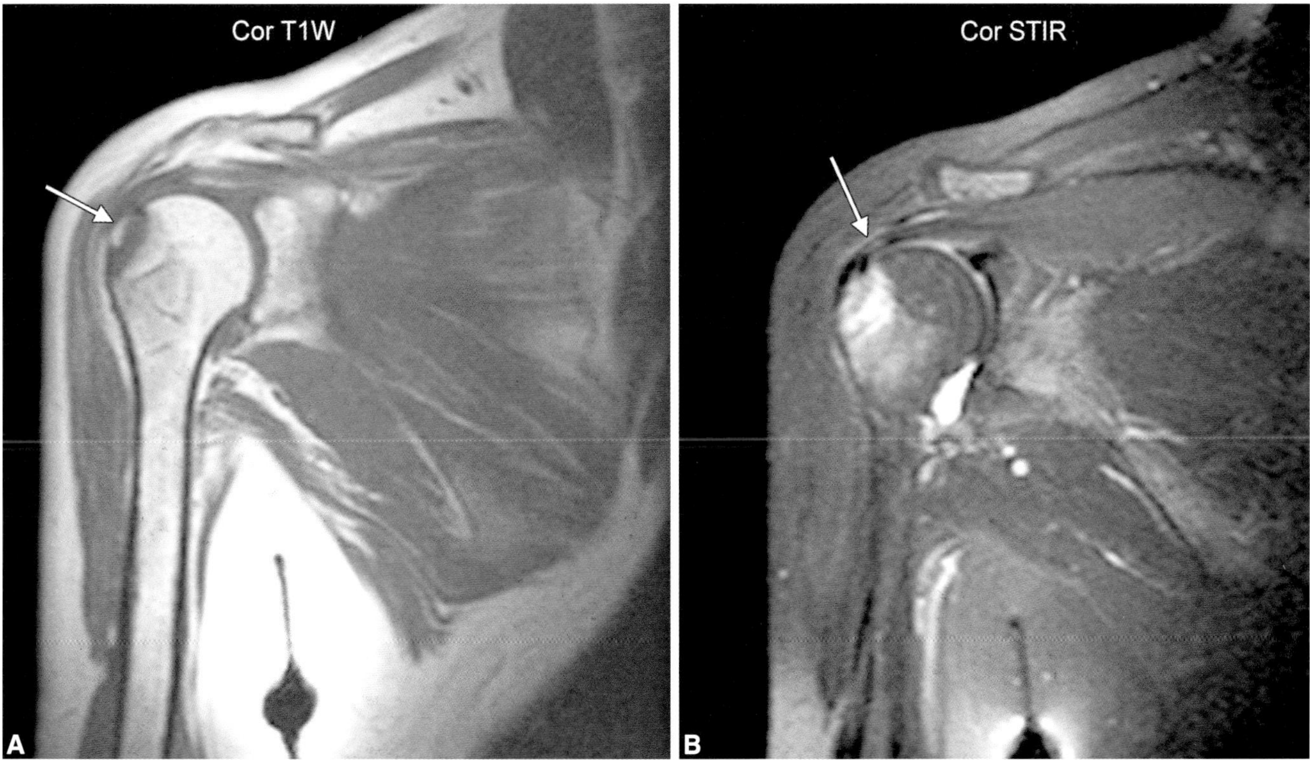

Figs 24A and B: Coronal T1W image (A) showing avulsion fracture (arrow) of the greater tuberosity and coronal STIR image (B) show partial tear of supraspinatus tendon (arrow)

Acromioclavicular Degeneration

The acromioclavicular (AC) joint is the synovial articulation between the acromion process of the scapula and the acromial facet of the clavicle in the shoulder; it is a common spot for osteoarthritis to develop in middle age.

Degeneration of the AC joint can be painful and can cause difficulty in using the shoulder for routine activities. The AC joint is under constant stress as the arm is used overhead. Weightlifters and others who repeatedly lift heavy weight overhead tend to have an increased incidence, and often at a younger age.

Acromioclavicular (AC) joint osteoarthritis may also develop following an injury to the joint, such as an AC joint separation. This injury is fairly common. A separation usually results from falling on the shoulder. The shoulder does heal, but many years later degeneration causes the AC joint to become painful. Degenerative changes or osteoarthritis occur almost universally in elderly persons. Joint space loss, sclerosis and marginal osteophytes are common radiographic features. MRI shoulder generally reveals hyperintense signal along the articular surfaces of the acromioclavicular joint with loss of joint space and degenerative osteophytes (Fig. 25).

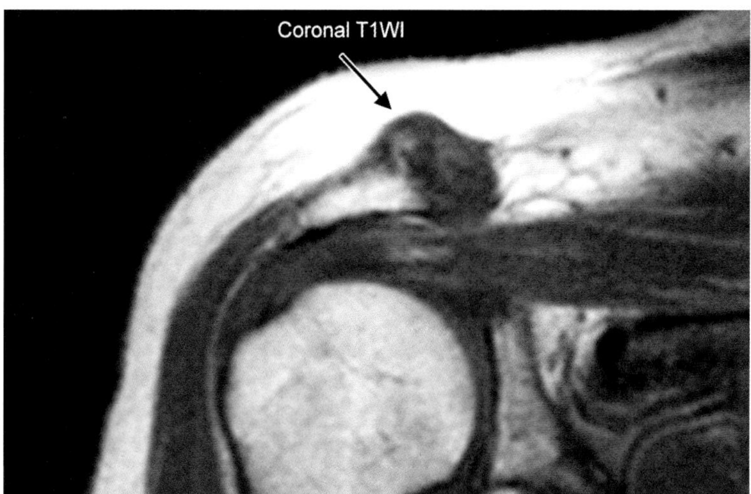

Fig. 25: A 42-year-old male patient with shoulder pain on T1W coronal image shows osteophyte formation at the acromioclavicular joint (arrow) suggestive of degeneration

Spinoglenoid Cyst

Paralabral cysts are common incidental findings on shoulder MR examinations. They arise from a torn glenoid labrum. The tear of the capsulolabral complex leads to extravasation of synovial fluid, which accumulates as either a unilocular or multilocular cystic structure. Paralabral cysts are classified as synovial cysts, ganglion cysts or pseudocysts. Synovial cysts occur through evagination of the joint capsule and contain a thin synovial cell lining. Ganglion cysts can arise from ligament, tendon, bone, joint capsule, or bursa. Pseudocysts are fluid-filled structures within the soft tissues that lack the cellular lining of a true cyst. Paralabral in spinoglenoid region are called spinoglenoid cyst (Figs 26A and B). Paralabral cysts in the suprascapular notch cause entrapment neuropathies of the suprascapular nerve alone or both the suprascapular and infrascapular nerves. If the ganglion expands in the supraspinous notch, it causes atrophy of both the supraspinatus and infraspinatus muscles. If the ganglion expands in the spinoglenoid notch, it leads to isolated atrophy of the infraspinatus muscle.

Magnetic resonance (MR) imaging findings include a thin-walled, rounded; sometimes multiloculated hyperintense structure on T2-weighted imaging and they appear hypointense on T1-weighted imaging. Electromyographic assessment and nerve conduction studies are helpful in determining the degree and site of nerve compression.

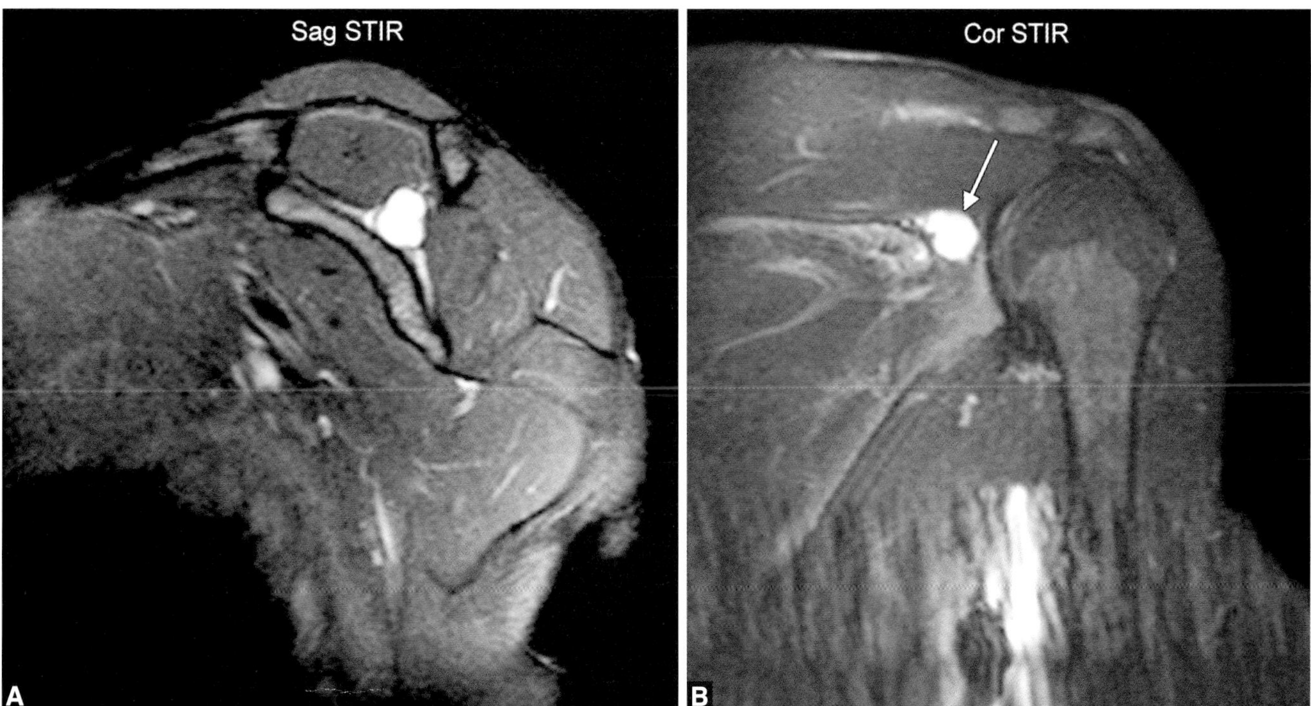

Figs 26A and B: Sagittal and coronal STIR images show a hyperintense cystic lesion in the spinoglenoid notch, a spinoglenoid cyst

Glenoid Labrum Tear

Glenoid labrum is a rim of fibrocartilaginous tissue attached to the edge of the glenoid cavity, which functions to add depth and greater stability to the glenohumeral joint.

Assessment of this structure is important in patients with shoulder instability. Arthroscopy provides accurate results but is invasive; consequently, conventional and computed arthrotomography are preferred. Using the latter methods, the Bankart lesion, Hill Sach's lesion, intra-articular osteocartilaginous bodies, and subluxation or dislocation of the bicipital tendon can be identified.

Magnetic resonance imaging, however, is the current imaging method of choice in assessing the glenoid labrum in patients with instability (Figs 27A to F). MR arthrography may also be employed.

The lesions involving the labrum are tears, anterior labroligamentous periosteal sleeve avulsion (ALPSA), glenoid labrum ovoid mass, humeral avulsion of the glenohumeralligament (HAGL), bony humeral avulsion of the glenohumeral ligament (BHAGL), and superior labral anterior and posterior (SLAP) tears.

In recurrent shoulder dislocations, disruption of the integrity of the glenoid labrum is the most frequent abnormality. In addition, with age the superior portion may become partially detached from the glenoid process.

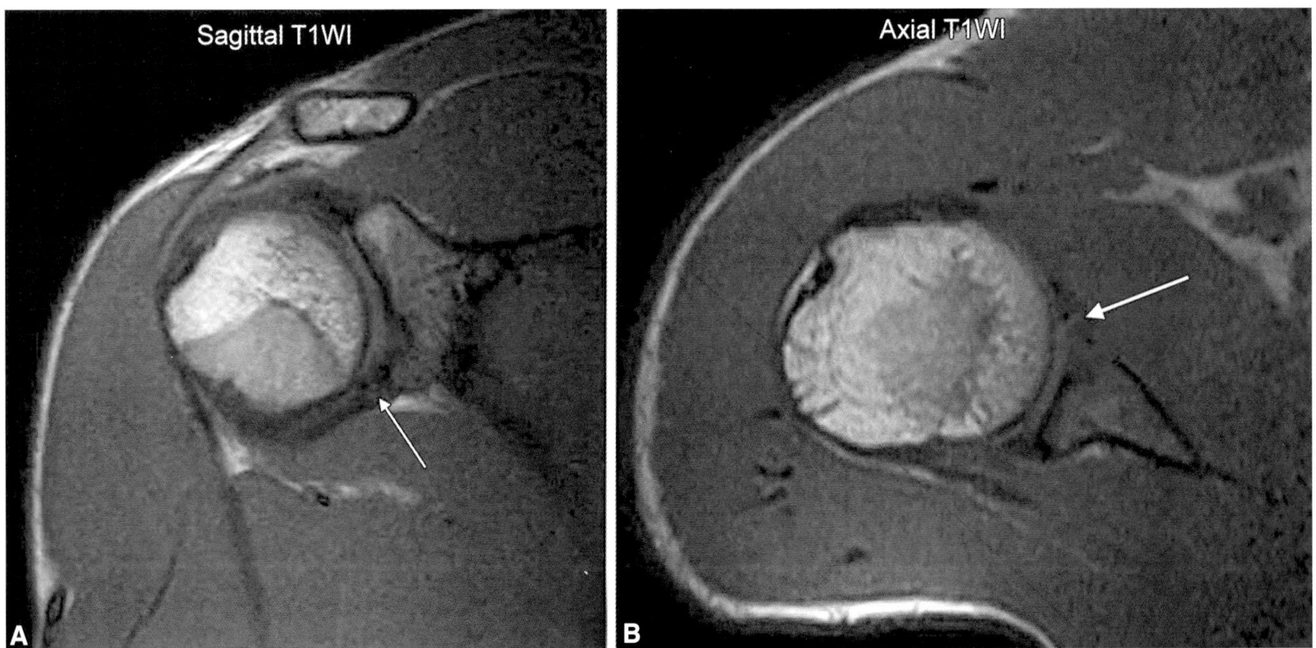

Figs 27A and B: Sagittal and axial T1-weighted images reveal abnormal hypointense signal in anteroinferior aspect of bony labrum

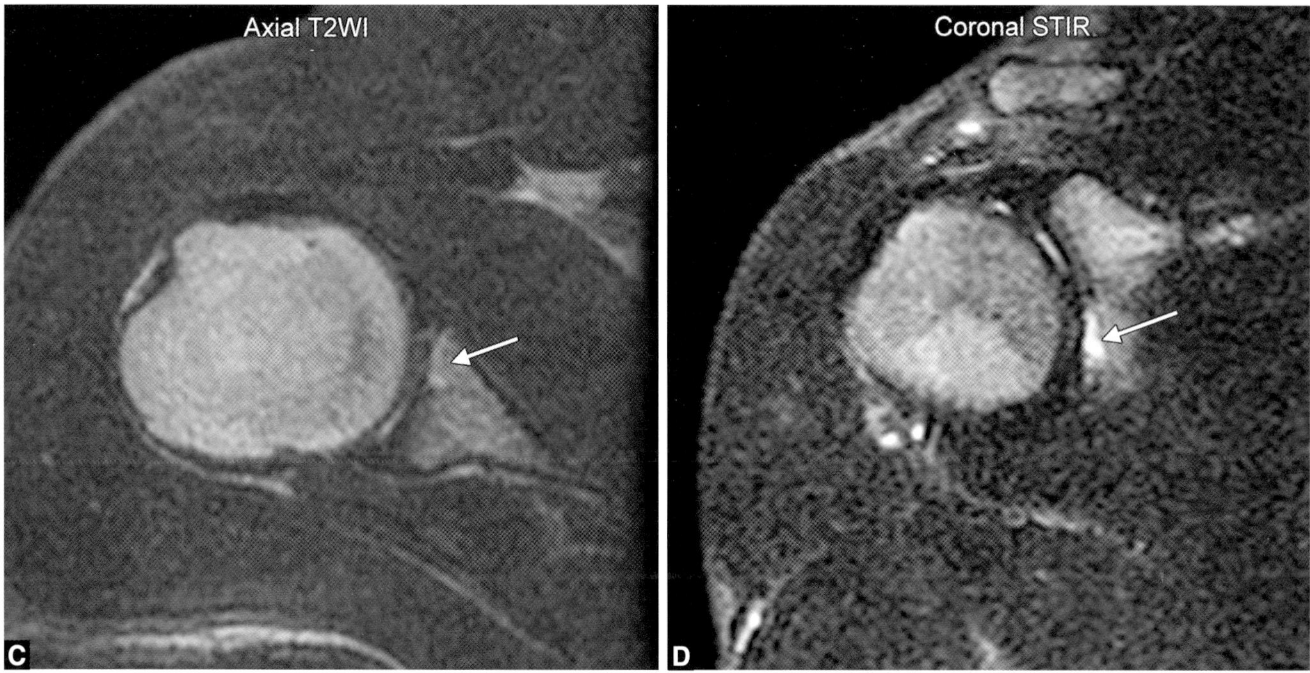

Figs 27C and D: Axial T2WI and coronal STIR images reveal abnormal hyperintense signal in anteroinferior bony labrum

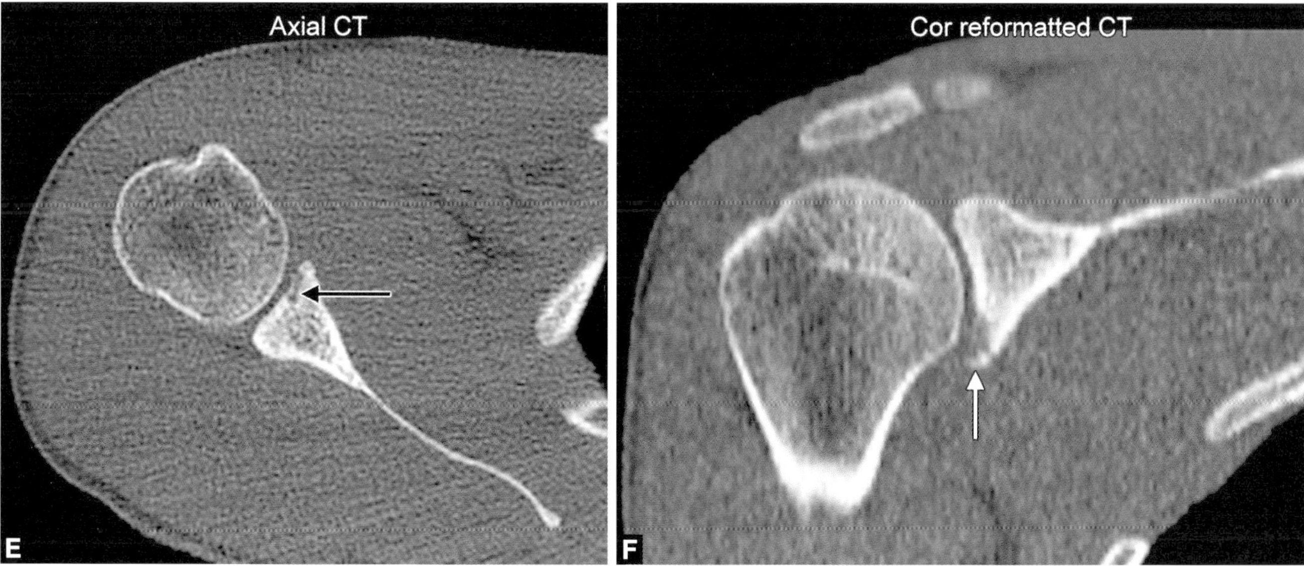

Figs 27E and F: Axial and coronal reformatted CT images show small subarticular erosive lesion in glenoid

Rotator Cuff Tears

The rotator cuff comprises of four muscles that stablize the shoulder joint: the supraspinatus, infraspinatus, teres minor and subscapularis. Tendons are fibrous tissue that connects muscle to bone. Tears in the rotator cuff can be within the muscle or at the site where the tendon attaches to the bone. Rotator cuff tears may be partial tears or full thickness tears. MRI is the investigation of choice for rotator cuff injuries (Fig. 28).

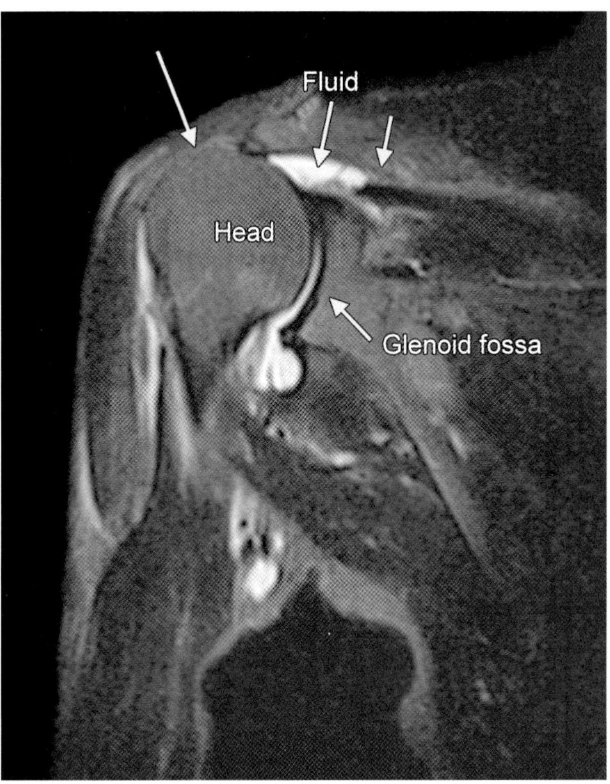

Fig. 28: STIR coronal image shows complete supraspinatus tendon tear with medial retraction of the tendon (short arrow) and superior displacement of the head of humerus (long arrow). Hyperintense signal due to effusion is seen in the subacromial space and joint cavity

Tuberculous Arthritis

Tubercle bacilli are deposited in the synovium via a hematogenous route or through direct penetration from a metaphyseal focus of osteomyelitis. A monoarticular presentation is most common and mainly large joints (hip, knee, shoulder or sacroiliac joint) are involved. Overt bony destruction is not usually evident on clinical presentation which, unlike acute septic arthritis, is characteristically slow and insidious with gradual onset of pain, stiffness and synovial swelling.

Initially joint effusion associated with a synovial hypertrophy is seen and is difficult to differentiate from other conditions including septic arthritis, Lyme disease, hemophilia, pigmented villonodular synovitis, and juvenile rheumatoid arthritis. Later on there is gradual proliferation of granulation tissue at the joint periphery which manifests clinically as a joint effusion with or without thickening of synovial tissue. Radiographically, there is soft tissue swelling and diffuse osteopenia, without a focal abnormality. Granulation tissue spreads across the joint, and the first bony changes are marginal erosions, which are evident radiographically. Over time, there is erosion of the articular cartilage and of the underlying bone, resulting in loss of joint space on plain radiographs. Later on secondary degenerative changes in the joint are observed. The early findings on magnetic resonance imaging are nonspecific, and include a joint effusion, marrow edema, and during the stage of arthritis—abnormalities within the articular cartilage and subchondral bone (Figs 29A to D).

Phemister's triad is a set of radiographic findings characteristic of tuberculous infection—juxta-articular osteoporosis, peripherally located bone erosions and gradual loss of joint space. Initially soft tissue swelling and osteoporosis may dominate the radiographic findings. Marginal erosions are characteristic of tuberculosis in 'tight' weight-bearing joints such as the hip, knee and ankle. These erosions produce corner defects simulating erosions of other synovial processes such as rheumatoid arthritis. The eventual outcome of tuberculous arthritis is a fibrous ankylosis of the affected joint. Bony ankylosis is seen occasionally but is more frequently observed with septic arthritis. The main differential diagnoses of tuberculous arthritis include erosive arthropathies (rheumatoid arthritis and gout), and other mono-articular processes (pigmented villonodular synovitis and osteochondromatosis).

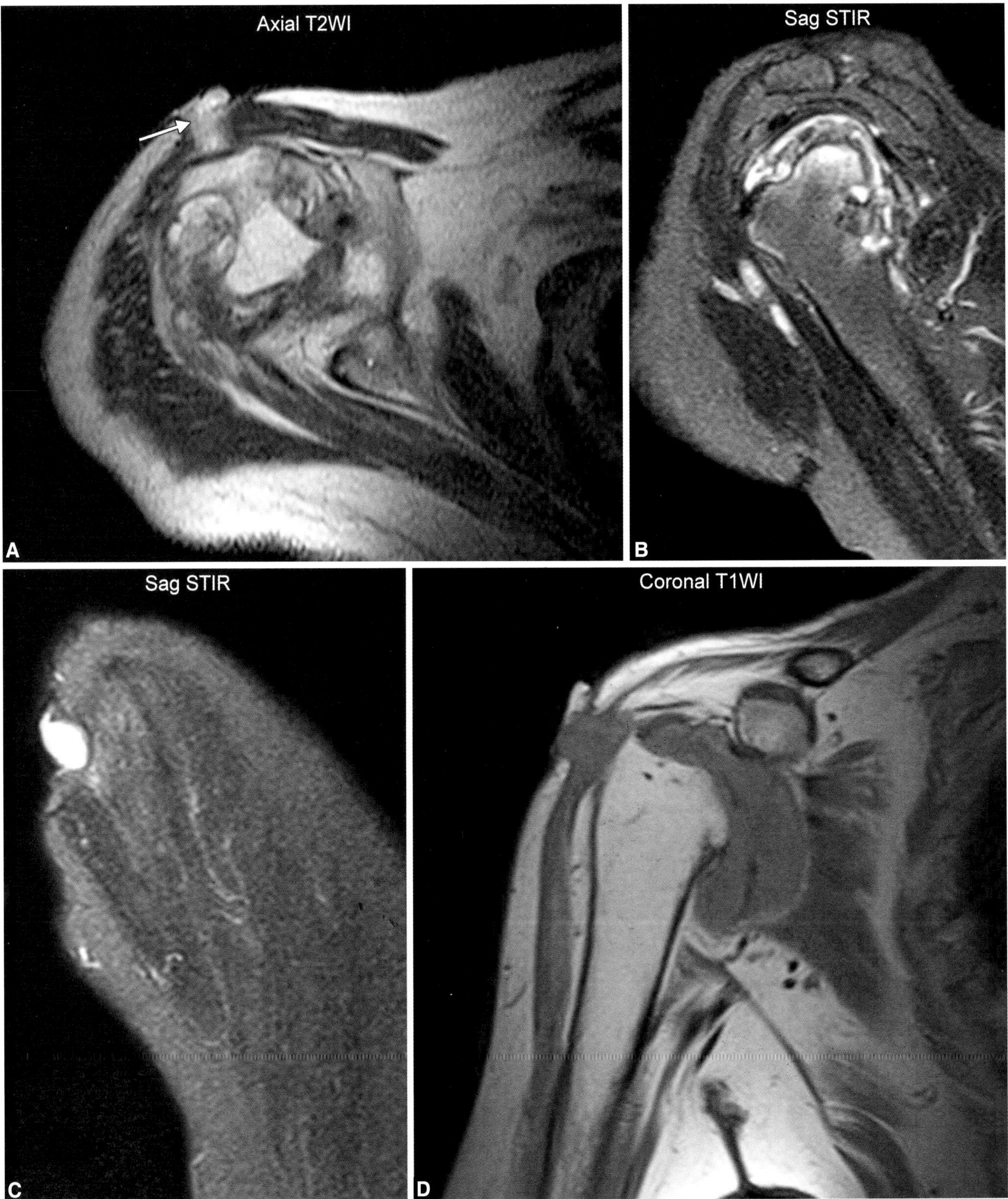

Figs 29A to D: A 57-year-old male presented with history of right shoulder discharging sinus since 5 months. No history of fever. MR shows loss of normal joint space with destruction of the articular surface involving the humerus and glenoid of right shoulder and moderate joint effusion with sinus tract extending anteriorly up to the skin surface (arrow). Atrophy of the rotator cuff muscles is seen, predominantly of the supraspinatus muscles. The effusion appears hyperintense on T2 and STIR (A to C) and hypointense on T1WI (D)

HIP JOINT

Anatomy Hip Joint

The hip joint is a multiaxial synovial joint (ball and socket joint). It engages the bony surface of the head of femur in the acetabulum of the hip bone. The stability of the joint is provided by the muscles and ligaments (Figs 30 to 52). The three parts of the hip bone (ilium, ischium and pubis) congregate at the acetabulum to form the triradiate synchondrosis.

The acetabular labrum is attached to the acetabular rim and the transverse acetabular ligament. It forms a complete ring encircling the head of femur which fits into the acetabular cavity. The transverse acetabular ligament bridges the acetabular notch.

At the site of the subtendinous bursa of psoas, where the capsule is partially deficient and weak, the joint is only supported by the psoas tendon. The inverted Y shaped iliofemoral ligament is attached superiorly deep to the rectus femoris muscle and becomes stiffer during medial rotation of femur at the hip joint.

The ligament of head of femur connects the head of femur to the acetabular cavity. Its fibers are also attached to the margins of acetabular notch. The ligament of the head of femur becomes stiffer during adduction movement of the hip joint, more so when the legs are crossed in front.

The fibrous capsule of the joint is strengthened by three ligaments—the iliofemoral ligament, the pubofemoral ligament and the ischiofemoral

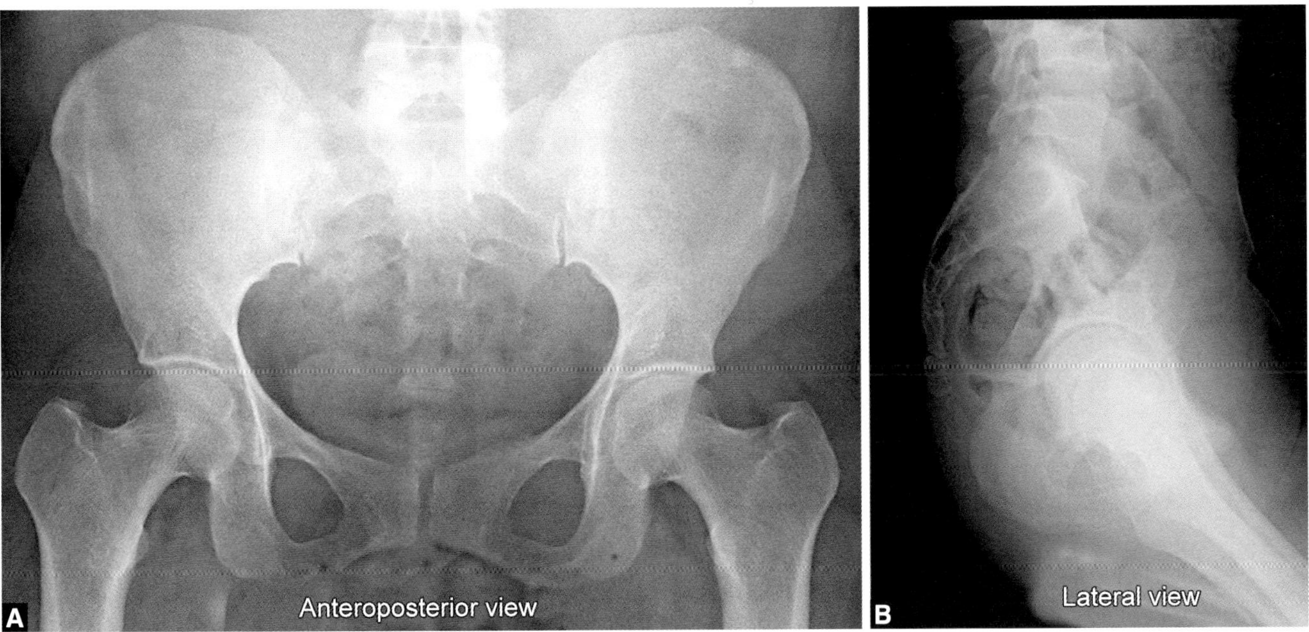

Figs 30A and B: Hip joint

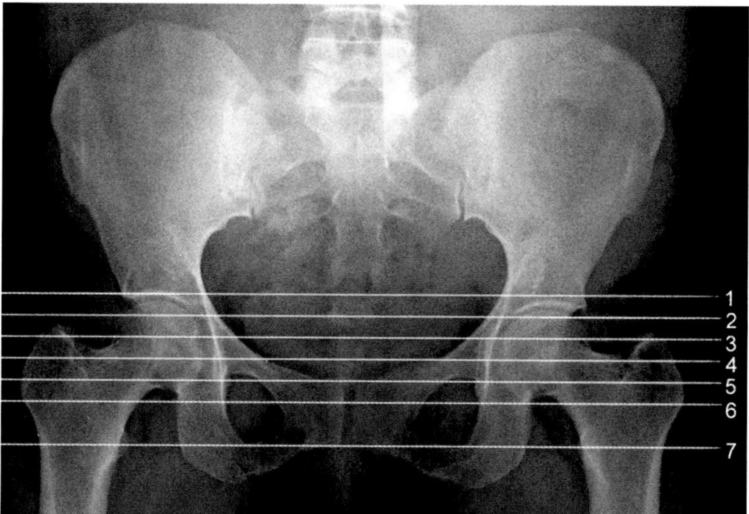

Fig. 31: Hip joint axial section plan

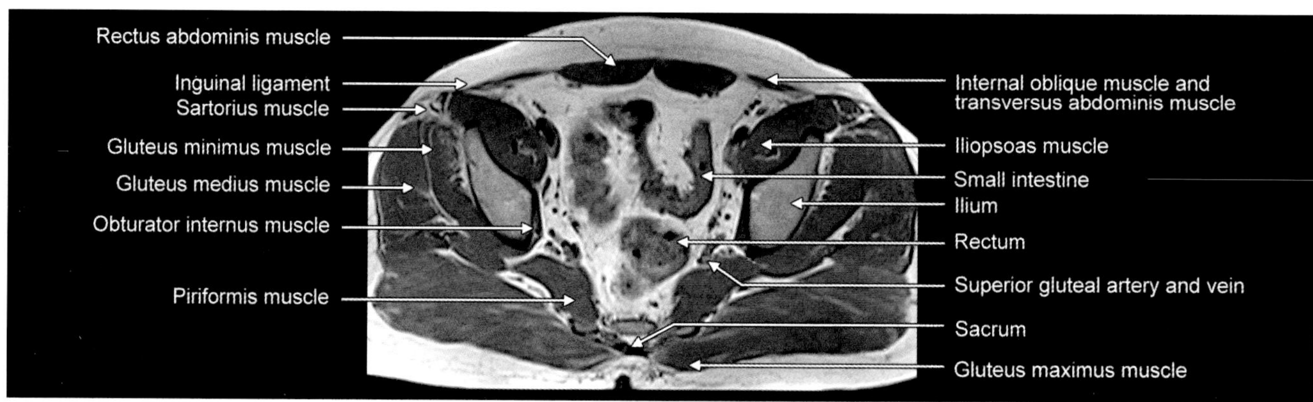

Fig. 32: Hip joint MRI: Axial T1WI (corresponds to level 1 in Fig. 31)

ligament. The fibrous capsule is thick where it forms the iliofemoral ligament and it is thinner posteriorly. The femoral sheath enclosing the femoral artery, femoral vein, lymph nodes and fat is loosely bound except posteriorly between the psoas and pectineus muscles, and is attached to the capsule of hip joint. The femoral nerve lies between the iliacus muscle and the fascia. The fibers of the capsule spiral to become stiffer during movements like extension and medial rotation of the femur.

The synovial membrane inferiorly forms a bursa for the tendon of obturator externus muscle. The subtendinous bursa of the obturator internus is seen at the lesser sciatic notch, where the tendon makes an angle of 90° to attach to the greater trochanter.

The obturator artery divides into anterior and posterior branches. The acetabular artery is a branch of the posterior branch of obturator artery. The acetabular branches pass through the acetabular foramen and enter the acetabular fossa where they diverge in the fatty tissue. The nutrient branches radiate to the margins of the acetabular fossa to enter the nutrient foramina. Major anastomosis occurs around the femoral neck involving branches from the femoral arteries (medial and lateral circumflex branches) and obturator artery branches. As the medial circumflex artery supplies a major portion of blood to the head and neck of femur, in fracture of femoral neck this blood supply is disrupted and the avascular necrosis femoral head is seen in many of these patients.

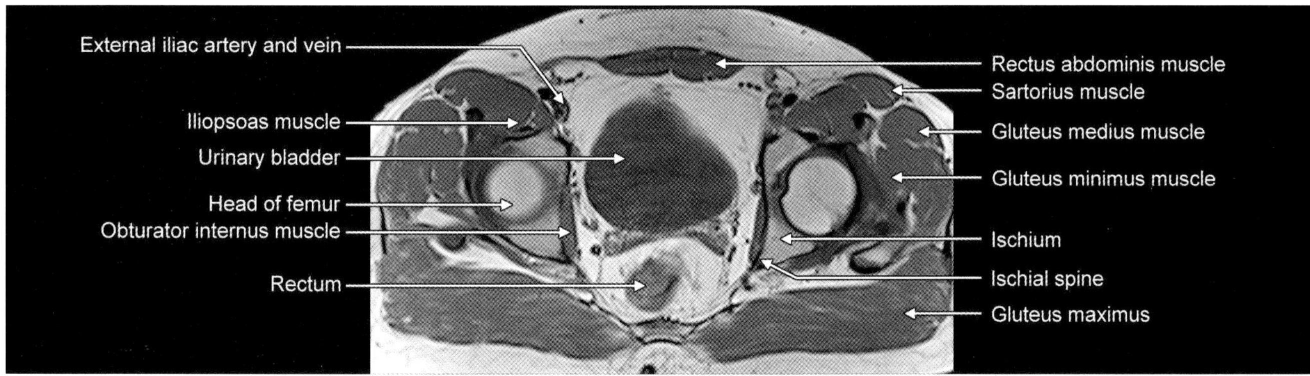

Fig. 33: Hip joint MRI: Axial T1WI (corresponds to level 2 in Fig. 31)

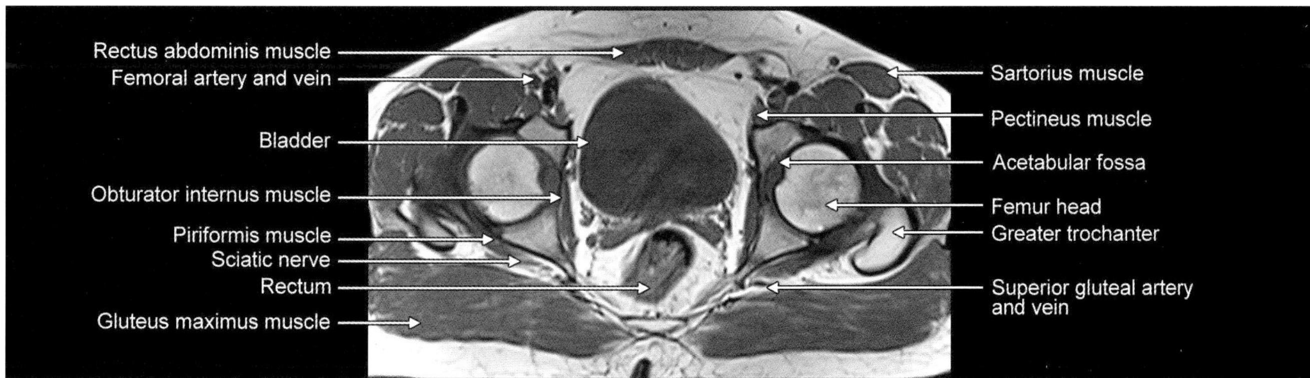

Fig. 34: Hip joint MRI: Axial T1WI (corresponds to level 3 in Fig. 31)

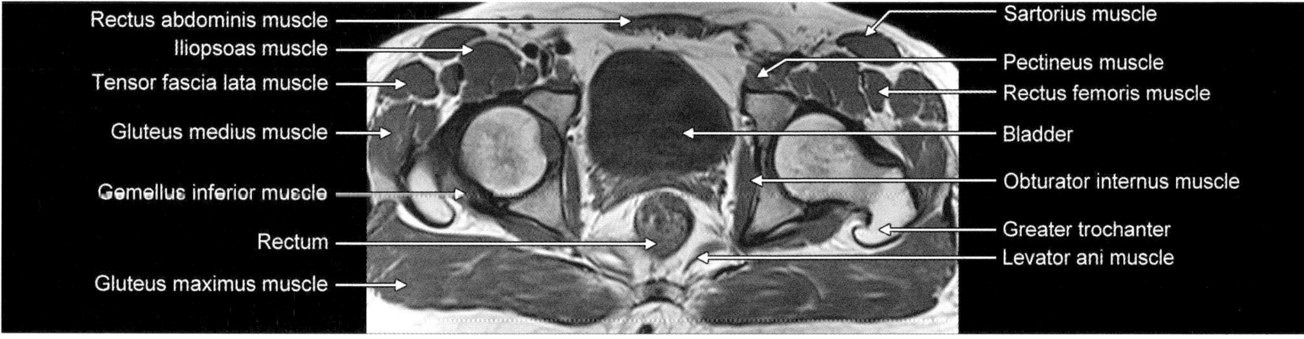

Fig. 35: Hip joint MRI: Axial T1WI (corresponds to level 4 in Fig. 31)

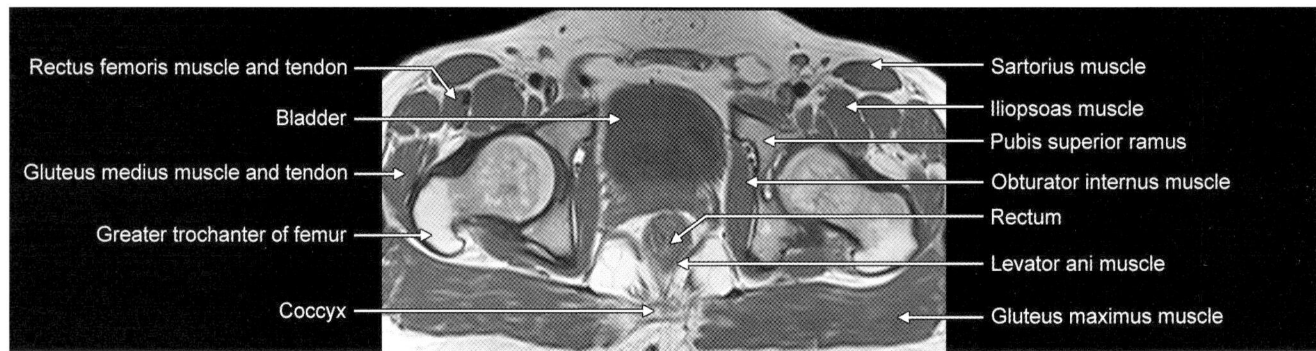

Fig. 36: Hip joint MRI: Axial T1WI (corresponds to level 5 in Fig. 31)

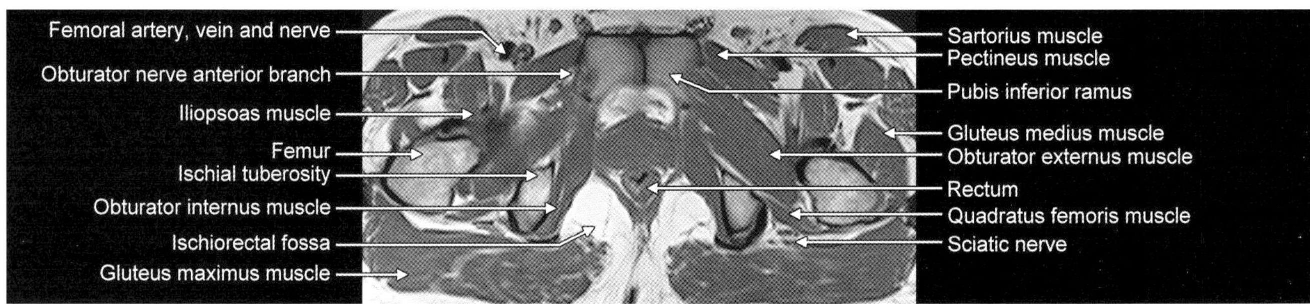

Fig. 37: Hip joint MRI: Axial T1WI (corresponds to level 6 in Fig. 31)

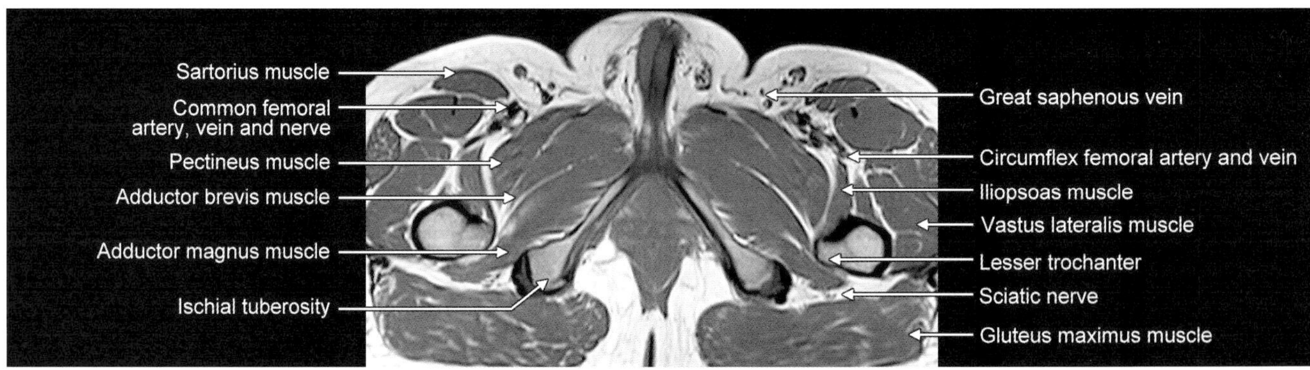

Fig. 38: Hip joint MRI: Axial T1WI (corresponds to level 7 in Fig. 31)

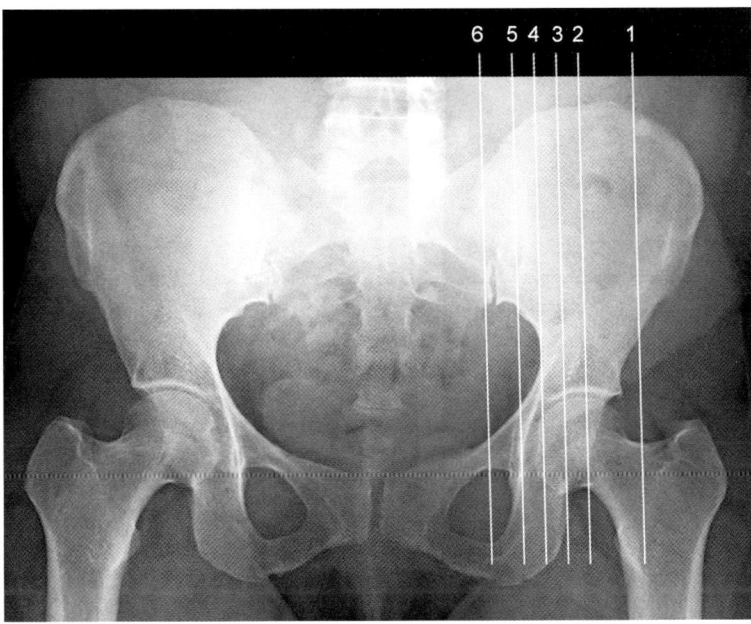

Fig. 39: Hip joint sagittal section plan

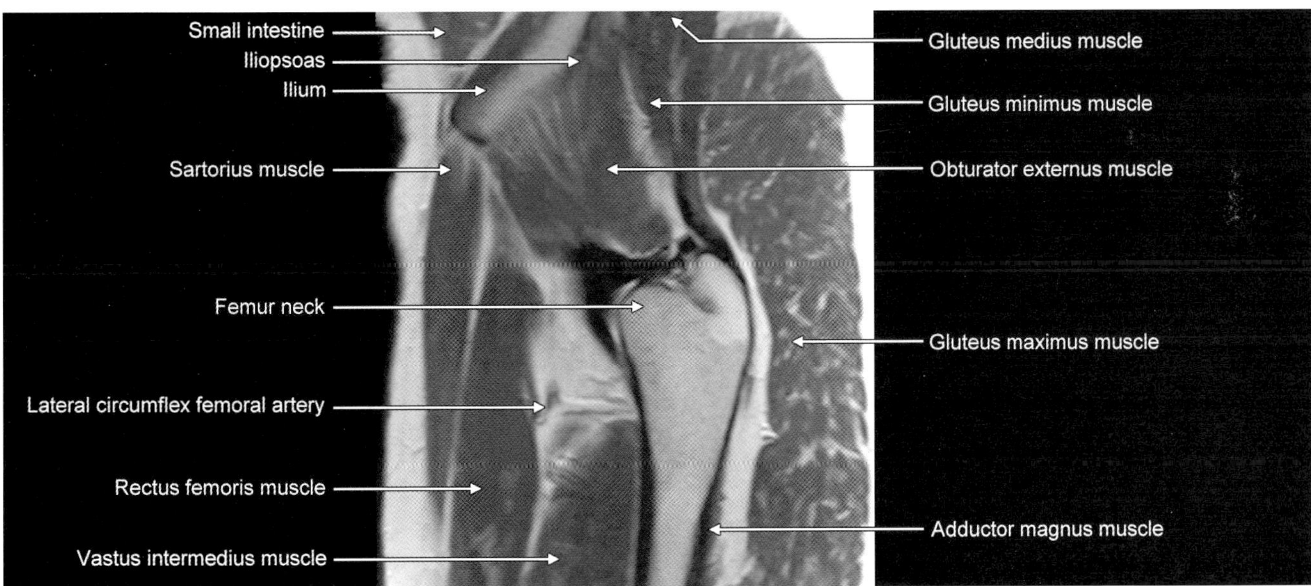

Fig. 40: Hip joint MRI: Sagittal T1WI (corresponds to level 1 in Fig. 39)

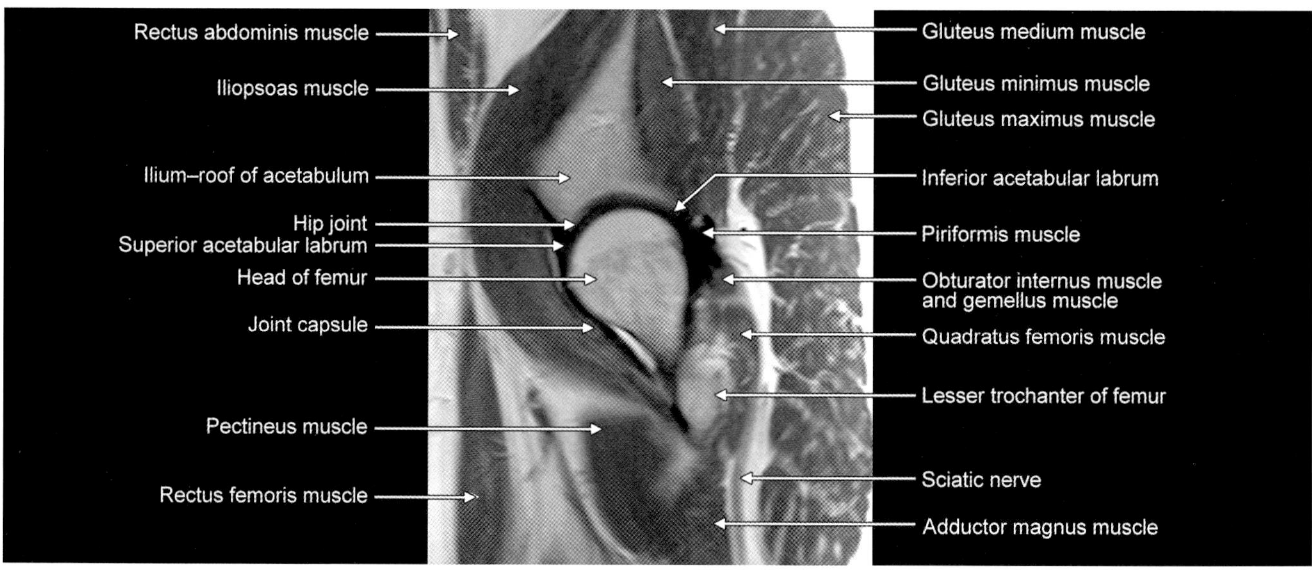

Fig. 41: Hip joint MRI: Sagittal T1WI (corresponds to level 2 in Fig. 39)

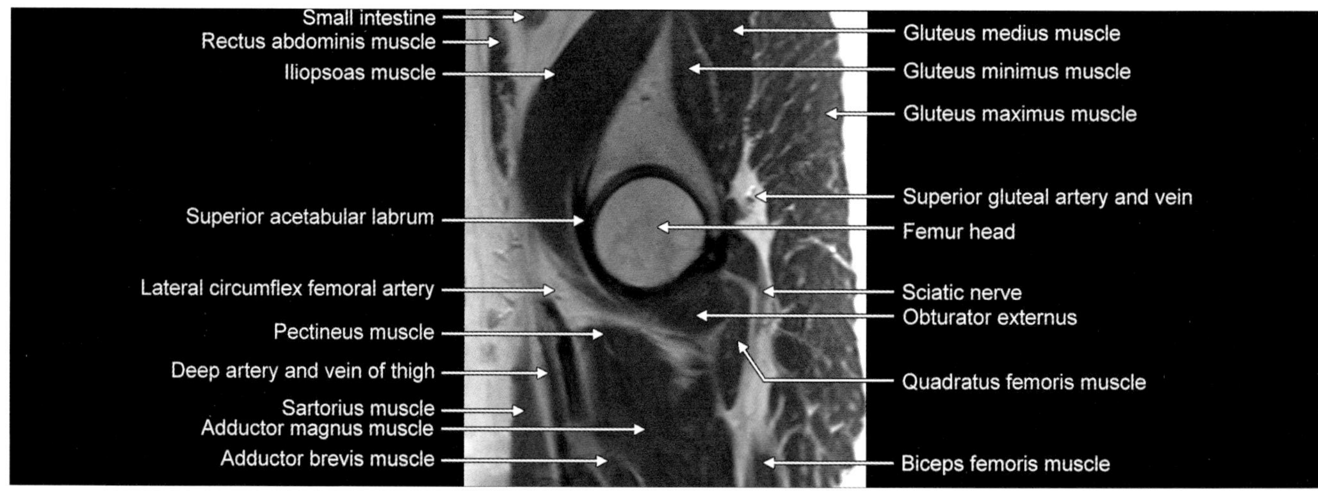

Fig. 42: Hip joint MRI: Sagittal T1WI (corresponds to level 3 in Fig. 39)

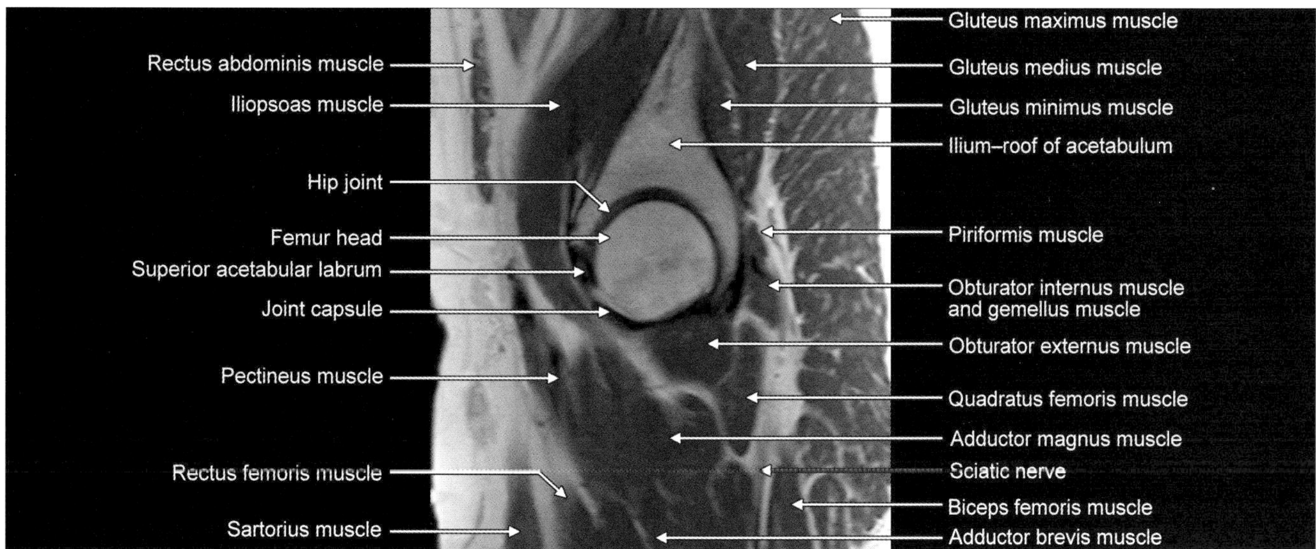

Fig. 43: Hip joint MRI: Sagittal T1WI (corresponds to level 4 in Fig. 39)

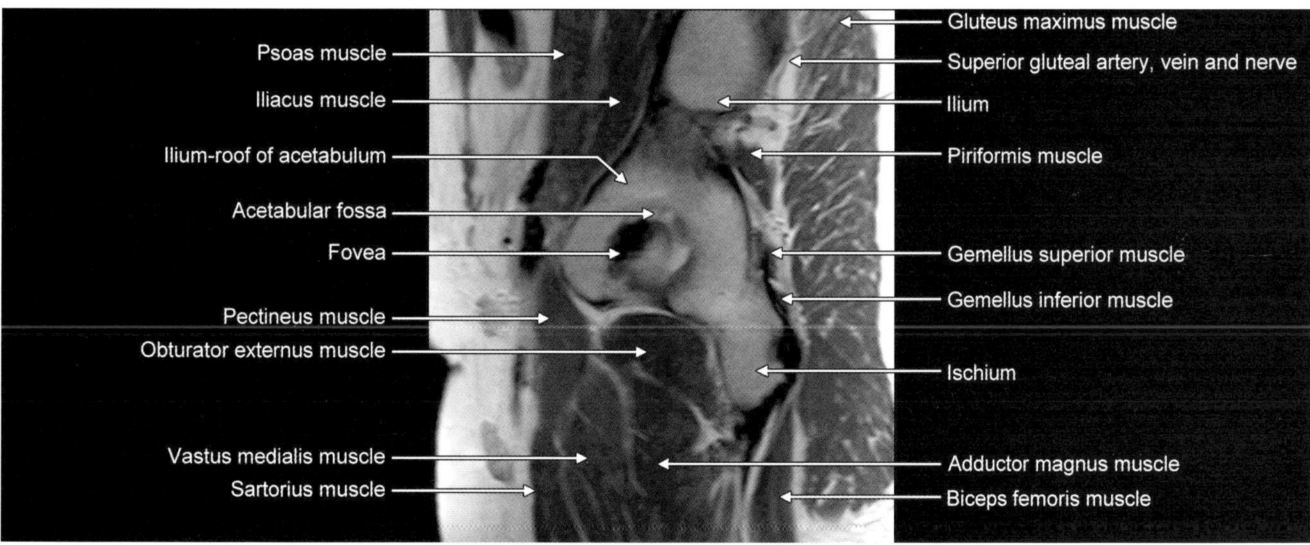

Fig. 44: Hip joint MRI: Sagittal T1WI (corresponds to level 5 in Fig. 39)

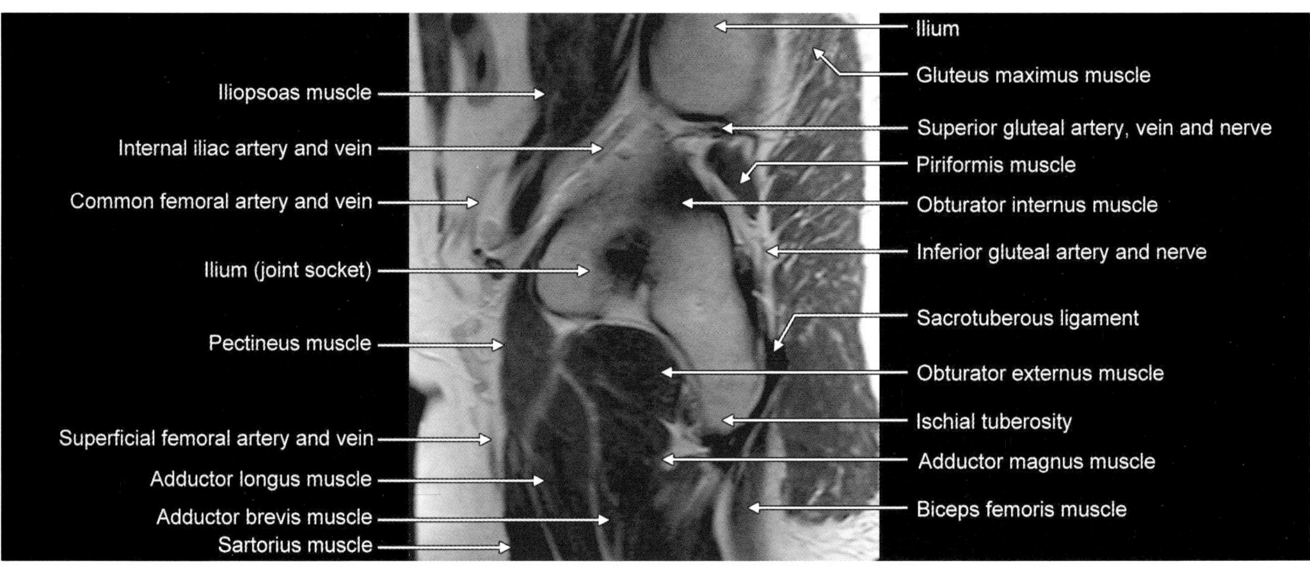

Fig. 45: Hip joint MRI: Sagittal T1WI (corresponds to level 6 in Fig. 39)

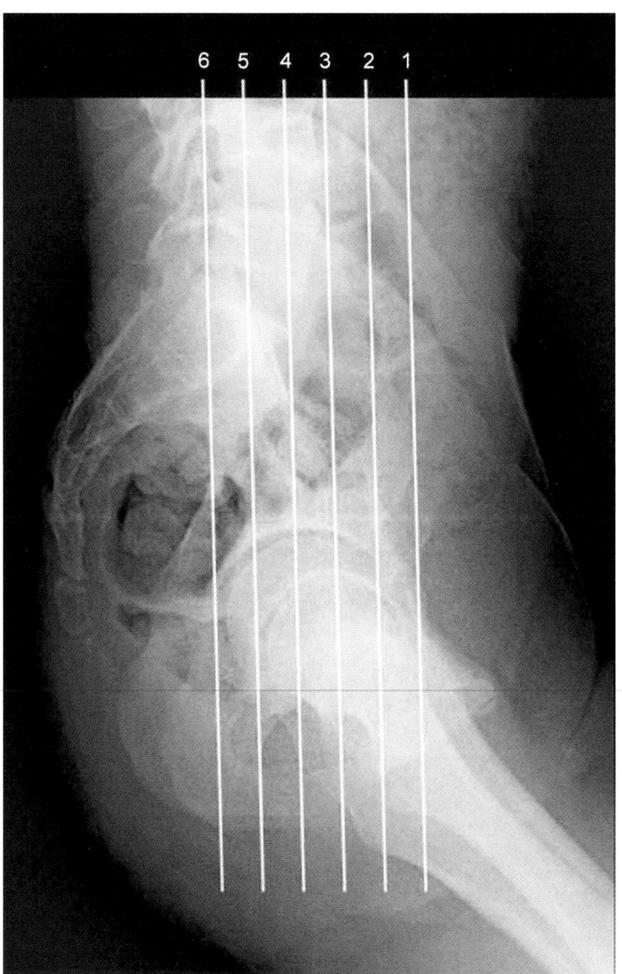

Fig. 46: Hip joint coronal section plan

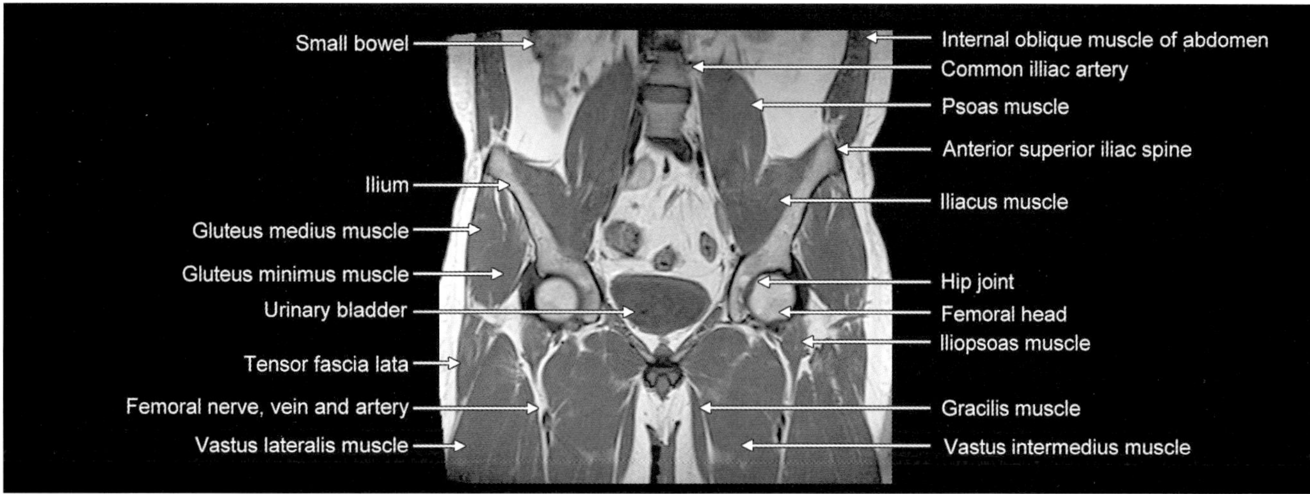

Fig. 47: Hip joint MRI: Coronal T1WI (corresponds to level 1 in Fig. 46)

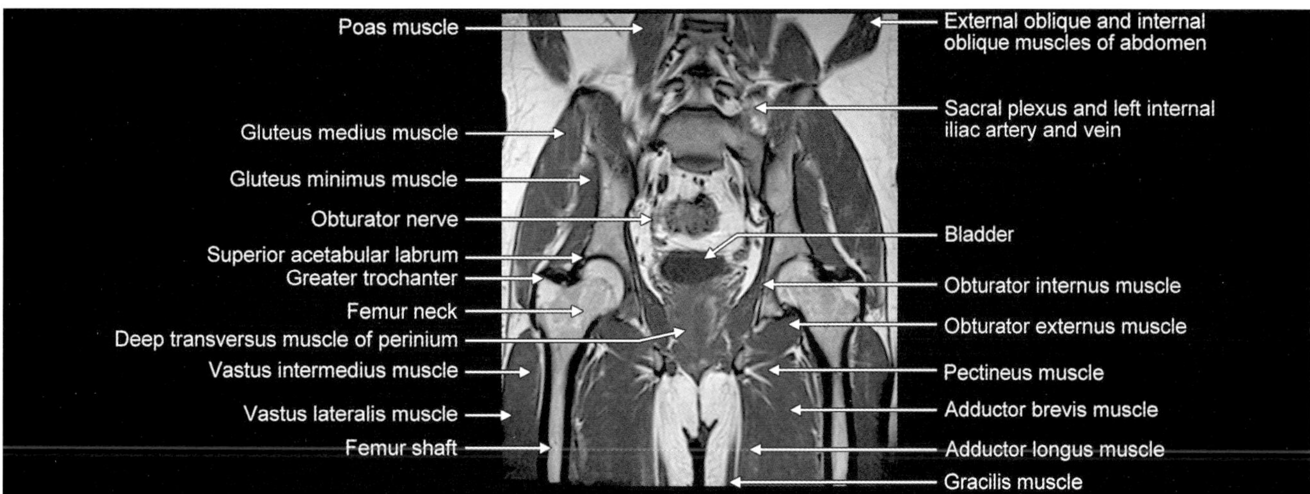

Fig. 48: Hip joint MRI: Coronal T1WI (corresponds to level 2 in Fig. 46)

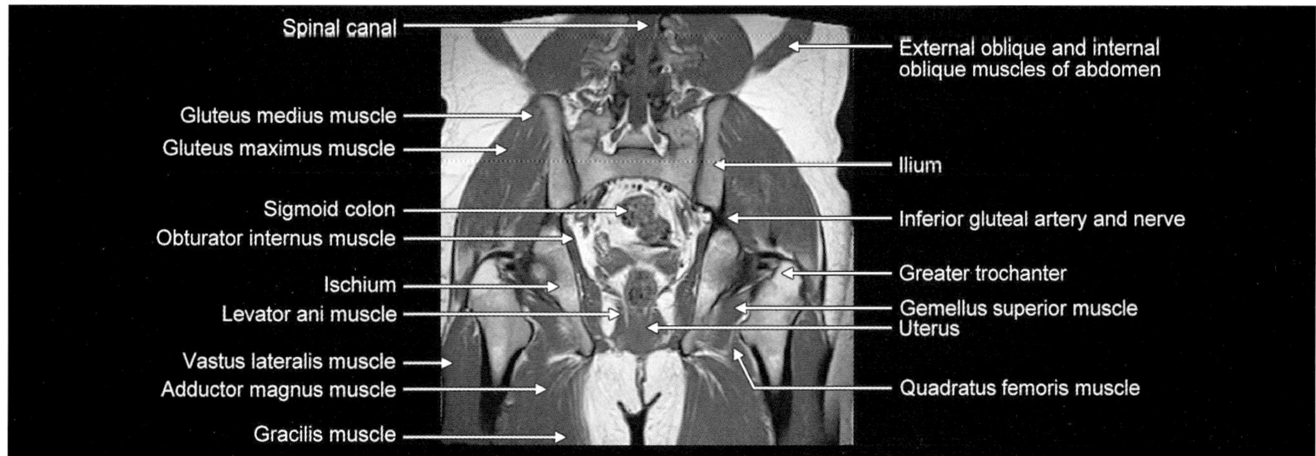

Fig. 49: Hip joint MRI: Coronal T1WI (corresponds to level 3 in Fig. 46)

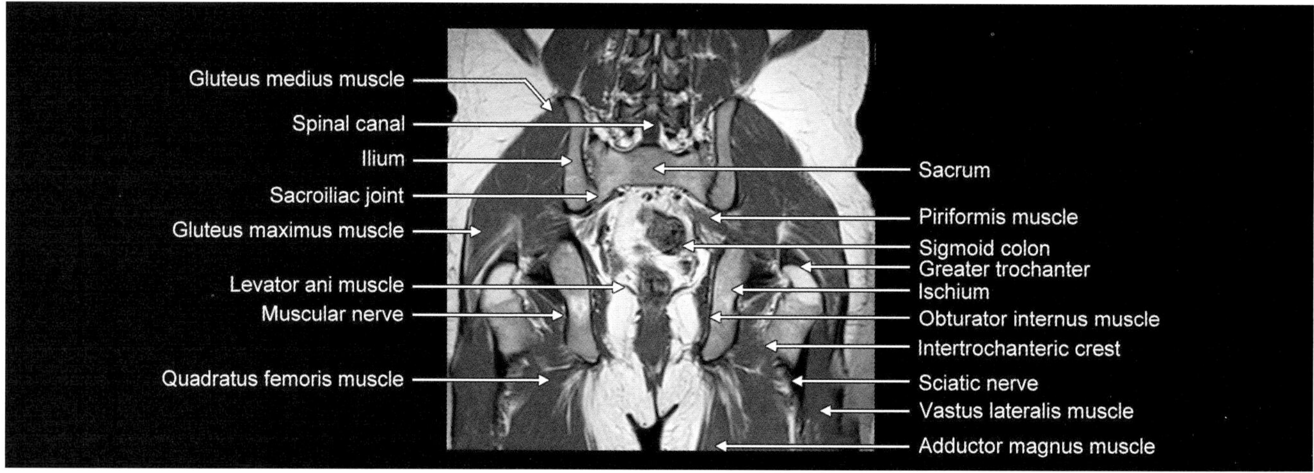

Fig. 50: Hip joint MRI: Coronal T1WI (corresponds to level 4 in Fig. 46)

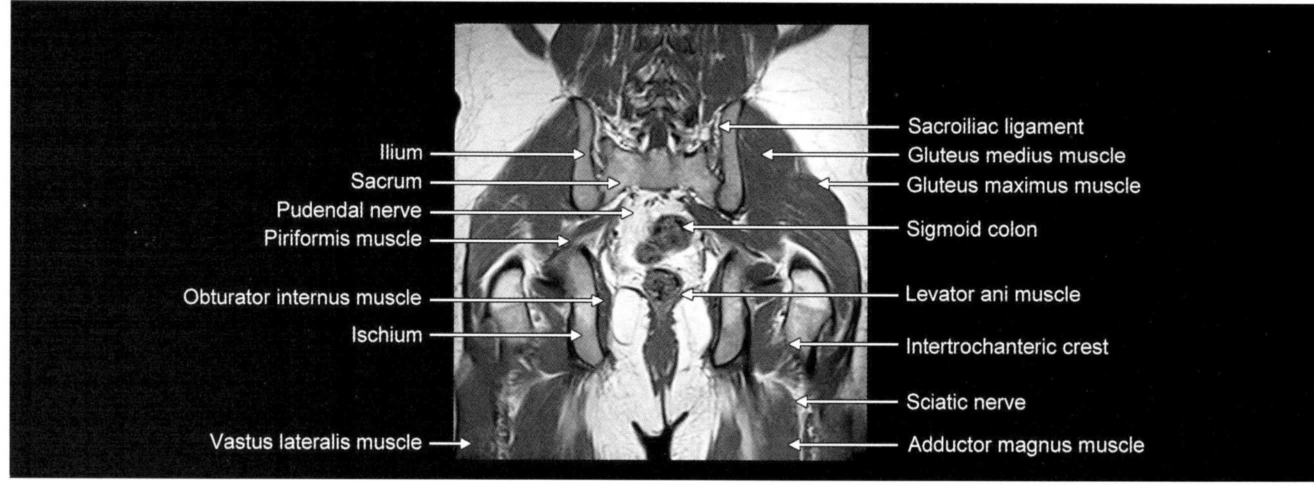

Fig. 51: Hip joint MRI: Coronal T1WI (corresponds to level 5 in Fig. 46)

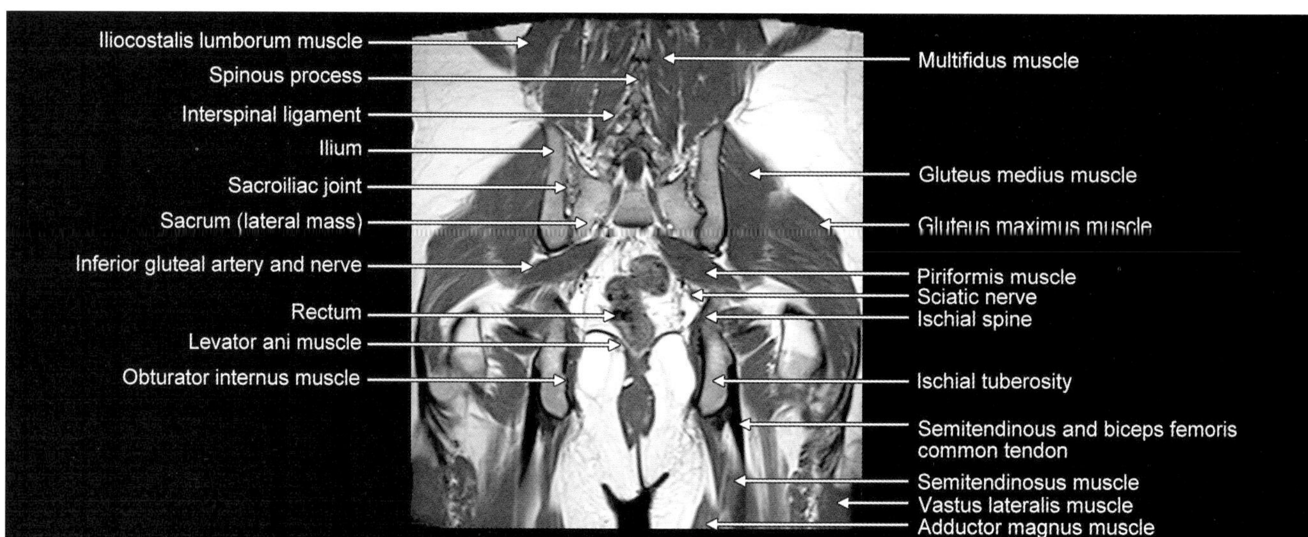

Fig. 52: Hip joint MRI: Coronal T1WI (corresponds to level 6 in Fig. 46)

Avascular Necrosis

Avascular necrosis (AVN) or osteonecrosis is the death of bone tissue due to a lack of blood supply leading to tiny breaks in the bone. It is the result of interruption of blood flow to the part of bone. It is seen if the bone is fractured or the joint becomes dislocated or with long-term use of steroids and excessive alcohol intake. Other common causes for avascular necrosis include sickle cell disease, pancreatitis, collagen vascular disease, Gaucher's disease, post infective and radiations. Hip is the most common joint affected by avascular necrosis and worsens with time.

Ficat and Arlet classification is used for AVN of the hip. It uses a combination of clinical features, plain film and MRI.

Grade 0

- *Clinical symptoms:* Nil
- *X-ray:* Normal
- *MRI:* Double line sign on the MR image in the asymptomatic hip in this stage.

Grade I

- *Clinical symptoms:* Pain typically in the groin
- *X-ray:* Trabeculae appear normal or minor osteopenia in femoral head.
- MR imaging may show a single line on T1 weighted images and the double line sign on FS PD FSE images. The double-line sign is specific and pathognomonic for AVN. The hyperintensity at the periphery of the necrotic focus is probably caused by hypervascular granulation tissue, a hyperemic response adjacent to thickened trabeculae.
- *Bone scan:* Central photon void area is noted in the femur head with peripherally increased tracer uptake in the femoral head (Fig. 53).

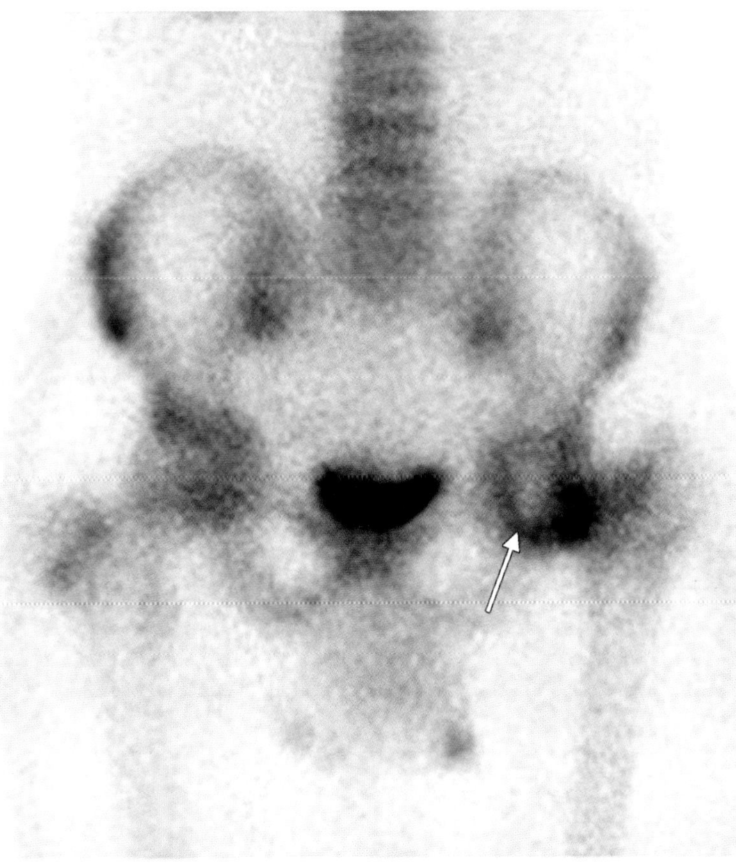

Fig. 53: Tc99m MDP—three phase bone scan shows central photon void area in the femoral head with peripherally increased (arrow) tracer uptake in the femoral head

Grade II

- *Clinical symptoms:* Pain and stiffness
- *X-ray:* Mixed osteopenia and/or sclerosis in the femoral head
- *MRI:* Geographic defect in femoral head as seen in stage I with associated marrow edema from the nonischemic region of the femoral head into the femoral neck (Figs 54A to C)
- *Bone scan:* Increased uptake in femoral head.

Grade III

- *Clinical symptoms :* Pain and stiffness+/- radiation to knee and limp
- *X-ray:* Stage III disease is marked by the loss of the spherical shape of the femoral head. The AP radiograph may appear normal, but the lateral view often reveals a crescent sign, or radiolucency, under the subchondral bone. This represents a fracture between the subchondral bone and

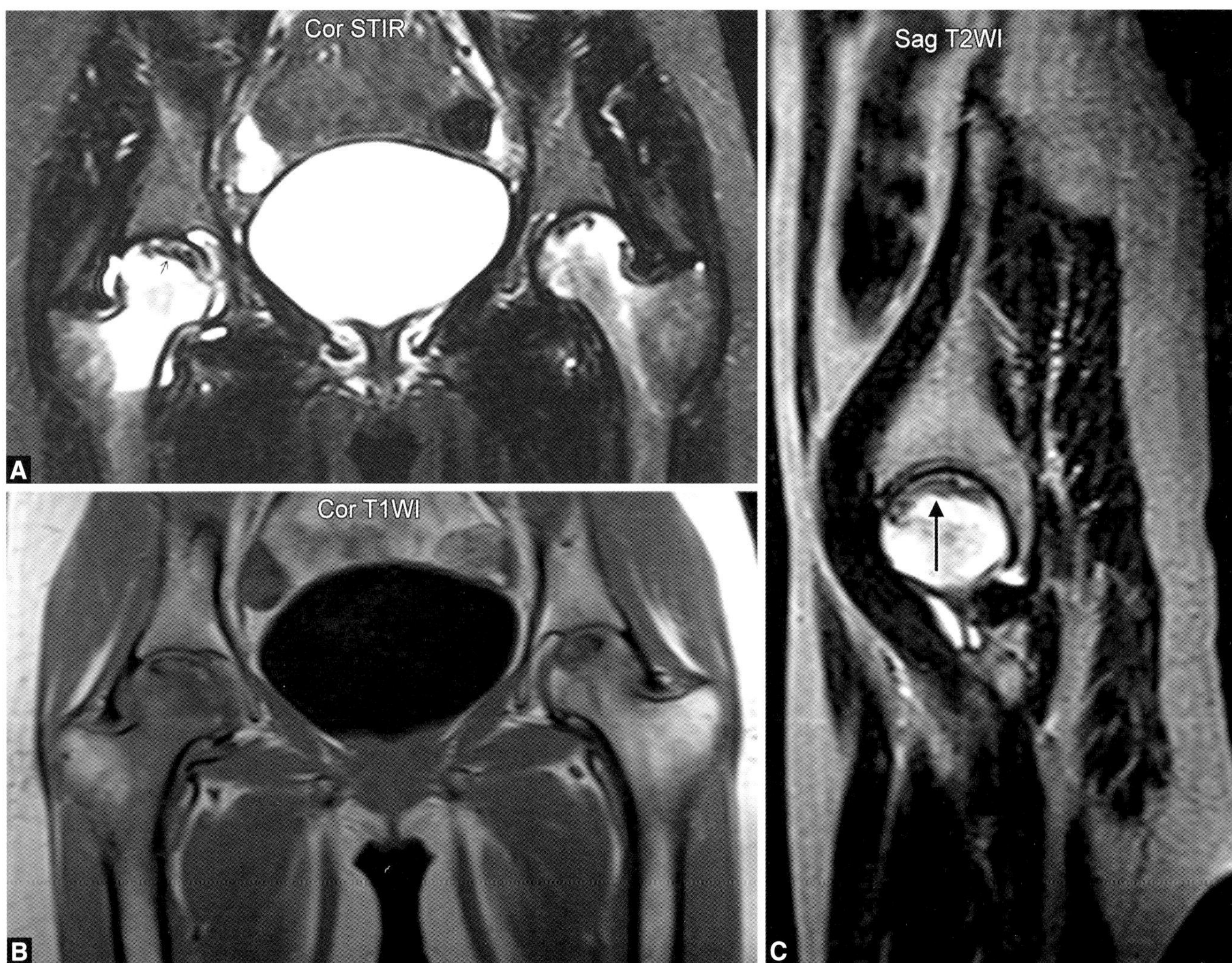

Figs 54A to C: Coronal STIR (A), coronal T1W (B) and sagittal T2W (C) images reveal well-defined crescents (arrow) of altered marrow signal in both femoral heads. The marrow within the crescent is predominantly hypointense on T1W, T2W and STIR images, suggestive of sclerosis. Normal contour of femoral head is maintained. These findings are suggestive of Grade II avascular necrosis

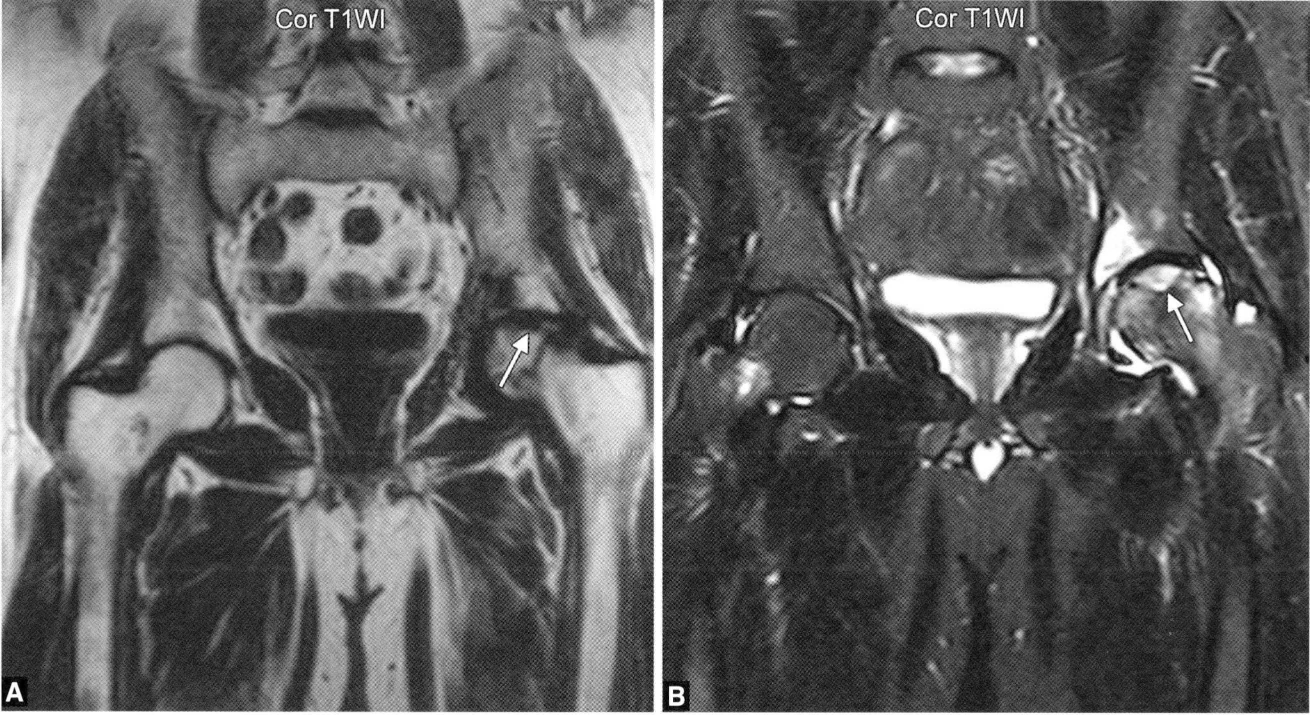

Figs 55A and B: Coronal T1WI (A) and STIR (B) shows evidence of altered signal changes seen in left femoral head with sclerosis and subchondral collapse (arrow). These findings are of Grade III AVN

the underlying femoral head. The crescent sign is the earliest indication of mechanical failure from accumulated stress fractures of nonrepaired necrotic trabeculae. The necrotic area becomes radio dense. The joint space remains preserved or may actually increase in height.

- *MRI:* Findings as seen in stage II with loss of the spherical shape of the femoral head. Subchondral collapse with crescent sign (Figs 55A and B).

Grade IV

- *Clinical symptoms :* Pain and limp
- *X-ray:* The femoral head undergoes further collapse, leading to articular cartilage destruction and joint space narrowing with evidence of secondary degenerative change in hip joint (Fig. 56A).
- *MRI:* Finding as seen in stage III with further collapse of femoral head and secondary degenerative change in hip joint (Figs 56A to E).

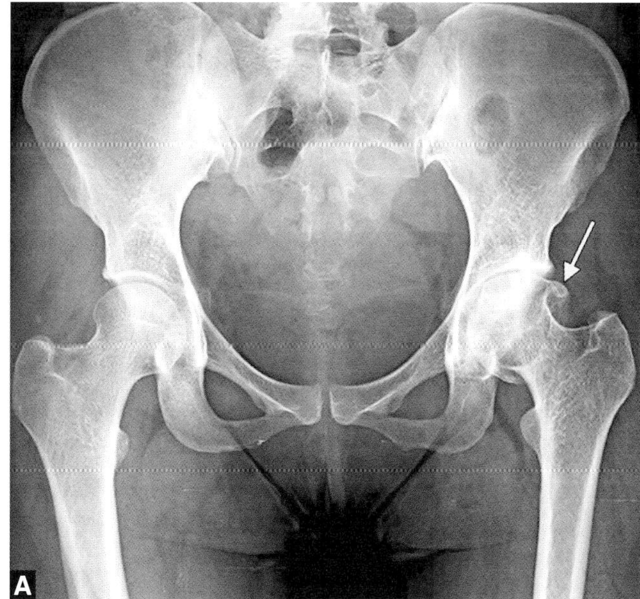

Fig. 56A: X-ray pelvis AP view shows a well-defined crescents of radiolucency with loss of normal contour of left femoral head with degenerative changes in the form of osteophytes

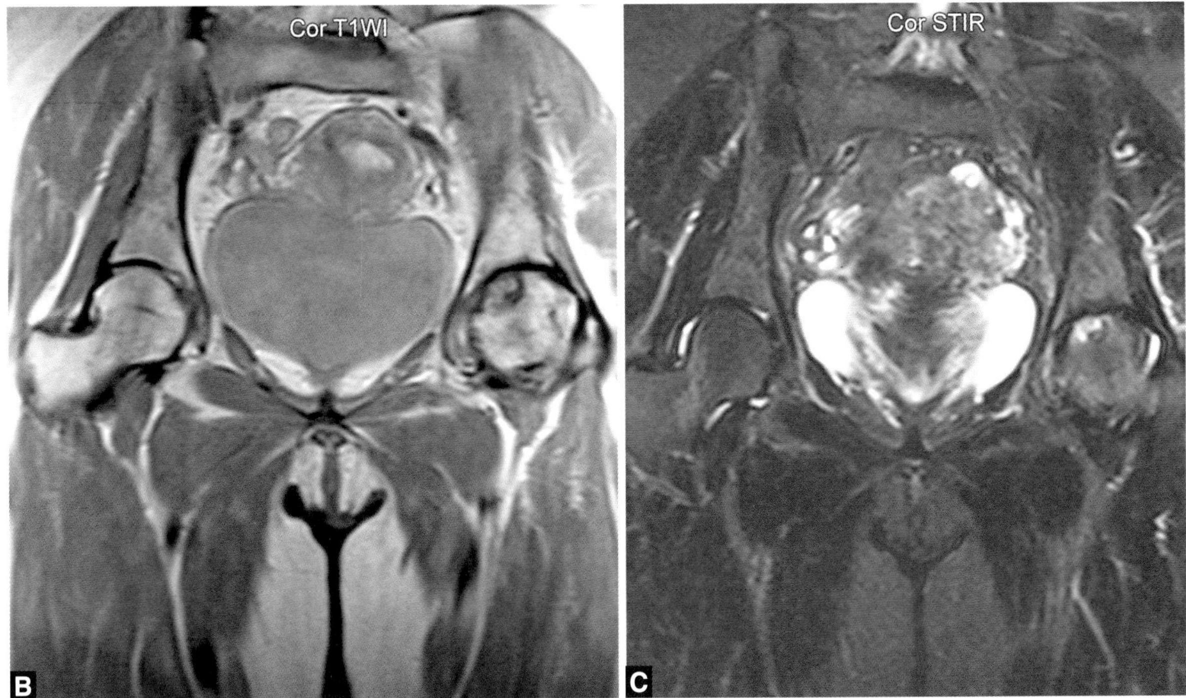

Figs 56B and C: Coronal T1WI (B) STIR (C) images show a well-defined crescents of altered marrow signal in the subchondral region of left femoral head

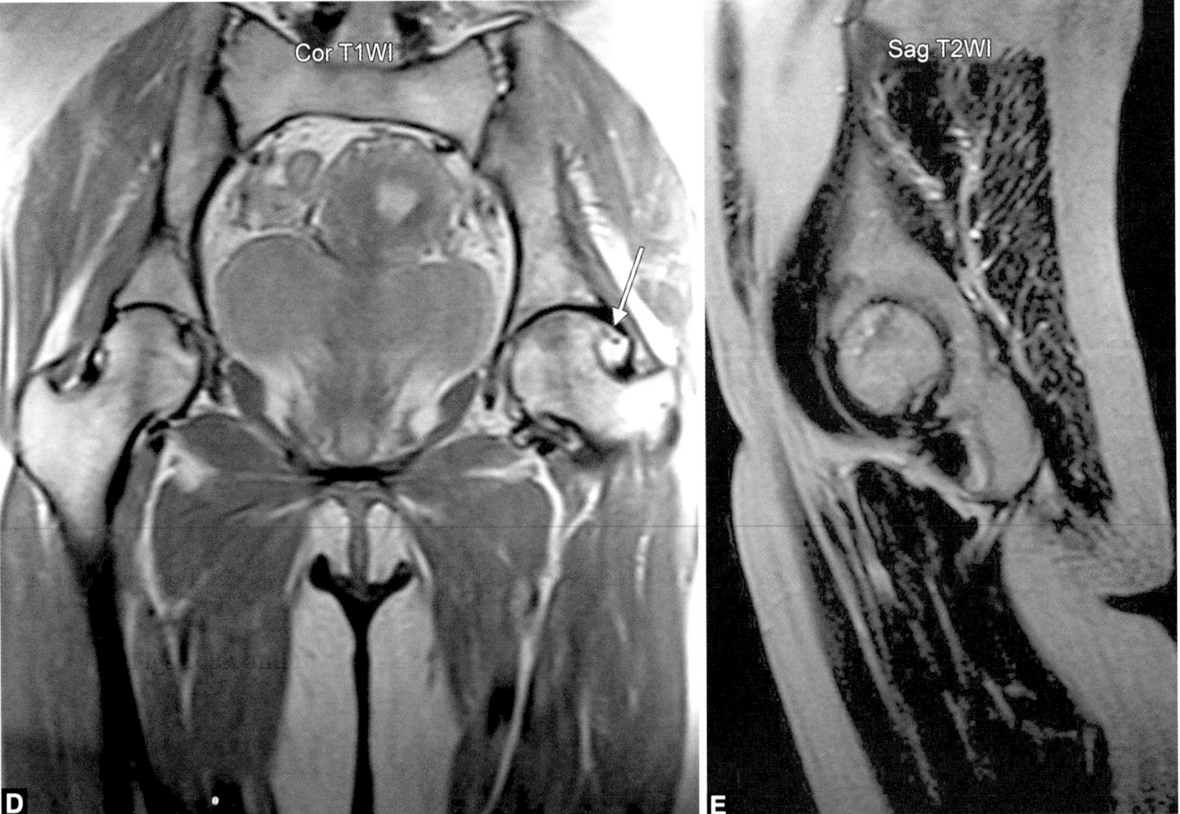

Figs 56D and E: Coronal T1WI (D) Sagittal T2WI (E) show loss of normal contour of left femoral head with secondary degenerative changes in the form of osteophytes (arrow)

Osteoid Osteoma

Osteoid osteoma is a benign lesion frequently found in the appendicular skeleton. The tumors produce excess bone and secrete pain-causing prostaglandins, resulting in intense pain especially at night. Patient usually presents with pain and tenderness, which is worst at night and is relieved by aspirins. Radiograph shows sclerosis and cortical thickening due to subperiosteal bone formation. The radiolucent nidus is visualized within. The location of the nidus, intranidal calcification, sclerosis, mature periosteal bone formation and location of original cortex are precisely demonstrated by CT (Figs 57A to C). MR signal of the nidus is variable and is usually has low to intermediate signal on T1WI depending on the mineralization in the nidus (Figs 57D and E). In addition, MR images also reveal marrow and soft tissue edema in the vicinity of the nidus, which is not demonstrated by CT.

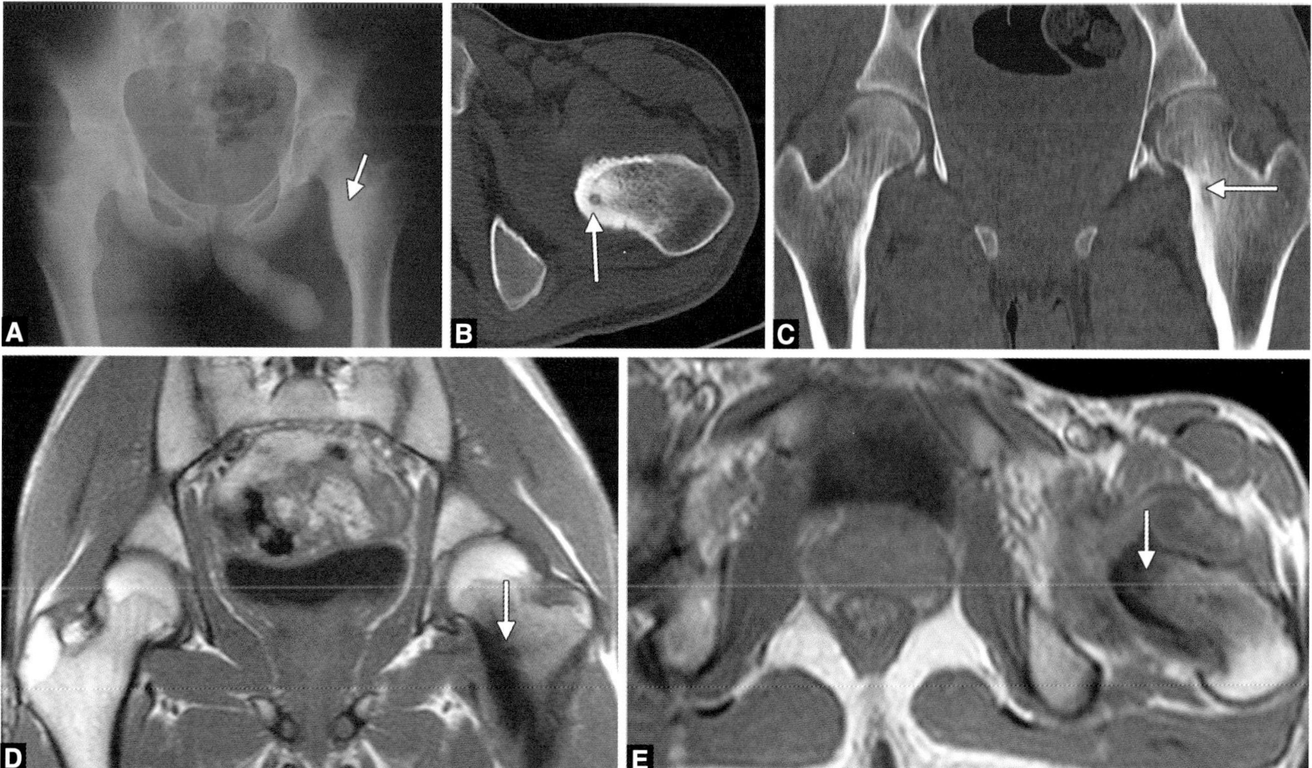

Figs 57A to E: Plain radiograph (A) reveals an ill-defined region of increased cortical thickness (arrow) and CT axial (B) coronal reformatted (C) reveals the presence small well-defined calcified nidus and dense cortical thickening near lesser trochanter. MRI coronal (D) and axial (E) reveals hypointense cortical thickening along lesser trochanter with well-defined small hypointense lesion adjacent to it (arrow)

ANATOMY KNEE JOINT

The knee joint is a modified pivotal hinge joint. It is the largest synovial joint in the body. It consists of two condylar joints between the femur and the tibia and a saddle joint between the patella and the femur (Figs 58 and 59). The intercondylar eminence of the tibia prevents sideway slipping of femur on tibia. The ligaments and muscles make knee a very stable joint.

The medial and lateral articular surfaces of the femur and tibia are asymmetrical. The distal surface of the medial condyle of the femur is narrower and more curved than the lateral condyle. The articular surface of lateral tibia is almost circular whereas the medial surface is oval in shape. The articular surface of patella has a larger lateral and a smaller medial surface.

Inferiorly, the capsule is attached to the margins of the tibial condyles posteriorly except where the popliteus tendon cross the bone. On either sides the capsule is attached to the margins of the tibial condyles, and laterally to the head of the fibula. On its deeper aspect the coronary ligaments connect the capsule to the rims of menisci. The capsule is attached to the tibial tuberosity anteriorly on the tibia.

The ligaments of knee joint include the cruciate ligaments, arcuate popliteal ligament, the oblique

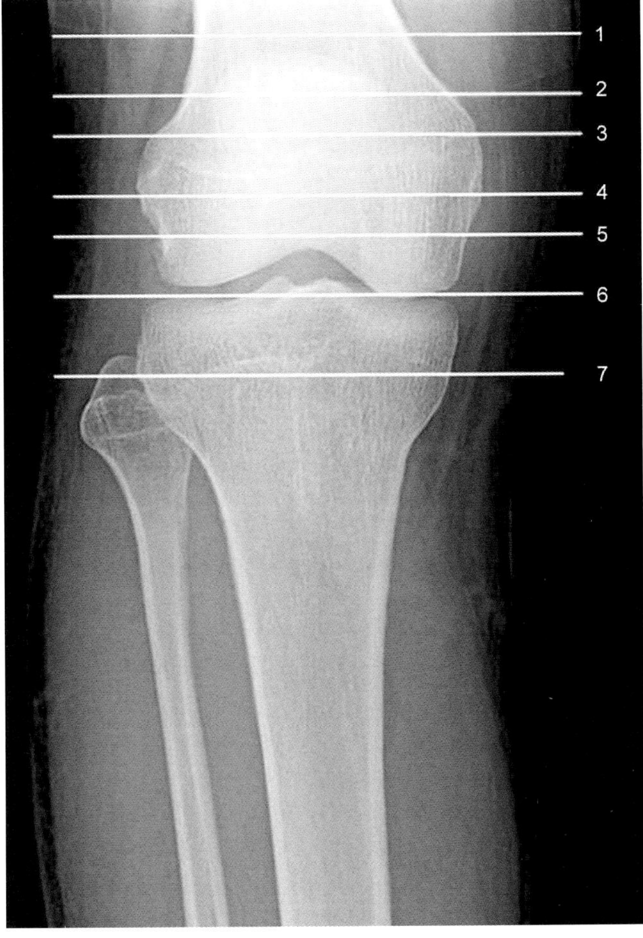

Fig. 59: Knee joint: Axial section plan

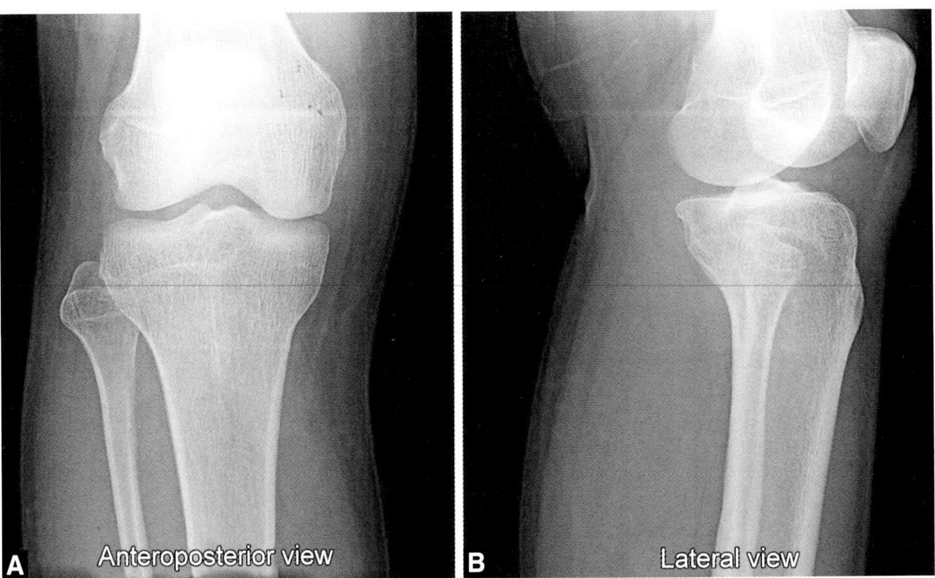

Figs 58A and B: Knee joint

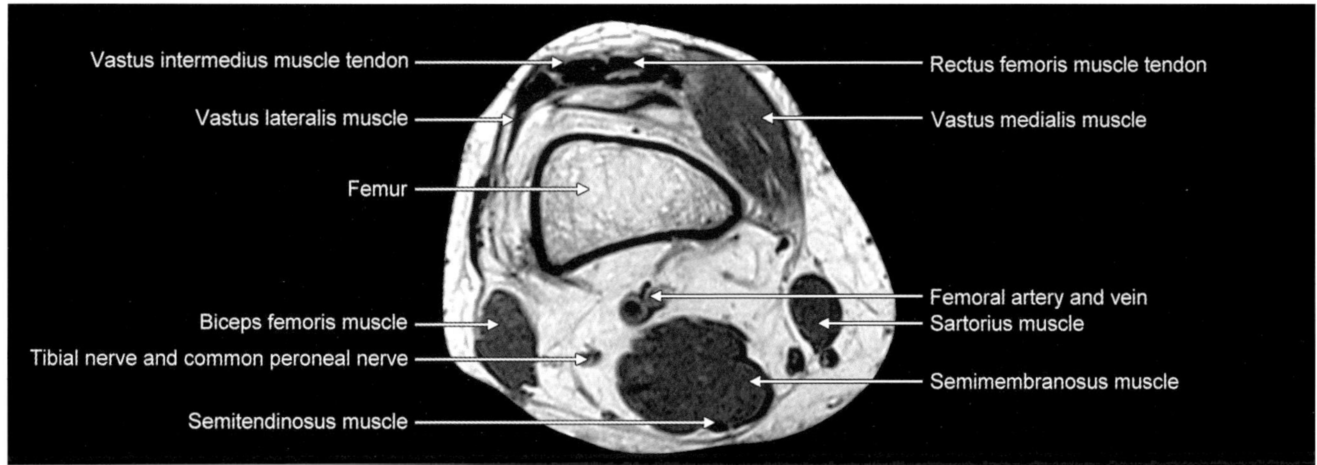

Fig. 60: Knee joint MRI: Axial T1WI (corresponds to level 1 in Fig. 59)

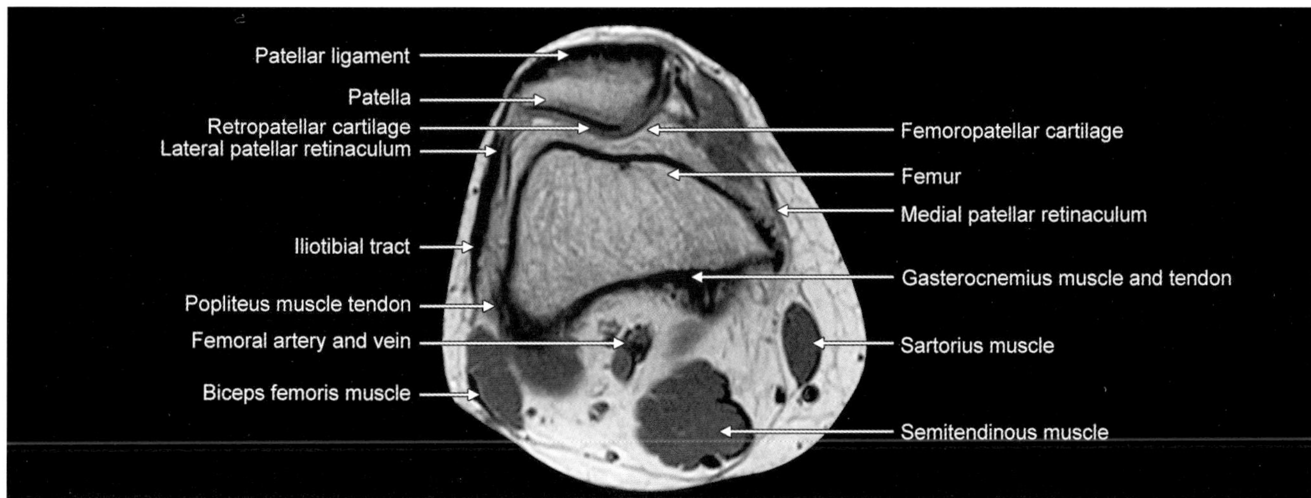

Fig. 61: Knee joint MRI: Axial T1WI (corresponds to level 2 in Fig. 59)

popliteal ligament, fibular collateral ligament and the tibial collateral ligament (Figs 60 to 81).

The cruciate ligaments are a pair of ligaments (anterior and posterior). They cross each other connecting the tibia to the femur and lie within the capsule of knee joint but outside the synovial membrane (Figs 62 to 65, 72 to 74 and 80). The anterior cruciate ligament is attached to the anterior part of the tibial plateau between the attachments of anterior horns of medial and lateral menisci. Posteriorly, the anterior cruciate ligament is attached to the posteromedial aspect of lateral femoral condyle. The anterior cruciate ligament appears as a fan shaped structure, it is 11 mm wide and 31 to 38 mm long. The posterior cruciate ligament is attached posteriorly to the intercondylar area on tibia and anteriorly it is attached to the anterolateral aspect of the medial femoral condyle. The posterior cruciate ligament is about 13 mm wide and 38 mm long. Both these ligaments stabilize the knee in a rotational fashion. Thus, if one of these ligaments is significantly damaged, the knee will be unstable when planting the foot of the injured extremity and pivoting, causes the knee to buckle and give way.

The arcuate popliteal ligament is a Y-shaped thickening of posterior capsular fibers, the stem of

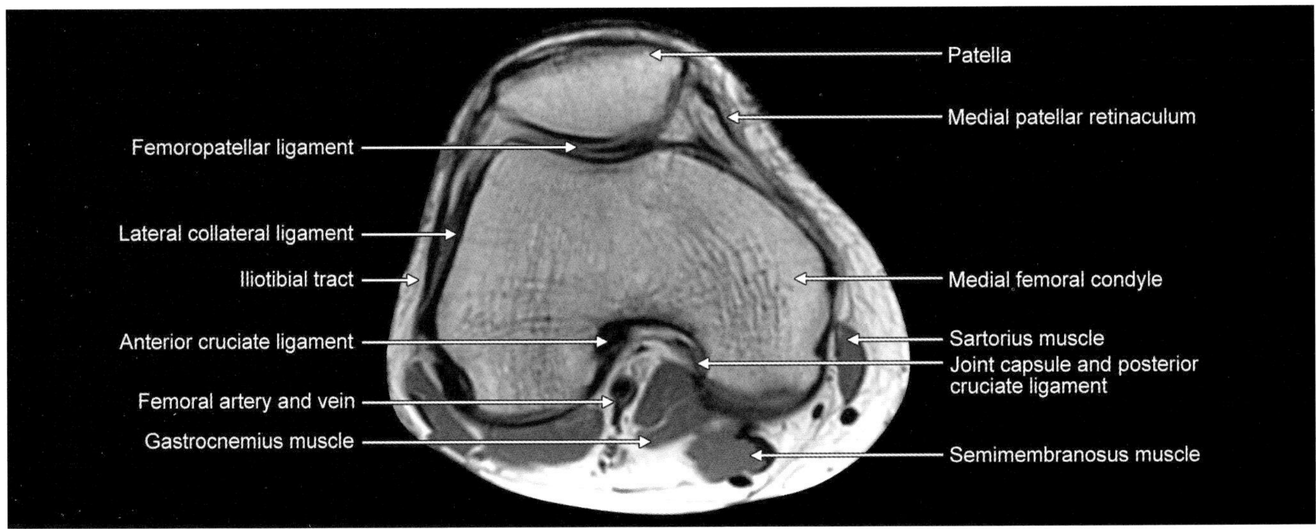

Fig. 62: Knee joint MRI: Axial T1WI (corresponds to level 3 in Fig. 59)

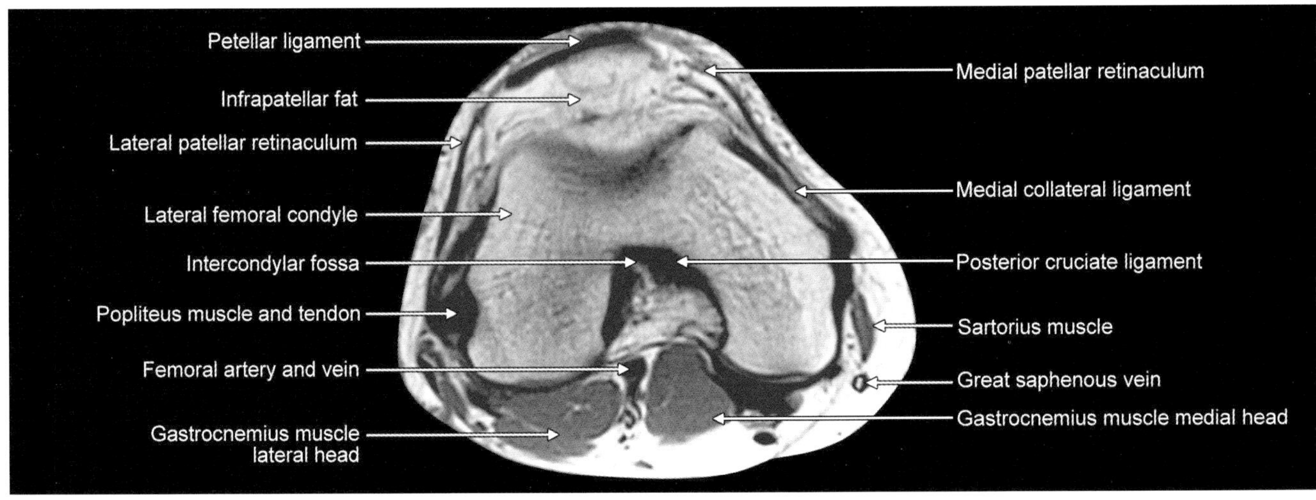

Fig. 63: Knee joint MRI: Axial T1WI (corresponds to level 4 in Fig. 59)

the Y is attached to the head of fibula. The medial limb of Y is attached to the posterior edge of the intercondylar area, while the lateral limb is attached to the lateral femoral condyle.

The oblique popliteal ligament is an expansion of the tendon of semimembranosus muscle that blends with the capsule posteriorly and ascends laterally.

The tibial collateral ligament is a triangular band 8 to 9 cm in length, attached above to the medial femoral epicondyle and below to the medial surface of tibia. Its anterior margin forms the vertical base of the triangle and is free except at its attached extremities. The posterior apex of the triangular ligament blends with the capsule and is also attached to the medial meniscus.

The fibular collateral ligament is 'cord-like' and is attached superiorly to the lateral epicondyle and inferiorly to the head of the fibula.

The patellar ligament (Figs 60, 61, 63 to 66 and 73) is a central band of the tendon of quadriceps femoris

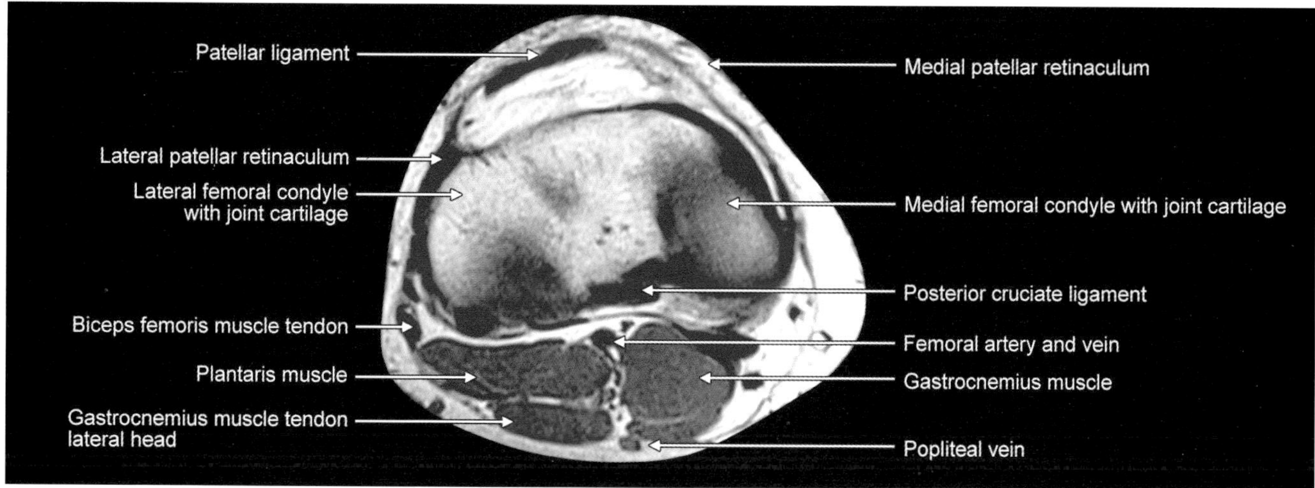

Fig. 64: Knee joint MRI: Axial T1WI (corresponds to level 5 in Fig. 59)

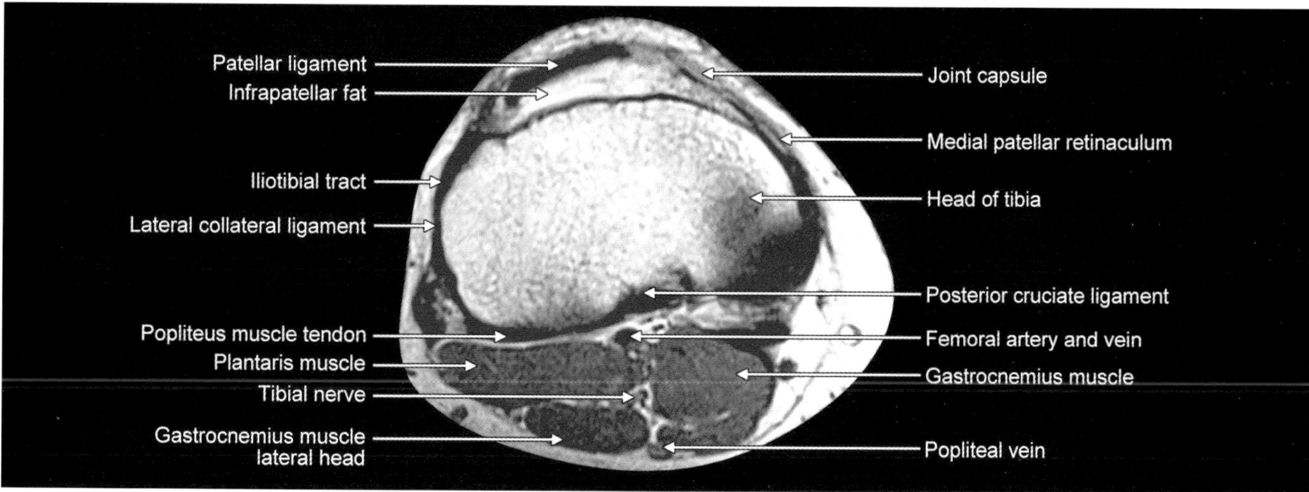

Fig. 65: Knee joint MRI: Axial T1WI (corresponds to level 6 in Fig. 59)

muscles; it is about 8 cm long. Proximally, it attaches to the anterior and posterior surfaces of patella including the apex. Distally it attaches to the smooth area of tibial tuberosity. The patellar ligament blends with the medial and lateral patellar retinaculum, which are aponeurotic expansions of vastus medialis and lateralis. The retinaculum supports the articular capsule of the knee laterally.

The menisci are called semilunar cartilages (Figs 68 to 73, 78 and 79). These are cresenteric disks of fibrocartilage that act as shock absorbers. The menisci are avascular structures comprising mainly of collagenous fibrous tissue attached to the tibial plateau. There are two menisci, the lateral and the medial meniscus. They are triangular in cross-section, being thicker at their convex periphery (5 mm in height). Their distal surfaces are flat while their proximal surfaces are concave and articulate with the convex femoral condyles. The menisci demonstrate diffusely low signal on all MRI pulse sequences because of their fibrocartilaginous nature.

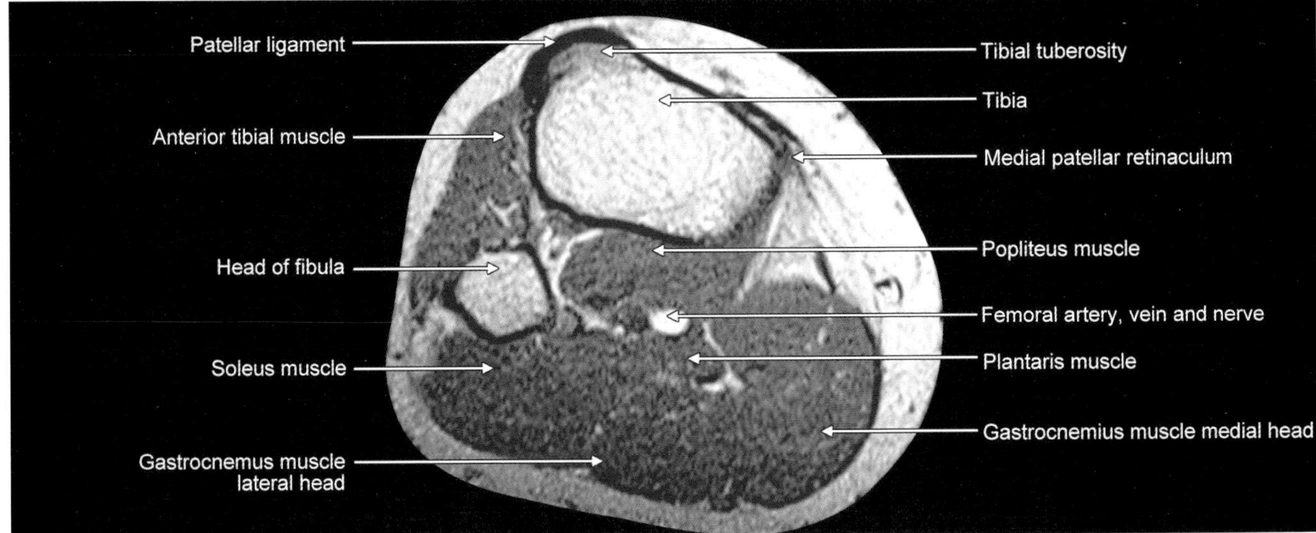

Fig. 66: Knee joint MRI: Axial T1WI (corresponds to level 7 in Fig. 59)

The medial meniscus is almost a semicircle in appearance and is broader posteriorly. Its anterior horn is attached to the intercondylar area in front of the anterior cruciate ligament; the posterior horn is attached in front of the posterior cruciate ligament in intercondylar area. The lateral meniscus is of uniform width and almost forms a complete circle. Its anterior horn is attached in front of the intercondylar eminence of the tibia behind the anterior cruciate ligament, while the posterior horn is attached in front of the posterior horn of the medial meniscus.

The synovial membrane lines the internal surface of the fibrous capsule and attaches to the periphery of the patella and the edges of the menisci. The synovial membrane is continuous with the lining of the suprapatellar bursa. Normal amount of synovial fluid is 0.5 mL.

Bursae of knee joint reduce the friction between tendon and bones. The suprapatellar bursa lies between the femur and the quadriceps femoris. The prepatellar bursa lies between the skin and the patella. The infrapatellar bursa lies between the skin and the tibial tuberosity. The deep infrapatellar bursa lies between the patellar ligament and the upper part of the tibia. The semimembranosus bursa lies between that muscle and the medial head of gastrocnemius.

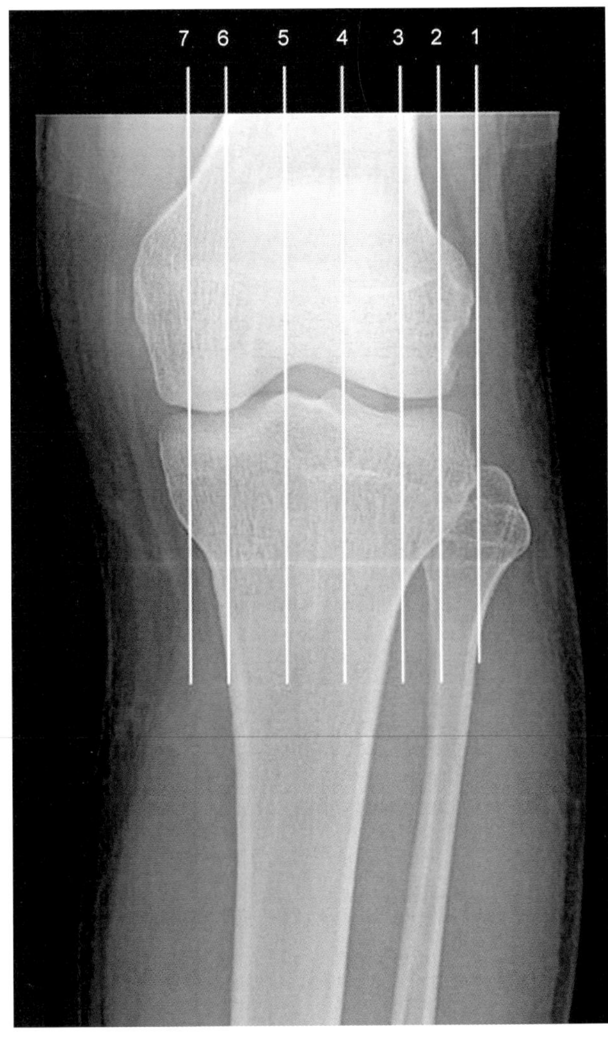

Fig. 67: Knee joint MRI: Sagittal section plan

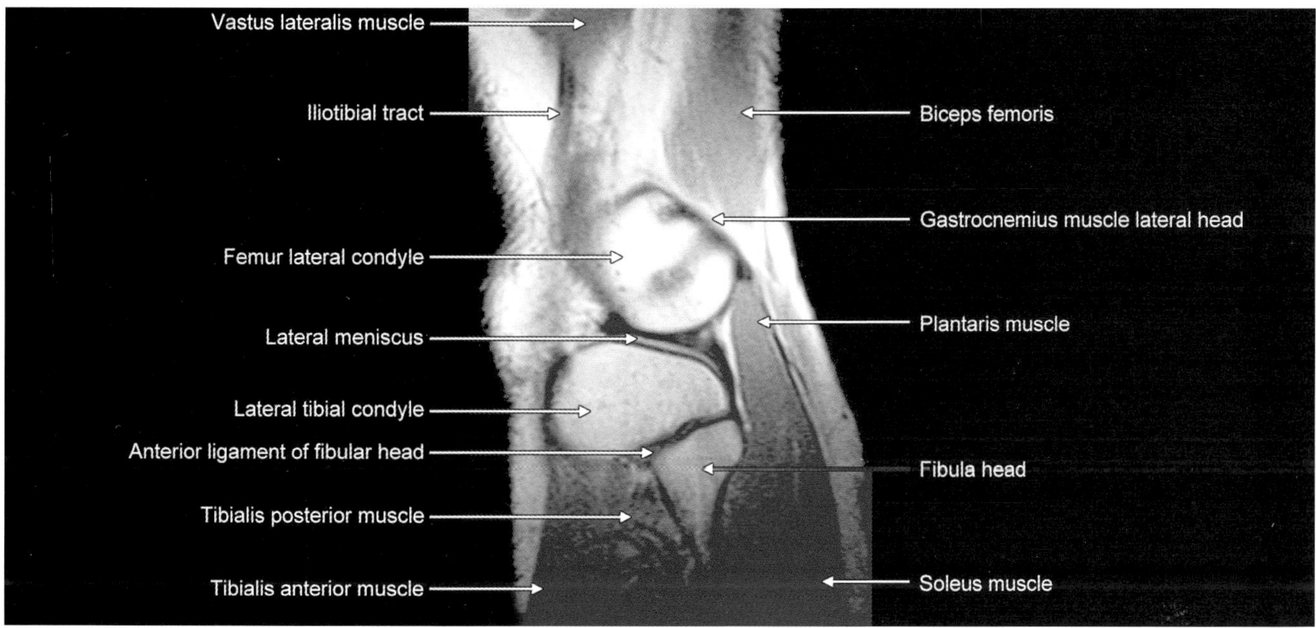

Fig. 68: Knee joint MRI: Sagittal T1WI (corresponds to level 1 in Fig. 67)

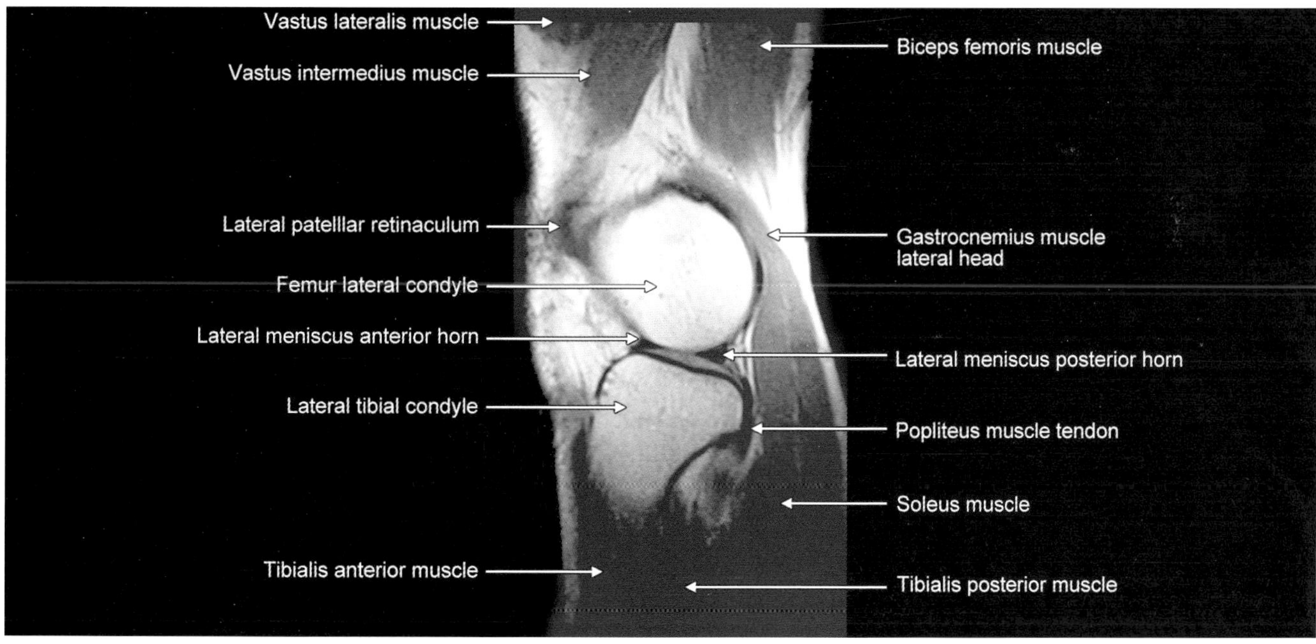

Fig. 69: Knee joint MRI: Sagittal T1WI (corresponds to level 2 in Fig. 67)

Blood supply to knee joint is by anastomosis of the genicular branches of the popliteal artery. The middle genicular branches supply the cruciate ligaments.

Movements at the knee joint are the flexion, extension and rotation. Flexion is limited to about 150 degrees due to soft tissue parts behind the knee. Flexion movements are primarily performed by the hamstring muscles. Extension is performed by the quadriceps femoris muscles assisted by tensor fascia lata. As the knee extends the shorter and rounded lateral femoral condyle completes its extension to about 30 degrees short of full extension. The rotation movement occurs during extension with the foot on ground. Passive medial rotation of the femur is a part of a 'locking' mechanism which secures the joint in 5-10 degrees of hyperextension when both the cruciate ligaments, the collateral ligaments and the oblique popliteal ligament are all taut. Lateral rotation is produced by the popliteus muscle when flexion occurs with the foot free.

The knee joint is stabilized by the surrounding muscles and their tendons. Anteriorly, it is the

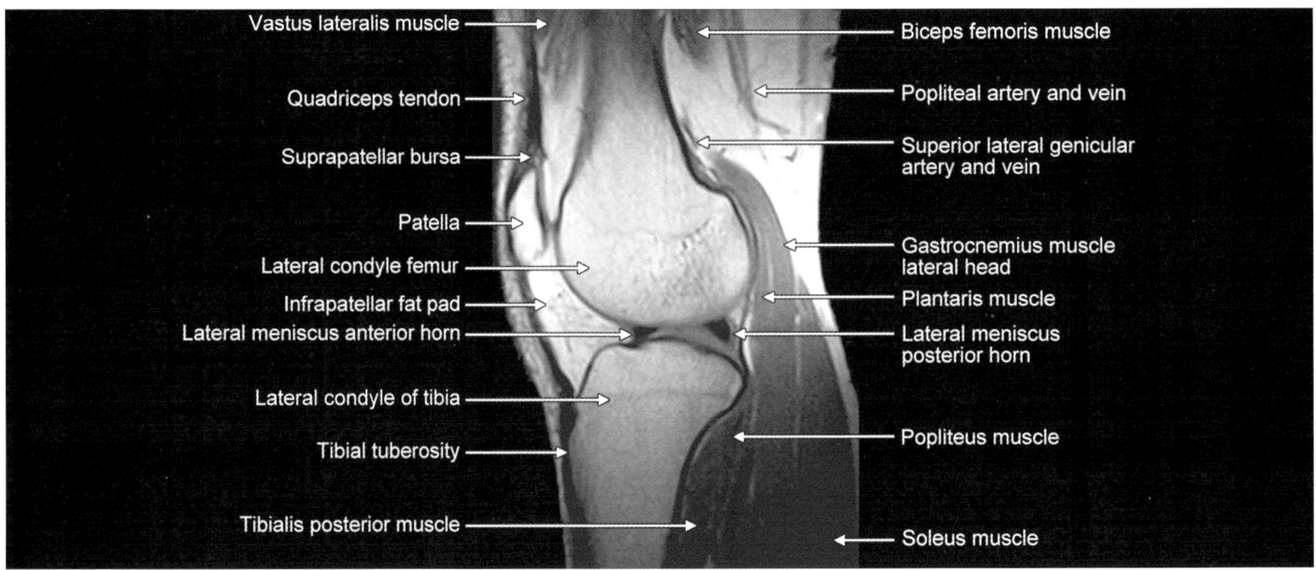

Fig. 70: Knee joint MRI: Sagittal T1WI (corresponds to level 3 in Fig. 67)

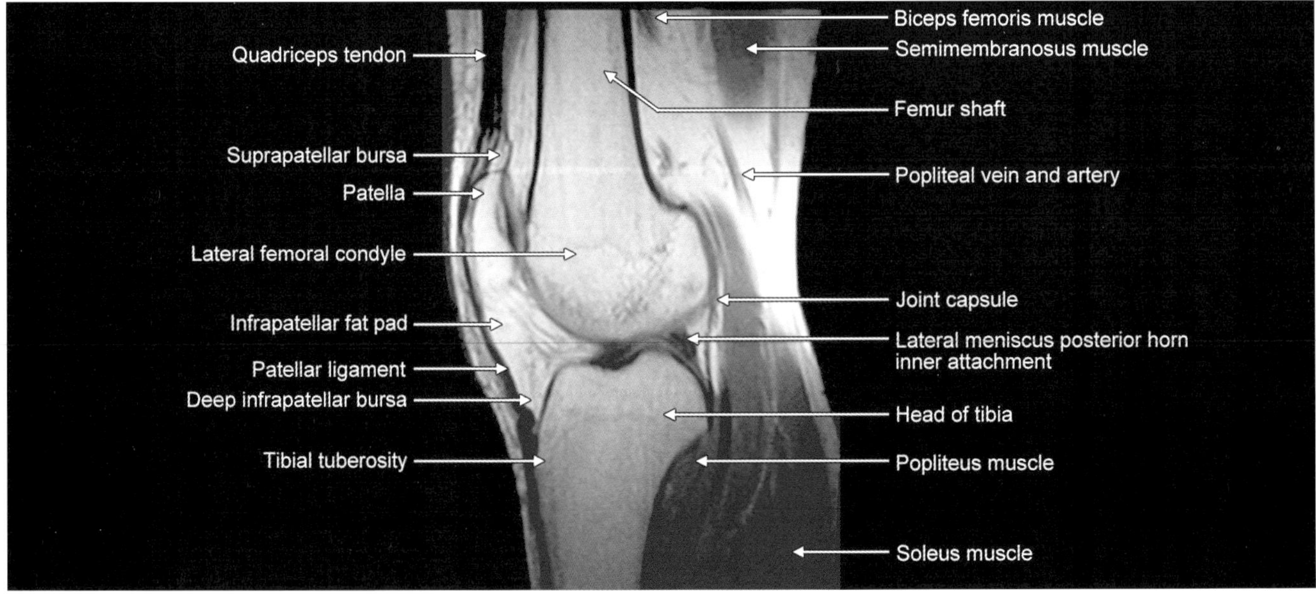

Fig. 71: Knee joint MRI: Sagittal T1WI (corresponds to level 4 in Fig. 67)

quadriceps tendon. This broad tendon attaches to and surrounds the patella and continues as the patellar ligament, which is attached to the tuberosity of the tibia. Posteriorly are the popliteus, plantaris and medial and lateral heads of gastrocnemius. Laterally are the tendons of the biceps femoris and popliteus. Medially by the sartorius, gracilis, semitendinosus and semimembranosus muscles are present.

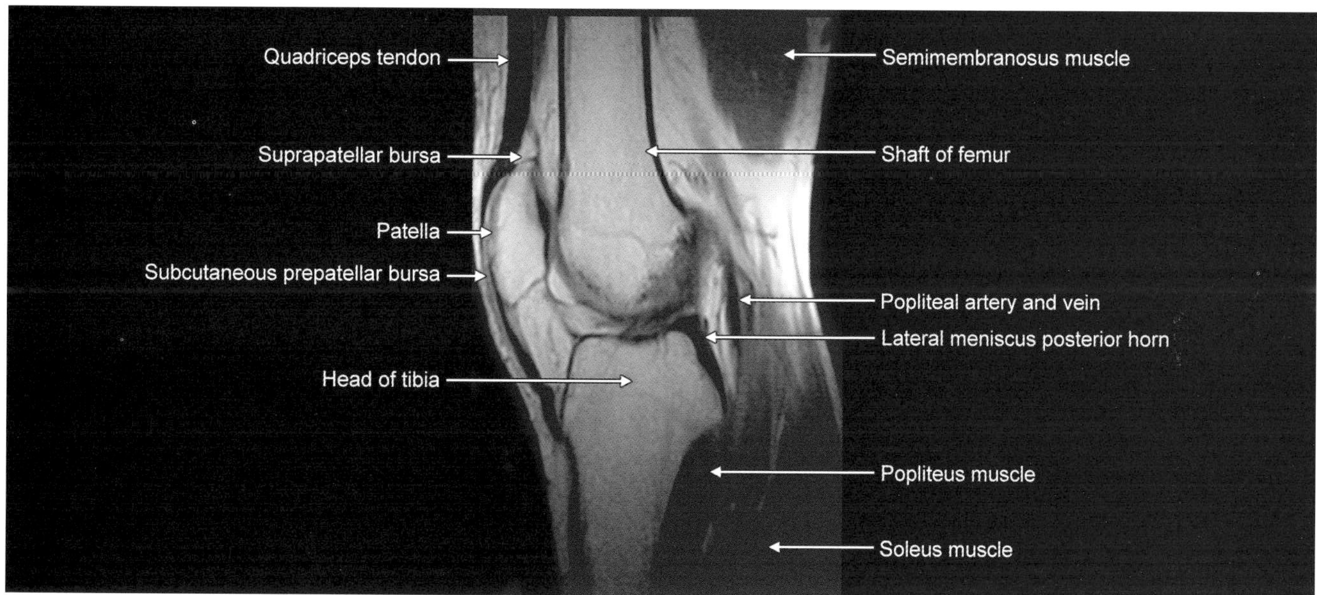

Fig. 72: Knee joint MRI: Sagittal T1WI (corresponds to level 5 in Fig. 67)

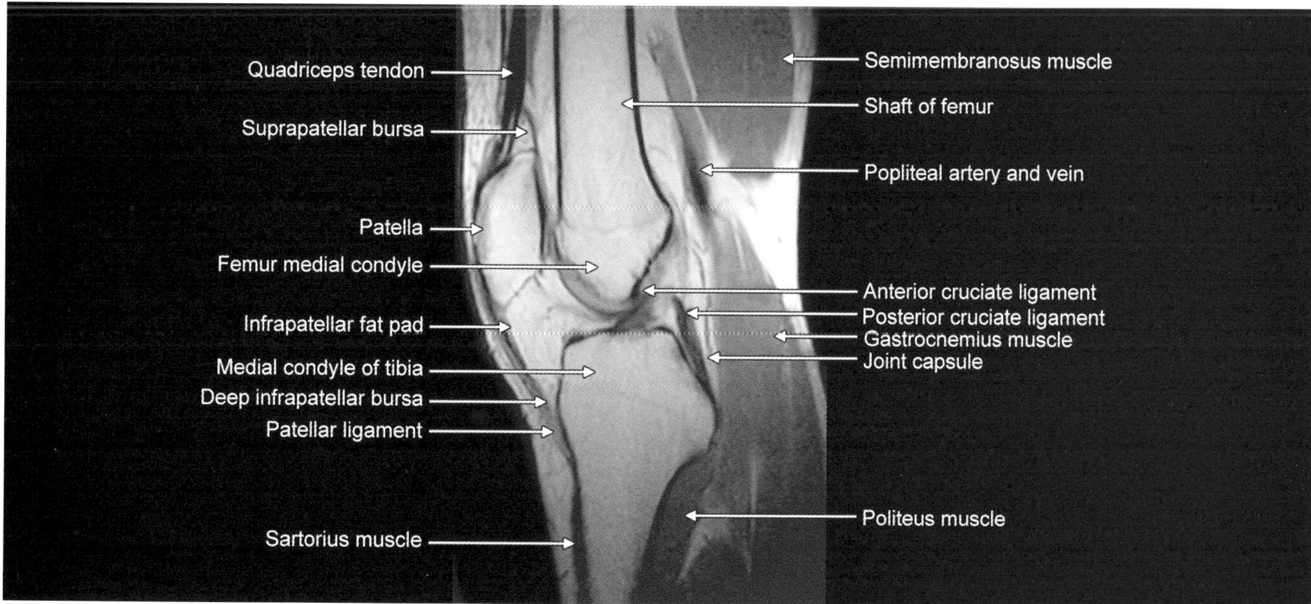

Fig. 73: Knee joint MRI: Sagittal T1WI (corresponds to level 6 in Fig. 67)

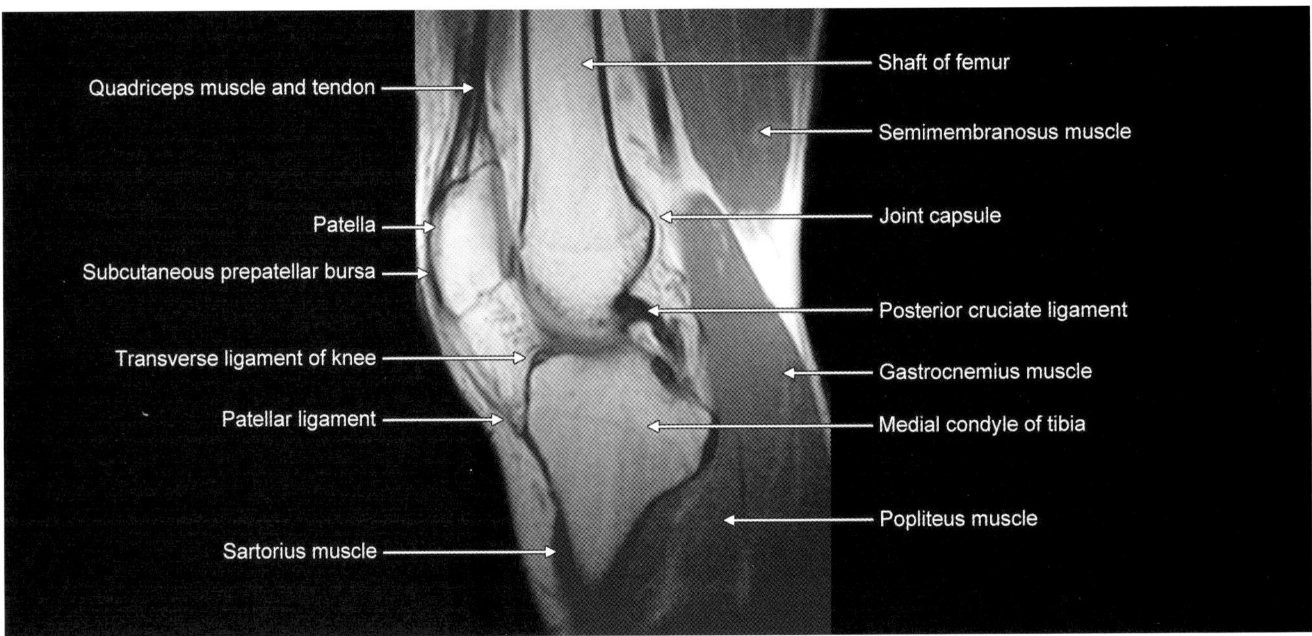

Fig. 74: Knee joint MRI: Sagittal T1WI (corresponds to level 7 in Fig. 10)

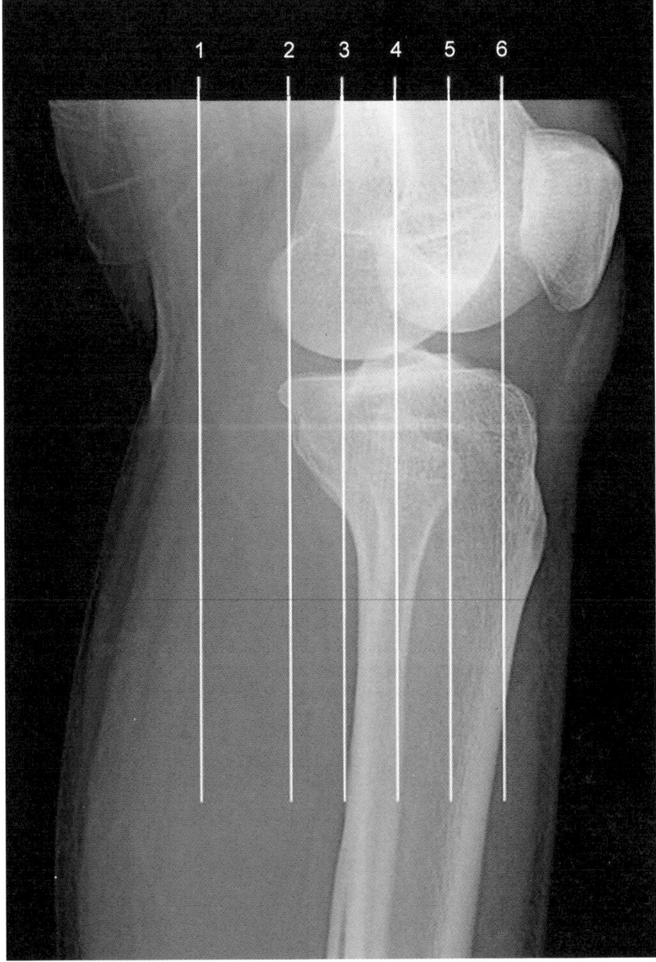

Fig. 75: Knee joint coronal section plan

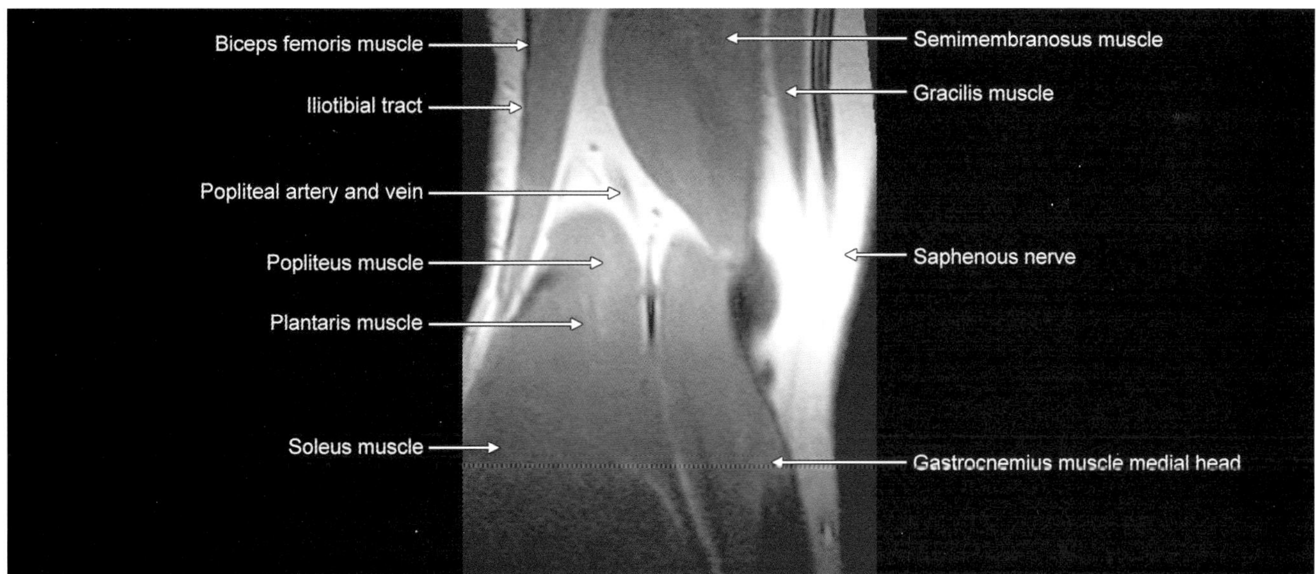

Fig. 76: Knee joint MRI: Coronal T1WI (corresponds to level 1 in Fig. 75)

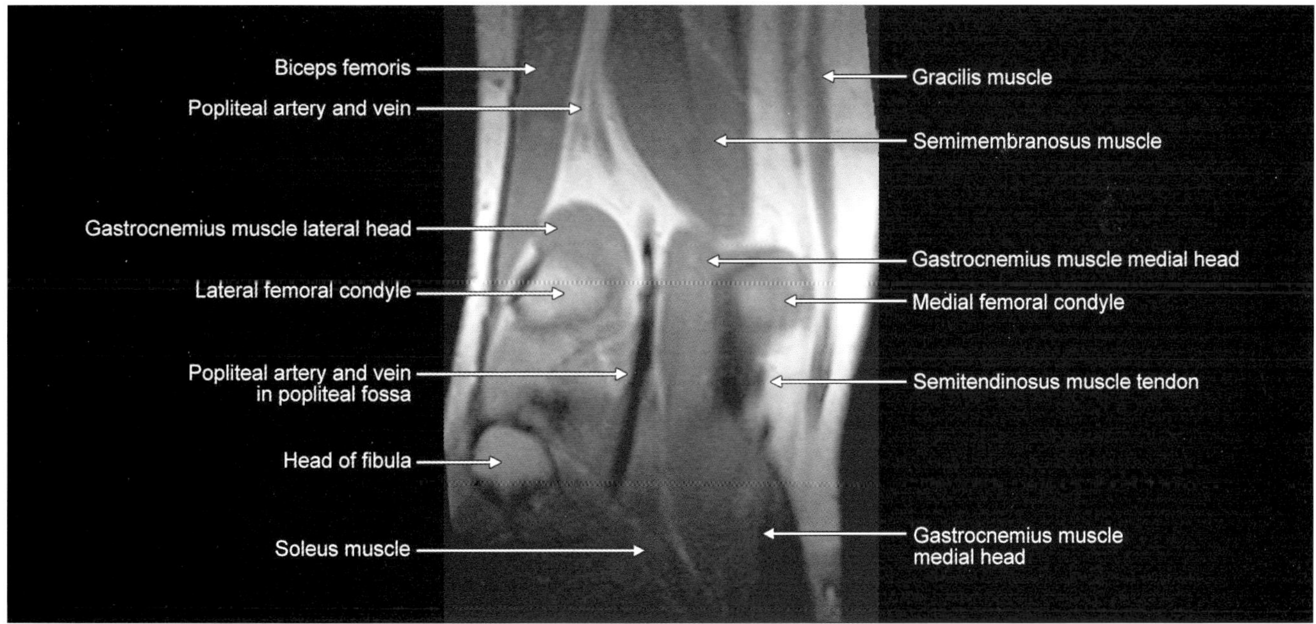

Fig. 77: Knee joint MRI: Coronal T1WI (corresponds to level 2 in Fig. 75)

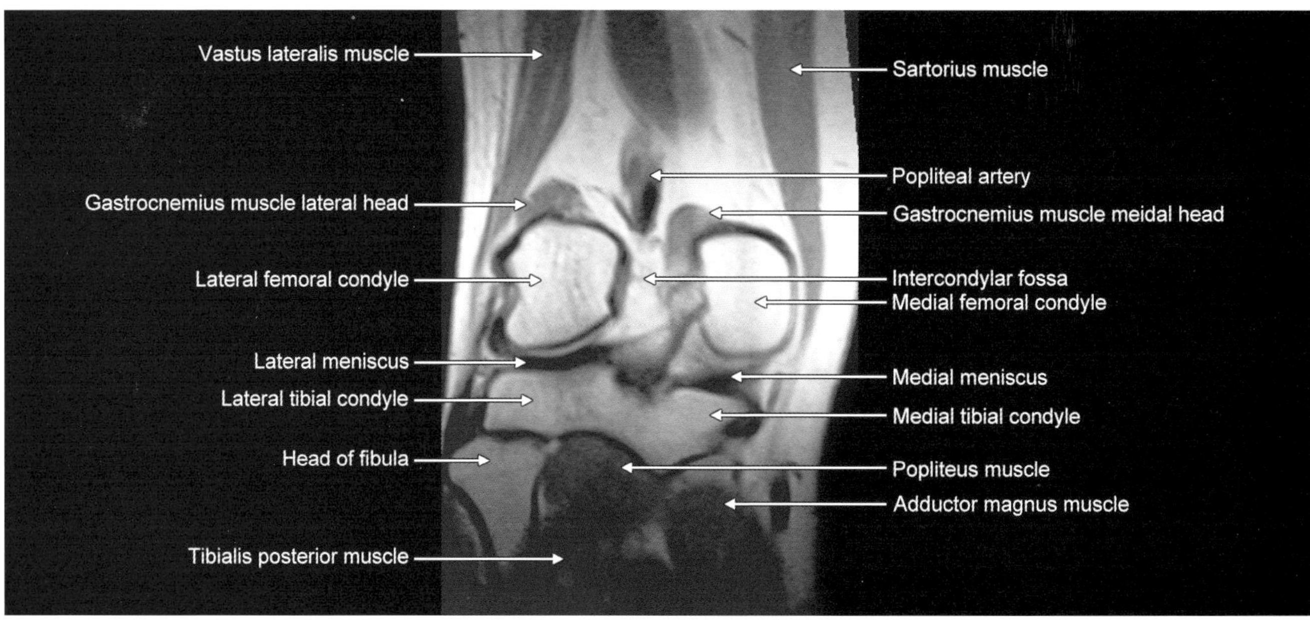

Fig. 78: Knee joint MRI: Coronal T1WI (corresponds to level 3 in Fig. 75)

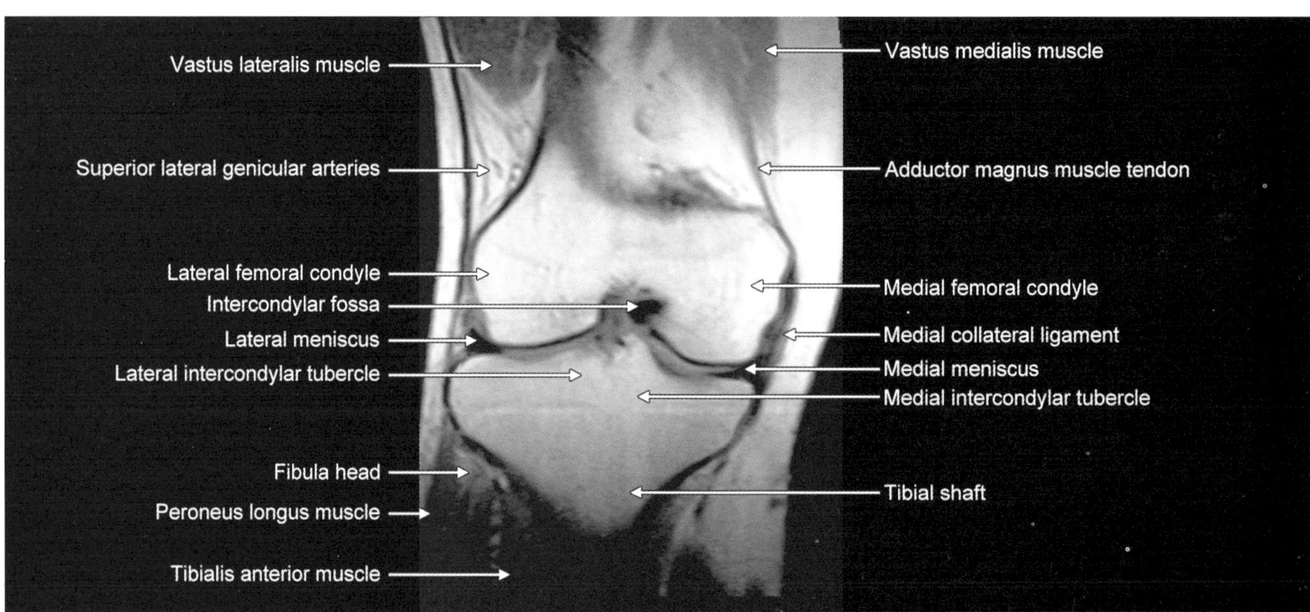

Fig. 79: Knee joint MRI: Coronal T1WI (corresponds to level 4 in Fig. 75)

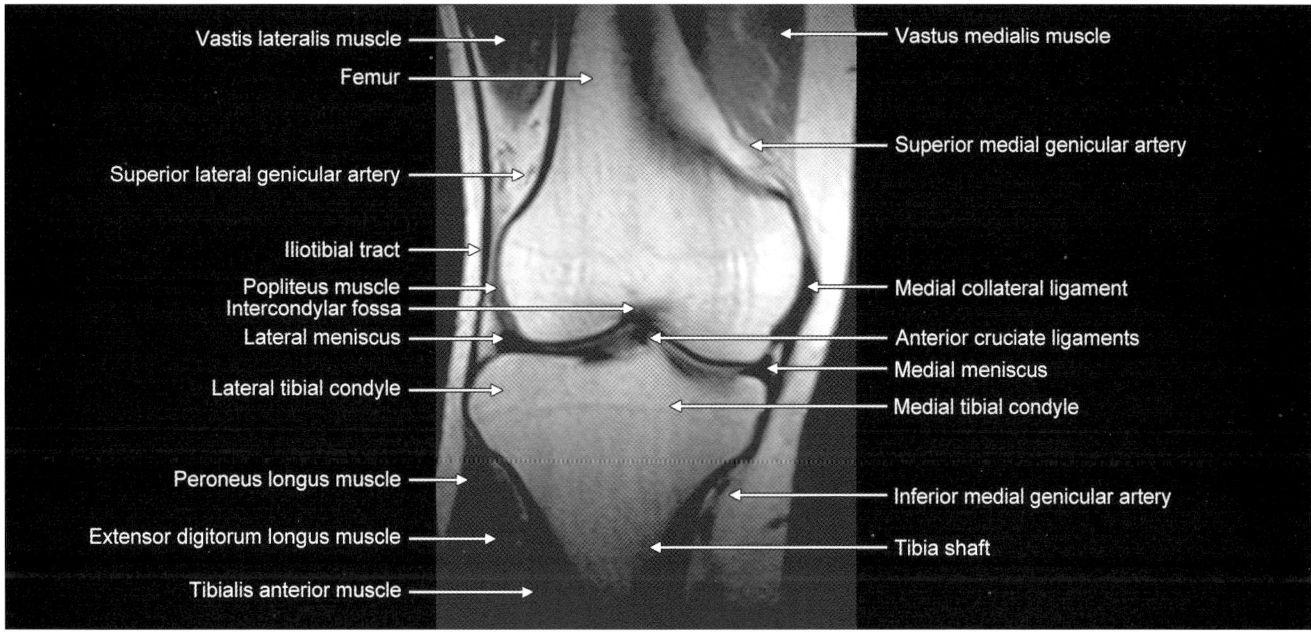

Fig. 80: Knee joint MRI: Coronal T1WI (corresponds to level 5 in Fig. 75)

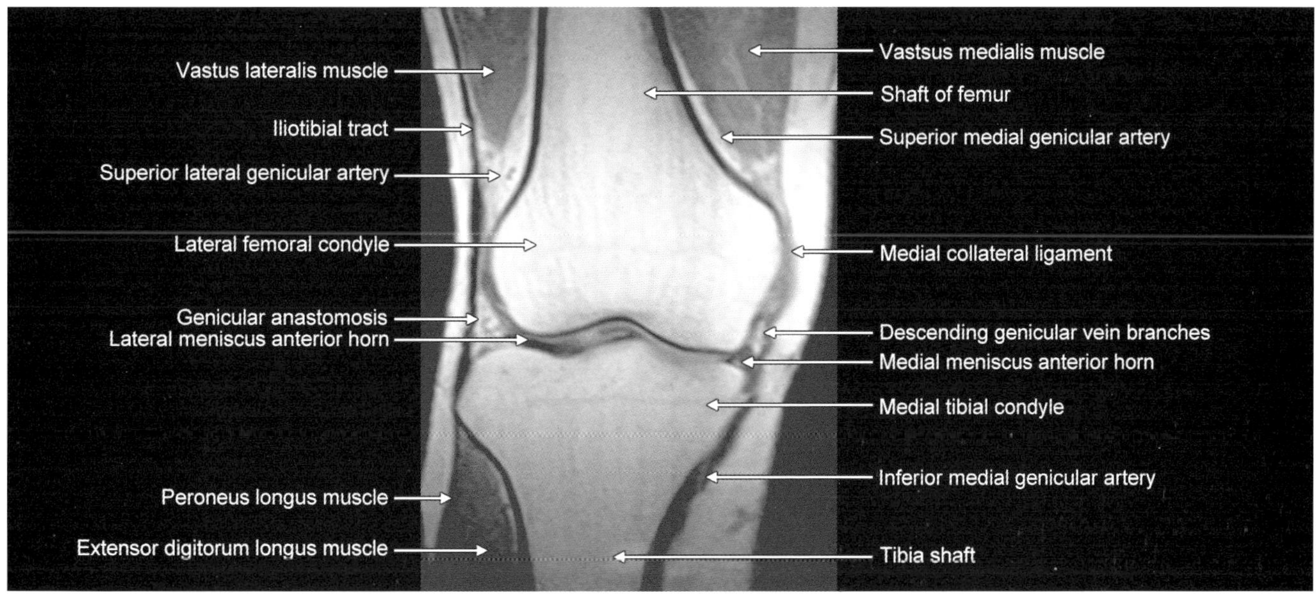

Fig. 81: Knee joint MRI: Coronal T1WI (corresponds to level 6 in Fig. 75)

Cruciate Ligaments

The anterior and posterior cruciate ligaments are two major ligaments of the knee. Their job is to maintain the anteroposterior relationship of the distal femur and proximal tibia to each other. This job is trickier by the fact that it needs to be done at all times during flexion or extension of the knee.

The anterior cruciate ligament (ACL) is linear band; fan shaped (Figs 82A to C). It attaches proximally at the internal aspect of the lateral femoral condyle, and runs distally to its broad attachment to the anterior tibia and the anterior aspect of the tibial spine. The anterior cruciate lies lateral to the posterior cruciate. The recognition of ACL is comparable to putting your hand inside the pocket of your trousers. This position represents ACL, i.e. the hand is positioned from posterior to anterior and from lateral to medial, so is ACL positioned. The reverse is true for PCL.

The posterior cruciate ligament (PCL) is a relatively simple band of tissue and attaches proximally on the internal aspect of the medial femoral condyle and runs distally to where it attaches to the posterior eminence of the tibia. It generally lies in the sagittal plane, and can usually be seen in its entirety on a single sagittal MR slice (Figs 88 A to C). Injuries to ACL and PCL are shown in Figures 83 to 87 and 89.

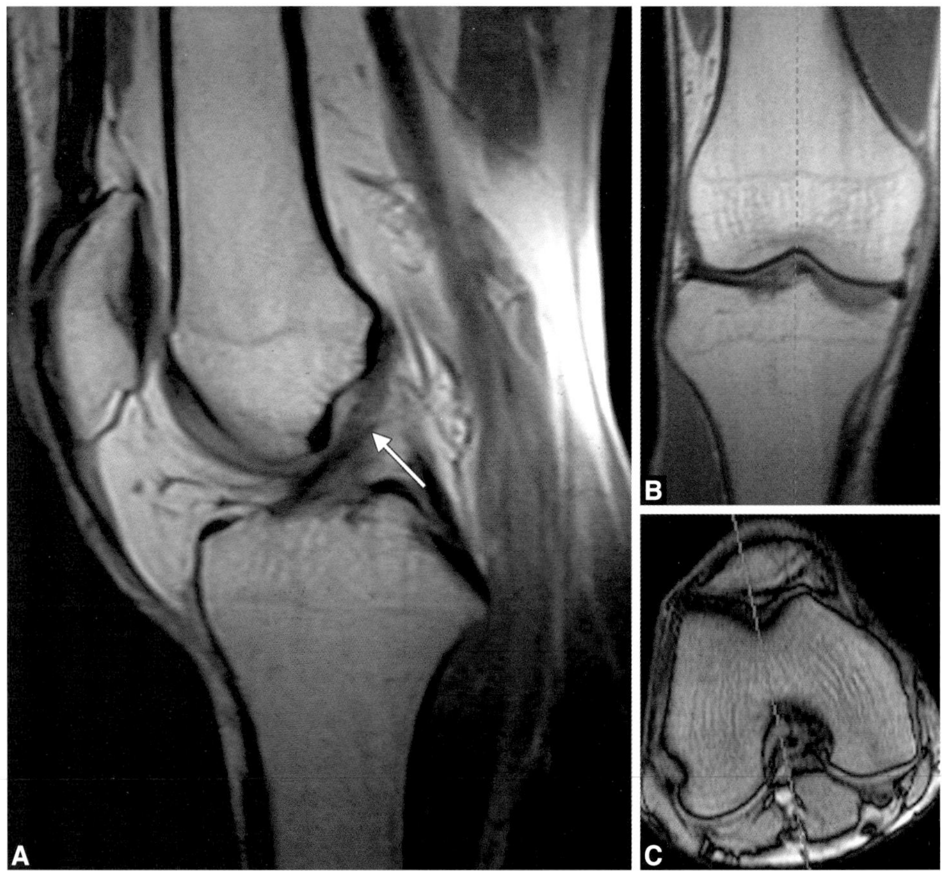

Figs 82A to C: Normal anterior cruciate ligament

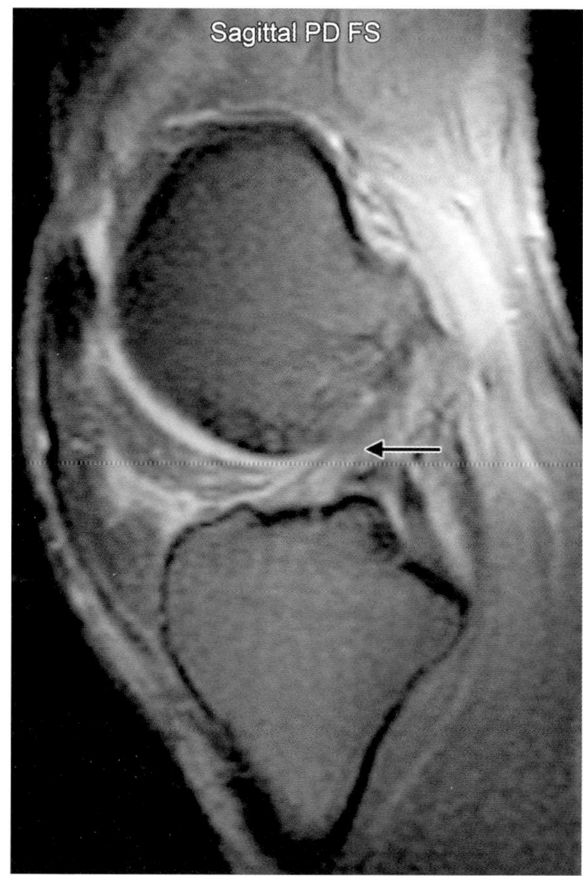

Fig. 83: Sagittal PD FS shows edematous (arrow) appearance of ACL with thinning of the fibers suggesting strain

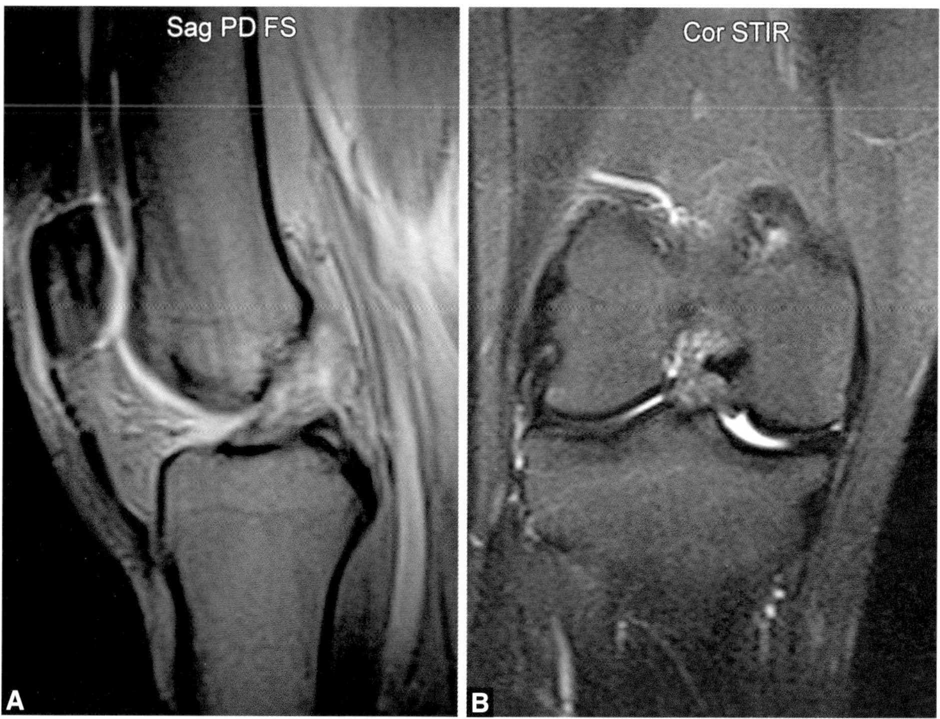

Figs 84A and B: Sagittal PD FS and coronal STIR image shows nonvisualization of the fibers of ACL suggestive of complete ACL tear

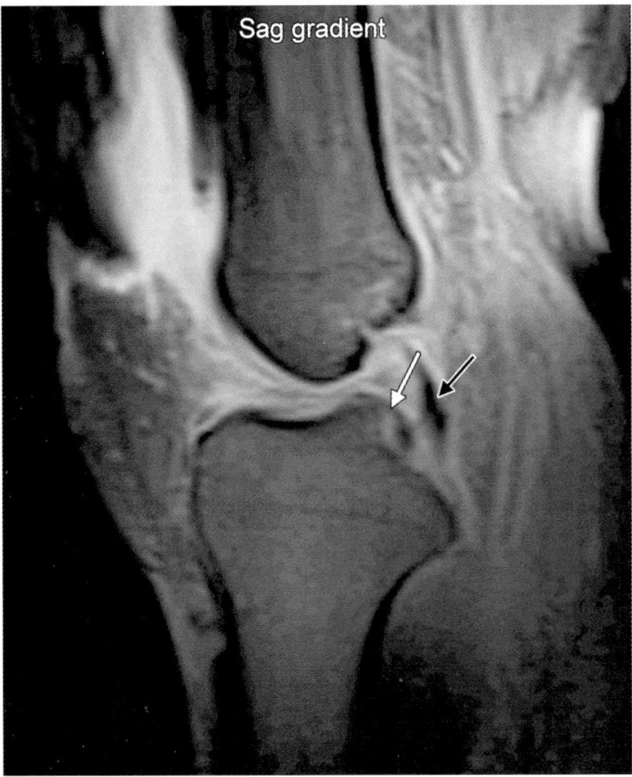

Fig. 85: Sagittal gradient image shows double PCL sign suggestive of Bucket handle meniscal tear (white arrow). Normal PCL is shown by black arrow

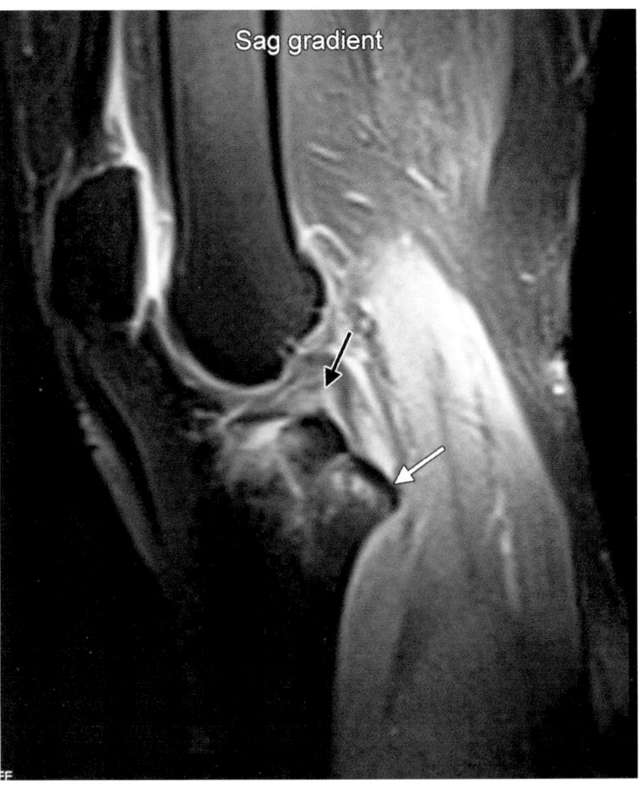

Fig. 86: Sagittal gradient sequence shows hyperintense signal seen in PCL at its tibial attachment with avulsion injury (white arrow) and also at ACL attachment with avulsion injury (black arrow)

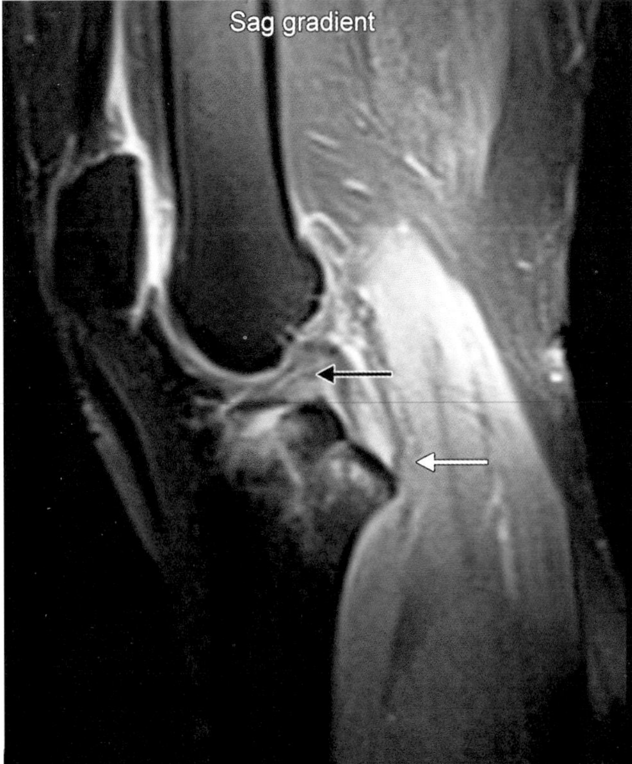

Fig. 87: Sagittal gradient sequence shows hyperintense signal seen in PCL at its tibial attachment with avulsion injury (white arrow) and also at ACL attachment with avulsion injury (black arrow)

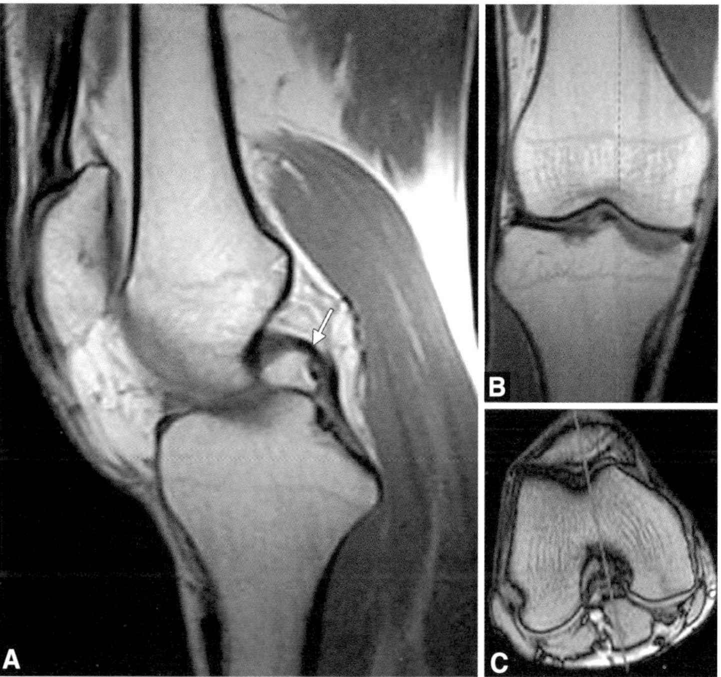

Figs 88A to C: Normal posterior cruciate ligament

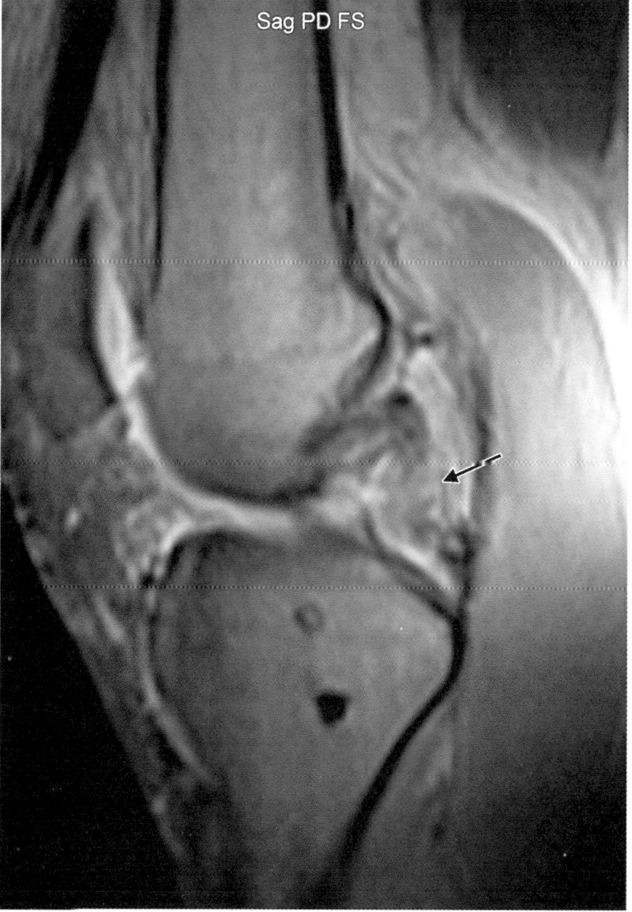

Fig. 89: Sagittal PD FS image shows interstitial tear of the fibers of PCL

Menisci

The articular discs of the knee joint are called menisci because they only partly divide the joint space. These two discs, the medial meniscus and the lateral meniscus consist of connective tissue with extensive collagen fibers containing cartilage like cells. Strong fibers run along the menisci from one attachment to the other, while weaker radial fibers are interlaced with the former. The menisci are flattened at the center of the knee joint, fused with the synovial membrane laterally, and can move over the tibial surface.

The menisci serve to protect the ends of the bones from rubbing on each other and to effectively deepen the tibial sockets into which the femur attaches. They also play a role in shock absorption, and may be cracked, or torn, when the knee is forcefully rotated or bent.

Meniscus knee anatomy is the key to understanding how injuries can affect the knee joint (Figs 90, 91 and 94 to 99). Menisci are small C-shaped structures of cartilage which sit in between the femur and the tibia. The cartilage sitting on the outside is known as the lateral meniscus (Figs 90A to C) and the one sitting inside is known as the medial meniscus (Figs 92 and 93). The posterior meniscus is just an extension of the medial cartilage. In between the knee joint is fluid which ensures that the meniscus stay lubricated and prevents any friction injury. Both menisci have a poor blood supply which is easily compromised during knee injury. The function of meniscus is to cushion the joint from any injury.

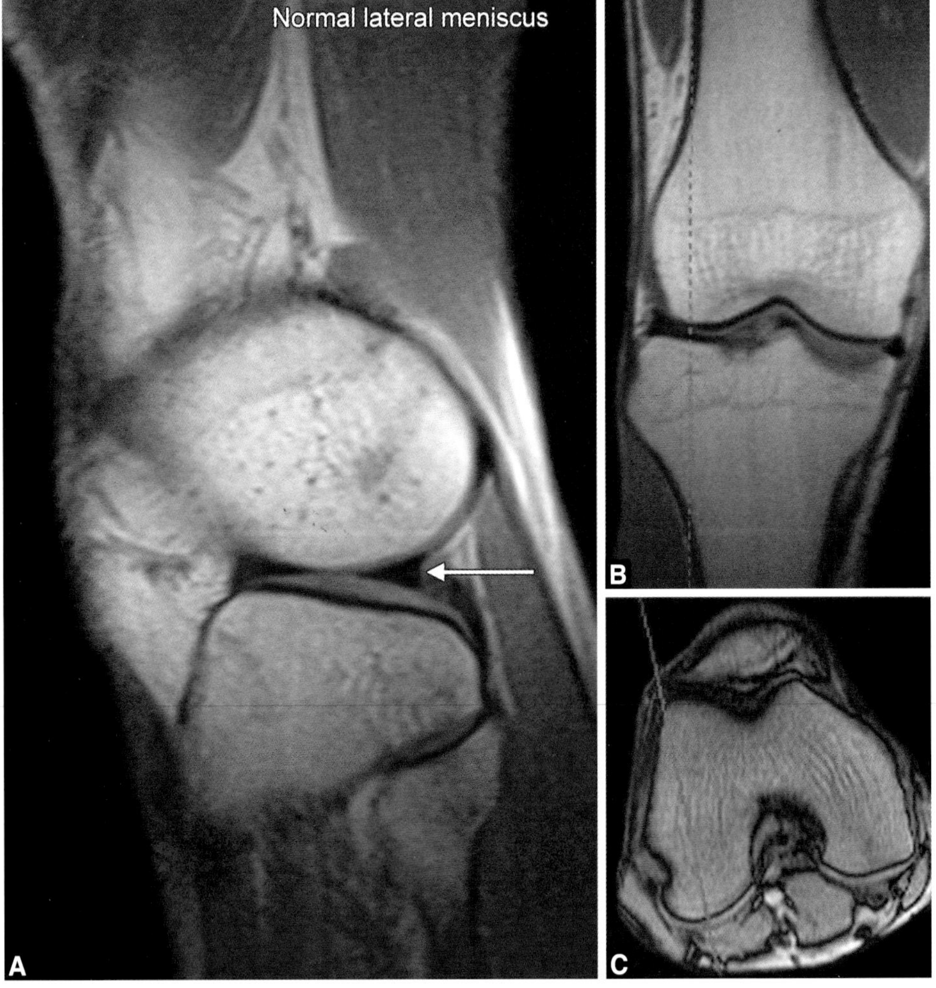

Figs 90A to C: (A) Sagittal section shows normal appearance of lateral meniscus;(B and C) Show scan planes

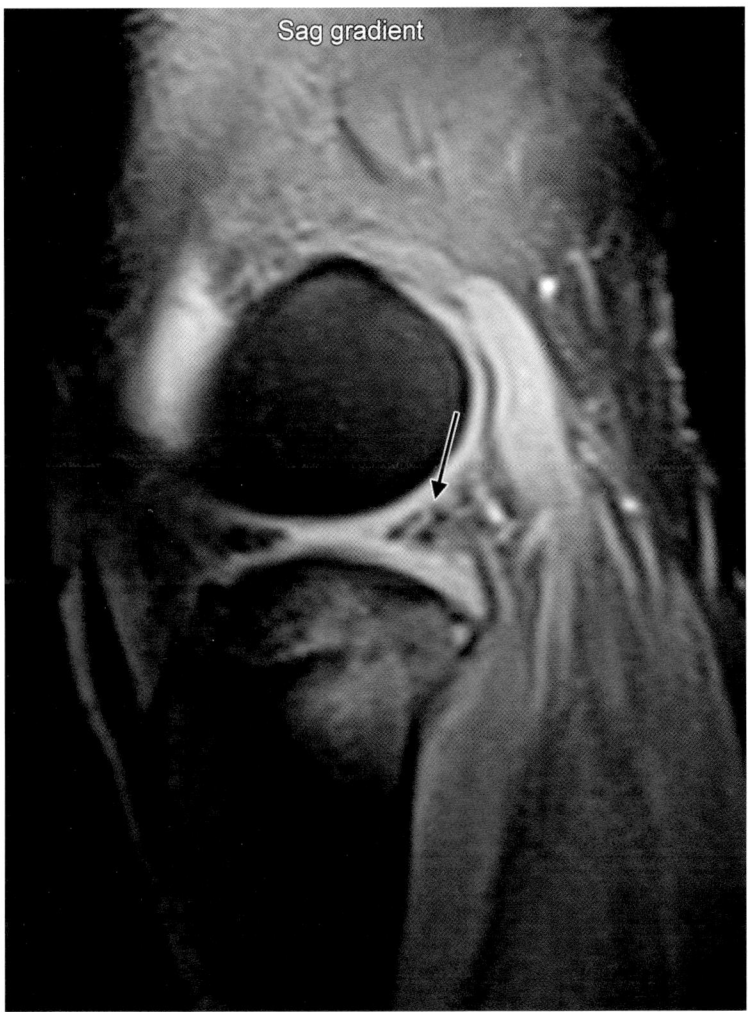

Fig. 91: Sagittal gradient sequence shows hyperintense signal in lateral meniscus of left knee extending into articular surface suggestive of grade III lateral meniscal tear (arrow)

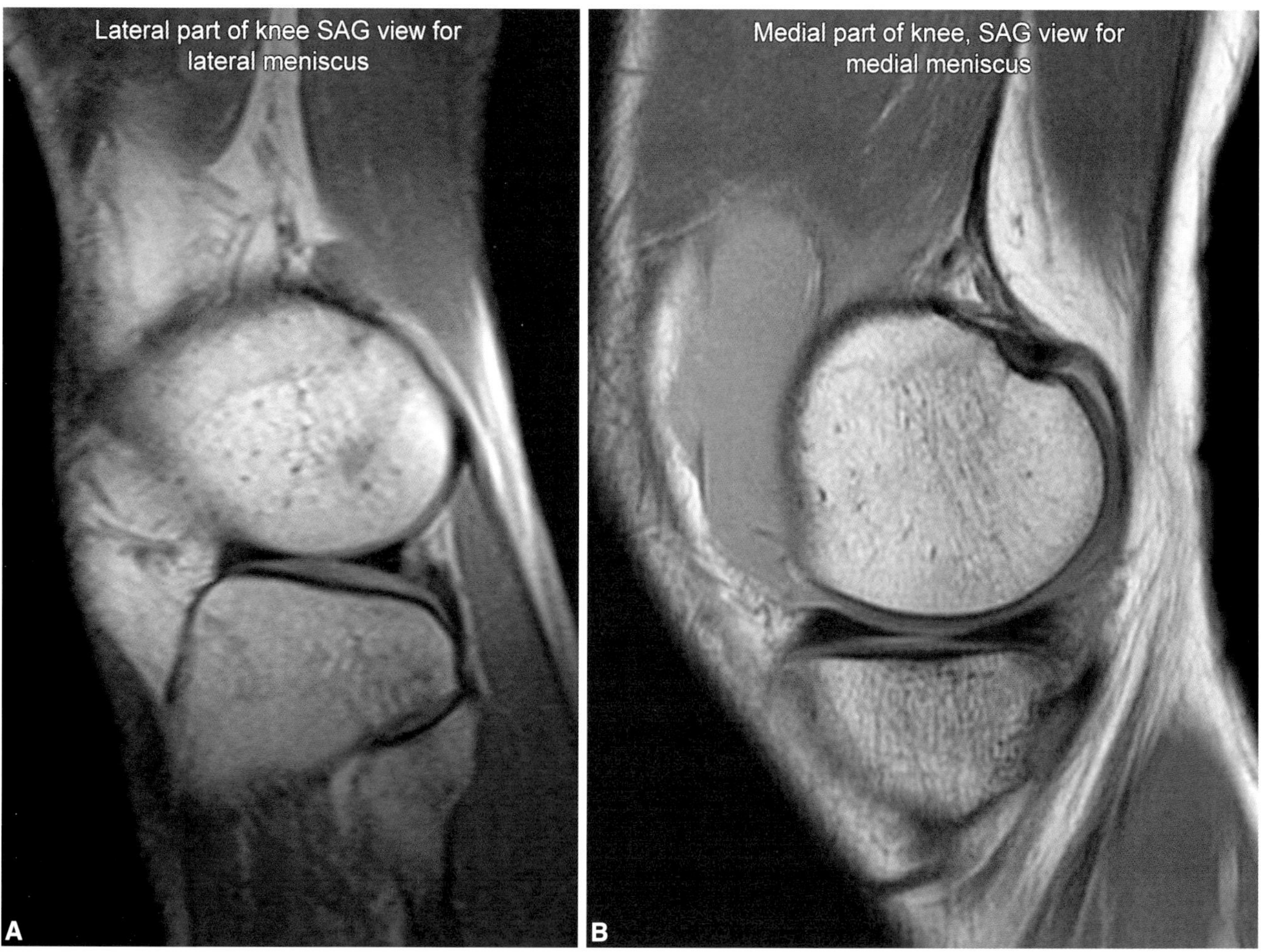

Figs 92A and B: Hint to recognize the medial or lateral meniscus on single sagittal section, when the fibular head is not included in the section. The tibial condyles always appear triangular in shape. The anterior margin of the lateral condyle is vertical and the medial condyle is almost an equilateral triangle in shape

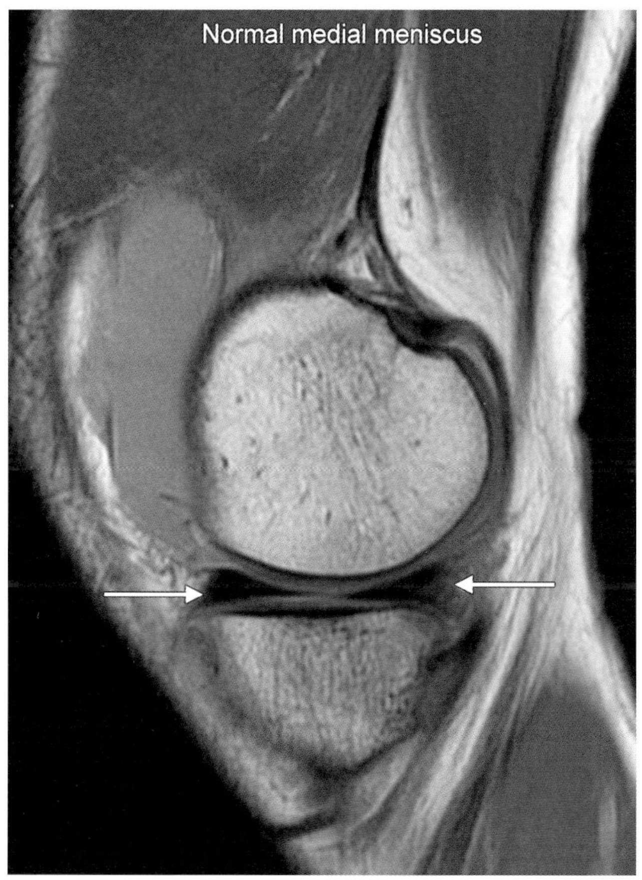

Fig. 93: Sagittal section shows normal appearance of medial meniscus

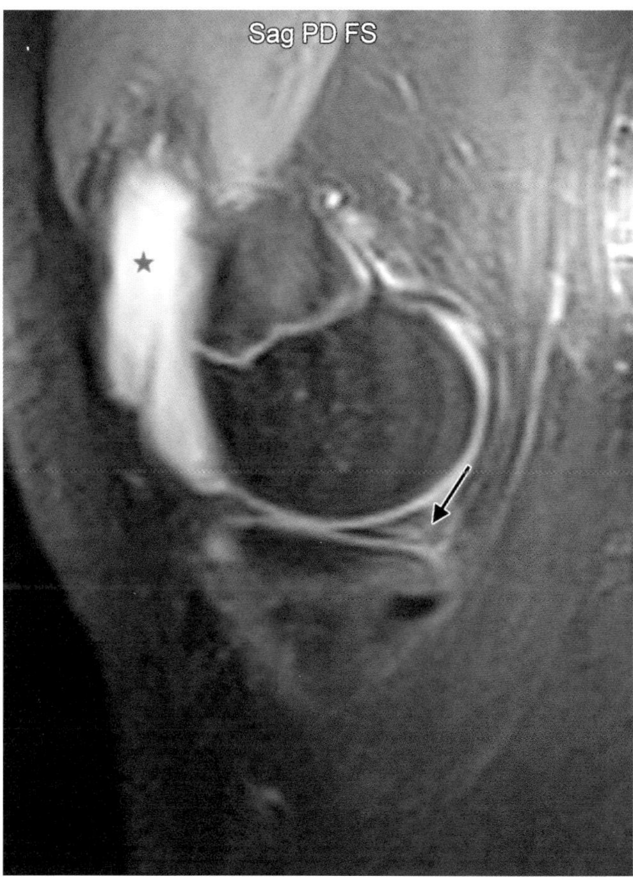

Fig. 94: Sagittal PD FS image reveals linear hyperintense signal in the posterior horn of medial meniscus not reaching upto articular surface suggesting grade II signal with joint effusion (*)

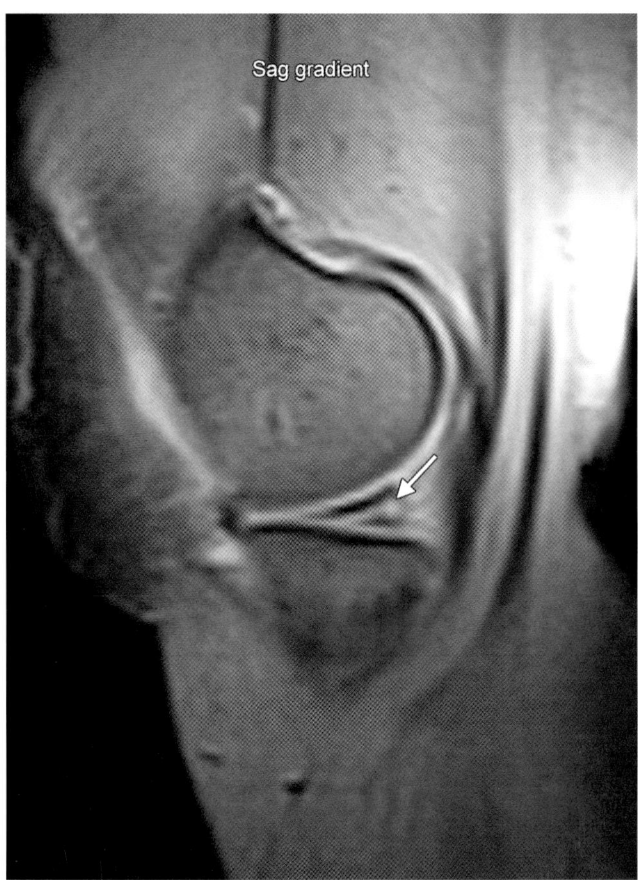

Fig. 95: Sagittal GRE sequence shows hyperintense signal in medial meniscus of left knee extending into inferior articular surface (arrow) suggestive of grade III lateral meniscal tear

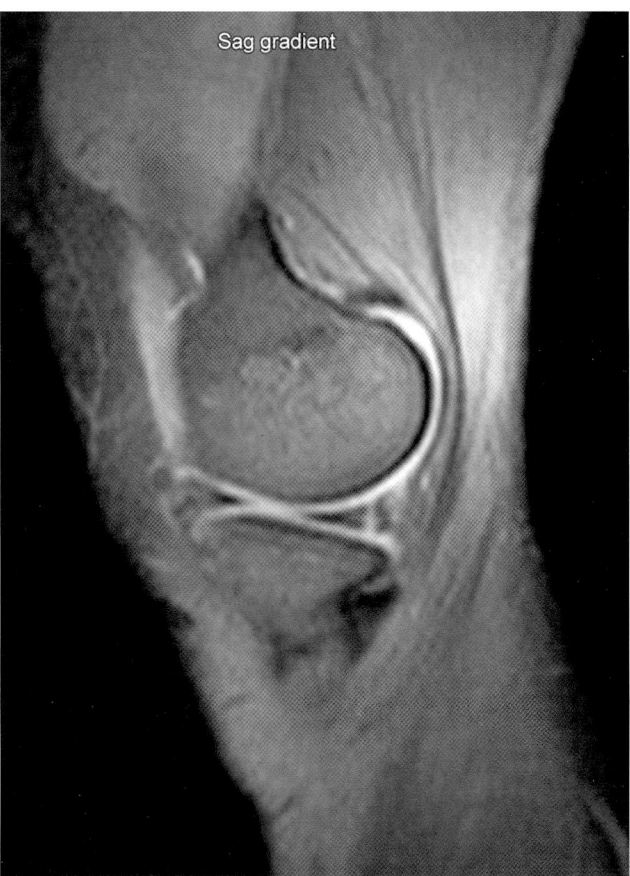

Fig. 96: Sagittal gradient image shows a meniscal tear as a vertical hyperintense signal in the posterior horn. It extends from the superior to the inferior articular surface and represents grade III medial meniscus tear

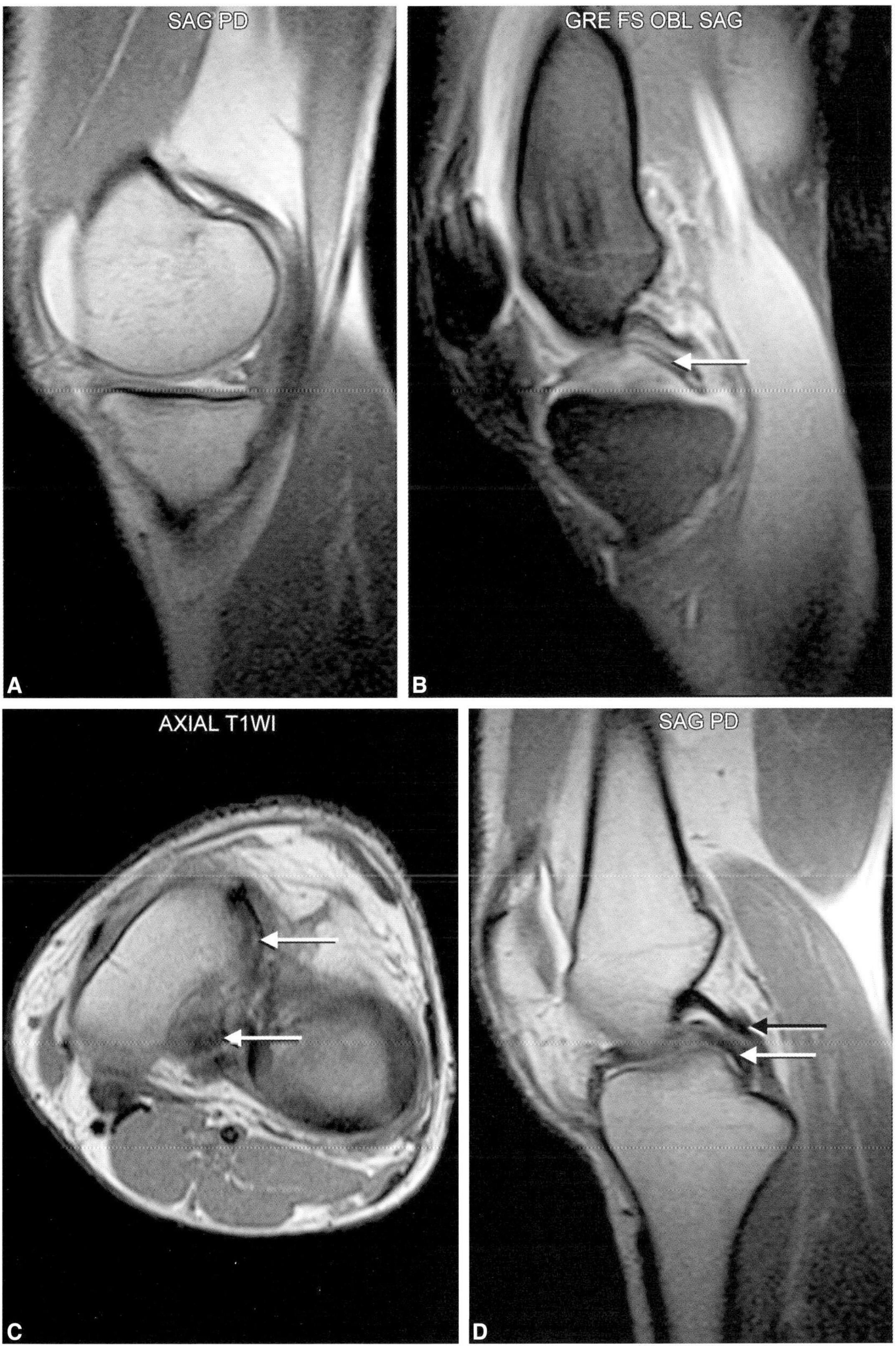

Figs 97A to D: Complex signal in posterior horn of medial meniscus extending in superior articular surface seen in sagittal PD image (A), suggestive of grade III tear. Axial T1WI, oblique sagittal GRE and sagittal PD images (B to D) show medially displaced medial meniscal fragment (white arrow) anteroinferior to PCL (black arrow) with 'double PCL' sign

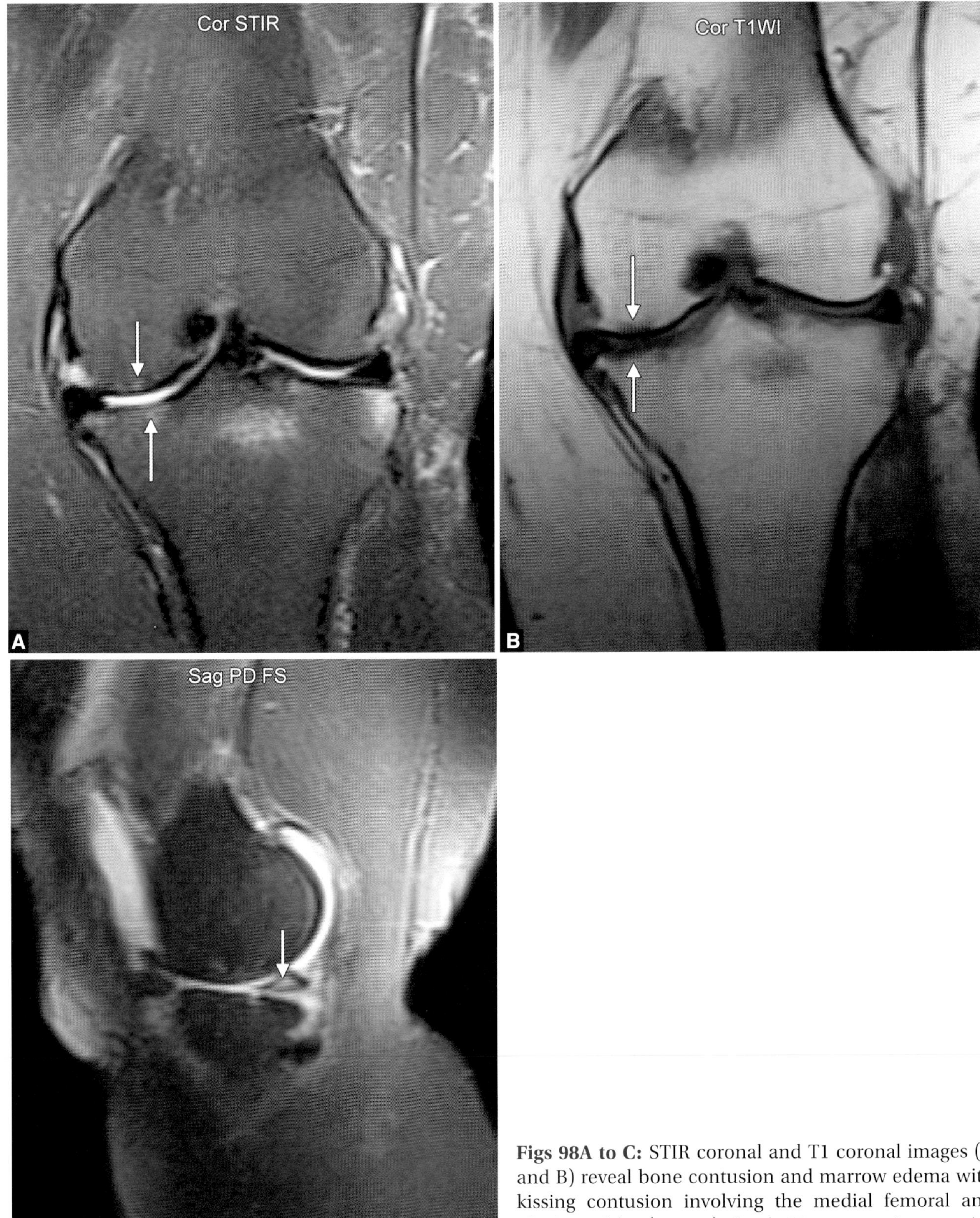

Figs 98A to C: STIR coronal and T1 coronal images (A and B) reveal bone contusion and marrow edema with kissing contusion involving the medial femoral and tibial condyles (arrows). Grade III tear seen in posterior horn of medial meniscus (C)

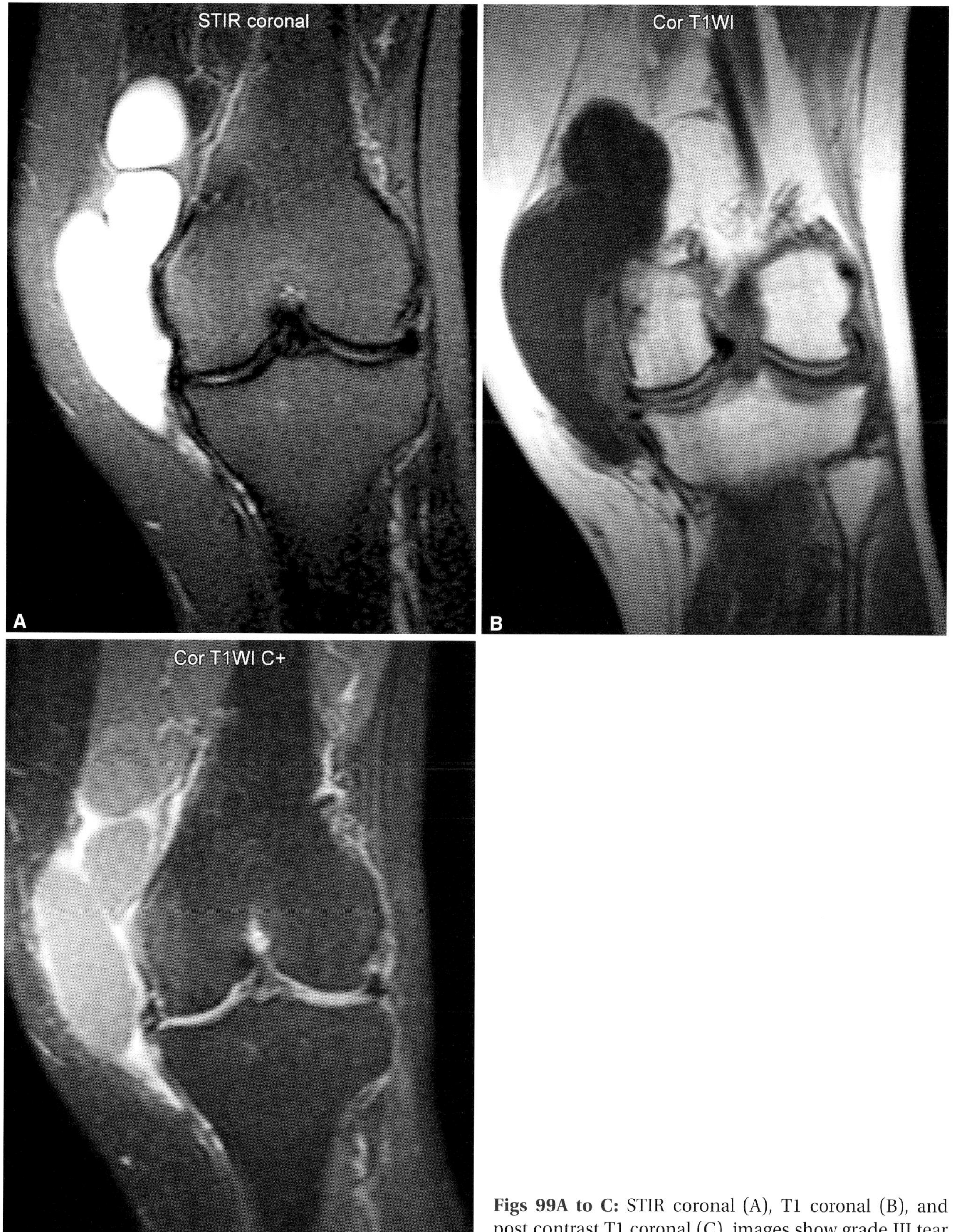

Figs 99A to C: STIR coronal (A), T1 coronal (B), and post contrast T1 coronal (C), images show grade III tear involving the medial meniscus with parameniscal cyst

Collateral Ligament

The collateral ligaments of the knees are found on the inside and outside of the knee joint. The medial collateral ligament and the lateral collateral ligaments are actually a series of much smaller ligaments that create a web of ligaments that go in many different directions and are comprised of different layers. The medial ligament is found on the interior facing side of the knee and connects the tibia to the femur (Figs 100A to C). The lateral ligament is located on the exterior facing side and connects the femur to the fibula in the lower leg (Figs 101A to C).

The function of these ligaments is to regulate the side to side movement of the knee and restrict it from making abnormal motions. Also, they prevent abnormal movement of the tibia backwards towards the femur. In some injury situations, the medial ligament also assumes responsibility of limiting the knee's rotation. In coordination with both the anterior cruciate ligament and the posterior cruciate ligament, proper knee motion and limitations are achieved.

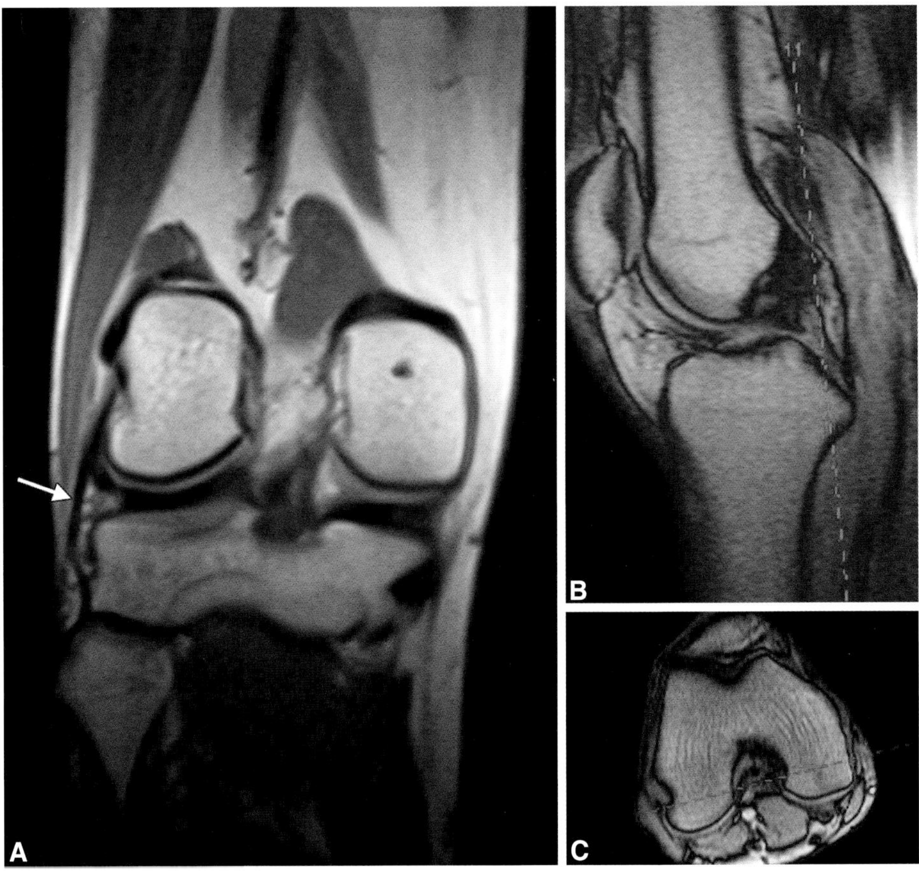

Figs 100A to C: (A) Normal lateral collateral ligament; (B and C) Show scan planes

In injuries involving these ligaments (Figs 102 and 103), the medial ligament is more susceptible to damage. Due to the complex nature of the knee's anatomy, most problems involving the lateral or medial ligaments also involve other parts of the knee. Most frequently, the injuries are caused by traumatic contact that forces the knee inwards and stretches or tears the ligament.

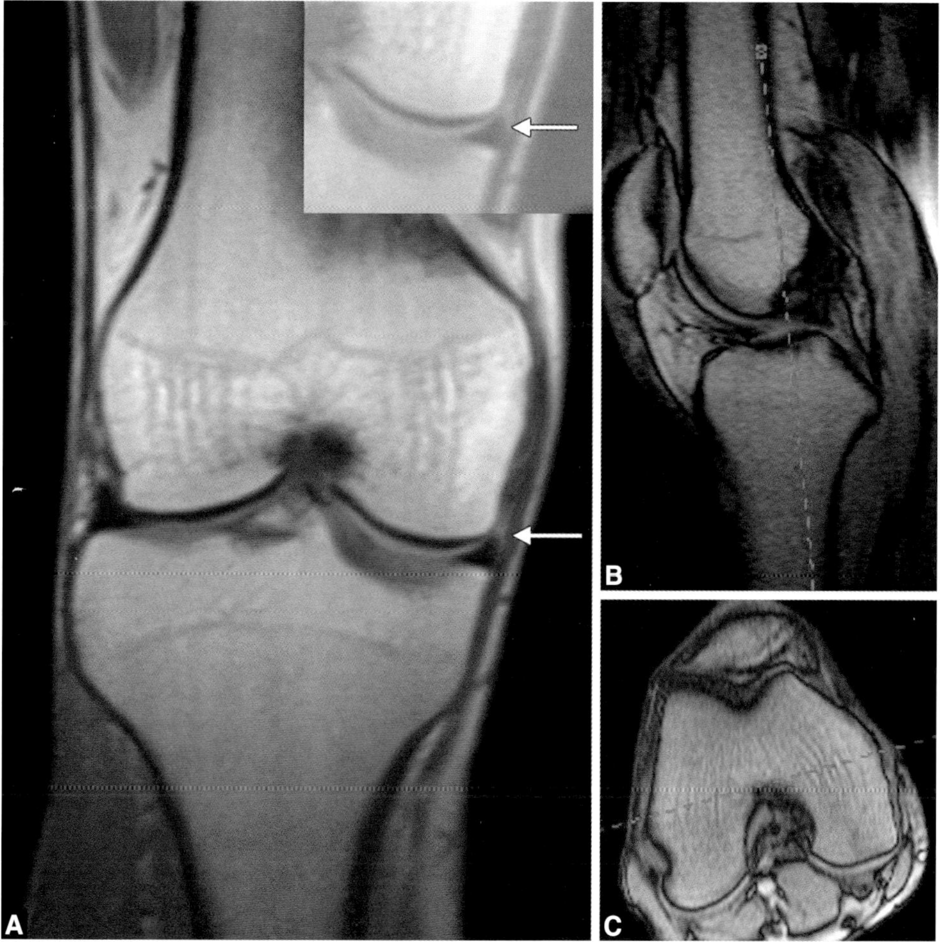

Figs 101A to C: (A) Normal medial collateral ligament; (B and C) Show scan planes

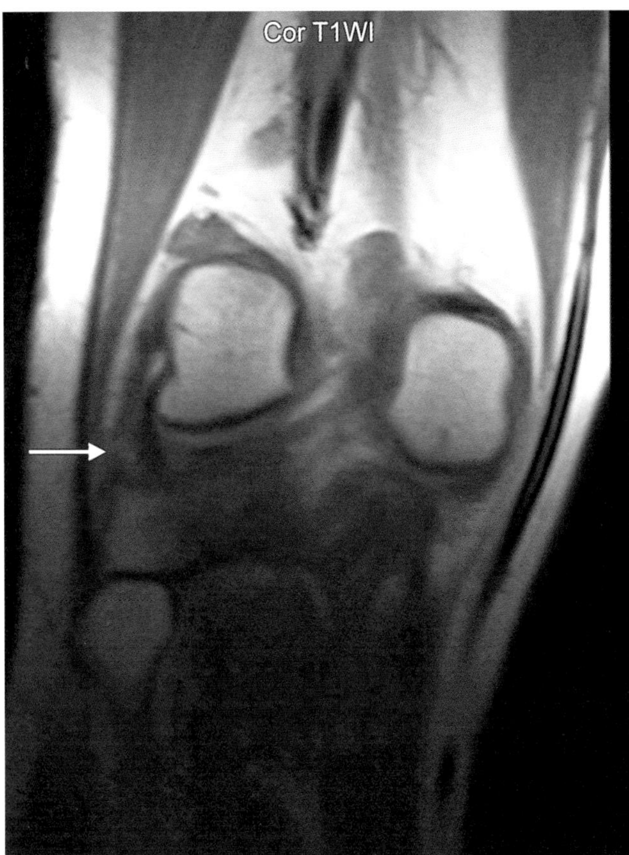

Fig. 102: T1 weighted coronal image shows edematous appearance of lateral collateral ligament in mid portion suggesting strain or partial tear of the lateral collateral ligament (arrow)

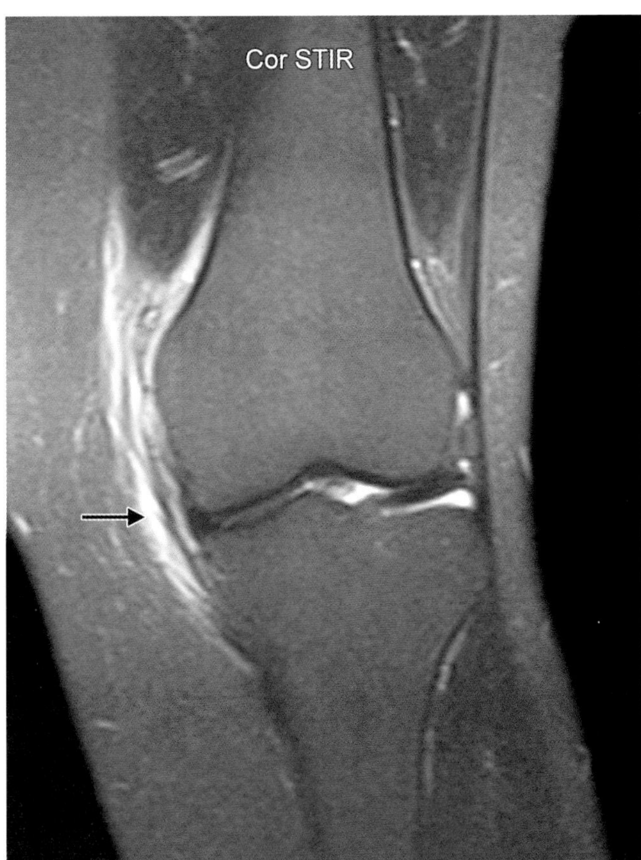

Fig. 103: STIR coronal image shows strain (arrow) with partial tear of the medial collateral ligament

Pigmented Villonodular Synovitis

Pigmented villonodular synovitis (PVNS) is a proliferative disorder of the synovial membrane that most commonly involves the knee, hip, elbow and ankle. A brown fluid can frequently be aspirated from the joint, which reflects hemosiderin deposits from chronic hemorrhage or fresh blood from acute hemorrhage. Radiographs often show the findings of joint effusion, preservation of joint space, the absence of osteoporosis and the presence or absence of bone erosions and cysts. Bone erosions and subchondral cysts can be prominent, particularly in the hip, ankle, elbow and wrist. Many of the radiographic features of diffuse intra-articular PVNS are identical to those of idiopathic synovial chondromatosis. In PVNS calcification is not seen.

A giant cell tumor of a tendon sheath represents a nodular lesion of tendon sheaths, usually in the hand or foot, which may sometimes be confused with some forms of PVNS because of similar histologic findings. In PVNS, a diffuse or localized soft tissue mass is observed, with adjacent erosion of bone (Figs 104 to 107).

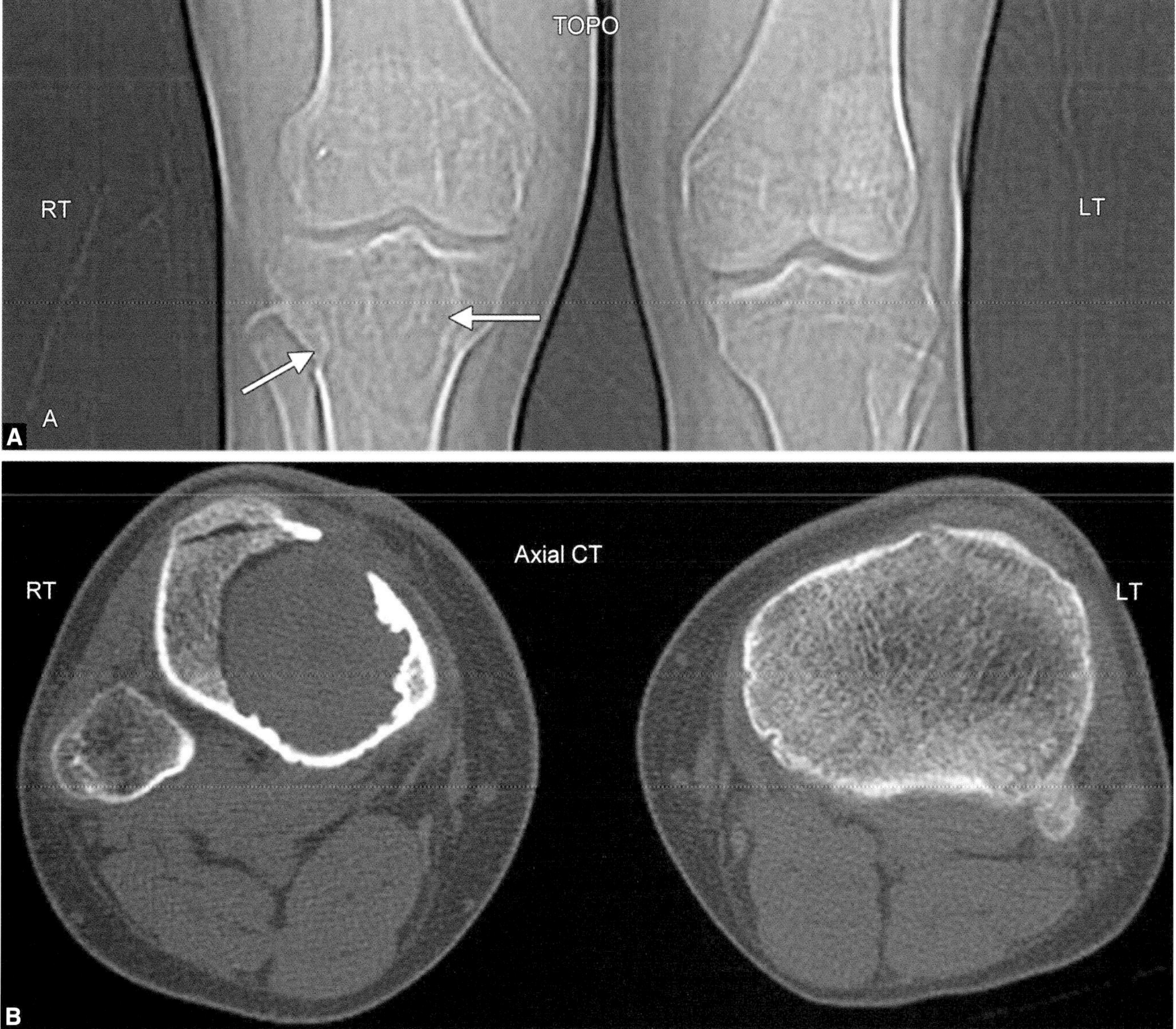

Figs 104A and B: Topogram (A) reveal lytic lesion in the right tibia proximal metaepiphysis. Axial CT (B) reveal lytic lesion with soft tissue in the right proximal tibial metaepiphysis

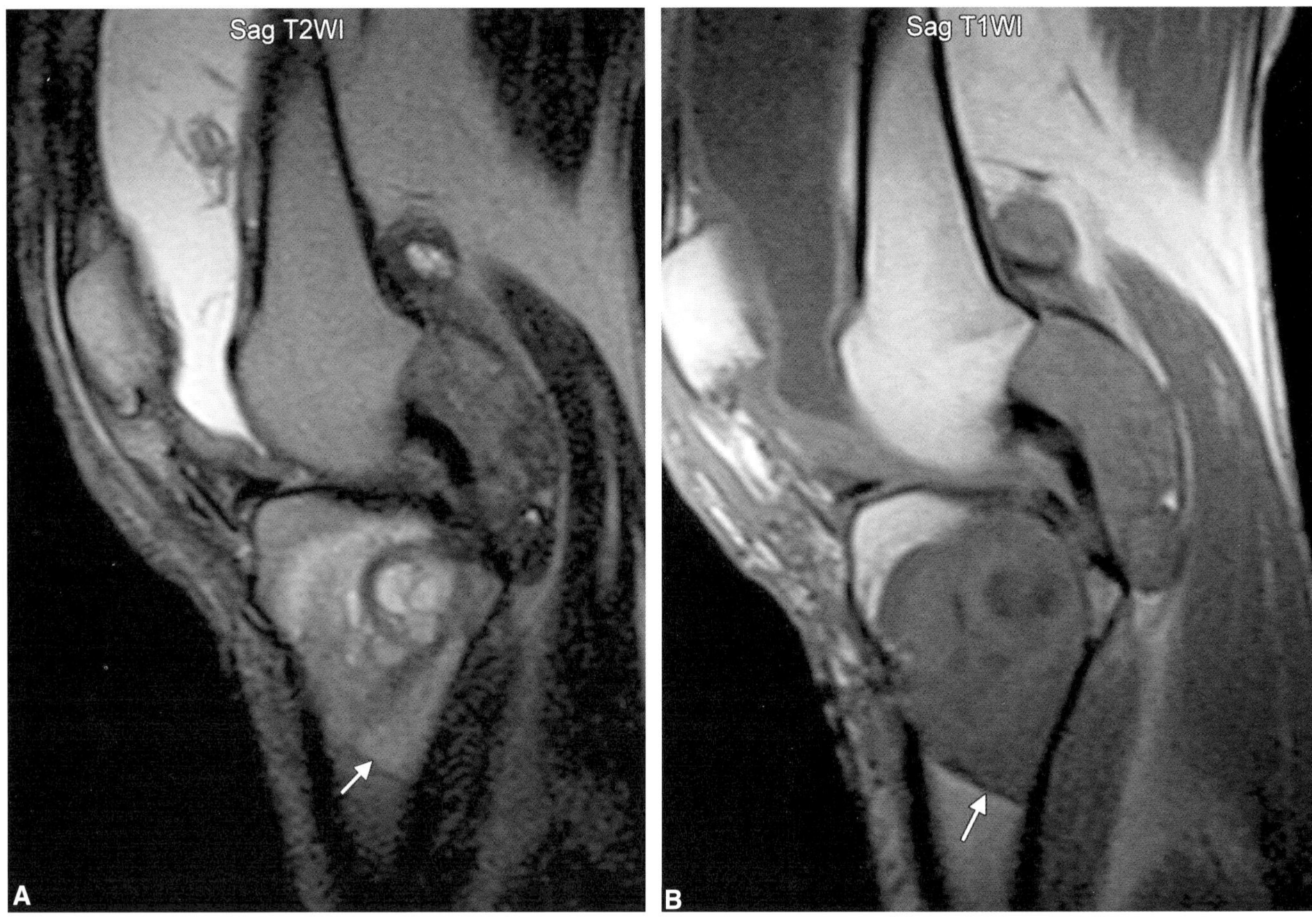

Figs 105A and B: Sagittal T2WI (A) heterogeneous hyperintense soft tissue intensity mass lesion in the proximal tibial metaepiphysis which is heterogeneous hypointense on T1WI (B) with moderate joint effusion

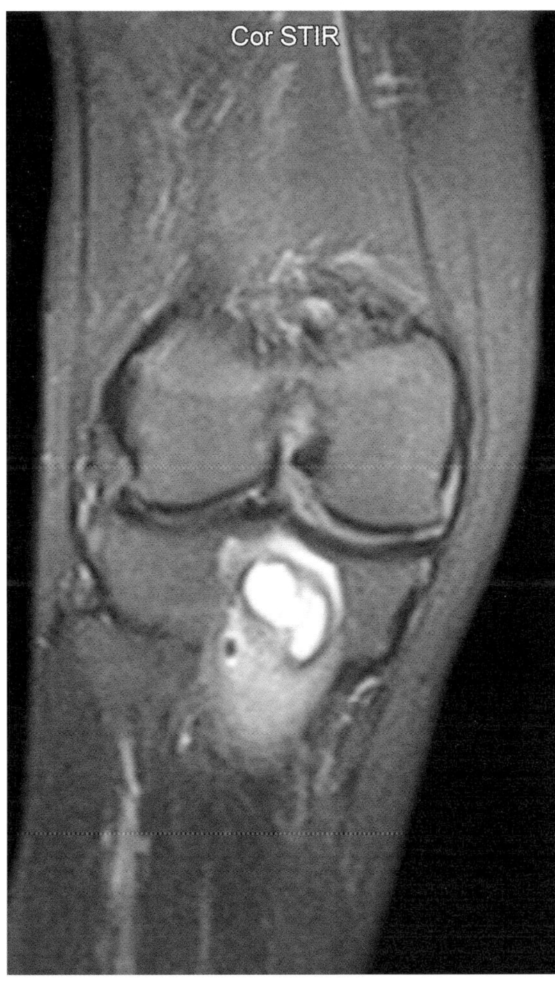

Fig. 106: Coronal STIR image reveal abnormal hyperintense mass lesion in the proximal tibial metaepiphysis with surrounding marrow edema

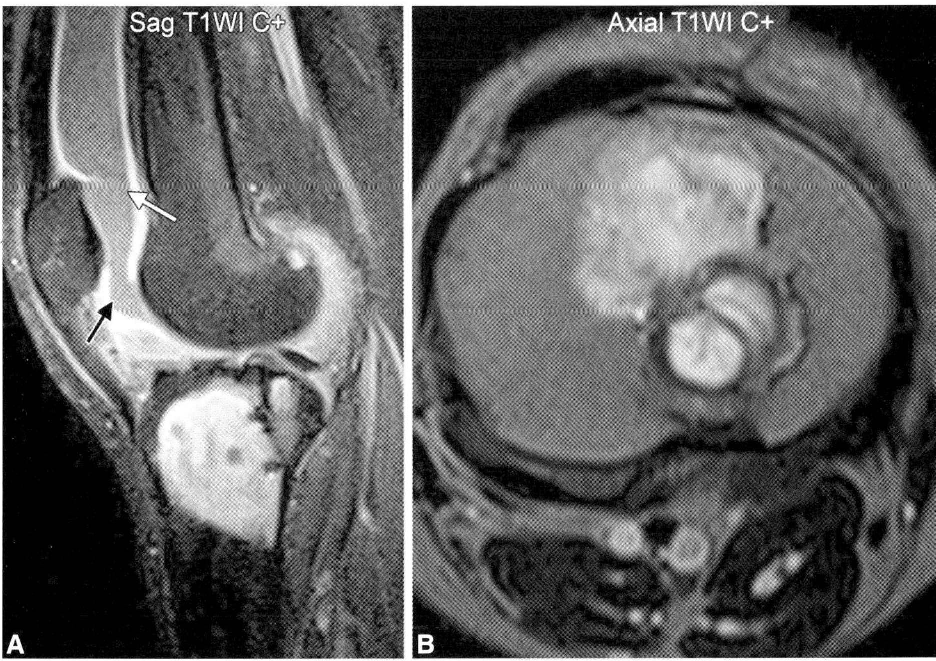

Figs 107A and B: Sagittal T1 and axial T1W post contrast images show abnormal post contrast enhancement in the soft tissue lesion with abnormal peripheral synovial enhancement with moderate joint effusion (arrow)

BONY LESIONS

Fracture Scaphoid

Trauma to the wrist may involve greater arc or lesser arc injuries to the carpal bones. In lesser arc injuries, usually only stage I (scapholunate dissociation) involves the scaphoid bone. Greater arc injuries represent fracture dislocations through the scaphoid and other bones of the carpus. Carpal fractures most frequently involve the scaphoid bone (Figs 108A and B); various sites may be affected (proximal pole, waist, distal part of the body, tuberosity). Often these fractures are associated with delayed union, nonunion or osteonecrosis (Figs 108C and D).

In scapholunate dissociation (also known as rotary subluxation of the scaphoid), the scaphoid and lunate carpal bones are separated, sometimes after a fracture of the scaphoid or of the proximal portion of the radius. This dissociation leads to dorsiflexion instability of the wrist, or dorsal intercalary segmental carpal instability (DISI). A distance between the scaphoid and lunate bones of 2 mm or more suggests the diagnosis, and a distance of 4 mm or more is unequivocal evidence of its presence.

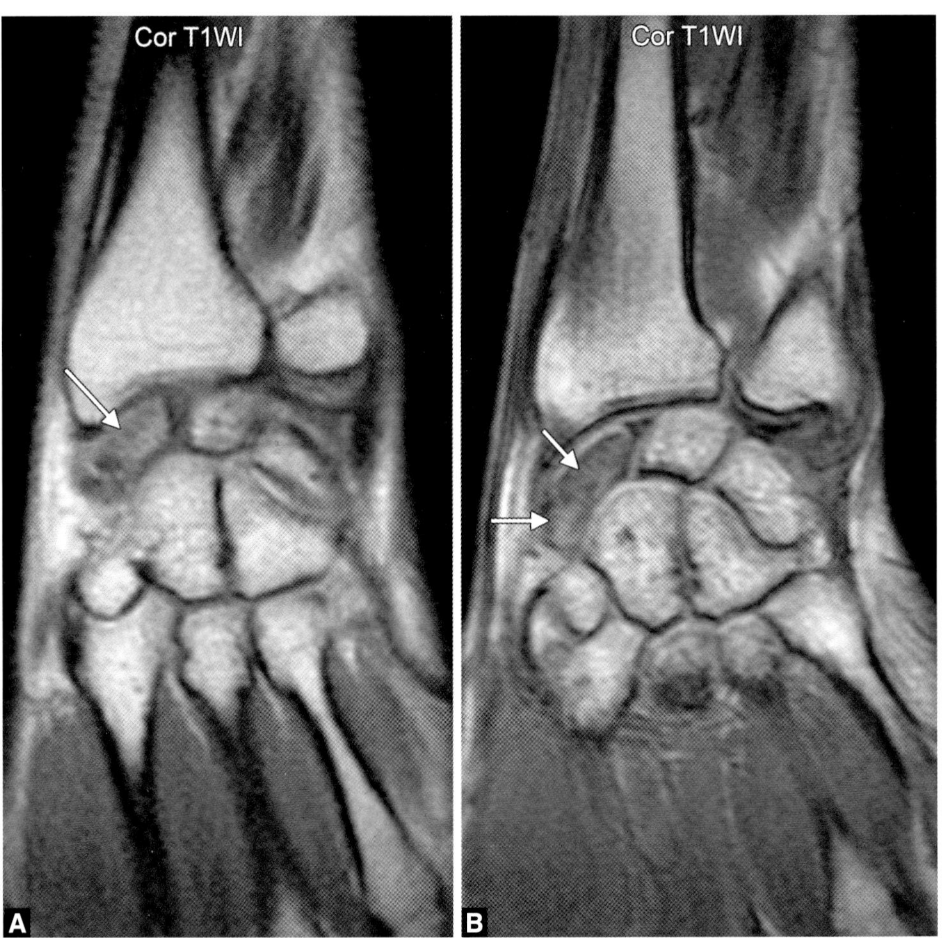

Figs 108A and B

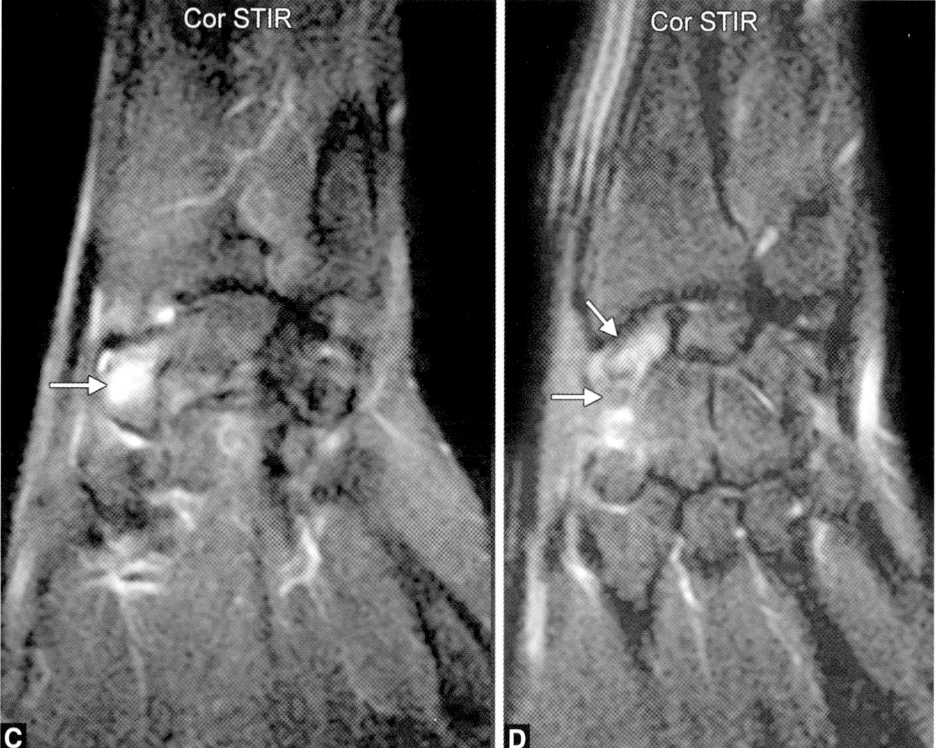

Figs 108C and D

Figs 108A to D: Complete oblique fracture is seen through the waist of scaphoid. There is hypointense signal (thin arrow) on coronal T1W images (A and B) suggestive of AVN and relatively less hypointense marrow signal (thick arrow) represents reactive marrow edema. The signal is hyperintense in scaphoid on STIR images (C and D)

Compression Fracture

A compression fracture occurs when the normal vertebral body of the spine is squashed, or compressed, to a smaller height. This injury tends to happen first, in patients involved in traumatic accidents commonly seen after a fall from height. Secondly when a load placed on the vertebrae exceeds its stability, it may collapse, which is much more common type. These patients are those with osteoporosis. Compression fracture is usually diagnosed by the history, physical examination and X-rays. In any patient over the age of 60 years with the acute onset of sudden low back pain, a compression fracture should be suspected. Physical exam will usually show tenderness directly over the area of pain as well as mild kyphotic deformity. Plain X-rays will demonstrate the wedge shape of the vertebral body on a lateral view. If osteoporosis is suspected, a bone mineral density test and thyroid function test may be requisitioned. They help determine the severity of the bone thinning. CT scan is occasionally needed to help differentiate a compression fracture from a burst fracture.

MR scan (Figs 109 and 110) is obtained to rule out disc herniation along with a compression fracture. MR also helps differentiate pathologic compression fractures, due to tumor or a typical osteoporotic compression fracture. In any patient with a known history of cancer, a compression fracture should tip off the physician to look for evidence of a metastatic lesion and pathologic fracture.

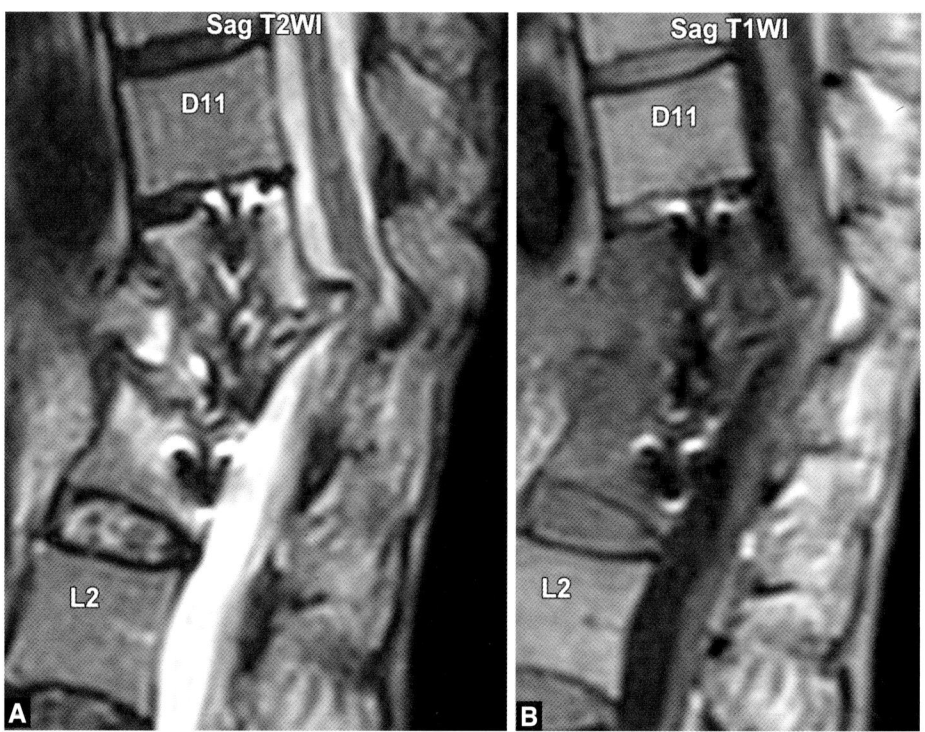

Figs 109A and B: Sagittal T2WI (A) and T1WI (B) wedge compression collapse fracture of the D12 vertebral body and break in the superior endplate of L1 vertebral body with retropulsion and compression of the lower end of cord at the same level

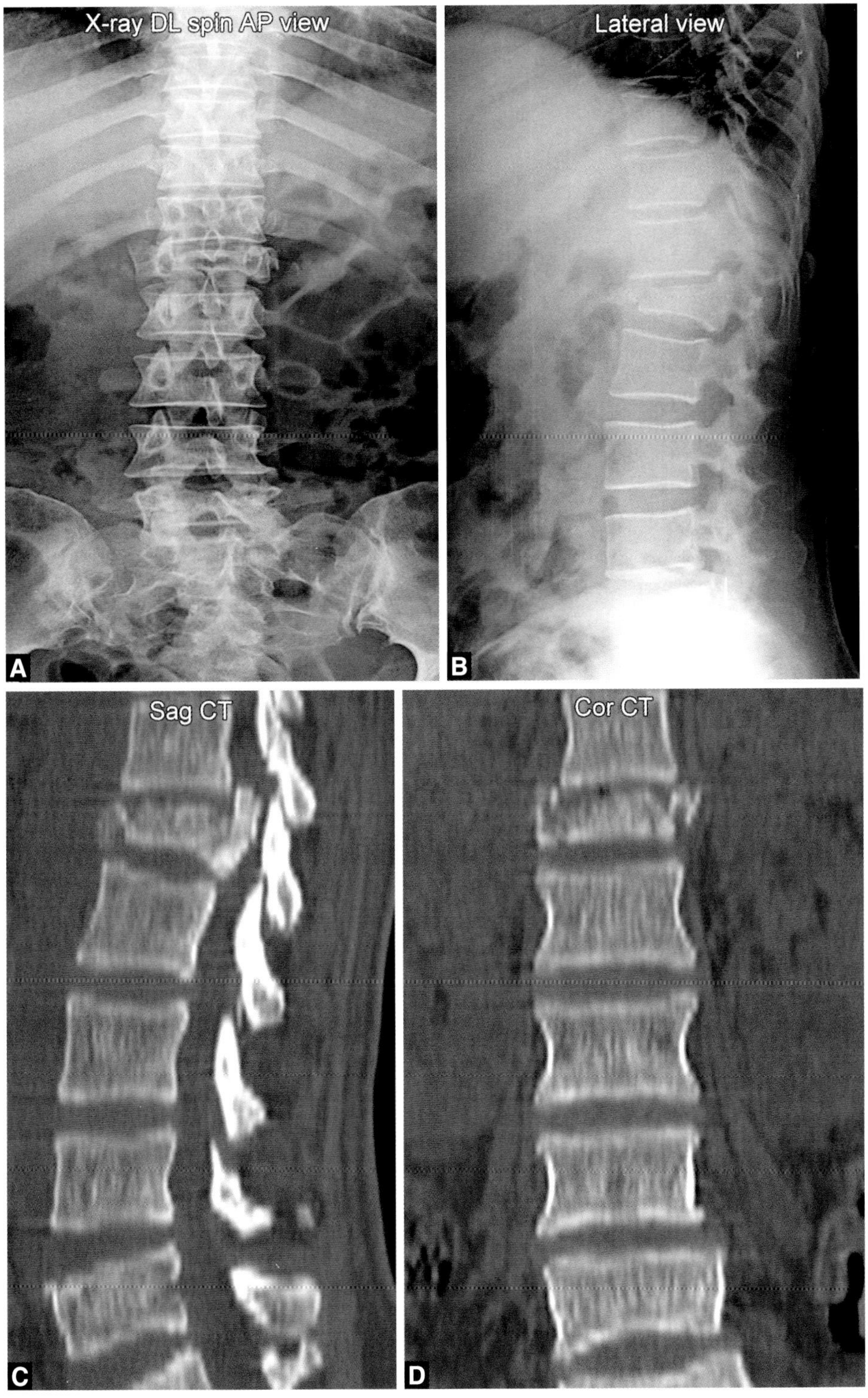

Figs 110A to D

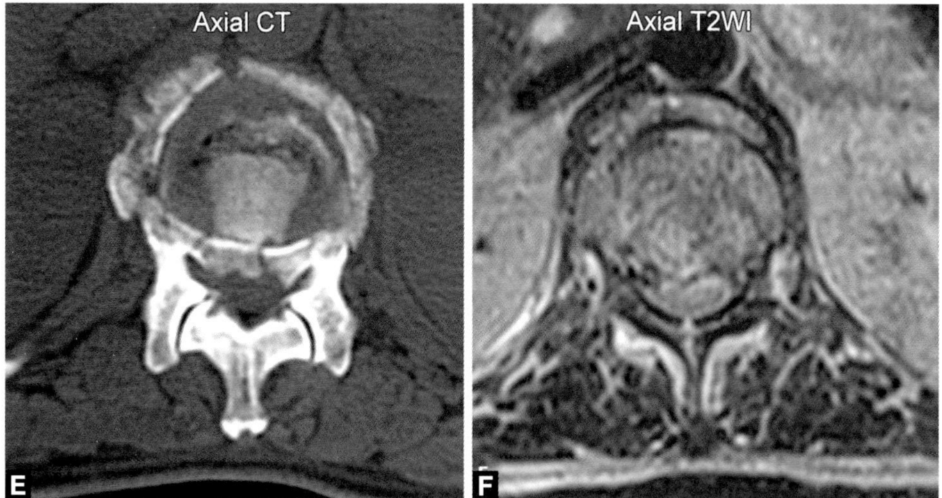

Figs 110E and F

Figs 110A to F: X-ray dorsolumbar spine AP and lateral views (A and B), sagittal and coronal reformatted CT image (C and D) wedge compression fracture collapse of L1 vertebral body with retropulsion of bone fragment with mild reduction in height of L5 vertebral body. Axial CT (E) MR T2WI (F) Fracture of the L1 vertebral body with retropulsion of the bone fragment in spinal canal

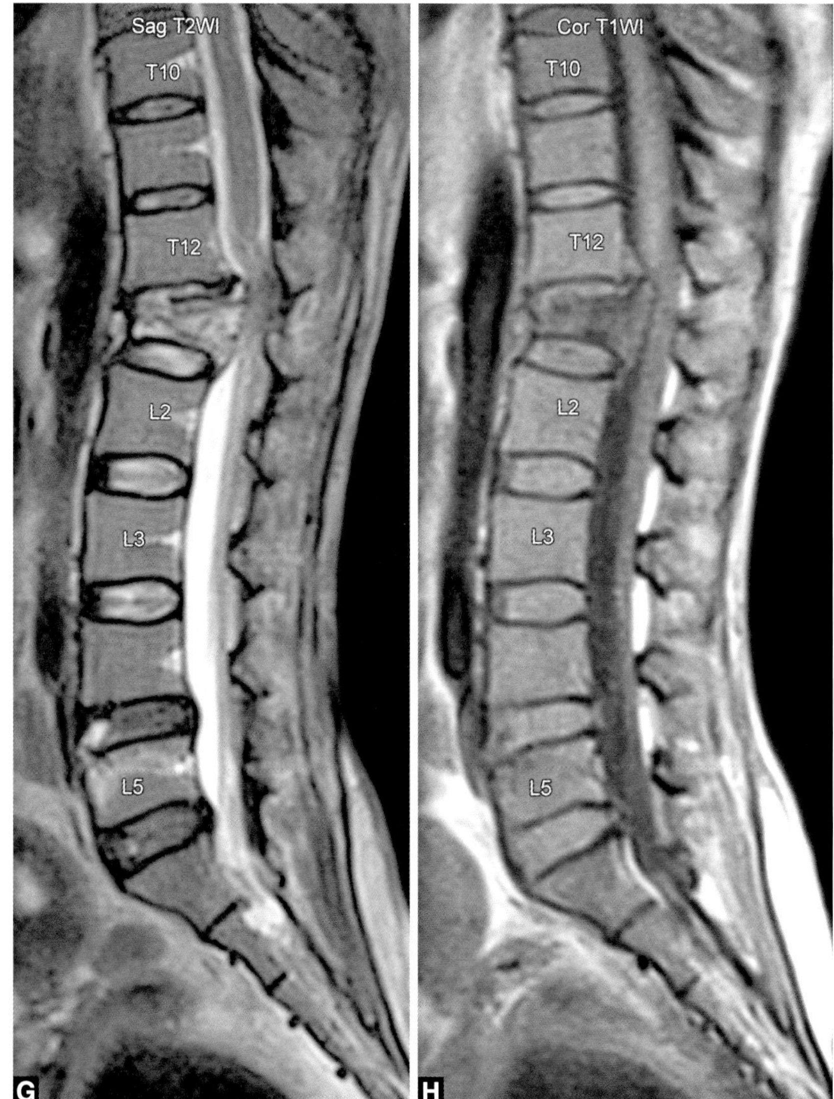

Figs 110G and H

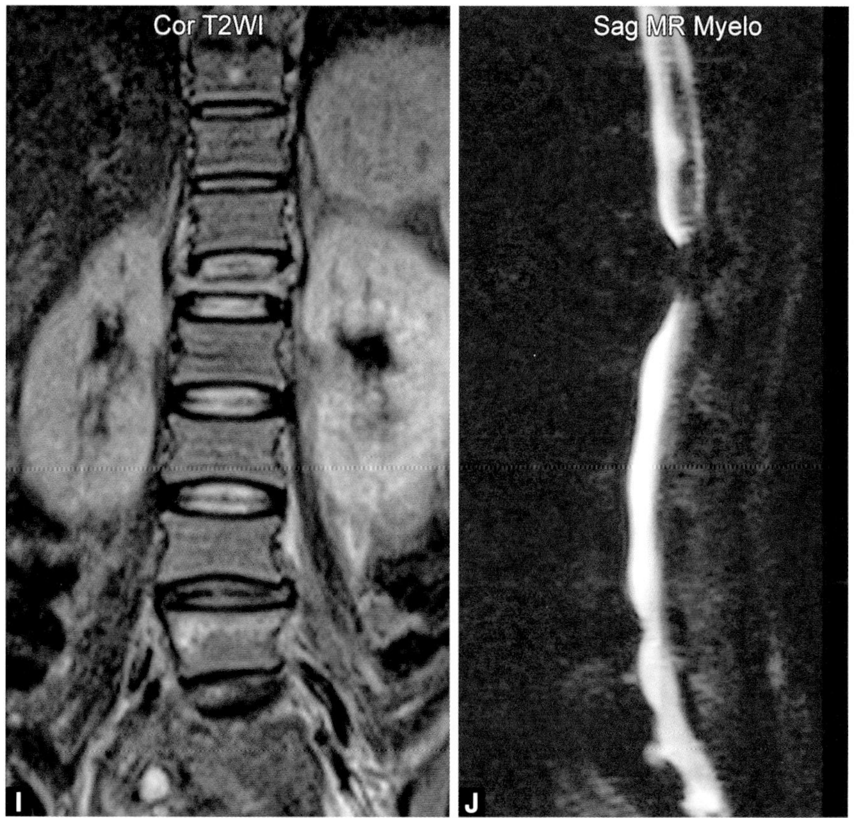

Figs 110I and J

Figs 110G to J: Sagittal T2WI (G) sagittal T1WI (H) coronal T2WI (I) wedge compression collapse fracture of L1 vertebral body with retropulsion of bone fragment with marrow edema. There is mild reduction in height of L5 vertebral body with marrow edema. Sagittal MR myelogram show severe compression with cut off thecal sac at L1 level (J)

Segond Fracture

The Segond fracture is a type of avulsion fracture of the lateral condyle of the tibia (Figs 111A to C), immediately beyond the surface which articulates with the femur. Segond fracture occurs in association with tears of the anterior cruciate ligament (ACL) and injury to the medial meniscus

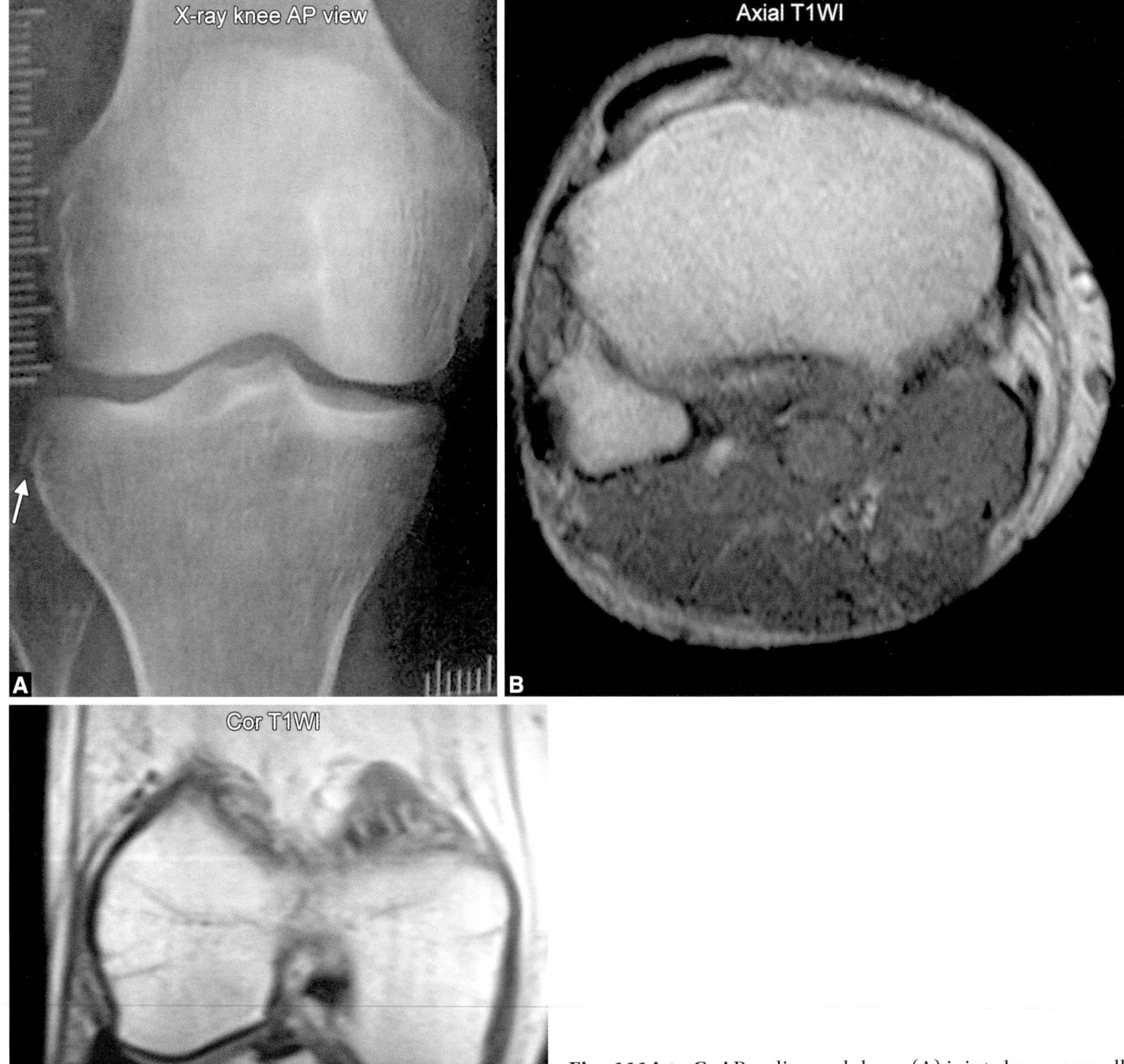

Figs 111A to C: AP radiograph knee (A) joint shows a small chip of bone at the lateral condyle of the tibia immediately beyond the surface which articulates with the femur. T1W axial image (B) shows a well-defined round hypointensity at the anterolateral corner of tibial condyle, which is an avulsion fracture. Coronal T1W image (C) shows a well-defined round hypointensity at the anterolateral corner of tibial condyle similar to the avulsion fracture seen on plain X-ray

Osteomyelitis

Osteomyelitis is an infection of bone and bone marrow, which may develop in acute, subacute and chronic clinical stages. All cases do not show progression through all these phases, and in some cases chronic osteomyelitis is present at the time of initial evaluation.

Four principal routes of contamination of bones and joints in osteomyelitis are from (a) hematogenous spread (b) spread from a contiguous source of infection (c) direct implantation of infectious material and (d) postoperative spread.

Owing to differences in vascular anatomy of tubular bones, haematogenous osteomyelitis may have different clinical and imaging patterns at different ages (infant, child, adult). Imaging finding include presence of sequestrum, a segment of necrotic bone separated from living bone by granulation tissue; involucrum, a layer of viable bone that has formed around necrotic bone; sinus tract, a tract leading to the skin surface from an infected site in bone; and Brodies abscess a sharply delineated focus of infection in bone.

Chronic osteomyelitis shows areas of osteolysis, periosteal reaction, sclerosis and sequestration. Scintigraphy and MR imaging are preferred methods in the early diagnosis of osteomyelitis, but MR imaging lacks specificity and bone abscesses cannot be distinguished from sterile fluid collections without intravenous contrast administration (Figs 112A to D). Scintigraphy is useful in differentiation of osteomyelitis from cellulitis and in the recognition of renewed activity in chronic osteomyelitis. CT has been used to identify single or multiple sequestra, bone or soft tissue abscesses, and sinus tracts.

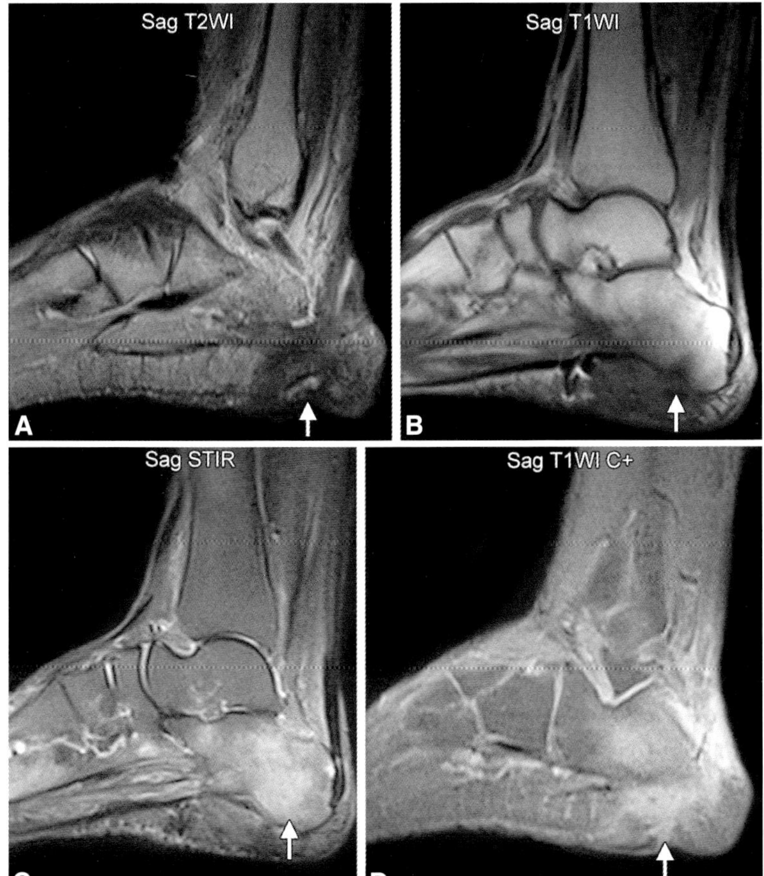

Figs 112A to D: Sagittal T2WI image (A) reveal abnormal hyperintense signal in the heel soft tissue region (arrow), appearing hypointense on T1WI (B) with hypointense marrow edema in the calcaneum (arrow), sagittal STIR image (C) shows abnormal hyperintense marrow edema in the calcaneum (arrow), (D) post contrast enhancement is seen (arrow)

Bone Cyst

Bone cyst is a cavitary lesion of bone. Various types of bone cysts may be identified: simple or unicameral, epidermoid, aneurysmal, subchondral and ganglion. Bone cysts may occur after trauma and in osteoarthritis, rheumatoid arthritis, neurofibromatosis and calcium pyrophosphate dihydrate crystal deposition disease. Simple bone cysts are lesions of unknown cause that may result from venous obstruction with failure of drainage of the interstitial fluid in rapidly growing or remodeling bones. These cysts occur more commonly in long tubular bones, especially the metaphysis, and in the bony pelvis. On X-ray these lesions appear radiolucent and are located centrally, with cortical thinning and mild expansion of the bone. Bone cyst in patella is uncommon (Figs 113 to 116). Pathological fractures are common. CT and MR imaging confirm the diagnosis of the bone cyst and shows no wall enhancement on post contrast images. Complications of simple bone cysts include fractures, cementomas, and rarely malignant transformation.

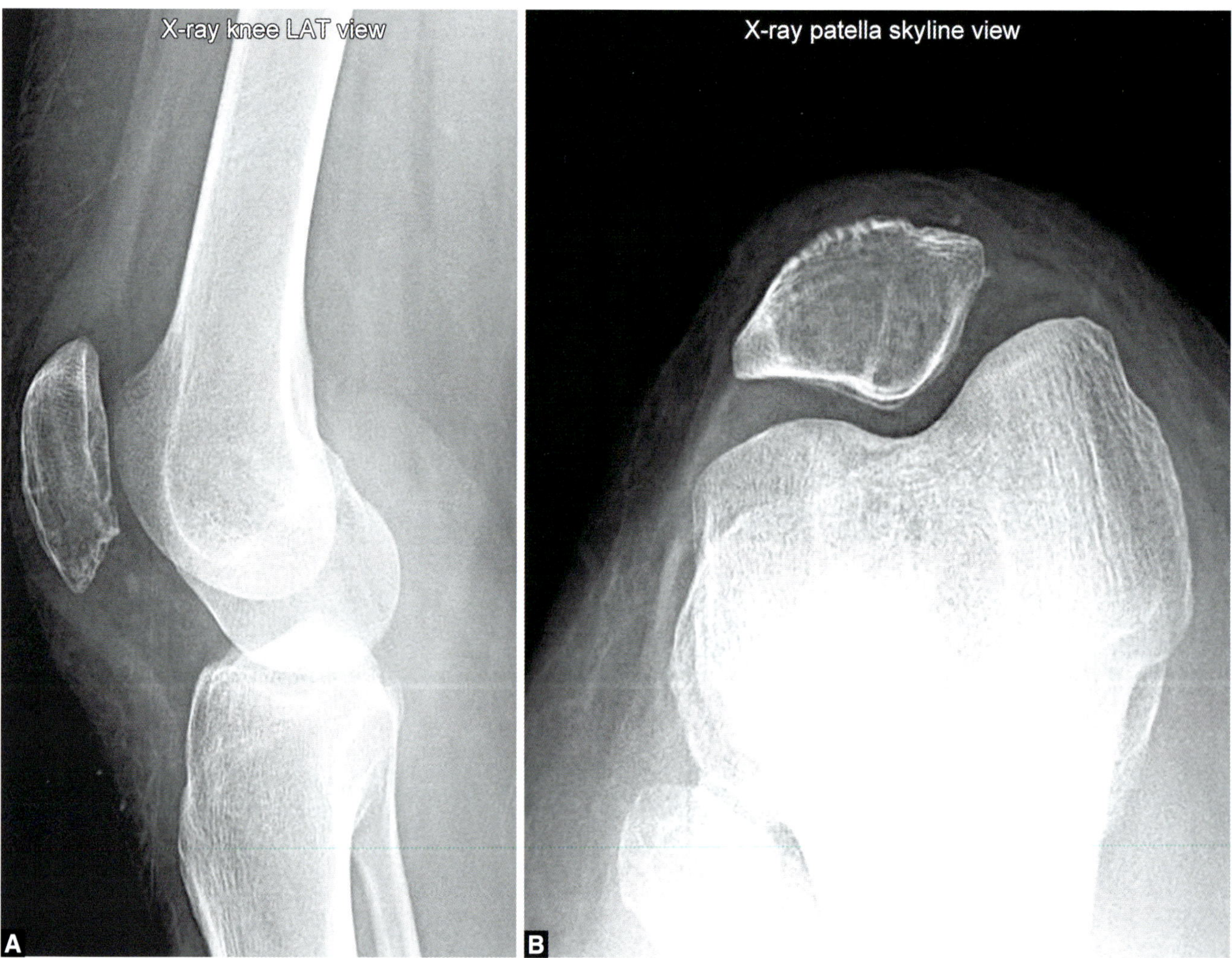

Figs 113A and B: X-ray lateral (A) skyline (B) views for patella shows a large lucency with thinning of cortical bone in left patella, cyst is better appreciated on skyline view

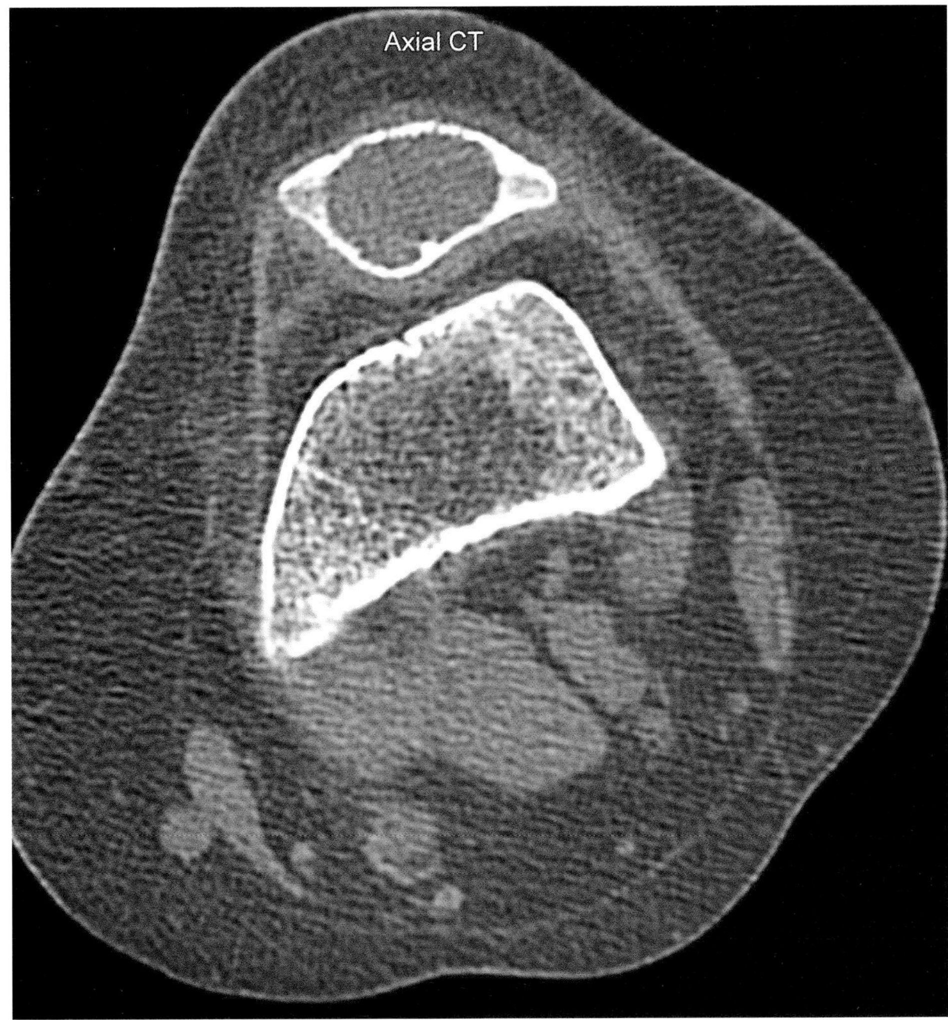

Fig. 114: Axial CT shows a large cystic lesion within the patella with a thin bony rim

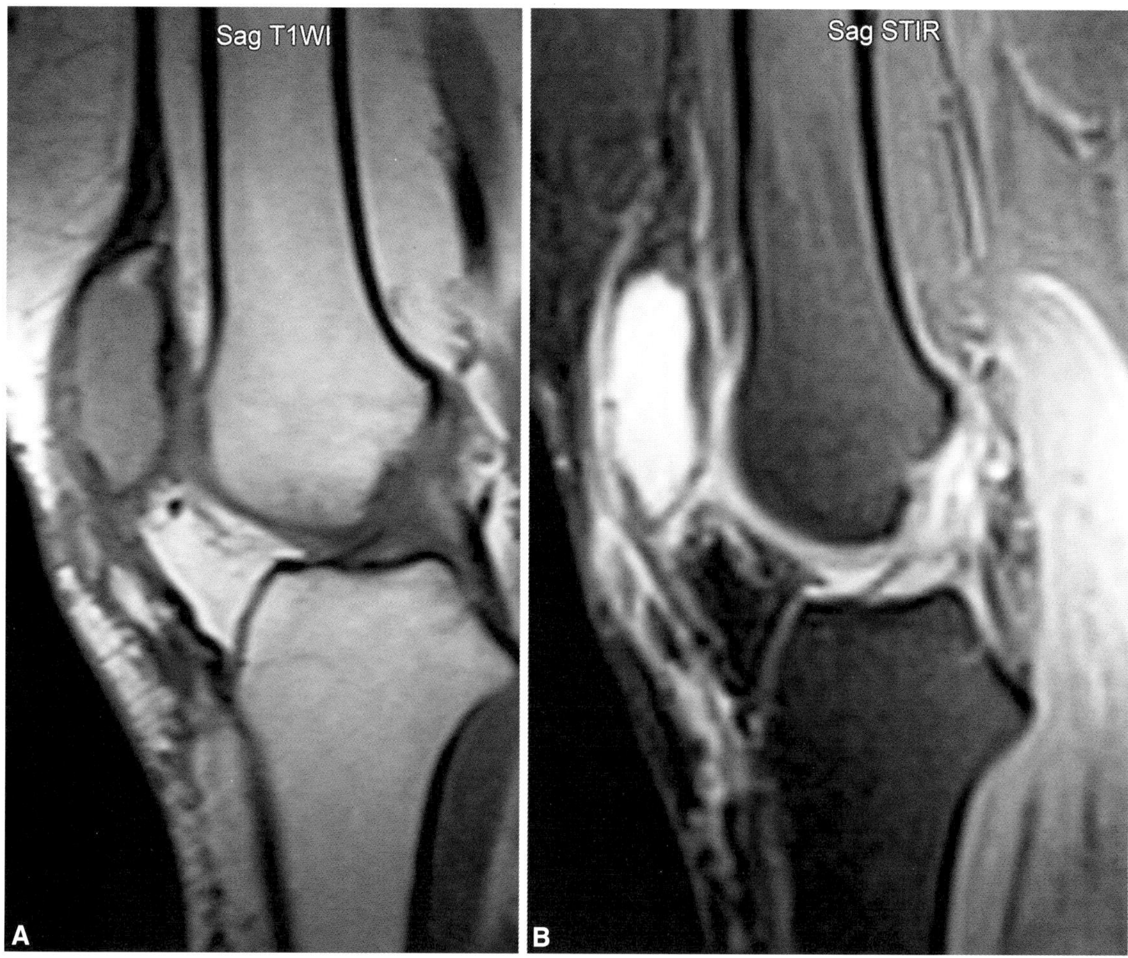

Figs 115A and B: Sagittal T1W image (A) reduced intensity in patella, appearing hyperintense on sagittal STIR image (B), confirms the finding of cyst

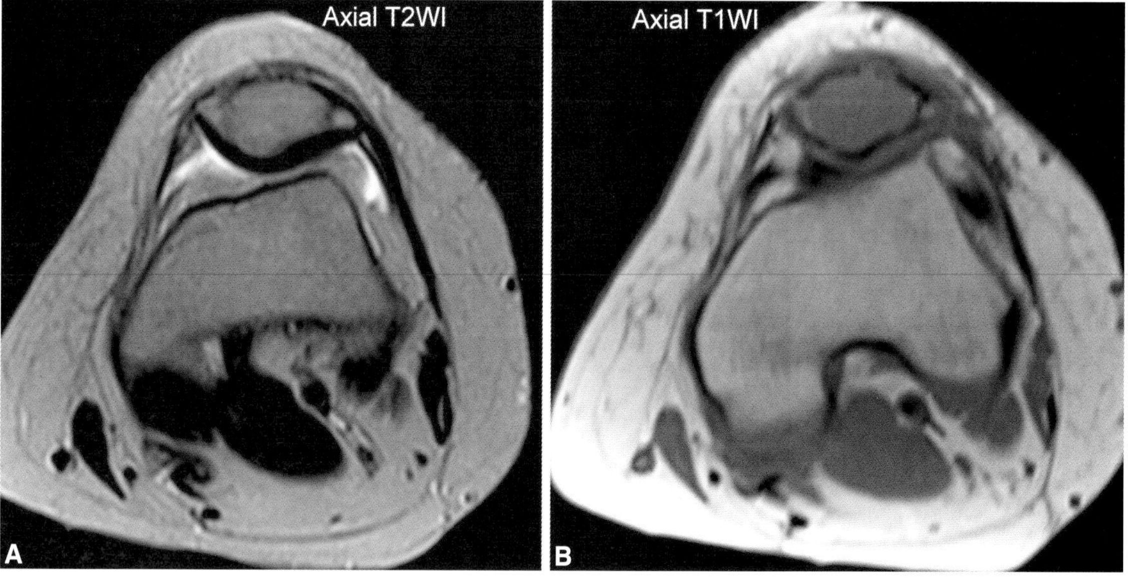

Figs 116A and B: Axial T2W image (A) iso to hyperintense signal in patella appearing hypointense on T1W image (B)

Avascular Necrosis (AVN) Scaphoid

Osteonecrosis frequently affects the proximal pole of the scaphoid bone after trauma to this region; the distal pole is less likely to undergo necrosis. Sometimes this condition is not apparent on radiographs until 4 to 8 weeks after injury. Delayed fracture union or nonunion, collapse of the necrotic segment, and secondary degenerative joint disease may complicate this process. Diagnosis may be facilitated by MR imaging or scintigraphy. A spontaneous osteonecrosis of the scaphoid, or Preiser's disease, has also been reported. The radiographic findings resemble those of Kienbock's disease.

MR imaging shows initial decreased signal on T1 and increased signal on T2 weighted or STIR sequences images reflecting edema (Figs 117A and B). Later on decreased signal or signal void on T1 and T2 weighted sequences are seen reflecting bone death or sclerosis.

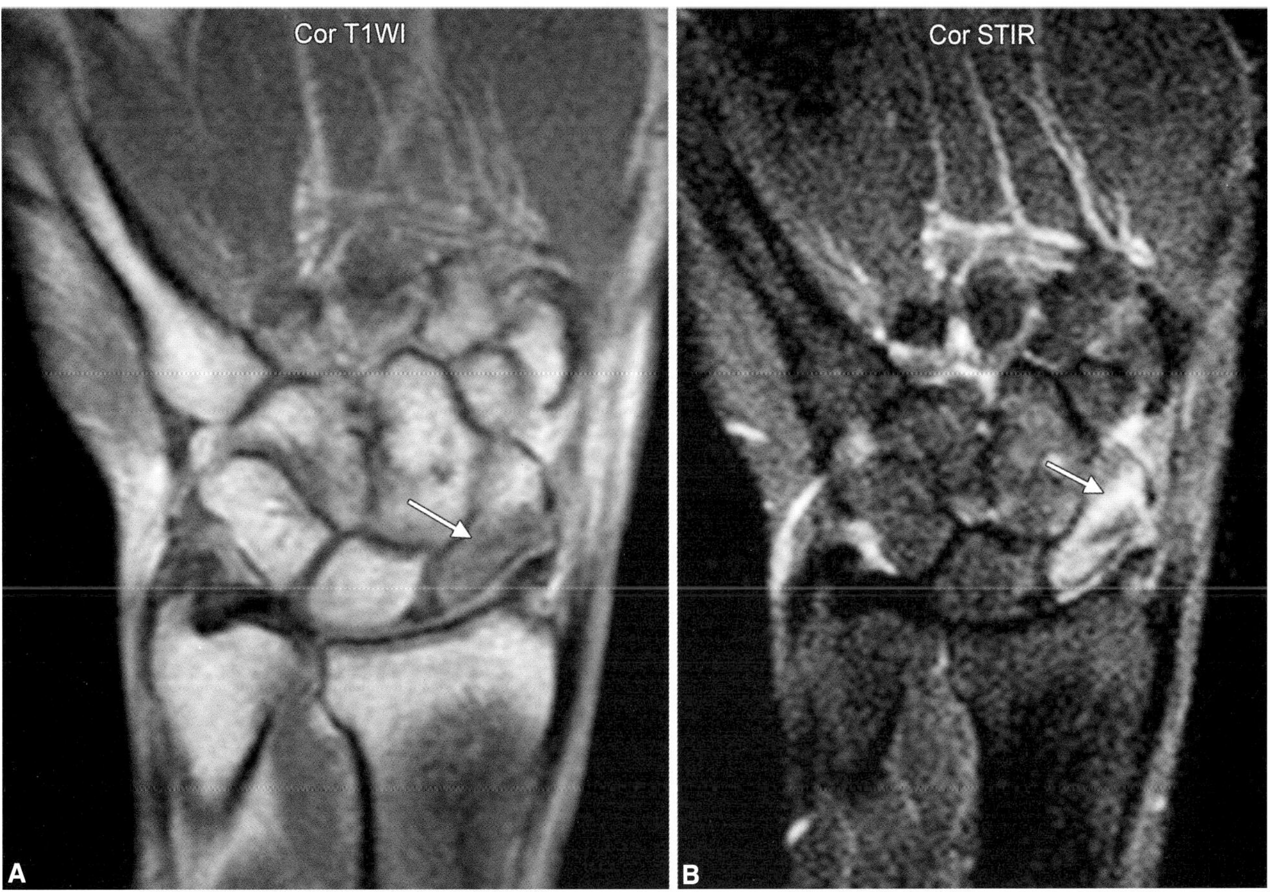

Figs 117A and B: Coronal T1W image (A) reveals hypointense signal in the scaphoid appearing hyperintense on coronal STIR (B) image features consistent with marrow edema

Bone Infarct

Bone infarct refers to a necrotic focus in the metaphyseal or diaphyseal regions, whereas osteonecrosis indicates the presence of ischemic cellular death of bone and bone marrow. Ischemic necrosis generally applies to areas of epiphyseal or subarticular involvement. Bone infarcts can be subdivided into four zones: (1) Central zone of cell death; (2) Zone of ischemic injury; (3) Zone of active hyperemia, and (4) Normal tissue.

In sickle cell anemia, diaphyseal infarction of larger tubular bones, the proximal aspect of the femur is common. Radiographically, bone infarction appears initially as a linear radiodense shadow adjacent to the cortex, which may extend along the entire shaft or may show no abnormality related to infarct (Fig. 118). Subsequently, the cortex becomes thickened. A bone within bone appearance is seen, which is diagnostic of osteonecrosis, is seen beneath the cortical bone. Other bones that may be infarcted include those of the pelvis, spine and thorax. Increased radiodensity of bone and a coarsened trabecular pattern are typical. In addition, epiphyseal infarcts in sickle cell anemia may involve the capital femoral epiphysis, leading to an appearance simulating that of Legg-Calvé-Perthes disease. Focal lucency and sclerosis, subchondral linear or curvilinear radiolucent shadows, collapse, and fragmentation are evident in involved epiphyses.

MR imaging is a very sensitive method for the early diagnosis of ischemic necrosis of bone (Figs 119A and B). It appears to be more sensitive in this regard than standard bone scintigraphy.

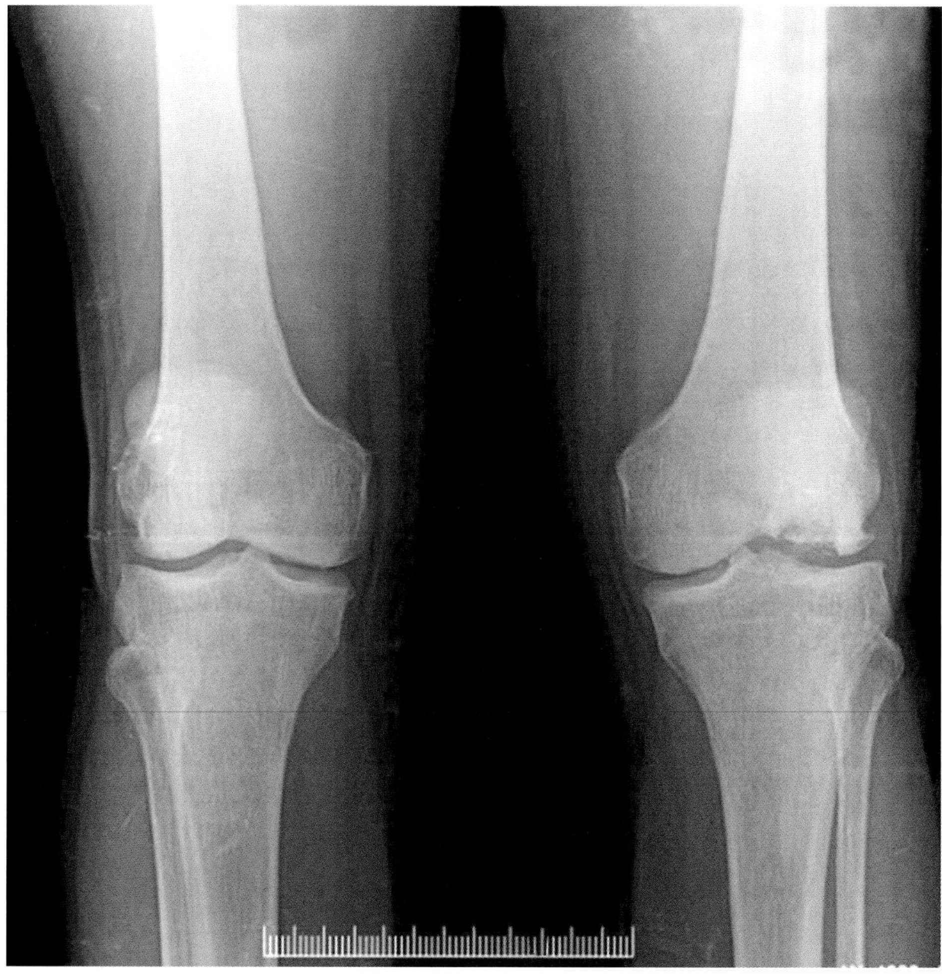

Fig. 118: X-ray both knee AP view shows fracture of the articular surface of lateral femoral condyle

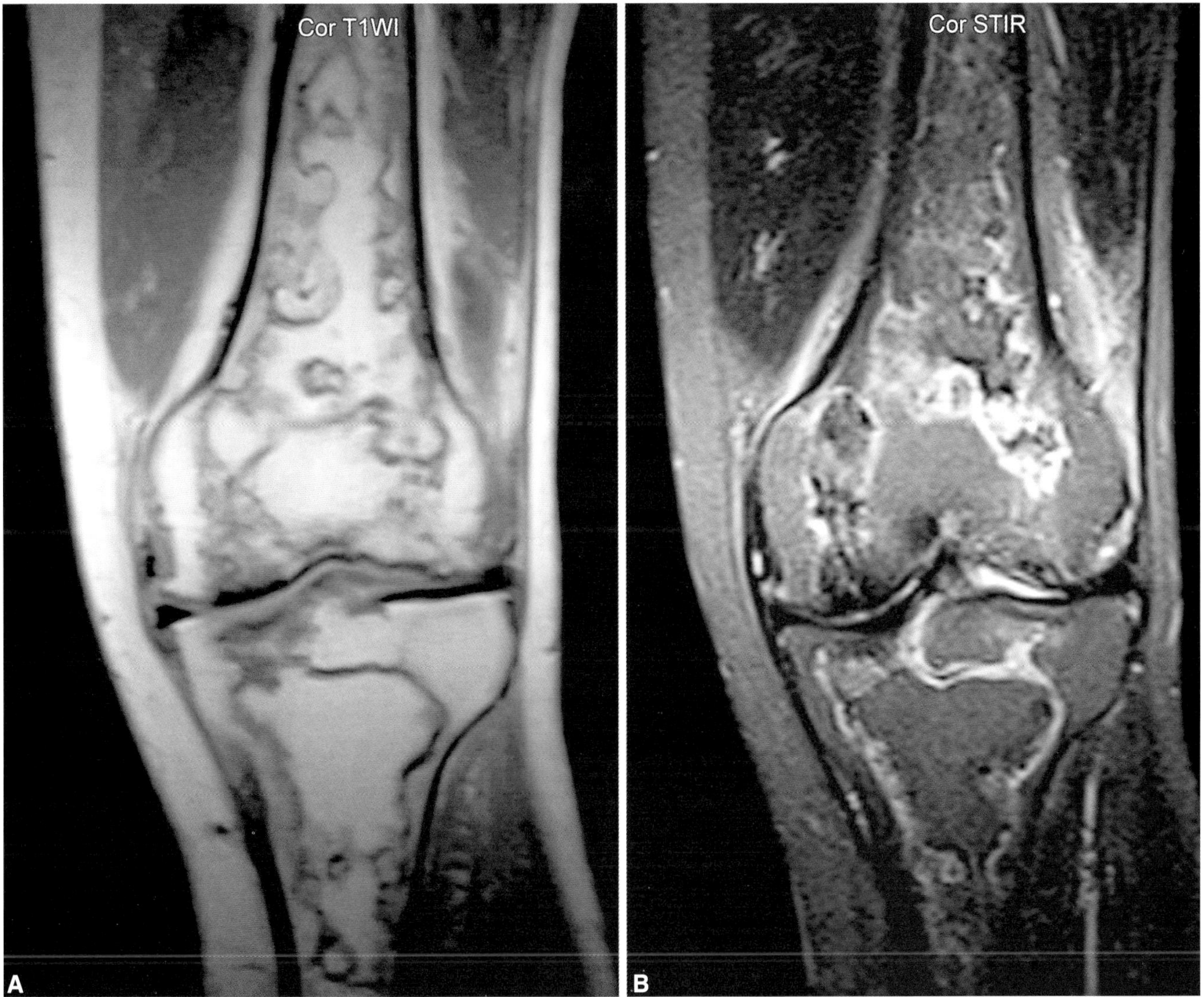

Figs 119A and B: T1W image (A) STIR images (B) Multiple geographic hyperintense lesions in the epiphysis, metaphysis and diaphysis of femur and tibia. The infarcts have sharply defined serpentine borders of low signal intensity on T1W images. Subchondral fracture in the lateral femoral condyle is seen

Fibrous Dysplasia

Fibrous dysplasia is an uncommon, benign disorder characterized by a tumor-like proliferation of fibro-osseous tissue. The cause of fibrous dysplasia is unknown. Fibrous dysplasia is usually found in the proximal femur, tibia, humerus, ribs, and craniofacial bones in decreasing order of incidence. Usually, only one bone is involved (monostotic fibrous dysplasia). Less often, multiple bones are involved (polyostotic fibrous dysplasia). The polyostotic form is generally more severe and is discovered earlier. This form can involve as few as two bones in the same limb or multiple bones throughout the skeleton. Males and females are equally affected by the disorder. Cases are usually diagnosed within the first three decades of life. It is usually asymptomatic, though pain and swelling may accompany the lesion.

Polyostotic fibrous dysplasia is known to have multiple associations with other disorders. The combination of polyostotic fibrous dysplasia, precocious puberty, and café-au-lait spots is called McCune Albright's syndrome. The association of fibrous dysplasia and soft tissue tumors has been given the name Mazabraud's syndrome. Other endocrine abnormalities including hyperthyroidism, Cushing's disease, thyromegaly, hypophosphatemia, and hyperprolactinemia have been associated with fibrous dysplasia.

Radiographically, fibrous dysplasia appears as a well circumscribed lesion in a long bone with a ground glass or hazy appearance of the matrix. There is a narrow zone of transition and no periosteal reaction or soft tissue mass. The lesions are normally located in the metaphysis or diaphysis with occasional focal thinning of the overlying cortex due to scalloping from within. The radiological appearance can also be cystic, pagetoid, or dense and sclerotic. Repeated fractures through lesions in the proximal femur can result in the formation of a shepherd's crook deformity. MRI scans or CT scans can be helpful in delineating the extent of the lesion (Figs 120A to I) and identifying possible pathological fractures and also sarcomatous change within the lesion.

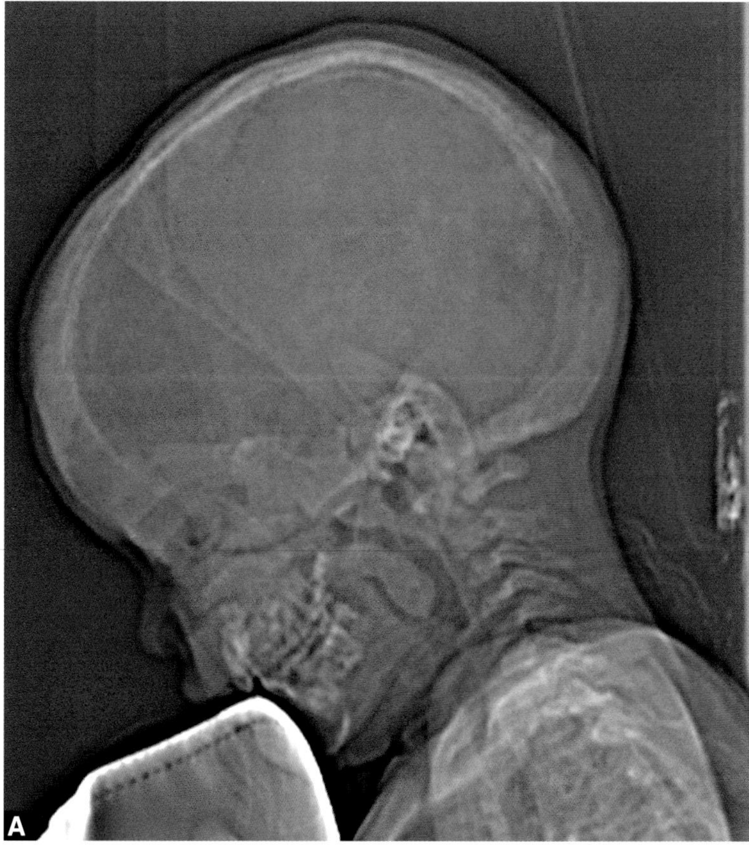

Fig. 120A: CT topogram reveals diffuse thickening of calvarium

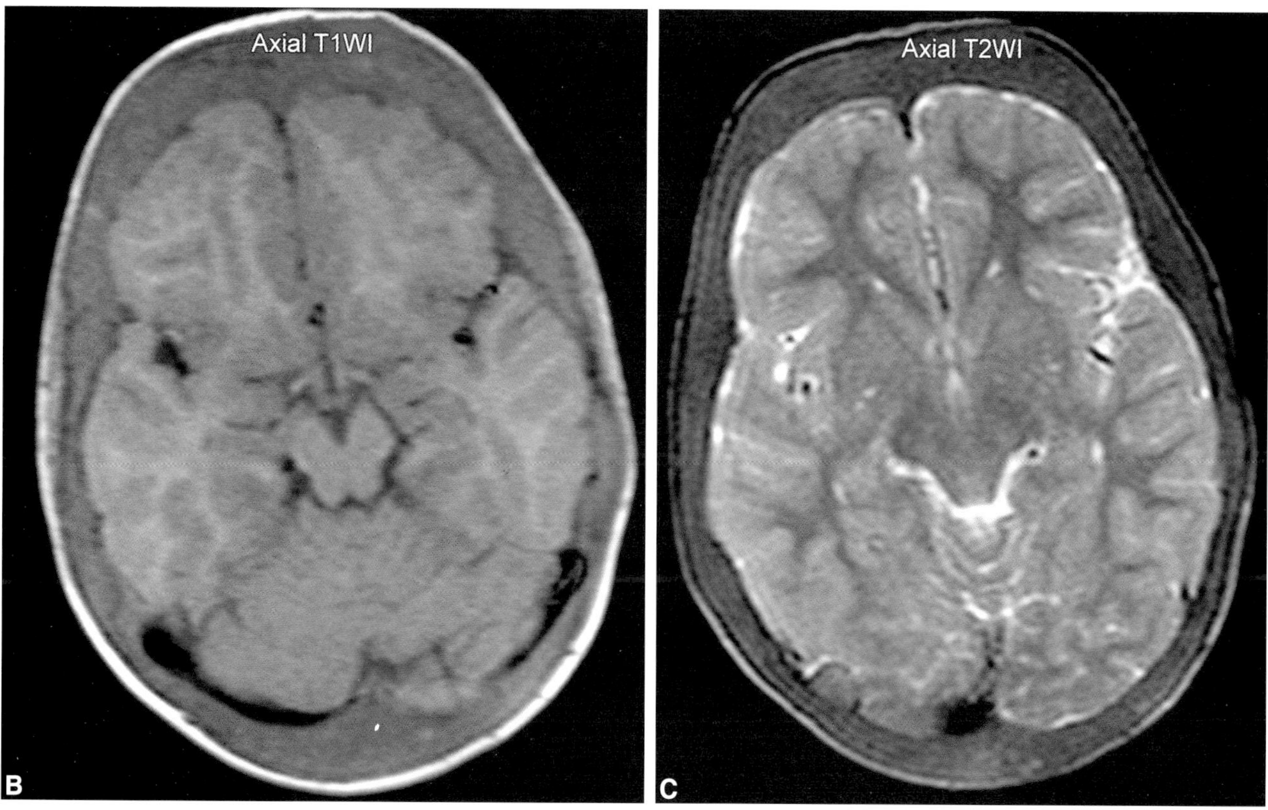

Figs 120B and C: Axial T1 (B) T2 (C) weighted images reveals diffuse calvarial thickening

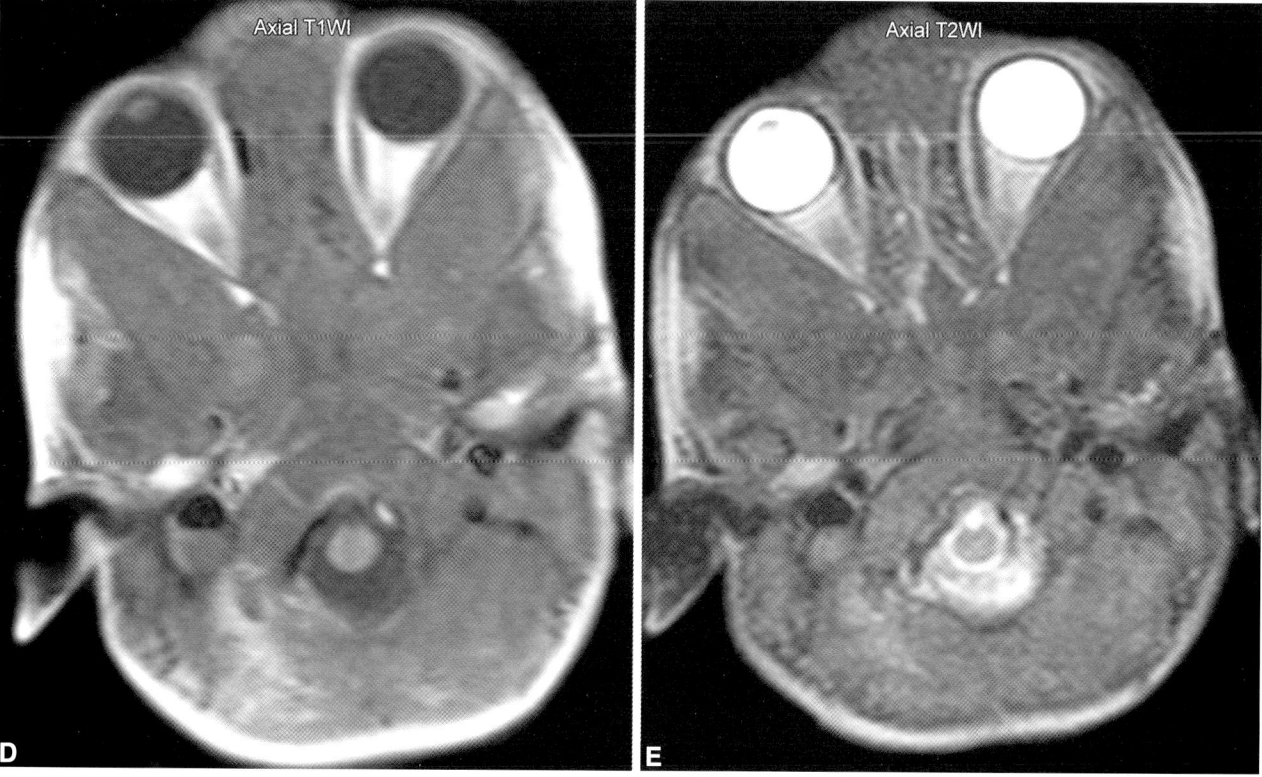

Figs 120D and E: Axial T1 (D) T2 (E) weighted images reveals diffuse thickening of calvarium and skull base

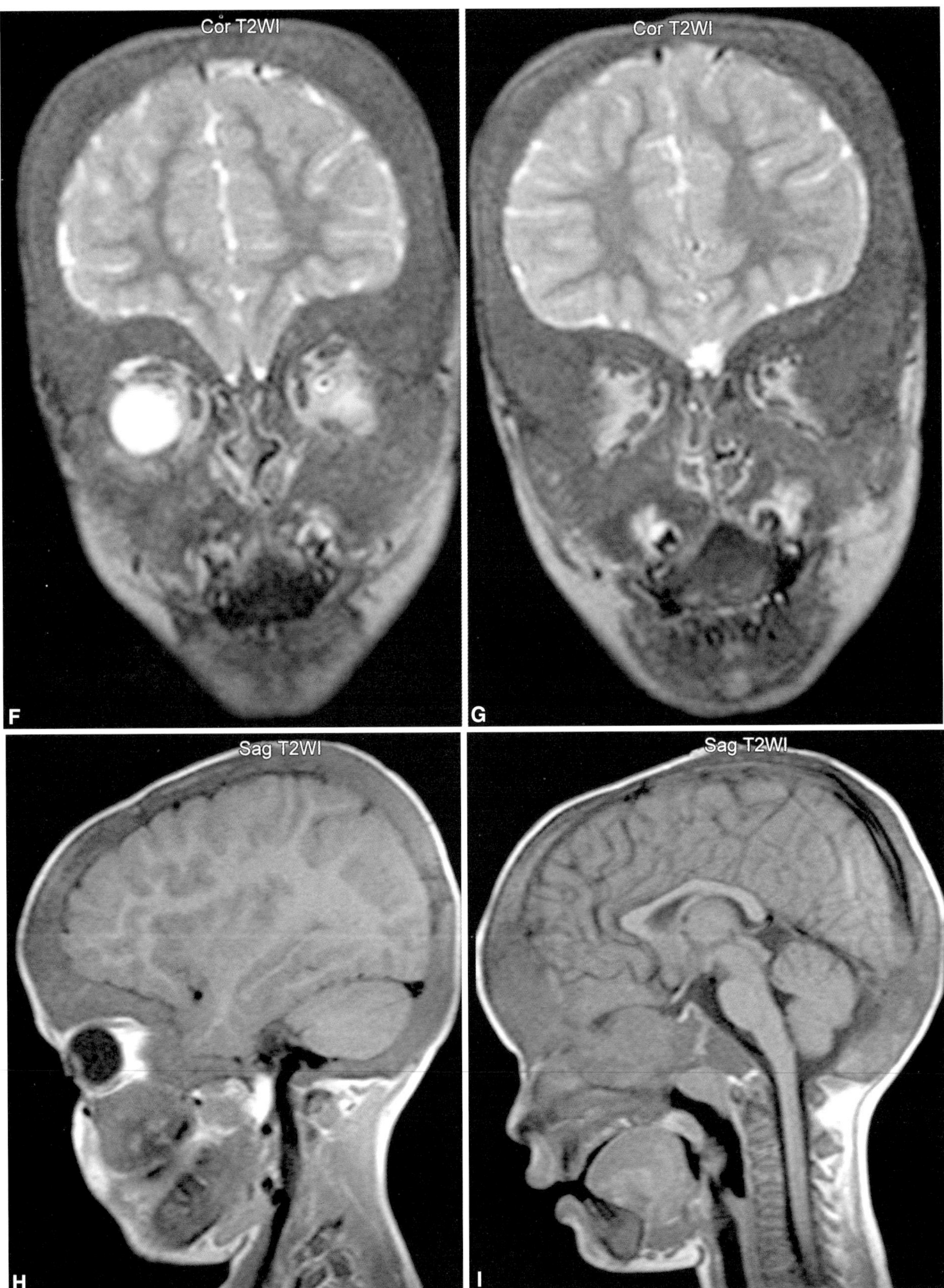

Figs 120F to I: Coronal T2 (F and G) Sagittal T1 (H and I) weighted images reveals diffuse thickening of calvarium, skull base and maxillofacial bones

Chondroblastoma

These rare cartilaginous tumor occurring in bone and seen in age range of 5 to 25 years. The tumor almost always arises in an epiphysis or apophysis but may extend into the joint or into the metaphysis, especially after skeletal maturity. Typical sites include the femur, humerus or tibia with approximately 50 percent occurring around the knee. Clinical presentation is usually with pain. There may be a joint effusion and reduced range of movement of the involved joint.

Radiographically the lesion appears as a well-defined eccentrically located intramedullary rounded lucency. The tumor shows a sclerotic margin, may expand and erode the cortex and often contains punctate calcification within the matrix. If the lesion extends into the metaphysis there may be associated periosteal new bone formation seen in the metaphyseal region. CT may better demonstrate the calcification within the lesion.

On MRI it shows low signal intensity on T1WI and variable signal intensity on T2WI. Surrounding marrow edema may be evident (Figs 121A to H).

Usually chondroblastomas are benign, but occasionally they exhibit a more aggressive course, invading soft tissues, adjacent bones and joint spaces. Metastases to the lung have been reported.

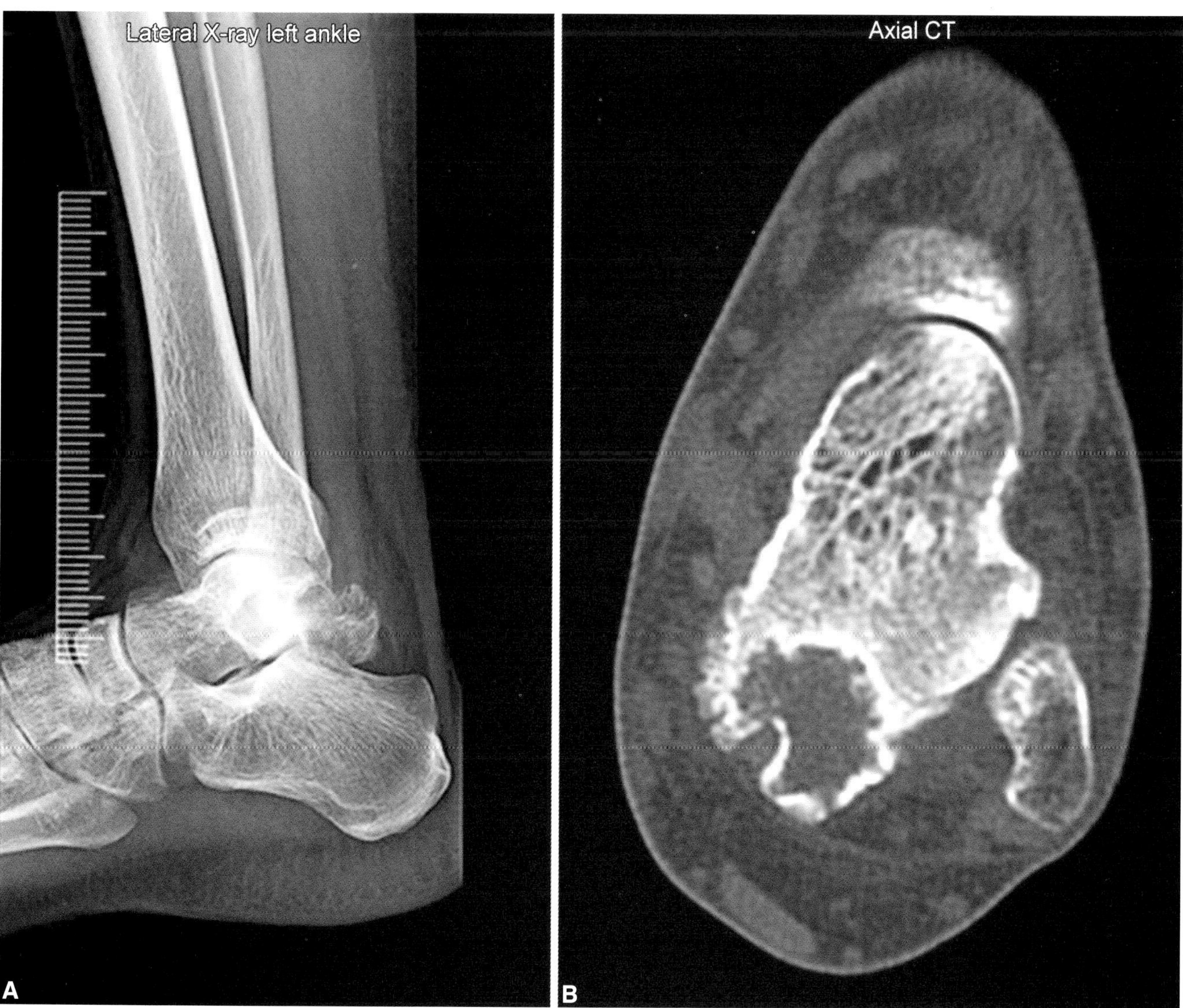

Figs 121A and B

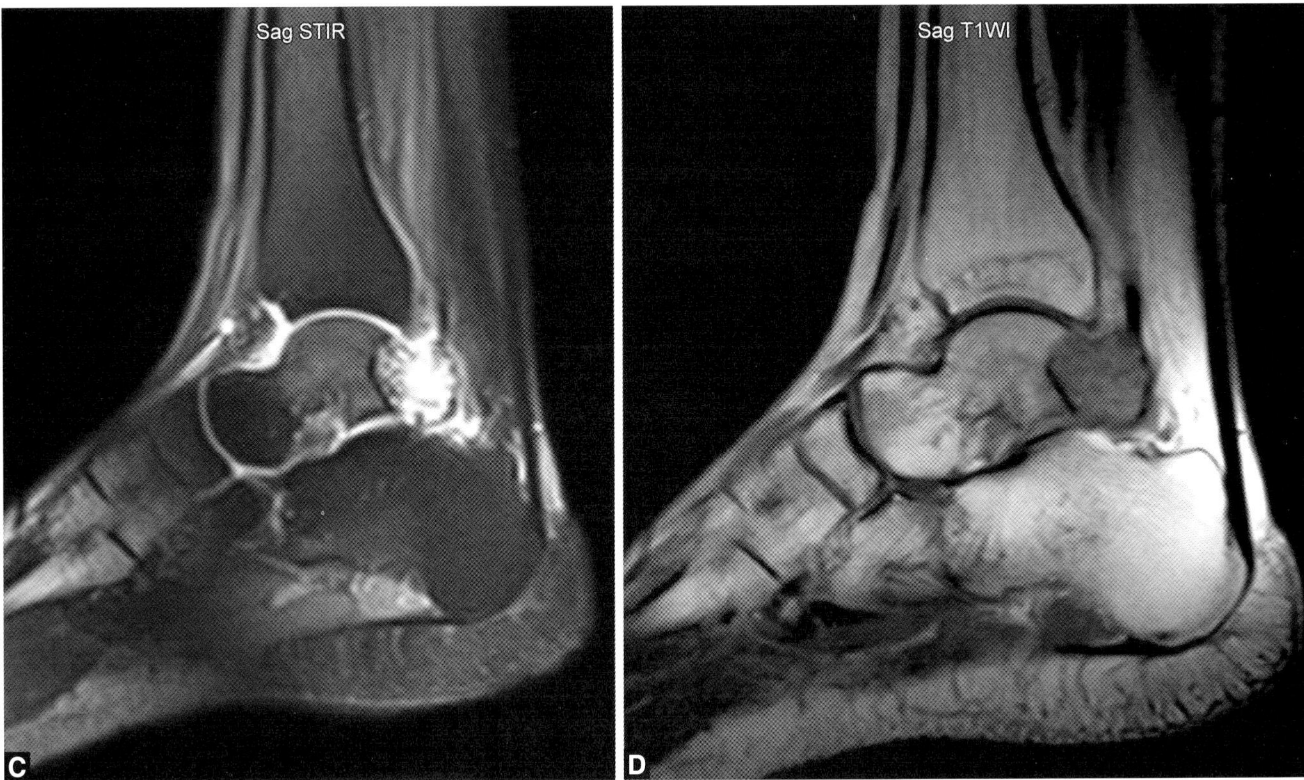

Figs 121C and D

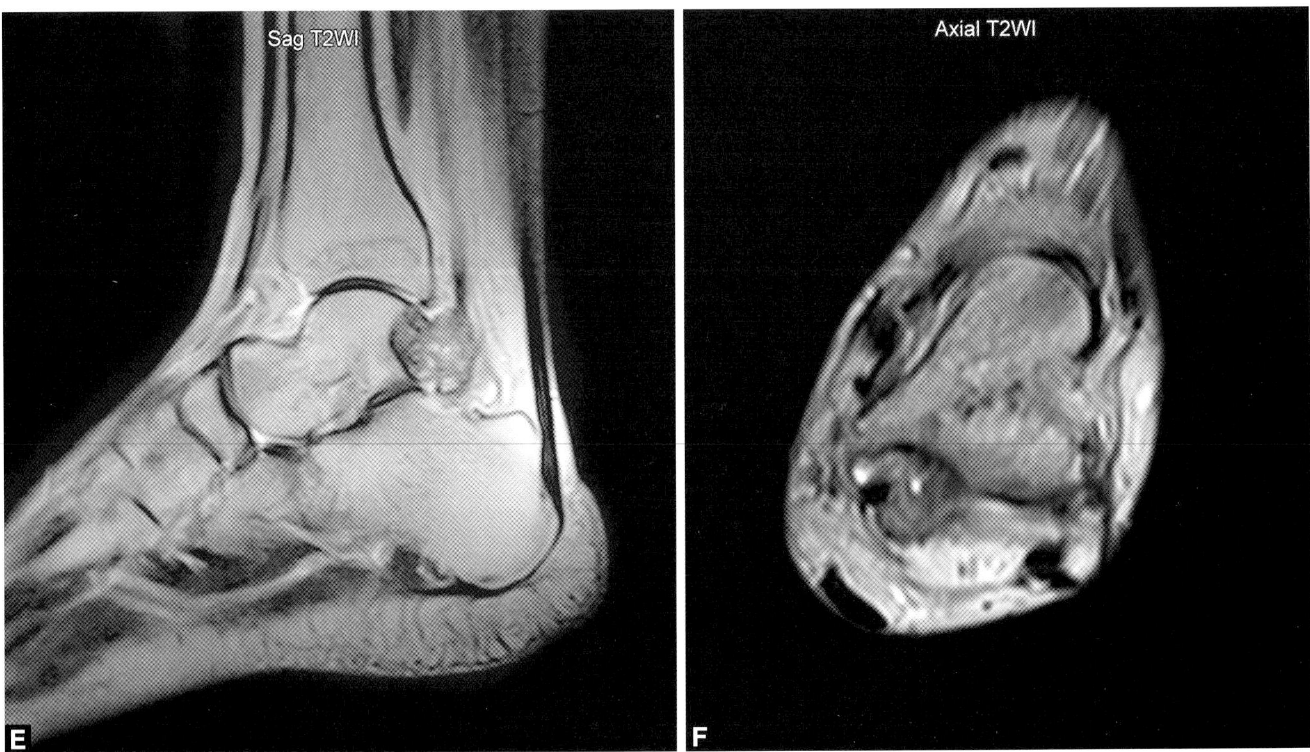

Figs 121E and F

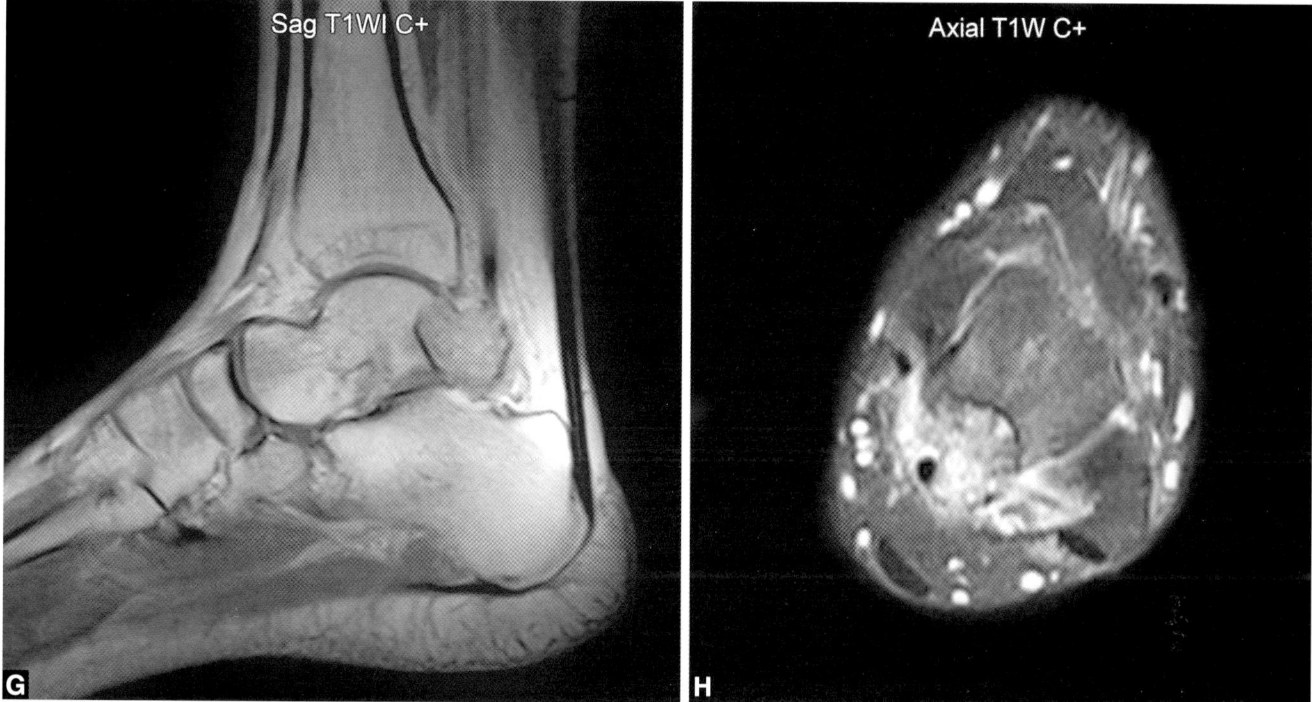

Figs 121G and H

Figs 121A to H: X-ray left ankle (A) in a 27-year-old male with hard swelling and pain in left ankle reveals a lytic lesion in posterior aspect of talus. Axial CT image (B) shows well-defined lytic lesion with sclerotic margin and cortical thinning. Sagittal STIR image (C) reveals well-defined lesion in posterior aspect of talus appearing hyperintense with associated mild marrow edema, it appears hypointense on T1WI (D). Sagittal (E) axial (F) T2W image reveals well-defined lesion in posterior aspect of talus appearing hyperintense with hypointense margin. Postcontrast T1W sagittal (G) and T1FS axial (H) images shows significant enhancement of the lesion

Adamantinoma

Adamantinoma is an extremely rare and locally aggressive or malignant lesion of bone composed of rows of epithelium-like cells in a dense fibrous stroma. Adamantinoma, fibrous dysplasia and ossifying fibroma share many radiographic and pathological features. Tibia is commonly involved. Other bones that may be involved are the humerus, ulna, femur, fibula and radius.

Adamantinoma is usually localized in the middle third of the tibia or other tubular bone. The lesion appears as a multilocular, slightly expansile, osteolytic lesion, with reactive bone sclerosis. Distinguishing adamantinoma from fibrous dysplasia and ossifying fibroma in the tibia may be very difficult. Fibrous dysplasia occurs in young persons and has a ground glass appearance radiographically. The radiographic features of adamantinoma and ossifying fibroma of the tibia are generally identical. On MRI these appear hypointense on T1 and hyperintense on STIR and T2WI (Figs 122A to D).

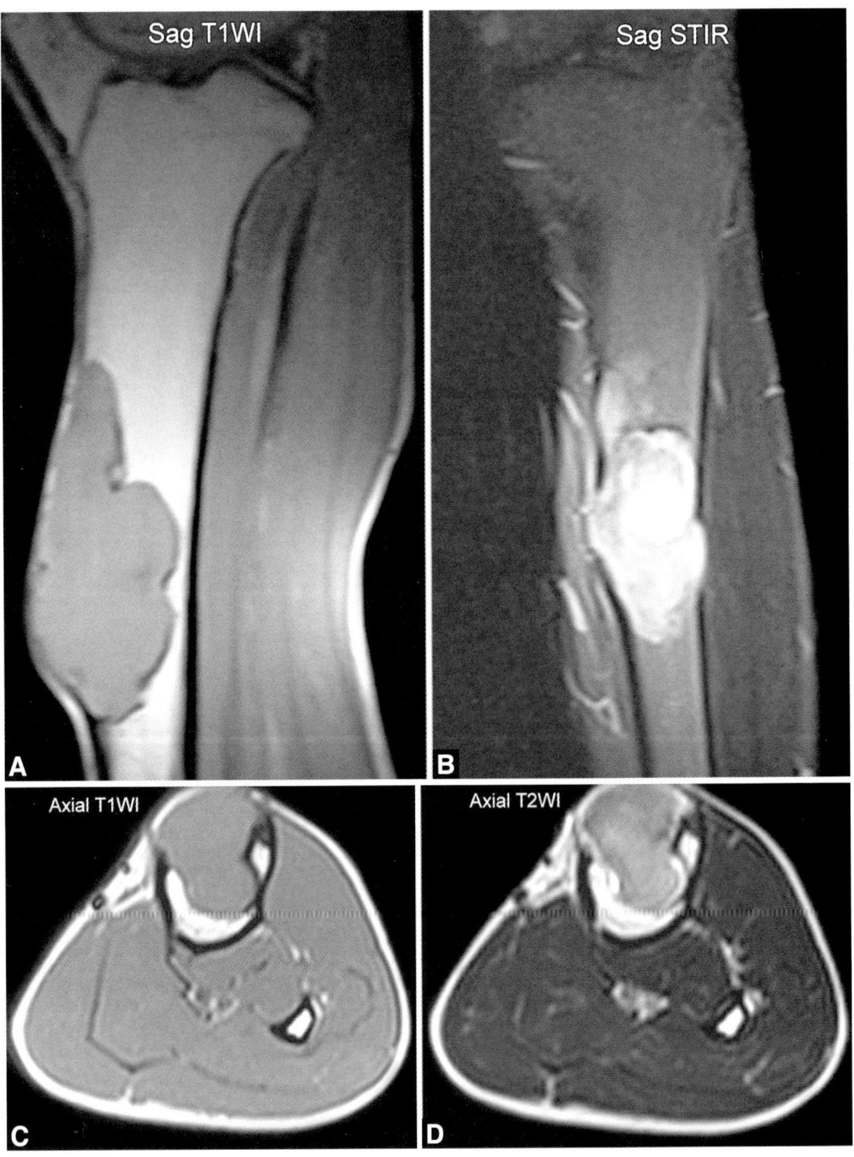

Figs 122A to D: In 21-year-old male with pain and swelling left leg, on MR shows a lobulated, expansile, well-defined soft tissue lesion seen in diaphyseal region of tibia. It appears hypointense on T1WI (A and C) and hyperintense on STIR and T2WI (B and D)

Osteosarcoma

Osteosarcomas is a malignant neoplasm of bone composed of proliferating tumor cells that in most instances produce osteoid or immature bone. Osteosarcomas can be classified according to location of the tumor within the bone (intramedullary, intracortical, surface, periosteal, or parosteal); degree of cellular differentiation (high or low grade); histologic composition, number of foci of involvement (single or multicentric); and status of the underlying bone.

Osteosarcomas generally involve the long tubular bones about the knee. A metaphyseal location predominates. The bone involvement shows a mixed pattern consisting of both osteolysis and osteosclerosis. Osteosarcomas in the tubular bones are usually evident as poorly defined intramedullary metaphyseal lesions that extend through the cortex and produce a sizeable soft tissue component. A periosteal reaction (Codmans triangle or sunburst pattern) and sometimes a pathologic fracture are additional features. In other skeletal sites the radiographic features of osteosarcoma are similar.

MR imaging is superior to CT scanning in defining the intraosseous and extraosseous extent of the tumor. On T1-weighted spin-echo images the tumor is typically of low signal intensity, whereas on T2-weighted images it is usually of high signal intensity (Figs 123A to C).

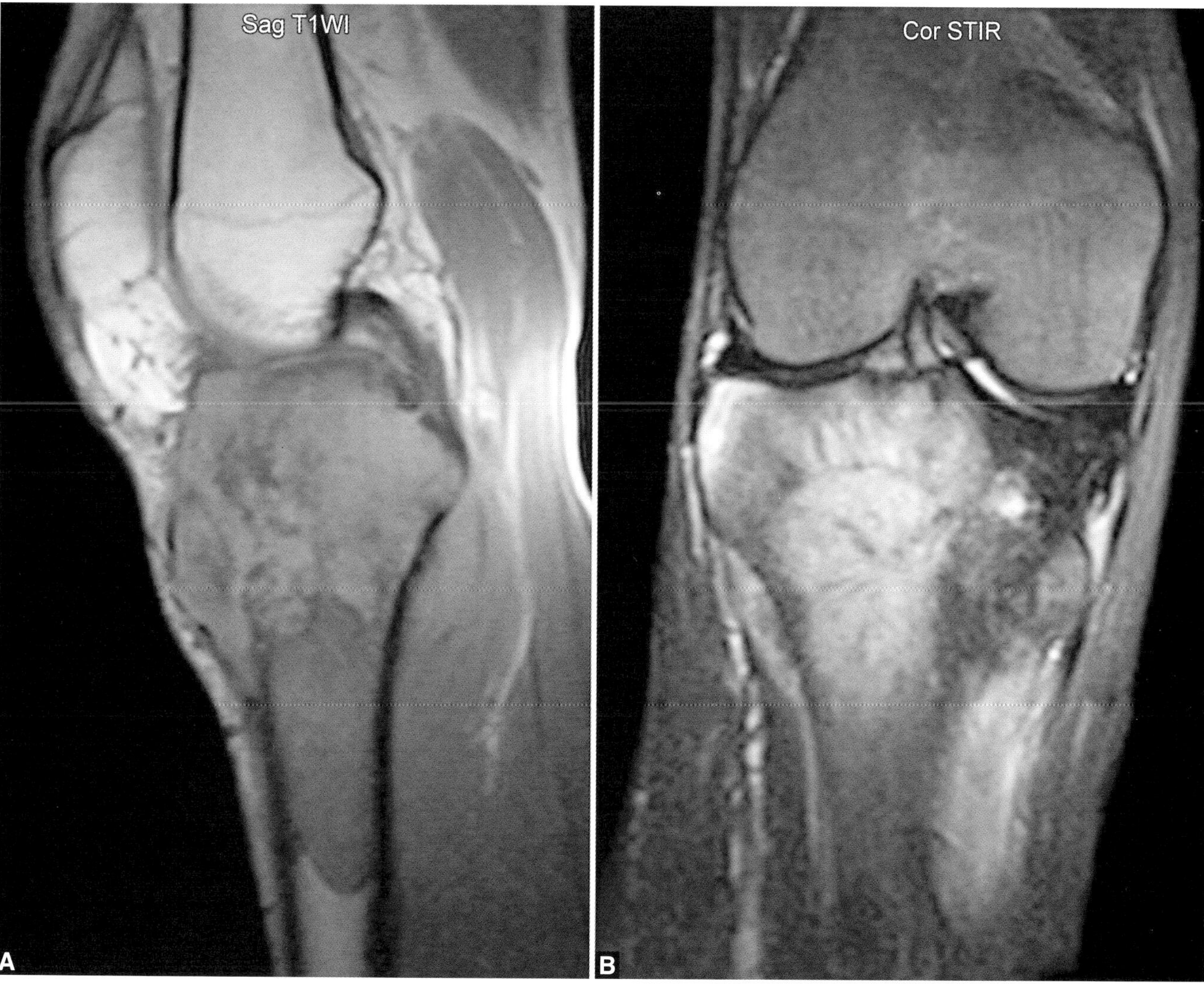

Figs 123A and B

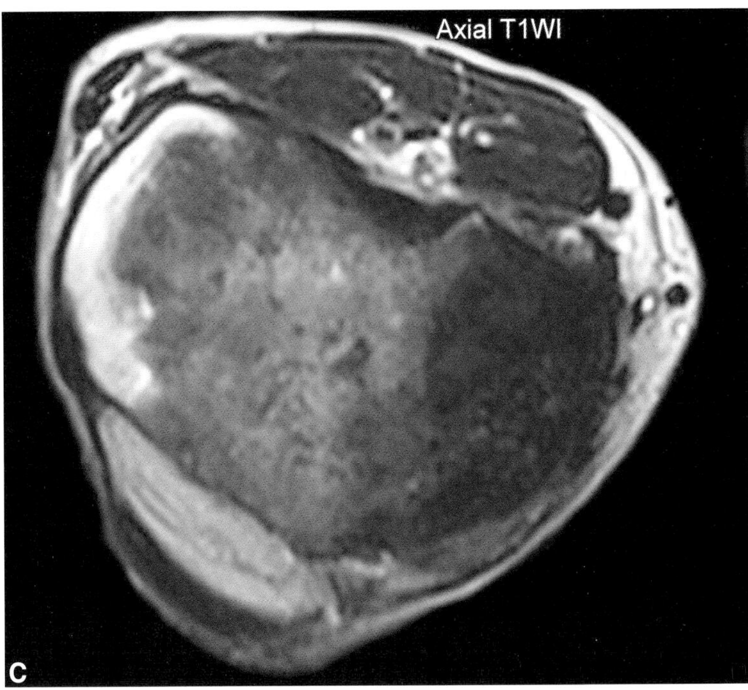

Figs 123A to C: Sagittal T1W (A) Heterogeneous signal intensity lesion appearing predominantly hypointense in proximal tibial epimetaphysis and hyperintense on STIR coronal images; (B) Axial T1W image; (C) Heterogeneous signal intensity lesion appearing predominantly hypointense

Sacrococcygeal Teratoma

A teratoma is a germ cell tumor, 40 percent of which are found in the sacrococcygeal region. A mature teratoma is benign, but on imaging it is impossible to exclude malignant components. In the neonate histological malignancy is present in up to 30 percent. The malignant component is usually due to embryonal carcinoma, yolk sac carcinoma or choriocarcinoma. Though histologically malignant, if the tumor is completely excised the prognosis is good. If elements are left behind, or the diagnosis is delayed, the incidence of malignancy increases. Elevated alpha fetoprotein levels can indicate malignancy but unfortunately in the neonatal period this is normally high and does not fall to normal levels until 9 months of age.

A sacrococcygeal tumor in the neonate usually presents as an external mass and where there is a presacral component the infant may also have urinary frequency or retention, or constipation. These are the symptoms in children who present later. Any intra-abdominal extent of disease renders the lesion more likely to be malignant.

The plain film will usually show a rounded mass extending externally in the buttock region. Calcification may be present and there are sometimes formed structures such as bone or occasionally teeth in solid lesions. The spectrum varies from being completely solid through mixed solid and cystic lesions to an almost completely cystic mass.

Full evaluation is best performed by MRI (Figs 124A and B). If there is invasion of the soft tissues or bone it implies malignancy, but the majority of the teratomas do not show this feature and the diagnosis has to be made by histology.

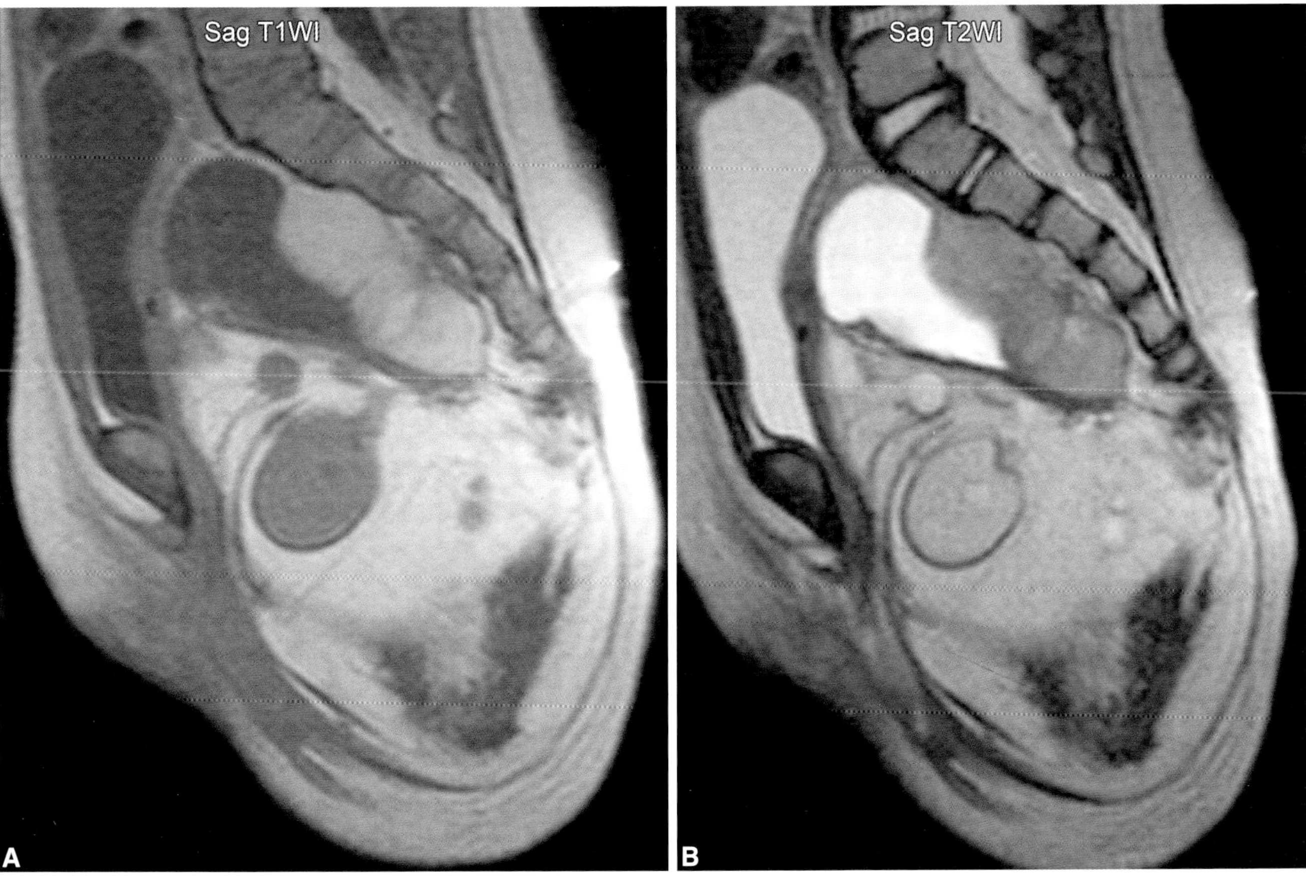

Figs 124A and B: In 1-year-female having buttock swelling since birth, and finds difficulty to walk on MR shows a large well-defined heterogeneous lesion in the pelvis posterior to the bladder. It is predominantly fatty with cystic and soft tissue component. Superiorly it extends upto the pelvic inlet, inferiorly into the right ischiorectal fossa and laterally extends upto the lateral pelvic wall. The coccygeal vertebrae reveal altered marrow signal with no intraspinal extension of the mass

SOFT TISSUE

Subcutaneous Lipoma

Lipoma, a benign tumor composed of mature fat cells, which may occur in any tissue that contains fat. Lipomas of soft tissue are seen more commonly in the subcutaneous tissues of the back, extremities and thorax. Lipomas are the most common soft-tissue tumor. Lipomas are slow growing, benign fatty tumors. They form soft, lobulated masses enclosed by a thin, fibrous capsule. Lipomas may rarely undergo sarcomatous change.

On MRI the lipomas show signal intensity characteristics similar to subcutaneous fat; hyperintense on T1-weighted images and moderately hyperintense on T2-weighted images. Fat suppression techniques are extremely useful in differentiating them from other soft tissue tumors (Figs 125A to D).

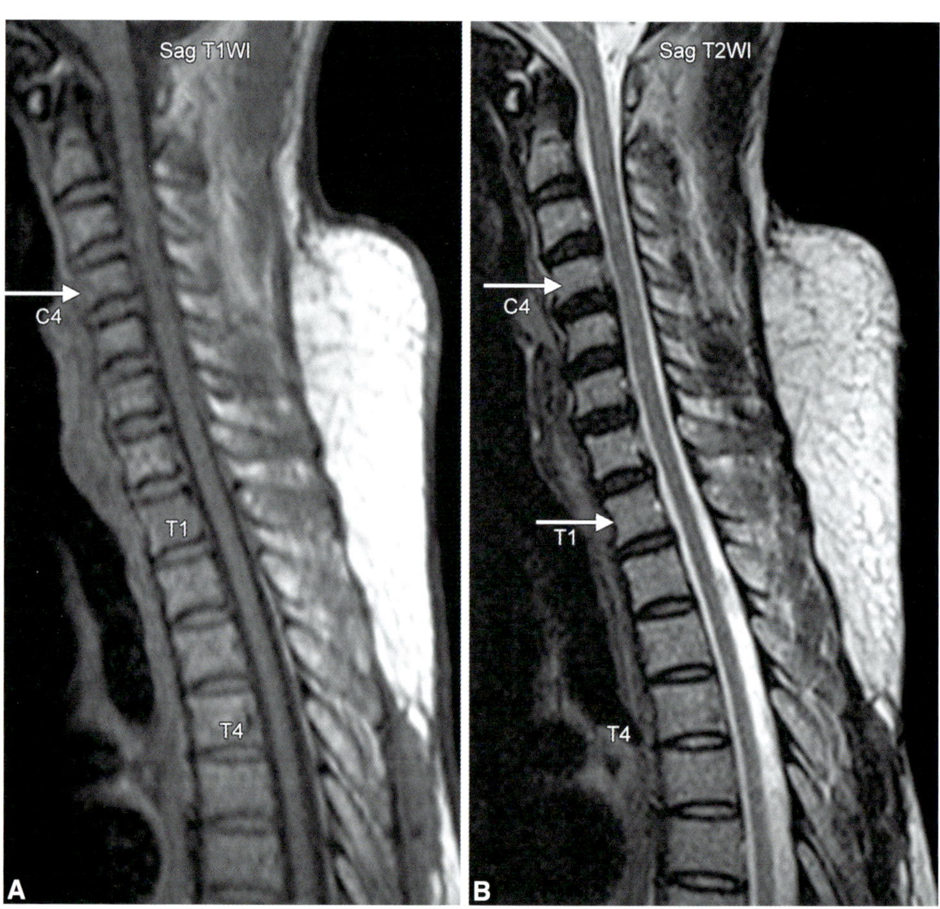

Figs 125A and B

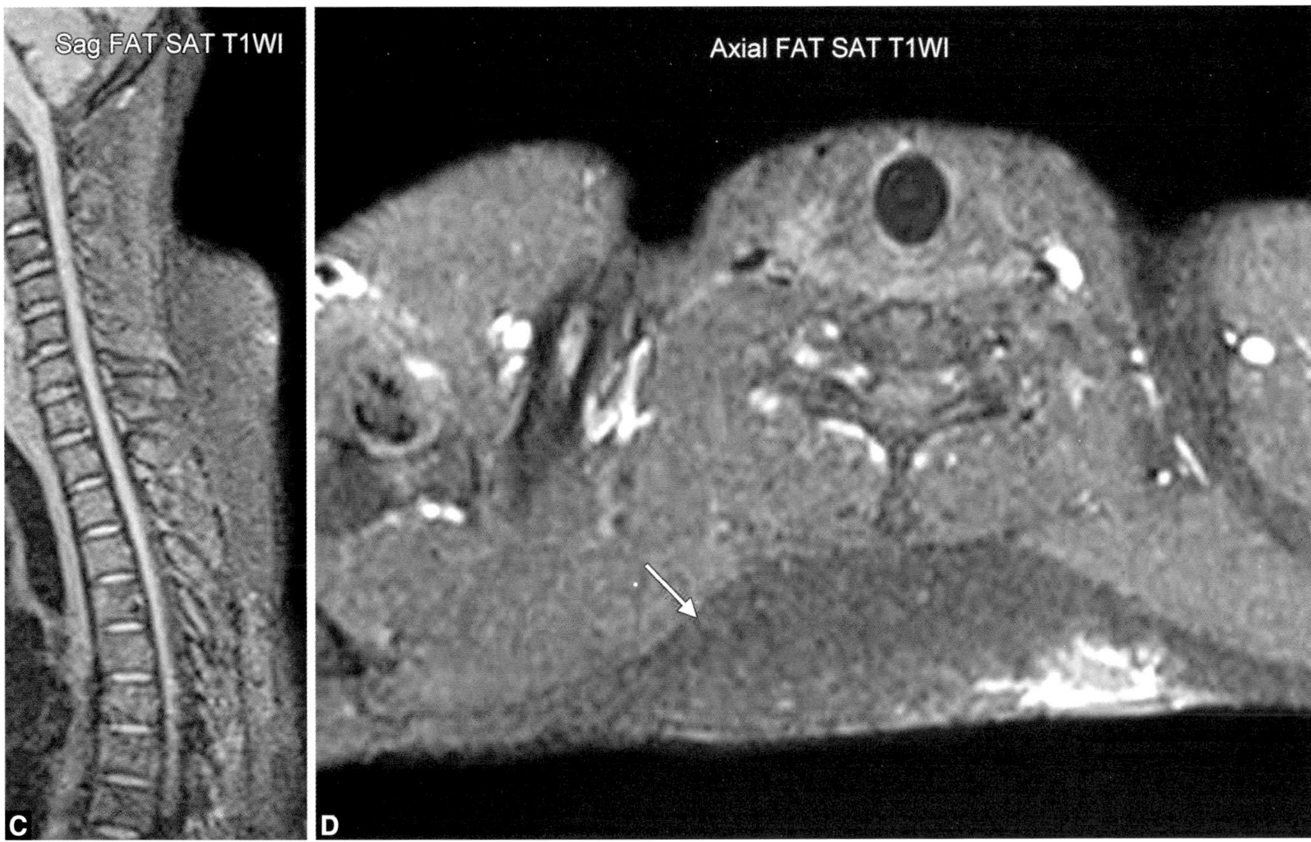

Figs 125C and D

Figs 125A to D: A large well-defined subcutaneous hyperintense lesion is seen on T1W and T2W images (A and B) in the posterior midline cervicodorsal region (14.2 x 3.8 x 8.7 cm). It gets suppressed on fat sat T1W images (C and D). Fat planes between the muscles and this lesion are well-maintained with no evidence of deep extension

Macrodystrophia Lipomatosa

Macrodystrophia lipomatosa is a congenital local gigantism of the hand and foot, characterized by proliferation of all mesenchymal components, particularly fibroadipose tissue (Figs 126 and 127). Macrodystrophia lipomatosa comes to clinical attention because of cosmetic reasons, mechanical problems secondary to degenerative joint disease or development of neurovascular compression.

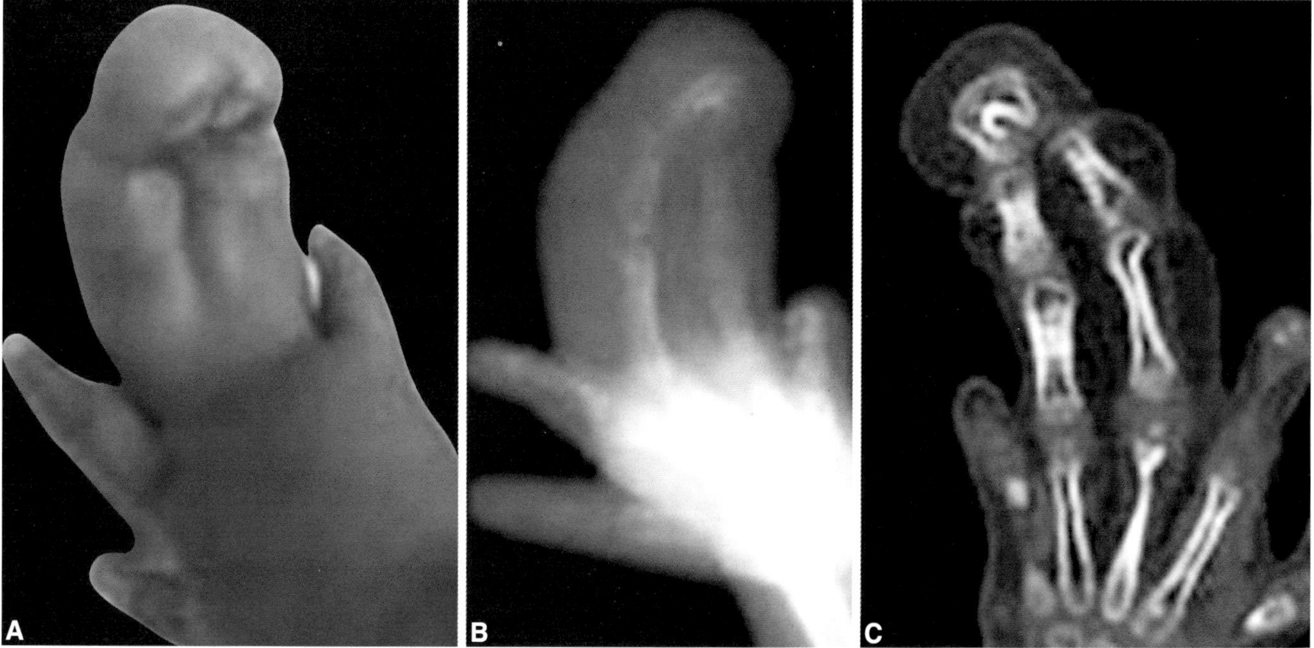

Figs 126A to C: (A) Clinical photograph of right hand shows enlarged, fused ring and middle finger; (B) Plain radiograph; (C) Coronal reformatted CT shows soft tissue swelling and proliferation of fat on palmar aspect of the ring and middle fingers, along with dorsal angulation and syndactyly

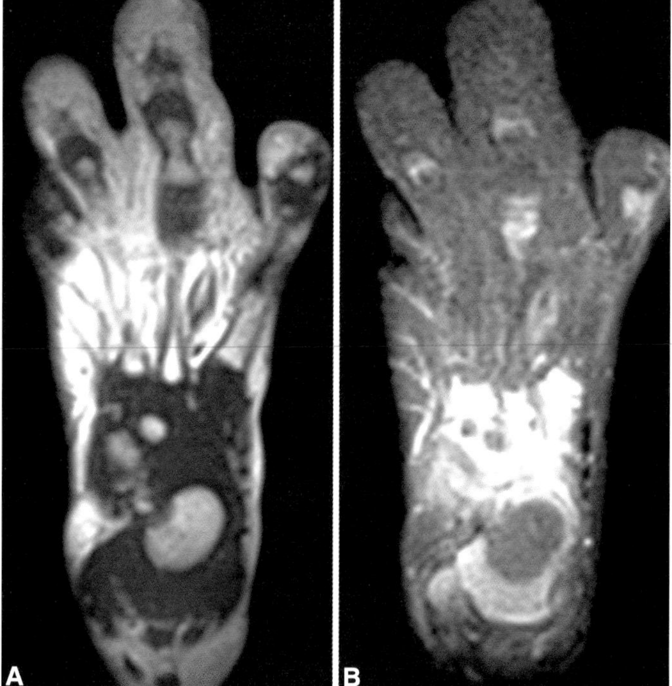

Figs 127A and B: T1 coronal MRI (A) reveals proliferation of fatty tissue on plantar aspect of the second and third toes of right foot with signal intensity similar to that of subcutaneous fat as seen by fat suppressed STIR coronal image (B)

Fibrolipomatous Hamartoma of Median Nerve

Fibrolipomatous hamartomas are benign tumors usually affecting infants and less commonly children and young adults. This uncommon lesion is also known as neural fibrolipoma, lipofibromatous hamartoma, perineural lipoma and intraneural lipoma. The median nerve is overwhelmingly the most commonly affected nerve (80% of cases), followed by the ulnar and radial nerves, and brachial plexus. The most common presentation is that of a soft, slowly enlarging and often asymptomatic mass on the volar wrist or forearm often present since infancy (Figs 128A and B). Occasionally nerve compression will lead to symptoms of pain, paresthesia or carpal tunnel syndrome. There is equal prevalence among males and females. Although the pathogenesis has not been definitively elucidated it is postulated that a congenital abnormality of growth of fibrofatty tissues causes infiltration of the endoneurium, perineurium and epineurium resulting in fusiform nerve enlargement.

CT and MRI imaging findings of fibromatous hamartomas show fusiform nerve enlargement which is caused by thickening of nerve bundles and fatty and fibrous proliferation (Figs 128C to G). Enlarged nerve bundles look like serpentine or tubular structures. The MRI characteristics of fibromatous hamartomas are pathognomonic presenting high signal intensity from fat on T1 and T2 weighted sequences (Figs 128E to G). which will drop out on fat suppressed images surrounding the bands of enlarged nerve fascicles.

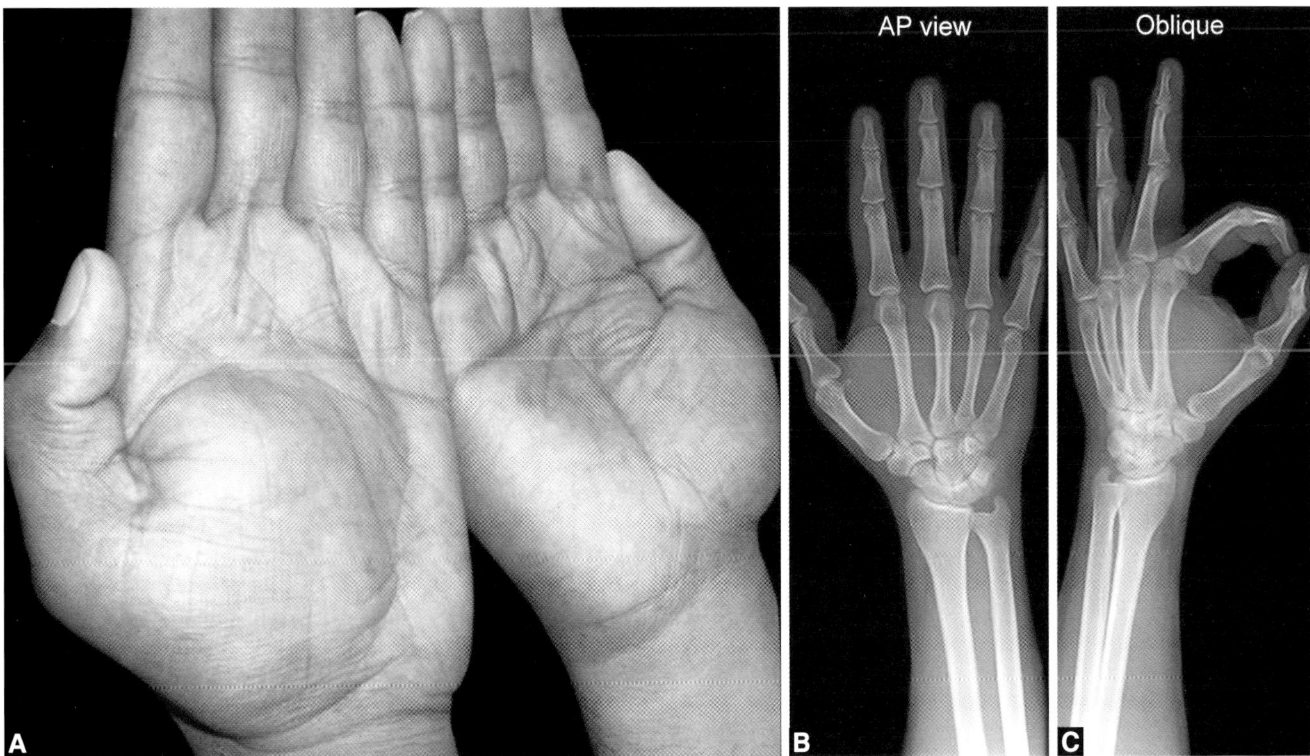

Figs 128A to C: 24-year-old male presented swelling of the left thenar eminence with pain on and off since 8 years, gradually increasing in size. Photograph of hands (A) X-ray AP and lateral views (B and C) of left hand shows soft tissue swelling in the region of thenar eminence *(For color version, see Plate 2)*

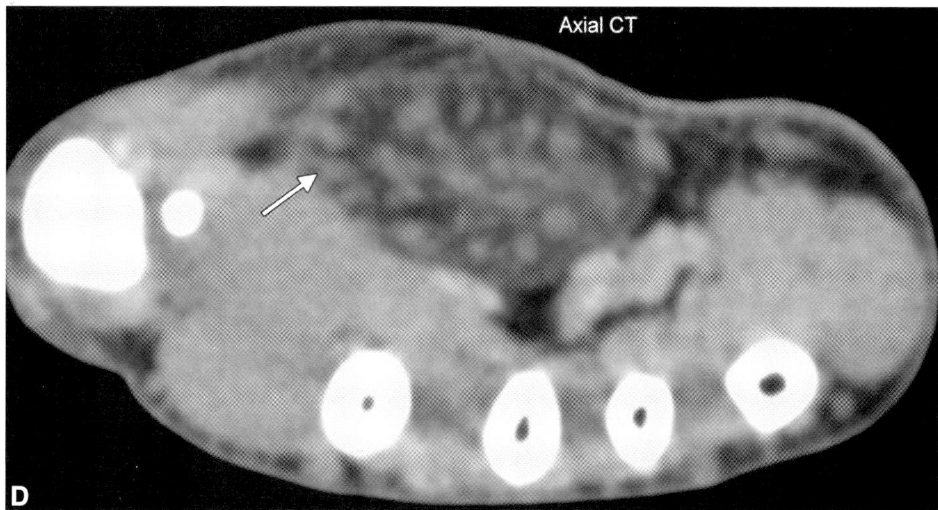

Fig. 128D: Axial CT section of hand shows a well-defined heterogeneous lesion seen in ventral aspect, anterior to the flexor tendons having fatty density within the lesion giving a polka dot appearance (arrow)

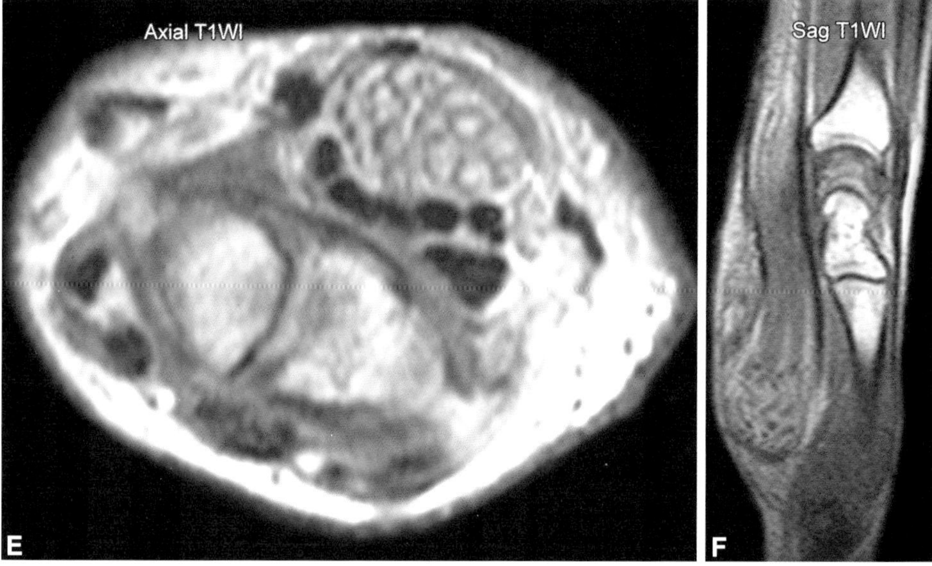

Figs 128E and F: Axial T1WI and SAG T1WI shows well-defined oval lesion on ventral aspect just distal to wrist appearing hyperintense on T1WI with flow voids within it

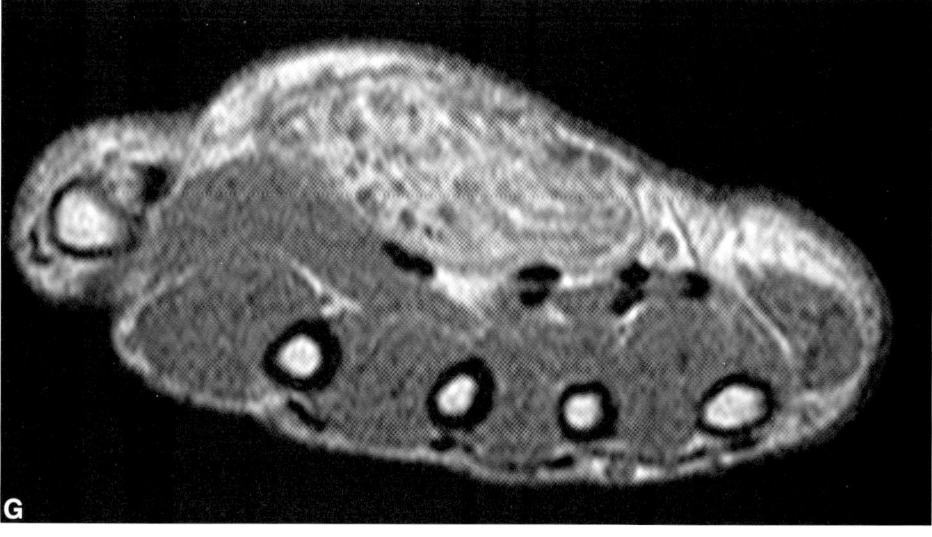

Fig. 128G: Shows fatty lesion with flow voids abutting the flexor tendons with polka dot appearance as seen in D because of enlarged median nerve with fat infiltration in between fascicles of median nerve

Liposarcoma

Liposarcoma is a malignant tumor that arises in fat cells in deep soft tissue, such as that inside the thigh or in the retroperitoneum. They are typically large bulky tumors which tend to have multiple smaller satellites extending beyond the main confines of the tumor.

Liposarcoma is a tumor derived from primitive cells that undergo adipose differentiation. It is largely a disease of adults, with peak incidence between 40 and 60 years of age, and it shows a slight predominance in men. When liposarcomas occur in the pediatric population, they tend to present in the second decade of life. In either event, the deep soft tissues of the extremities, particularly those of the thigh, are the most common location, accounting for more than 50 percent of liposarcomas. Its presentation in this location is most commonly that of a slow growing, painless mass. Often these tumors are first noticed following a minor trauma.

MRI is obtained, both with and without contrast enhancement. The MRI (Figs 129A to D) findings in liposarcoma can be quite distinct, and suggest the diagnosis even before biopsy report. This largely depends on how closely the tumor resembles normal fat and how well-differentiated it is.

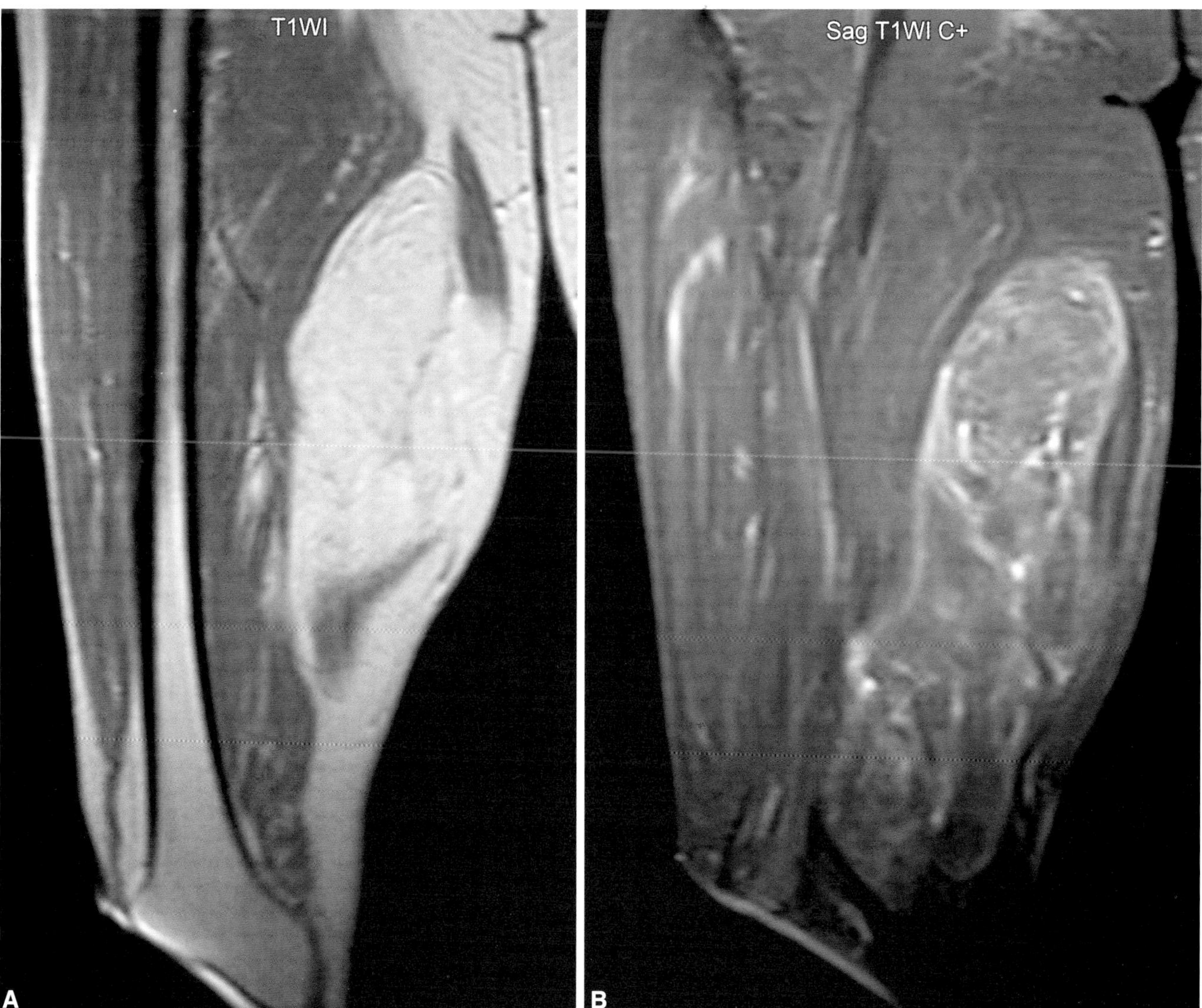

Figs 129A and B

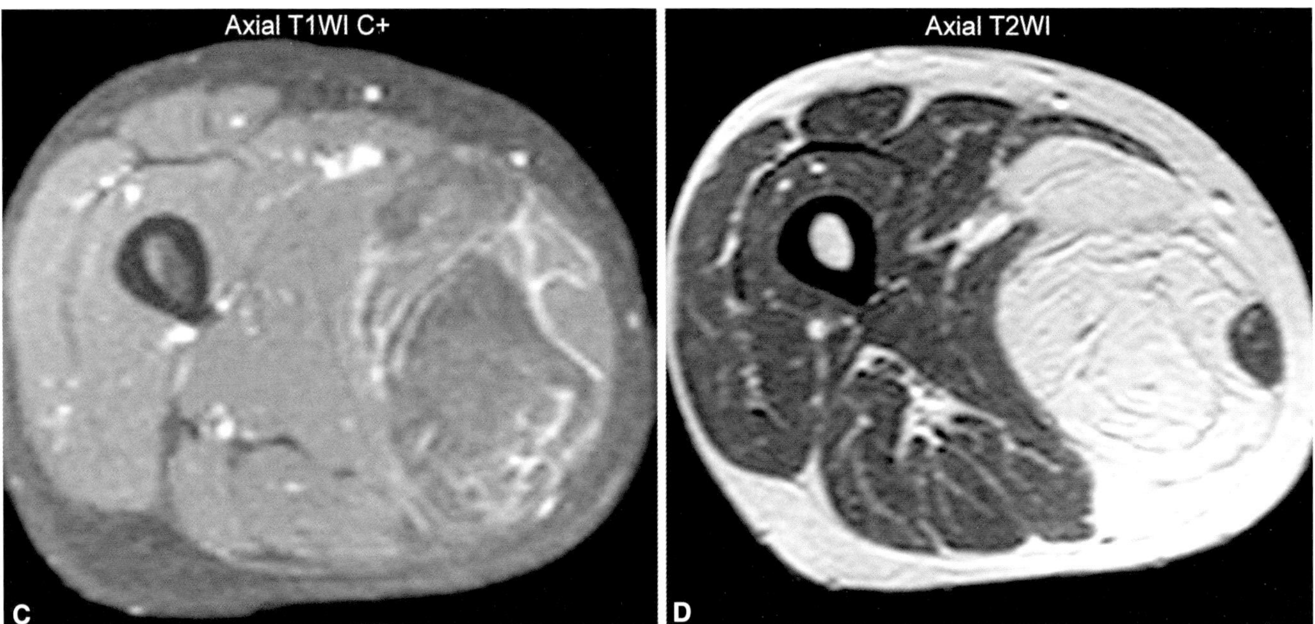

Figs 129C and D

Figs 129A to D: Large well-defined T1 hyperintense lesion is seen along the medial aspect of thigh between the adductor group muscles and the gracilis muscle on T1WI (A) T2WI (D) Multiple septae are seen within it. No evidence of fluid component or calcification. Postcontrast images (B and C) Shows mild patchy and septal enhancement

Neurogenic Tumors

Neurogenic tumors are relatively common and account for approximately 12 percent of all benign and 7 to 8 percent of all malignant soft tissue neoplasms. These characteristic imaging findings include a specific clinical presentation or location, relationship to a nerve, and certain lesion shape and signal intensity patterns. Schwannoma (neurilemmoma, neurinoma) is a slow-growing neurogenic tumor that is believed to arise from the Schwann cells of a peripheral nerve. Therefore, the lesion usually develops eccentrically to the nerve fibers and is encapsulated by the perineurium. Schwannoma most frequently affects patients 20 to 50 years of age and accounts for approximately 5 percent of all benign soft tissue neoplasms. Men and women are affected equally. Although the head and neck, the flexor surfaces of the extremities (particularly the ulnar and peroneal nerves), and the mediastinum and retroperitoneum represent the most common sites of involvement, schwannomas can occur almost anywhere. Pain and neurologic symptoms are uncommon unless the lesion is large. Long-standing tumors that are relatively large can undergo degenerative changes such as cyst formation, calcification, hemorrhage, and fibrosis.

STIR and T2W images (Figs 130A to C) show fusiform hyperintense mass in continuity with the neurovascular bundle, a finding that is virtually

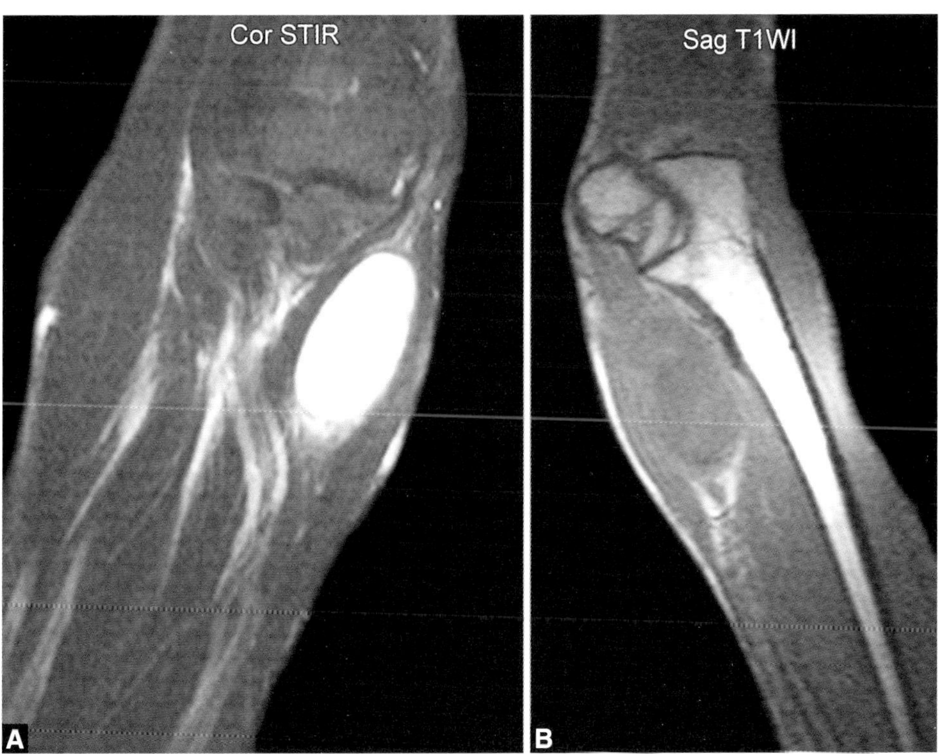

Figs 130A and B

diagnostic of peripheral nerve sheath tumor. A sagittal T1-weighted image (Fig. 130B) shows the fusiform mass is surrounded by a thin margin of fat (Split fat sign). This appearance results as the mass within the neurovascular bundle enlarges and displaces the adjacent intermuscular fat. On contrast-enhanced images (Fig. 130D), small nerve sheath tumors often show intense and relatively homogeneous enhancement. Large lesions may demonstrate predominantly peripheral, central or heterogeneous nodular enhancement.

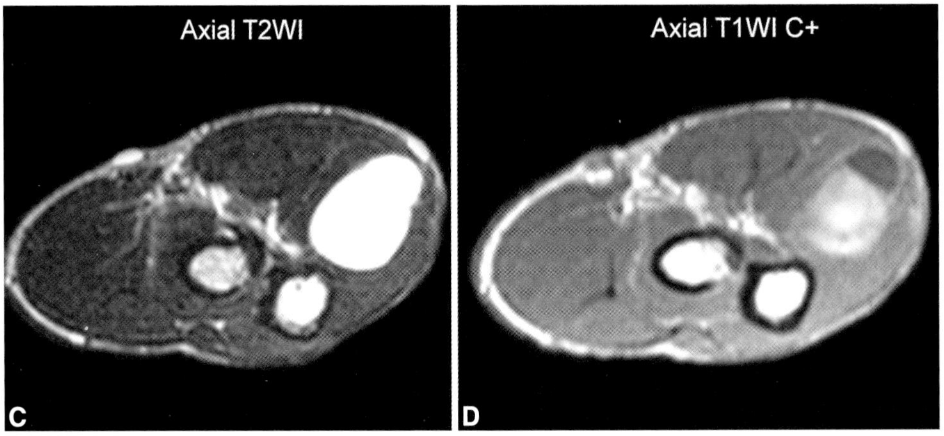

Figs 130C and D

Figs 130A to D: An oval well-defined hyperintense lesion on STIR and T1WI (A and D), appearing isointense on T1WI (B) is seen in the anterior aspect of right forearm in the intermuscular fat plane and shows moderate postcontrast enhancement (C)

Miscellaneous 7

Sikandar Sheikh

BRONCHOGENIC CYST

Bronchogenic cysts are congenital in nature and represent part of the spectrum of congenital abnormalities of the lung, including pulmonary sequestration, congenital cystic adenomatoid malformation, and congenital lobar emphysema.

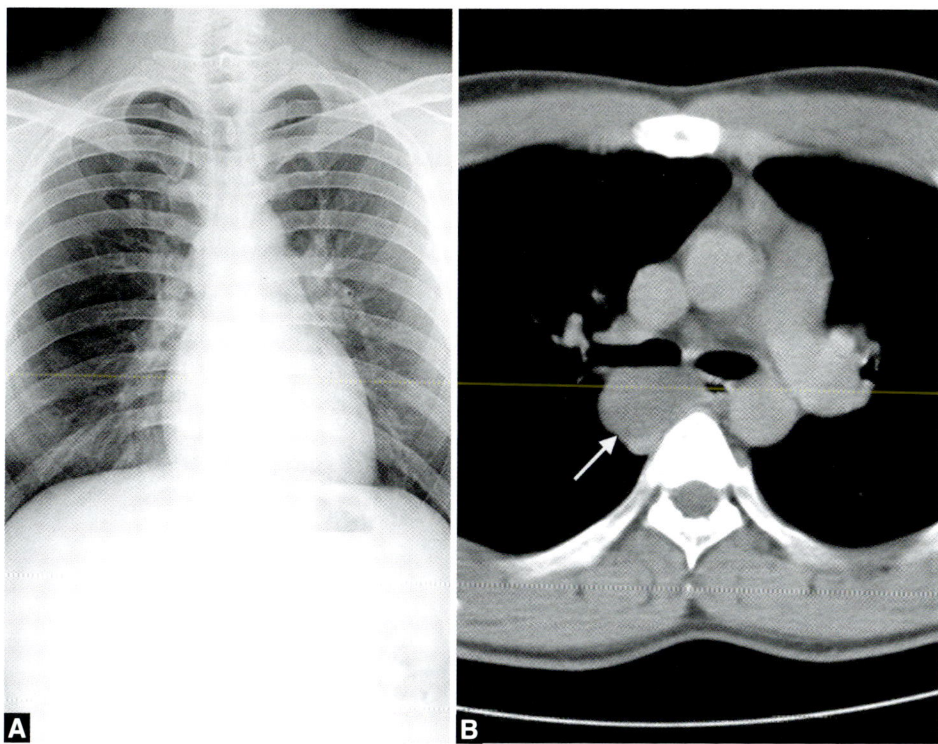

Figs 1A and B: (A) X-ray chest PA view reveals a subtle opacity along right tracheobronchial angle with broad base towards mediastinum. CT chest axial section (B) in mediastinal window, shows a well-defined nonenhancing lesion posterior to carina in midline and to right side, abutting esophagus and carina, having CT value of 14 HU, suggesting a benign cystic lesion

Bronchogenic cysts are usually an incidental finding, and differentiating them from other pathologic conditions is important. On conventional radiographs (Fig. 1A), the appearances of mediastinal or lung masses are nonspecific and it is limited in its ability to differentiate solid masses from fluid. Mediastinal cysts are visualized as a mediastinal mass on conventional radiographs. Intrapulmonary cysts usually present as a solitary pulmonary nodule unless the cyst contains air.

Bronchogenic cysts are sharply marginated masses demonstrating water or soft-tissue density. Differences in attenuation result from the amount of proteinaceous fluid within the cysts. Cysts do not enhance after administration of IV contrast. The appearance of cyst may be of water density, soft-tissue density, containing milk of calcium or may be completely air filled or containing an air-fluid level.

CT scan (Fig. 1B) findings are characteristic when the lesion demonstrates water density. If the lesion demonstrates soft-tissue density, differentiating the cyst from lymph nodes or other solid lesions is difficult.

MRI findings are usually diagnostic for mediastinal cysts. Bronchogenic cysts are usually bright on T2-weighted images and dark on T1-weighted images (Figs 1C to E). Cysts do not enhance after administration of IV gadolinium.

In addition to intrapulmonary and mediastinal locations, bronchogenic cysts are located in infradiaphragmatic, intrapericardial areas and intramural areas of the esophagus. Intrapulmonary cysts are difficult to diagnose and must be aspirated to confirm the diagnosis.

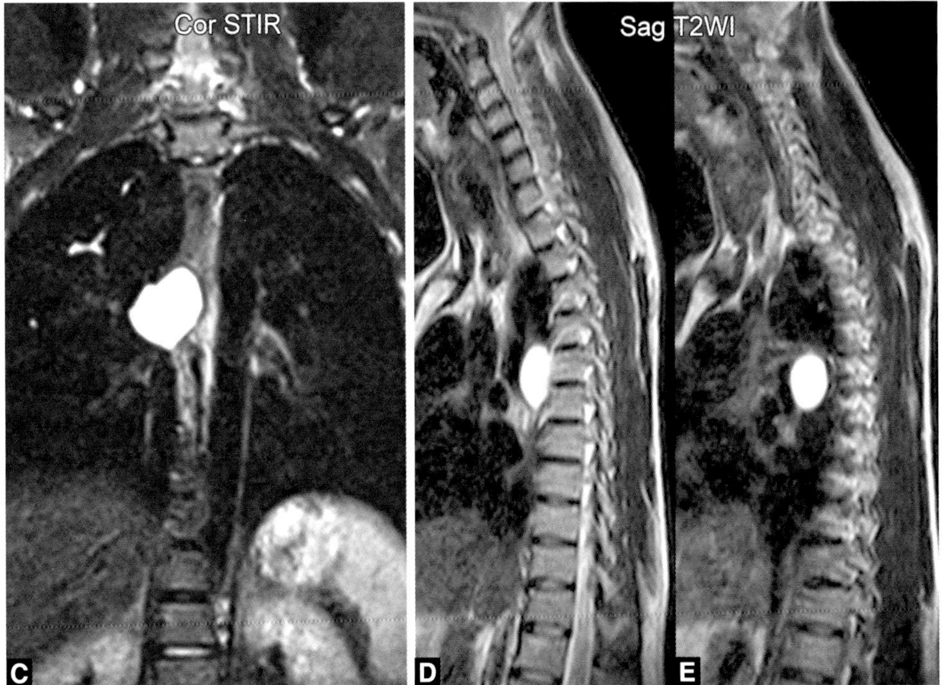

Figs 1C to E: Coronal STIR (C) image reveals hyperintense homogeneous lesion posterior to distal trachea and carina in midline and to right side. Sagittal T2 weighted images (D and E) demonstrate the craniocaudal extent of the hyperintense lesion posterior to distal trachea and carina in midline and to right side, confirmed as bronchogenic cyst

PANCOAST TUMOR

Carcinoma of the apex of the lung is termed as Pancoast tumor or superior sulcus tumor that may involve the brachial plexus and sympathetic ganglion of the lower neck and upper mediastinum. Bronchogenic carcinoma or metastatic lesion are the most common causes of Pancoast tumors, other causes are lymphoma, mesothelioma, and multiple myeloma.

Pancoast syndrome is a clinical triad of: (1) Horner's syndrome—ptosis, miosis, anhidrosis, and enophthalmos, (2) Ipsilateral arm pain, (3) Wasting of the hand muscles. Pancoast tumors are best depicted on the coronal and sagittal MR images (Fig. 2).

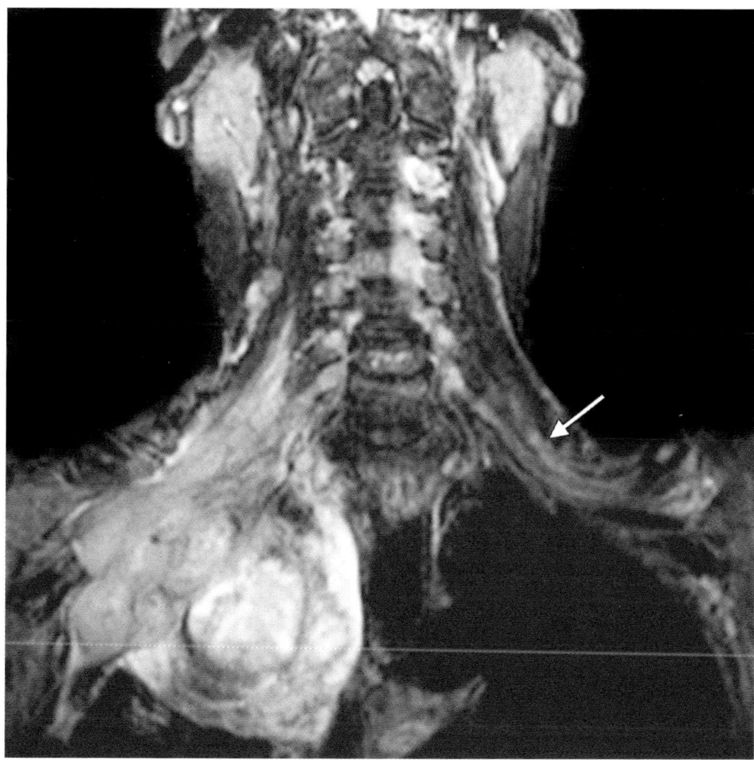

Fig. 2: MRI shows a large heterogeneous lesion is seen in the apex of right lung involving the ribs, brachial plexus and adjacent soft tissues. Brachial plexus is normal on left side (arrow)

HEPATOCELLULAR CARCINOMA

Hepatocellular carcinoma (HCC) is the most common primary malignant tumor of the liver occurring predominantly in patients with underlying parenchymal liver disease. The main etiological factors of HCC are cirrhosis, hepatitis B and C infection and carcinogens. Other risk factors are primary hemochromatosis, glycogen storage disease and thorium dioxide deposition in the liver. Alcohol related cirrhosis is considered the most frequent cause of HCC in the Western world.

HCC can be expansive (solitary, multifocal or more rarely diffusely infiltrating). Multifocal tumors may present as dominant massive masses with satellite nodules or as multiple nodular structures of similar size. The expansive type of tumor displays a slower and less aggressive growth pattern than the infiltrative one, and may be surrounded by a capsule.

On T1-weighted images HCC has been reported as iso- or hyperintense in 47 to 62 percent of patients. The capsule, as well as the central scar, is usually markedly hypointense on T1-weighted images. Hyperintensity on T1-weighted images has been related to fatty metamorphosis, recent hemorrhage, excessive glycogen or copper deposition. On T2-weighted images the majority of HCC are hyperintense (Figs 3A and B). Frequently the signal intensity is inhomogeneous due to localized hyperintense foci which correspond to dilated sinusoids and necrosis within the tumor. The central scar is high in signal intensity on T2-weighted images.

Dynamic contrast enhanced MRI with gadolinium DTPA, which is able to detect more lesions than unenhanced MRI, shows an enhancement pattern similar to that observed on contrast enhanced dynamic CT. While (Figs 3C and D) undifferentiated HCC does not take up specific liver contrast agents directed to the reticuloendothelial system, well-differentiated HCC may show a distinct uptake. Quantitative evaluation of the percentage signal intensity loss after contrast administration may be the most useful approach to distinguish well-differentiated HCCs from benign liver neoplasms. It has also been shown that malignant liver tumors frequently show ring enhancement after administration of contrast.

MRI may be specifically helpful in differentiating regenerative nodules, siderotic nodules and

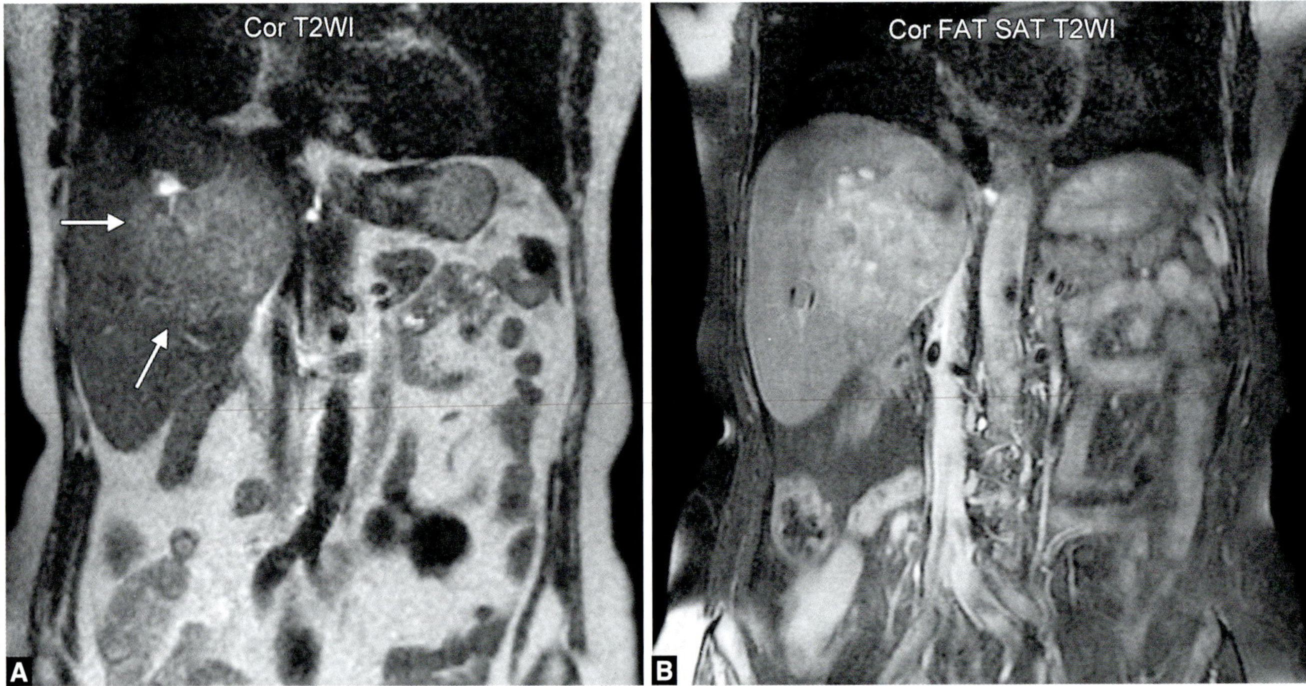

Figs 3A and B

dysplastic nodules that are frequently present in cirrhosis from HCC. Regenerative nodules tend to be hypo-, iso-, or hyperintense on T1-weighted images and hypo- or isointense on T2-weighted images. Most dysplastic nodules are hyperintense on T1-weighted and hypointense on T2-weighted images.

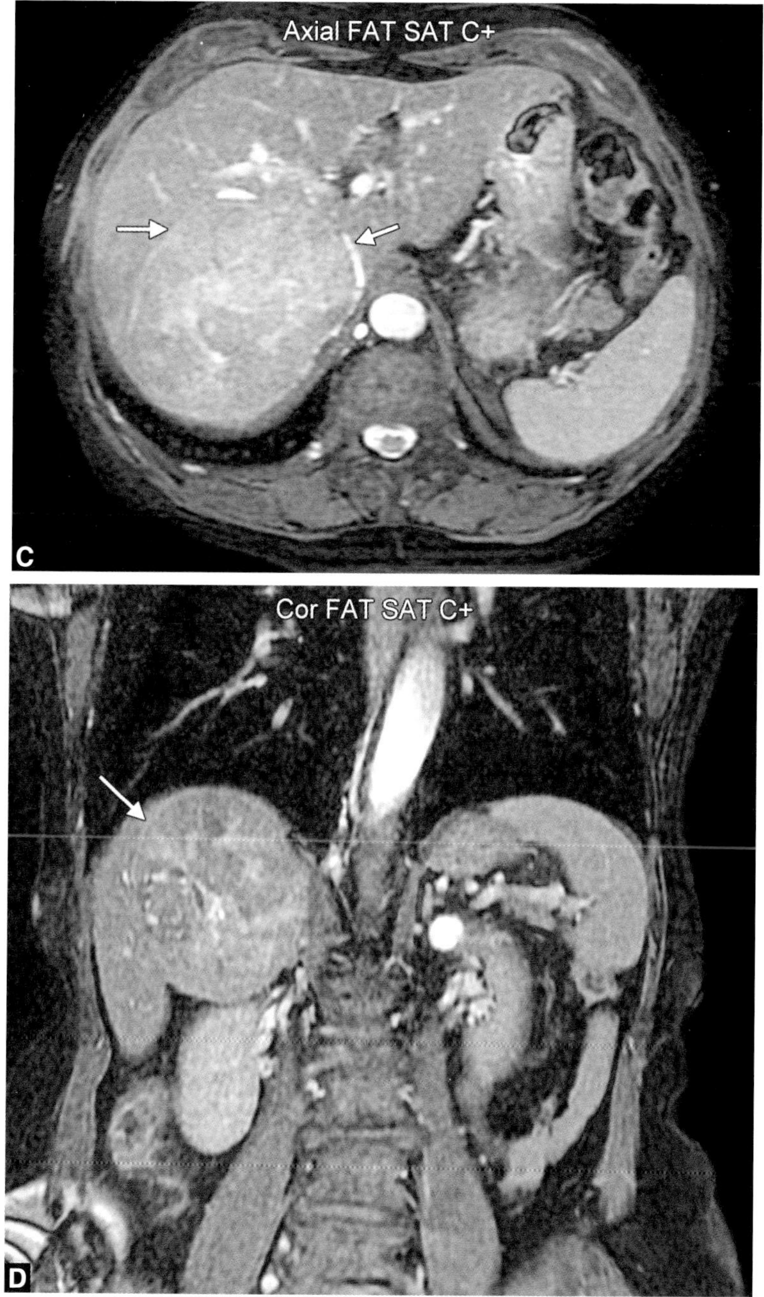

Figs 3C and D

Figs 3A to D: Coronal T2WI (A) shows ill-defined hyperintense lesion in right lobe of liver. Coronal fat saturated T2WI (B) also shows few small necrotic areas within the lesion. Postcontrast axial (C) and coronal (D) fat saturated FIESTA sequence shows heterogeneous enhancement with ring like pattern

HEPATIC METASTASIS

The liver is second only to lymph nodes as a site of metastatic disease, and liver metastases are 20 times more common than primary liver tumors. Most hepatic metastases are solid, but some have a complete or partially cystic appearance. Metastases that become necrotic will appear cystic at imaging, which is most commonly seen in hypervascular metastases for example, from a neuroendocrine tumor, sarcoma, melanoma, and certain subtypes of lung and breast carcinoma. Mucinous primary tumors such as colorectal or ovarian tumors frequently give rise to cystic metastases. In the case of a cystic ovarian primary tumor, metastases have been reported to evolve into cystic lesions, even if they were initially solid. Also, metastases may undergo cystic change with response to treatment. On imaging, cystic liver metastases may show variable wall thickness, (Figs 4A to D) and on MRI, enhancement and fluid-fluid levels may be seen. Their imaging appearance will vary depending on the primary tumor and the stage of treatment.

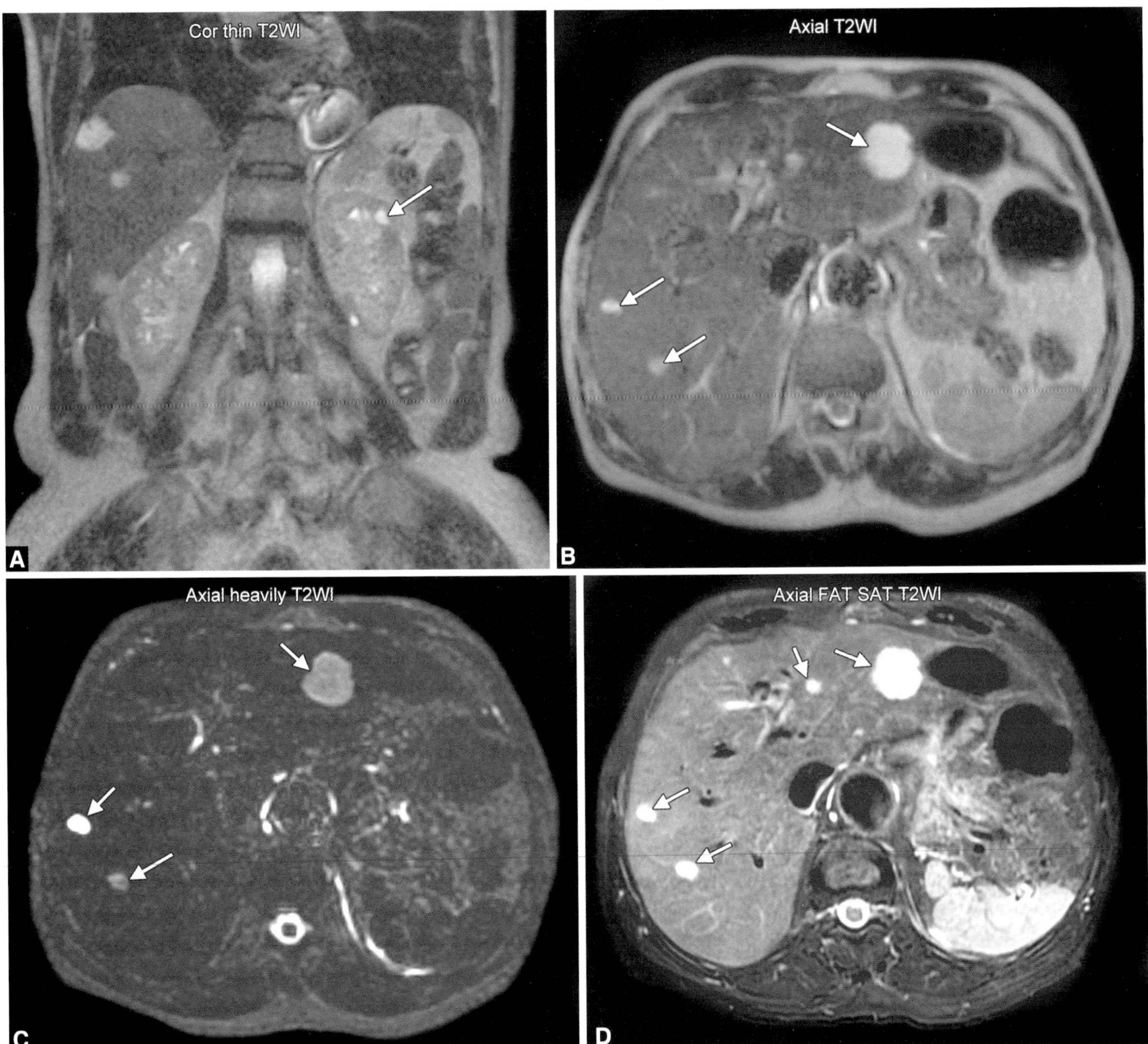

Figs 4A to D: MR abdomen of a 74-year-old male, a known case of carcinoma lung with anorexia and weight loss. On coronal T2WI (A) and axial T2WI (B) show multiple variable sized hyperintense lesions in both lobes of liver. A small hyperintense lesion is also seen in upper pole cortex of left kidney (B). Axial T2WI (C) and axial fat sat T2WI (D) also shows variable sized hyperintense lesions in both lobes of liver representing as cystic metastases in liver from carcinoma lung

CHOLELITHIASIS

Gallstone disease is common worldwide. Common risk factors for development of gallstone are obesity, diabetes, hemolytic anemia and increasing age. A common saying for risk factors is a fat fertile female of forty years.

Most patients are asymptomatic, about 20 percent present with biliary colic and another about 2 percent present with acute cholecystitis.

Composition of gallstone or type of gallstones

- Cholesterol stone (70%)
- Pigment stone (30%)
- Gas containing gallstone

The ultrasound is the most sensitive in detection of the biliary calculi. The ability to detect stones on CT depends on the difference in density of the stone with respect to bile. The reported sensitivity of CT for detection of gallstones is approximately 79 percent with 100 percent specificity. Calcified stones are readily identified on CT as they are denser than bile. Stones with high concentration of cholesterol may also be readily identified as these stones are less dense than bile. When stones degenerate, nitrogen gas may collect in central fissures and create the "Mercedes-Benz" sign. This sign may be the only visual evidence of gallstones and appears as a focal collection of gas in the nondependent gallbladder lumen. Noncalcified pigment stones are soft tissue density attenuation. Small stones are frequently missed on CT unless their density differs markedly from bile.

T2 weighed MR imaging shows calculi as hypointense foci in gallbladder and common bile duct (Fig. 5). MRCP is better option to delineate a calculus in a biliary tree and show biliary dilatation proximal to it.

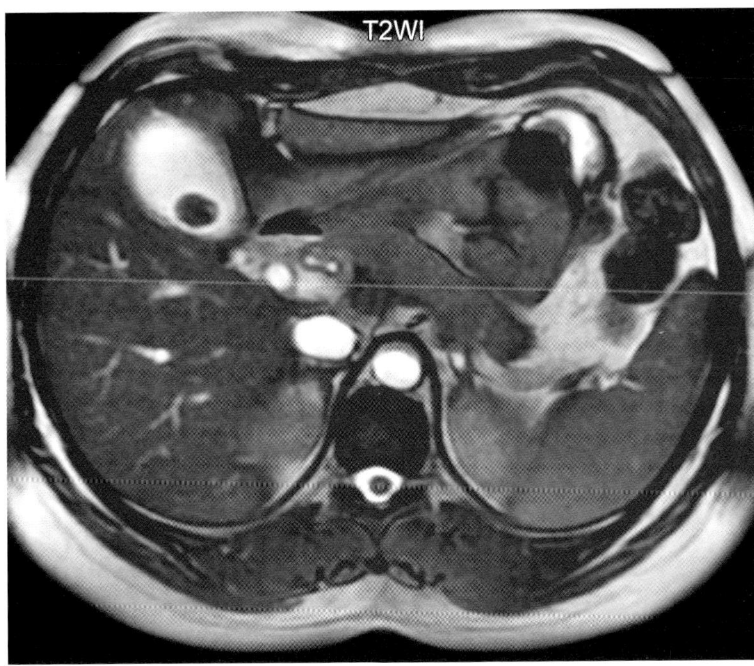

Fig. 5: Axial T2 weighed image shows a hypointense single round calculus lying within hyperintense gallbladder sac

GALLBLADDER SLUDGE

Gallbladder sludge is debris formed in the bile and seen as echogenic material in the gallbladder which moves with position on ultrasound examination. The debris has low level echoes which do not cast an acoustic shadow. Occasionally, sludge balls may form. It is a nonspecific finding and most often relates to biliary stasis which may be due to obstruction but more commonly due to decreased bile production and flow, a common accompaniment of many debilitating acute or chronic illnesses. Gallbladder sludge may be a precursor to stone formation but in most instances it disappears without forming stones. It is seen in parenteral nutrition, cholecystitis, and sickle cell disease.

On MRI it is seen as layering in the gallbladder, in which thick dependent debris is seen as hypointense on T2WI and hyperintense on T1WI (Figs 6A and B). Whereas normal nondependant bile shows fluid characteristics signal.

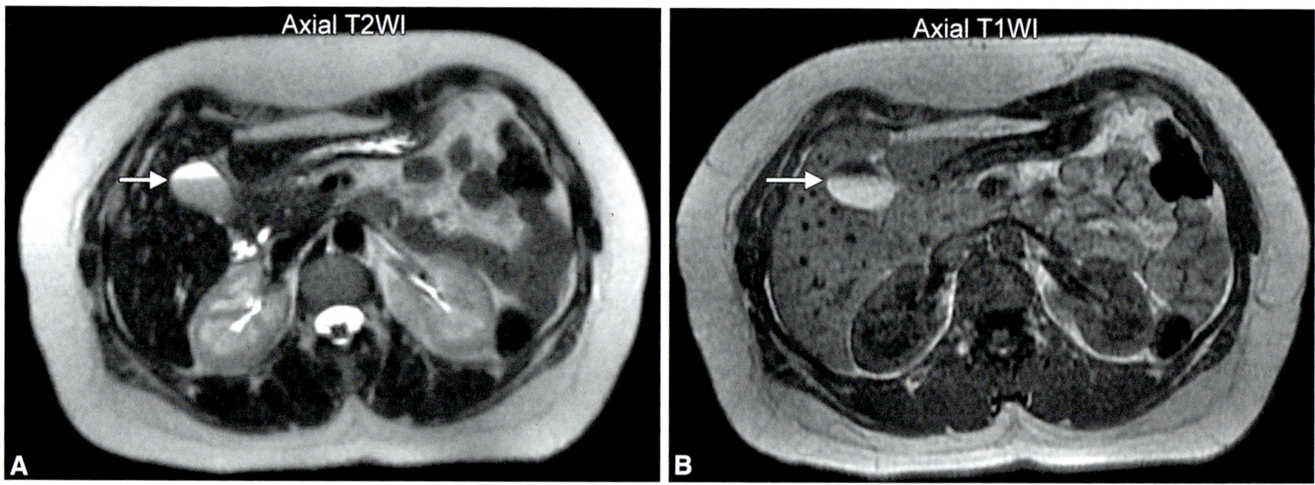

Figs 6A and B: In 43-year-old fat female with pain in right hypochondriac region and nausea, MR axial T2WI shows layering in the gallbladder, in which thick dependent debris is seen as hypointense and clear fluid superiorly as hyperintense and in axial T1WI the thick dependent debris is seen as hyperintense and clear fluid above is hypointense. The fluid sludge level is shown by arrow

MR CHOLANGIOGRAPHY

MR cholangiography provides precise diagnostic accuracy to evaluate biliary disease, especially for calculi measuring greater than 4 mm in size, biliary strictures and dilated intrahepatic biliary radicles. MR cholangiography is useful in planning of interventional procedures or understanding of complex relationships between pathologic and normal duct anatomy. The examination is ideally done on a 1.5 Tesla or higher system.

MR cholangiography is based on a heavily T2 weighted pulse sequence which shows stationary fluids, such as bile, giving high signal intensity whereas the surrounding liver and flowing blood generates little signal (Fig. 7).

With long effective echo times, only fluid-filled compartments are observed with nearly complete background suppression and minimal sensitivity to motion and signal loss due to magnetic susceptibility. Patient cooperation is very important for MR cholangiography sequences as respiratory motion can blur the images. Respiratory gating with free breathing sequences can also be obtained. Ghosting and blurring could be noted with fluids affected by peristalsis and heart pulsation. Ghosting from pulsation of cerebrospinal fluid could be suppressed by means of a presaturation band over the spinal canal. Slow moving blood does not interfere with image quality as the signal from fluid is higher.

As a result of this MR cholangiography provides optimal contrast between the hyperintense signals of the bile duct and the hypointense signal of surrounding tissue (Figs 8 and 9).

Fig. 7: Normal MR cholangiography

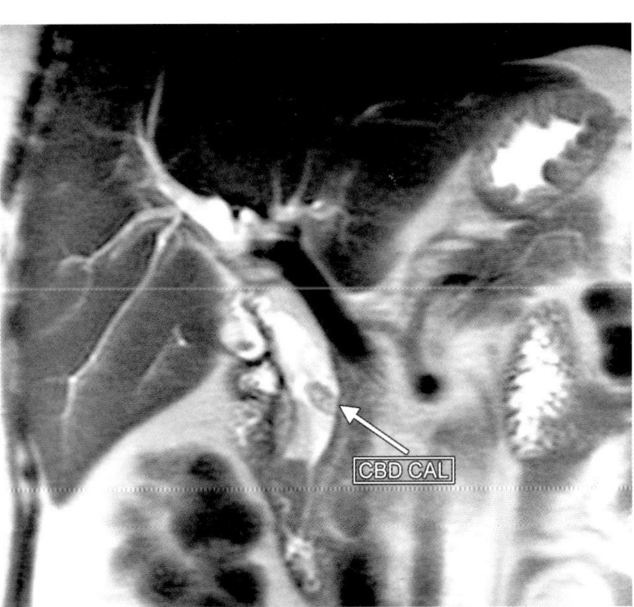

Fig. 8: MR cholangiography in 3D MIP image shows a well-defined oval filling defect (arrow) in the distal common bile duct (CBD) with dilatation of the proximal common bile duct (CBD) and intrahepatic biliary radicles

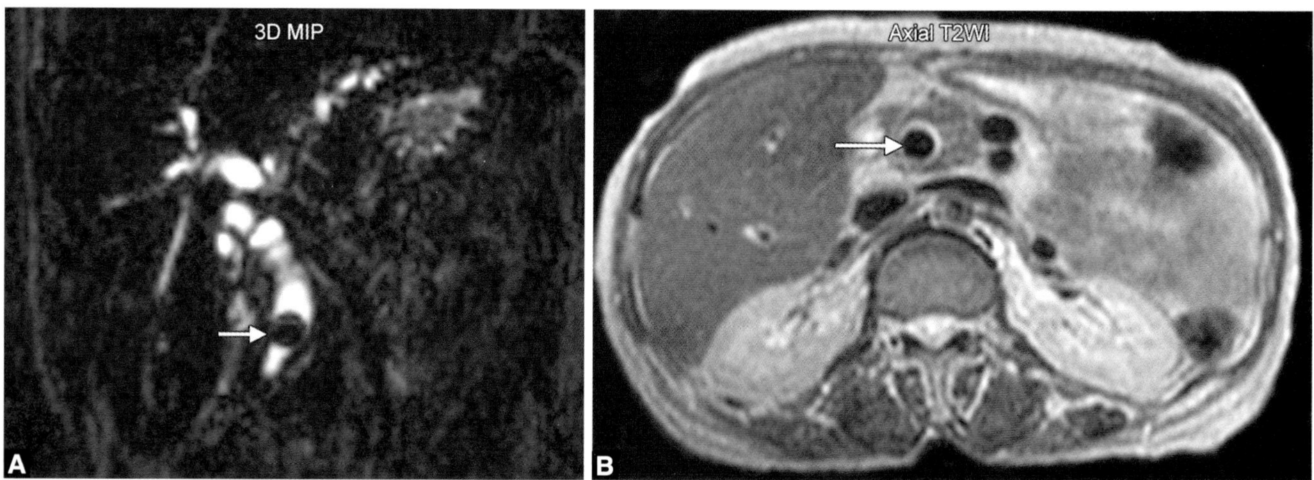

Figs 9A and B: MR cholangiography in 3D MIP images (A) shows a well-defined round filling defect (arrow) in the distal CBD with dilatation of the proximal CBD and intrahepatic biliary radicles. Axial T2WI (B) reveals a hyperintense rim of bile around the hypointense filling defect (CBD calculus)

PSEUDOCYST OF PANCREAS

Pseudocyst of pancreas is a circumscribed collection of fluid rich in pancreatic enzymes, blood, and necrotic tissue, typically located in the lesser sac of the abdomen. Pseudocyst of pancreas is usually complication of pancreatitis. MR and magnetic resonance cholangiopancreatography (MRCP) are sensitive diagnostic modalities for pancreatic pseudocysts. They are generally not routinely used because CT scanning typically offers all the diagnostic information that is required (Figs 10A and B). MR or MRCP is superior to CT in depicting debris within fluid collections and pseudocysts (Figs 10C and D). MRCP techniques can also depict subtle branch-chain dilatation in chronic pancreatitis. They are also highly sensitive to blood products, such as those seen in complex hemorrhagic fluid collections or pseudocysts.

MR is more expensive, but has no ionizing radiation, its multiplanar capabilities has the ability to depict choledocholithiasis far superior to that of CT or US.

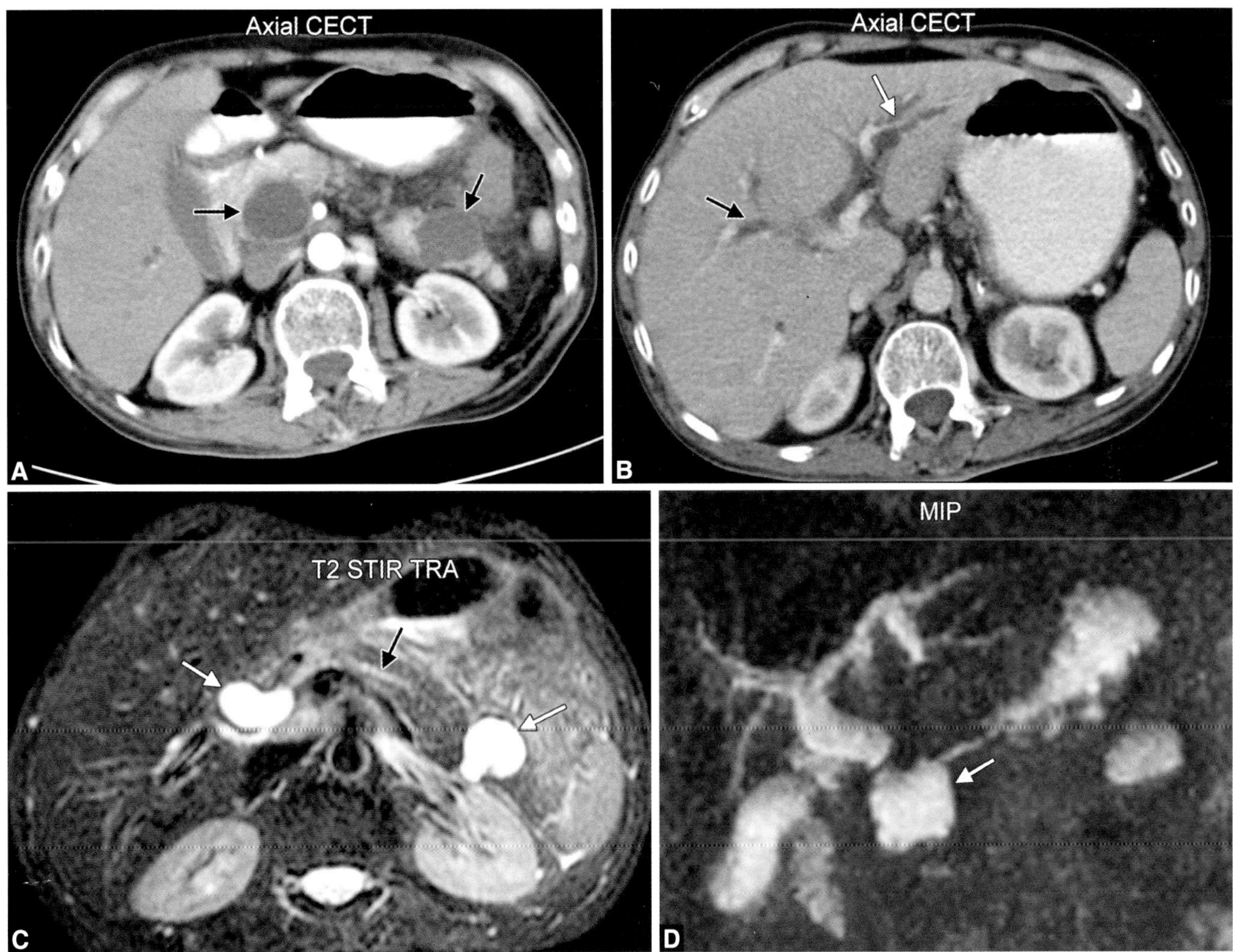

Figs 10A to D: Axial CECT sections (A and B) of a 48-year-old male patient with history of jaundice reveal dilatation intrahepatic biliary radicles. A well-defined peripherally enhancing cystic lesion (arrows) is seen in the head and another in the tail region of pancreas with compression of CBD and dilatation IHBR, right and left hepatic ducts and CBD (arrow). Axial T2 STIR image (C) shows a well-defined cystic lesion in the head (white arrow) and another in the tail region of pancreas, pancreatic duct is dilated. Magnetic resonance cholangiopancreatogram MIP image (D) shows CBD dilatation (black arrow) due to compression by pseudocyst in the head (white arrow)

ADRENAL ADENOMA

Adrenal adenoma is common benign tumor of the adrenal cortex. Adenomas measuring 5 mm or more are found in approximately 1 percent of routine autopsies, and measuring 3 mm or more in approximately 3 percent. The vast majority are nonfunctional and finding is incidental. The incidence increases with age, so that adenomas are found in 5 percent of patients over 60 years. Associations with hypertension, diabetes mellitus, renal cell carcinoma and hereditary polyposis coli is seen. Occasionally the tumors are functional, and cause an endocrinopathy (Cushing's syndrome, Conn's syndrome or adrenogenital syndrome). Pathologically, adrenal adenomas consist of clear cells arranged in cords between fibrovascular stroma. The clear cells are derived from the adrenal cortex, and contain abundant intracytoplasmic lipid, reflecting the steroid synthetic function of the adrenal cortical cells.

The typical imaging features of an adrenal adenoma are those of a small homogeneous mass. The masses are small and surrounded by fat, so that they are often not detected at ultrasound. At CT, adrenal adenomas have a smooth rounded appearance with a low density on noncontrast-enhanced scans, due to intracytoplasmic lipid. Immediate post-contrast CT is unhelpful in the characterization of adenomas. However, delayed contrast-enhanced CT may be helpful, because adenomas demonstrate a more rapid washout of contrast than other causes of adrenal masses.

On MRI, adenomas are usually isointense or hypointense to liver on both T1 and T2 weighted images (Fig. 11). Adenomas demonstrate significant signal loss on opposed phase gradient-echo T1 weighted images, when compared to in-phase images. This finding is due to signal cancellation between intracytoplasmic fat and water protons. A signal loss of at least 45 percent, using the spleen as an internal reference, has a sensitivity of 80 percent and a specificity of 100 percent for the diagnosis of adrenal adenoma. A rim of high signal intensity has been described as a specific sign on fat-suppressed T2-weighted spin-echo images, and may represent a capsule or compressed adjacent parenchyma. The tumors enhance after intravenous gadolinium. MR angiography can clearly show the vascular supply of adenomas.

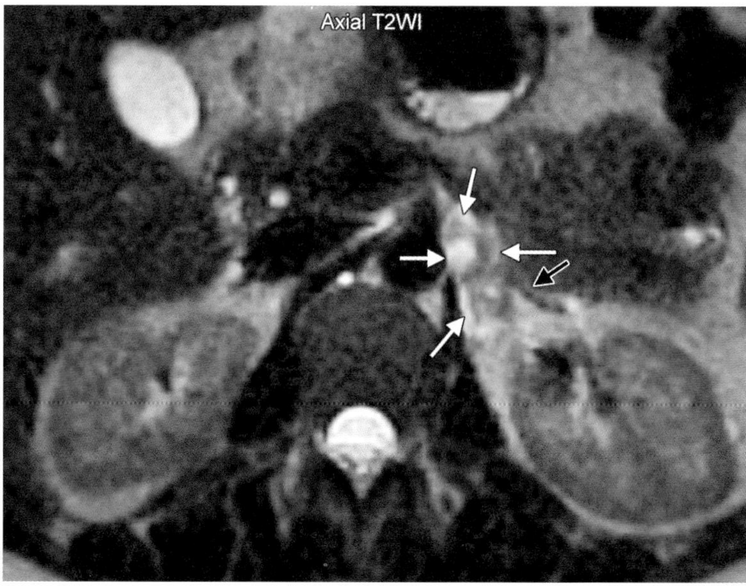

Fig. 11: In 25-year-male, a young hypertensive on axial T2WI shows bulky enlarged isointense medial limb of left adrenal (white arrows) with well-defined rounded hyperintense lesion within (elbow arrow). The lateral limb is normal (black arrow)

Self Assessment 8

Amol Sasane

A 35-year-old male patient reported with history of mild pain left knee for 2 months.

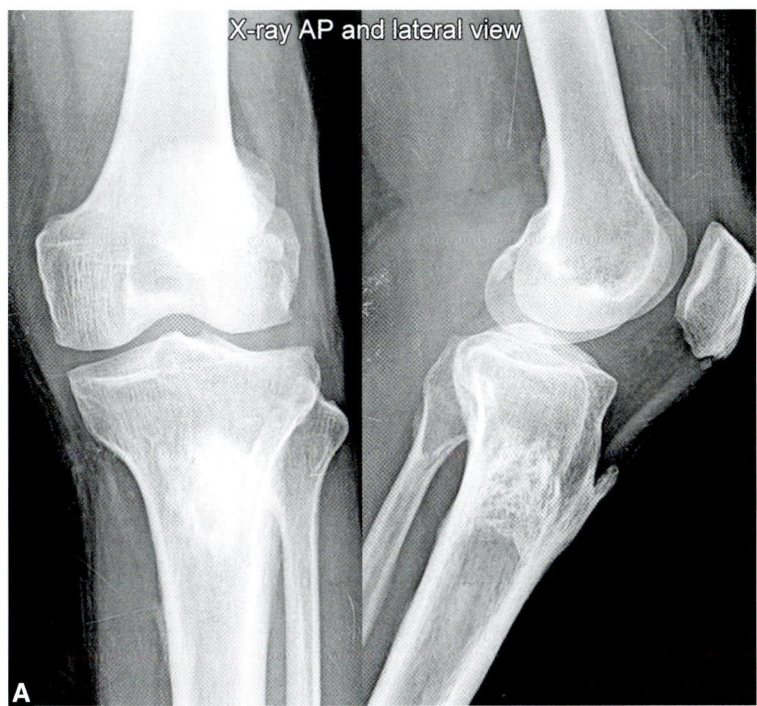

Fig. 1A

Answer: Hemangioma proximal tibial.

X-ray knee joint AP and lateral (Fig. 1A) view shows heterogeneously dense intramedullary lesion in proximal tibial diaphysis. T1W coronal image shows a well defined iso to hypointense lesion with irregular margins in proximal tibial diaphysis. This lesion appears hyperintense on STIR images. There is no perilesional edema or medullary widening (Fig. 1B). On post-contrast T1W weighted image the lesion shows moderate heterogeneous enhancement (Fig. 1C).

Bone hemangiomas are benign, malformed vascular lesions, overall constituting less than 1 percent of all primary bone neoplasms. They occur most frequently in the vertebral column (30-50%)

and skull (20%), whereas involvement of other sites (including the long bones, short tubular bones, and ribs) is rare. Hemangiomas are largely asymptomatic, usually found incidentally. On plain radiographs hemangiomas are seen as dense lesions with prominent trabecular pattern. On MRI hemangiomas are iso to hyperintense on T1W images and appear hyperintense on STIR images. Post-contrast images show heterogeneous enhancement.

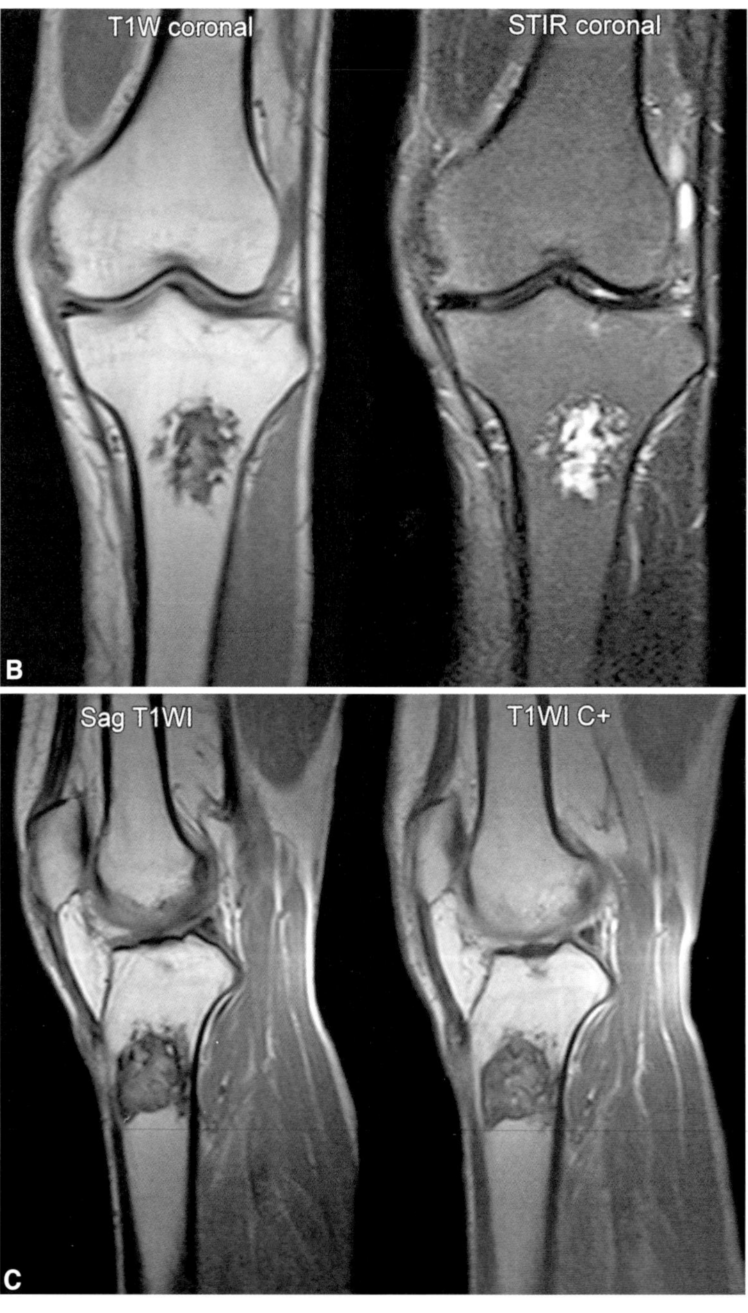

Figs 1B and C

A 10-year-old boy, presented with history of two episodes of convulsions with mild fever and weight loss since two months.

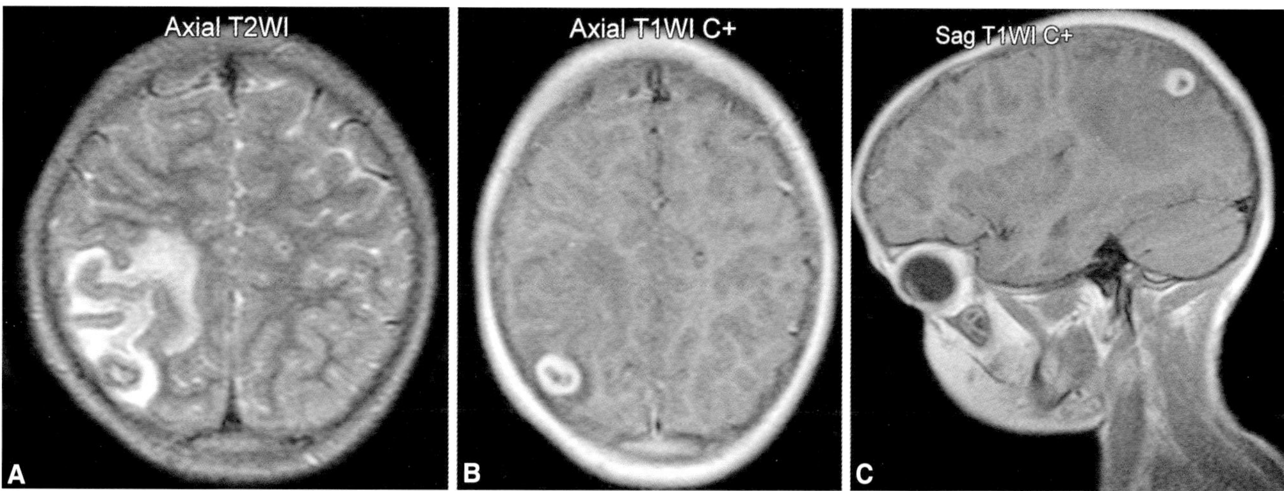

Figs 2A to C

Answer: Tuberculoma.

Small subcentimeter sized peripherally enhancing lesions are seen in the right high parietal parenchyma. The enhancing walls are thick (Figs 2B and C) and appear hypointense on T2W image (Figs 2A). The central nonenhancing portion is hyperintense on T2W images. There is moderate perilesional white matter edema.

The tubercular focus starts off as an area of cerebritis. The cerebritis then progresses to a focal non-caseating granuloma, which will be surrounded by perilesional edema. The word 'caseation' refers to conversion of tissues into a cheese-like substance. As caseation progresses, the central part of the tuberculomas undergoes necrosis. This is seen as central non enhancing hyperintense area. Perilesional edema remains. On MR spectroscopy it shows increased choline peak.

Tuberculomas may be solitary or, more commonly, multiple. They are of variable sizes. They tend to lie superficially in the brain, most characteristically adjacent to the Sylvian fissure. The frontal and parietal lobes are the most commonly affected regions. They may or may not be associated with TB meningitis.

A 19-years female with history of low backache since 6 months. No history of fever or any other significant history.

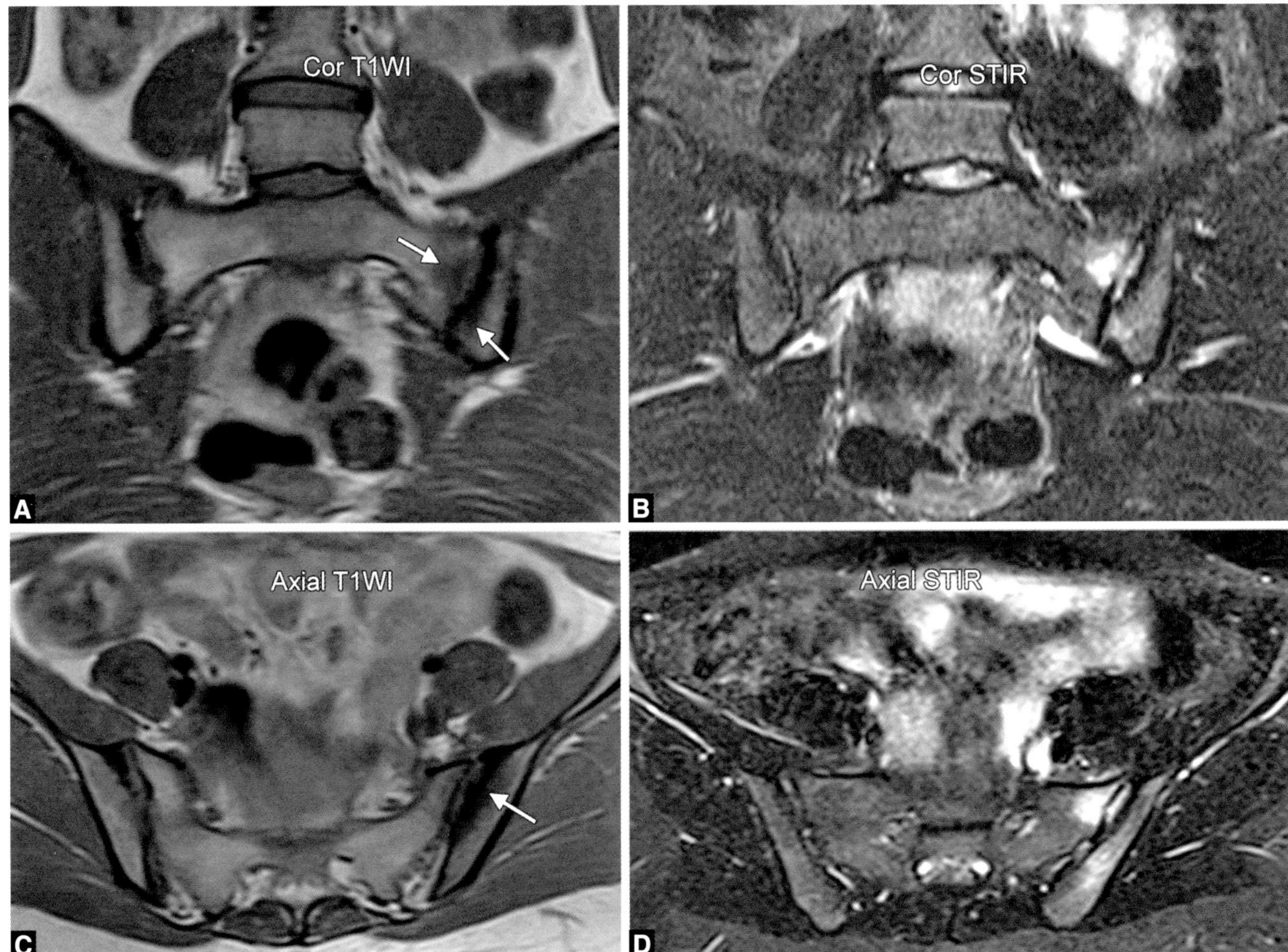

Figs 3A to D

Answer: Sacroiliitis.

Abnormal hypointense signal is seen on T1W images (Figs 3A and C) involving the articular surface of the left sacroiliac joint. STIR images (Figs 3B and D) show hyperintense signal involving the articular surface of the left sacroiliac joint. Imaging findings are suggestive of left sacroiliitis.

Sacroiliitis is inflammation of the sacroiliac joint. Characteristic radiographic features include joint space narrowing, sclerosis, and erosions of the ilium and sacrum. Sacroiliitis is the hallmark of ankylosing spondylitis. The inflammation is evident early in the course of the disease. In later stages, the radiographic changes are almost invariably bilateral and symmetric. The alterations occur in both the synovial and the ligamentous (anterior and posterior) portions of the joint and predominate in the ilium. Periarticular osteoporosis and loss of definition, superficial erosion, and focal sclerosis of subchondral bone are present initially.

MRI may have a role in the early diagnosis of sacroiliitis. Detection of synovial enhancement on MRI has been found to correlate with disease activity, as measured by laboratory inflammatory markers. Advantages of MRI include direct visualization of cartilage abnormalities, detection of bone marrow edema, improved detection of erosions, and the absence of ionizing radiation.

A 2-year-old girl presented with a sacral dimple.

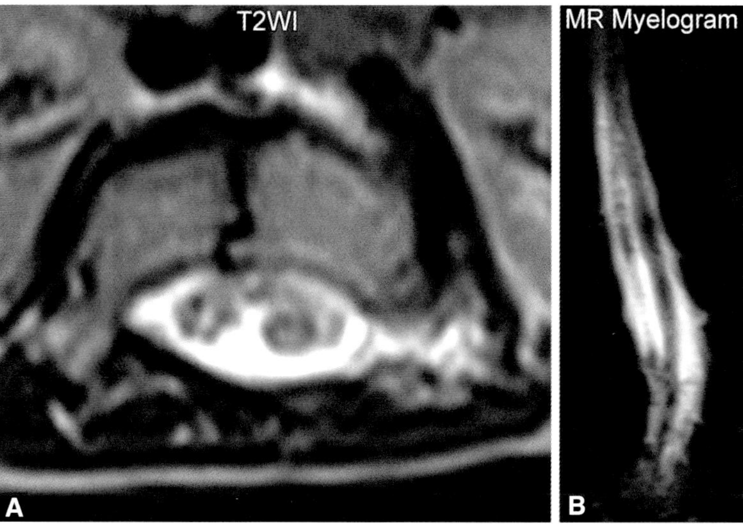

Figs 4A and B

Answer: Diastematomyelia.

Axial T2WI (Fig. 4A) and MR myelogram (Fig. 4B) shows split cord extending from L1 level caudally with low lying cord suggestive of diastematomyelia. Plain films and nonenhanced scan usually show abnormal osseous spine in diastematomyelia. The hemicords and subarachnoid spaces are well delineated on MR and MR myelography.

Diastematomyelia refers to a pathologic longitudinal splitting of the spinal cord and the intradorsal nerve roots into two columns. Separation into the two hemicords may be due to a bony spur, cartilaginous separation or fibrous band with a usual asymmetry in size of the hemicords.

Two types of diastematomyelia have been described. Each accounts for roughly 50 percent. Type I refers to a split cord that is surrounded by a normal undivided arachnoid-dural sleeve without a septum. Type II refers to a split cord in which each hemicord is invested by a separate dural sleeve that is divided by a fibrous, cartilaginous, or bony septum.

Diastematomyelia usually occurs in the lower thoracic and upper lumbar regions and 85 percent of the time is associated with bony abnormalities including spina bifida, widened interpediculate distances, hemivertebrae, and scoliosis. There are also associated cutaneous manifestations of the dorsal midline including telangiectasias, atrophic skin, hemangiomas, and subcutaneous lipomas.

A 35-year-old male with history of fall from a horse onto his outstretched arm, with pain at shoulder joint and anterior dislocation of shoulder joint.

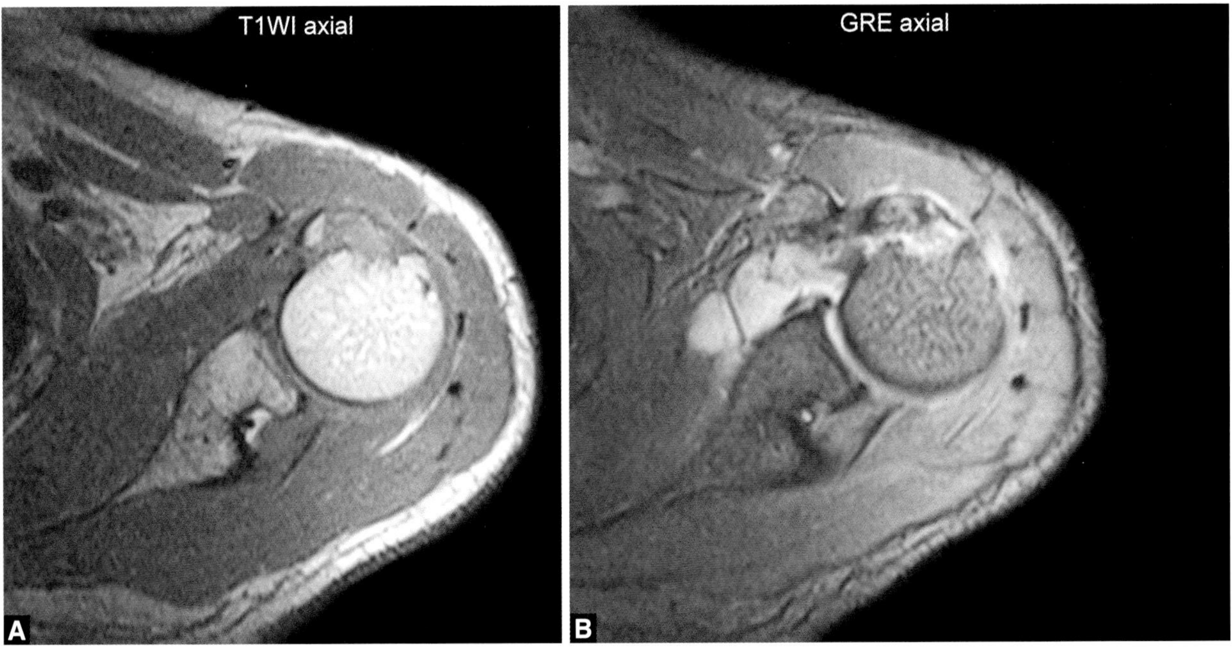

Figs 5A and B

Answer: Avulsion fracture of greater tuberosity of humerus.

Coronal T1W (Fig. 5A) and gradient weighted (Fig. 5B) axial images show medially displaced avulsion fracture of the greater tuberosity of humerus at the attachment of the subscapularis tendon. Joint effusion is present.

Acute avulsion injuries result from extreme, unbalanced, and often eccentric muscular contractions, and patients with such injuries present with severe pain and loss of function. In contrast, chronic avulsion injuries are the result of repetitive microtrauma or overuse and usually occur during organized sports activities, such as athlete.

Most often the injury is abrupt and a clear history is available as in this case, which makes clinical and radiographic diagnosis easy. Sometimes, however, there is no history of a specific traumatic event and radiographic findings are confusing. Such findings can lead to excessive imaging, biopsy, and incorrect diagnosis because post traumatic bone changes can simulate osteomyelitis or even malignancy at radiography.

It is difficult to distinguish between isolated humeral avulsion fractures of the greater tuberosity and rotator cuff tears at clinical examination. The distinction is crucial, however, because treatment of the two injuries is different. At radiography, the fracture may not be readily apparent.

Most of these sites the fracture plane is through the physis of an apophysis as an apophysis acts as the insertion site for muscle and the physis represents a weak link in the immature skeleton. Radiographs generally confirm the diagnosis by demonstrating a bony fragment displaced at variable distance from the parent bone. Ultrasound can show displacement of the apophysis and dynamic examination allows confirmation that this corresponds with the site of tenderness. Ultrasound may also demonstrate associated hematoma within the adjacent muscle.

MRI shows the fracture to greater advantage. MR imaging is often requested in cases of suspected rotator cuff tear in which marrow edema is incidentally seen surrounding the greater tuberosity and denoting the margins of the occult avulsion fracture. It will demonstrate reduced signal on T1 and increased signal on T2-weighted or STIR sequences, particularly within the fatty marrow of the secondary ossification centre. It is important to recognize the fracture by its characteristic site and radiographic appearance so as to avoid misdiagnosis.

A 69-year-old female patient presented with history of fall.

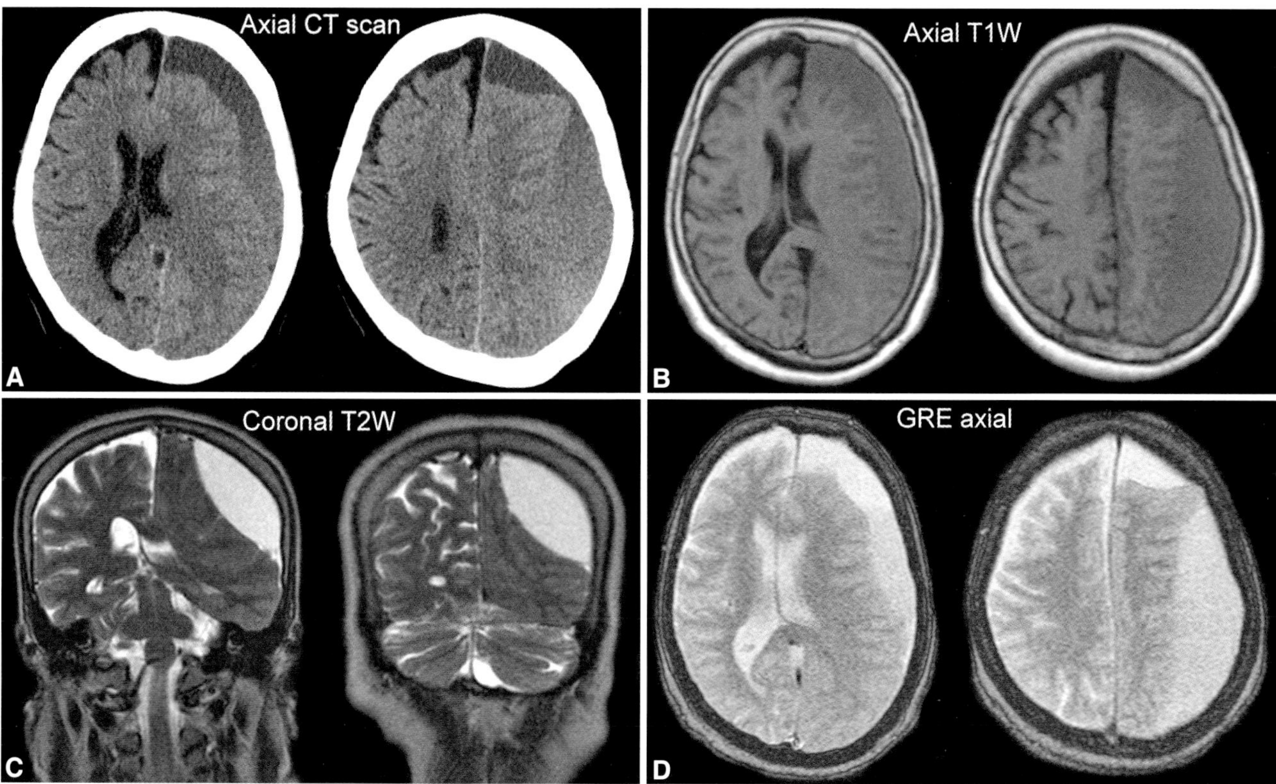

Figs 6A to D

Answer: Subdural hemorrhage.

Axial CT images of brain at the level of lateral ventricles and centrum semiovale (Fig. 6A) shows a large extra-axial collection along the left frontoparietal region which is hypodense to brain parenchyma. There is significant mass effect of the lesion causing effacement of sulcal spaces and compression over the underlying brain parenchyma with mild midline shift towards right side. On axial T1W images (Fig. 6B) the lesion appears iso to hyperintense to gray matter of brain. Also there is generalized cerebral atrophy and prominent extracerebral CSF spaces in right fronto-parietal region. On coronal T2W images (Fig. 6C) the lesion appears hyperintense as compared to gray matter, less intense than cerebrospinal fluid and on axial gradient images (Fig. 6D) the lesion appears hyperintense.

Subdual hemorrhage occurs in between dura and arachnoid mater. It has a concavo-convex appearance and does not cross the midline. It occurs due to injury to bridging cortical veins.

Table 1 shows staging of hematomas according to time on MR examination. Hyperacute and acute hematomas contain oxyhemoglobin and deoxyhemoglobin respectively and are isointense to gray matter on T1 sequence. After 3 days methemoglobin forms which shows high signal on T1 sequence. Methemoglobin continues to be hyperintense on T1 even when it is released from the hemolyzed red blood cells and seen as hyperintense

Table 1: MR staging of hematomas according to time

Stage	*Time*	*Hemoglobin*	*T1*	*T2*
Hyperacute	<24 hours	Oxyhemoglobin	Iso	Hyper
Acute	1–3 days	Deoxyhemoglobin	Iso	Hypo
Early subacute	3–7 days	Methemoglobin in RBCs	Hyper	Hypo
Late subacute	>7 days	Methemoglobin free	Hyper	Hyper
Chronic	>14 days	Hemosiderin	Iso, hypo	Hypo

on T2 sequence. Chronic hemorrhage on MR is seen as a hypointense rim of hemosiderin deposits along brain parenchyma. Gradient echo T2* sequences show hemorrhage as hypointense. T2* is decay of transverse magnetization because of spin-spin relaxation and inhomogeneity of the magnetic field. T2* is associated with GRE (gradient-echo) imaging only, as 180° pulse in spin echo imaging eliminates the magnetic field inhomogeneties. In GRE T2* sequence is the main determinants of image contrast and forms the basis of MR applications including perfusion imaging, functional imaging and susceptibility weighted imaging. A low flip angle, long echo time and long repetition time makes the GRE T2* sequence.

Susceptibility-weighted imaging uses phase information in addition to T2* to develop the magnetic susceptibility differences in blood, iron, and calcium in various tissues.

Motor vehicle accident of a 20-year-old male reported with neck pain and loss of function at the wrists, hands, shoulders and upper arms.

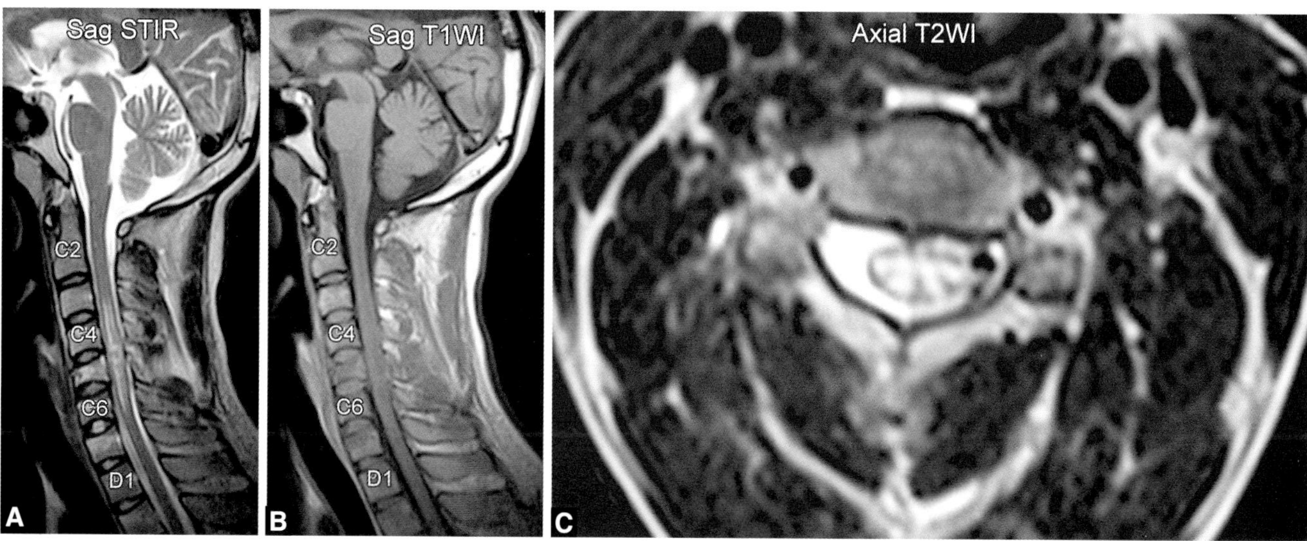

Figs 7A to C

Answer: Compression fracture of fifth cervical vertebra with cord hematoma and edema.

Sagittal STIR (Fig. 7A), T1W (Fig. 7B) and axial T2W (Fig. 7C) images reveal compression fracture of C5. Hyperintense signal is seen in the C4 to C7 vertebral bodies on STIR images. It appears hypointense on T1W images and represents edema. Focal cord hematoma is seen at C4-5 level with surrounding edema.

Flexion compression fracture is the result of a combination of flexion and compression, which is usually the result of a motor vehicle accident. With a pure flexion injury, a longitudinal pull is exerted on the nuchal ligament complex which because of its strength usually remains intact. The anterior vertebral body bears most of the force, sustaining simple wedge compression anteriorly without any posterior disruption.

In some cases, the larger posterior part of the vertebral body is displaced backward into the spinal canal of these over 70 percent of patients have neurological deficit. The MR-images demonstrate the spinal injury.

There is a strong correlation between the length of the spinal cord edema and the clinical outcome. The most important factor however is whether there is hemorrhage, since hemorrhagic spinal cord injury has a poor outcome.

A 46-year-old male patient presented with left sided weakness since 3 weeks.

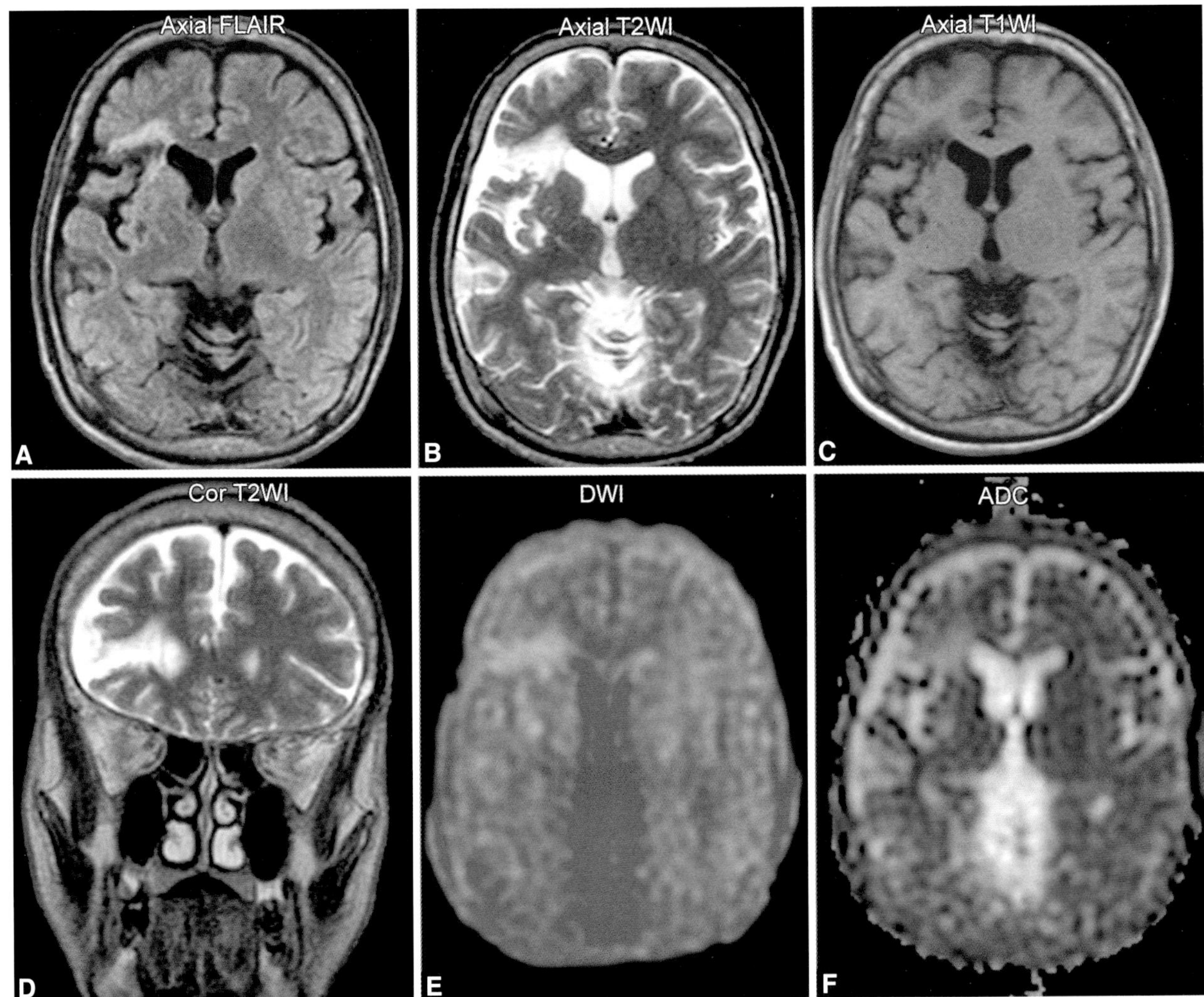

Figs 8A to F

Answer: Perisylvian infarct.

MRI brain reveals hyperintense signal on T2W and FLAIR images (Figs 8A, B and D) without any restricted diffusion (Figs 8E and F) in the right perisylvian region appearing hypointense on T1W image (Fig. 8C) with ex vacuo dilatation of the right lateral ventricle.

A cerebral infarction is the ischemic stroke due to a disturbance in the blood vessels supplying blood to the brain. It can be atherothrombotic or embolic. A cerebral infarction occurs when a blood vessel that supplies a part of the brain becomes blocked or leakage occurs outside the vessel walls. This loss of blood supply results in the death of that area of tissue. Cerebral infarctions vary in their severity.

Ischemic infarcts in the perisylvian region involving the insular cortex or corticobulbar tracts can cause opercular syndrome. It is characterized by a loss of voluntary control of facial, lingual, pharyngeal and masticatory muscles. There is a preservation of reflexive and automatic function of the same muscles.

Diffusion weighted MRI can detect ischemia much earlier than standard CT scan or MRI and provides useful data in stroke and TIA patients outside of the initial management window. Diffusion weighted magnetic resonance imaging provides potentially unique information on the viability of brain tissue. It provides image contrast that is dependent on the molecular motion of water, which may be substantially altered by disease.

Acute infarct is bright on DWI image and old infarct (encephalomalacia) is low signal intensity on DWI.

A 15-year-old female patient with history of recurrent episodes headache, giddiness and loss of consciousness over last three years.

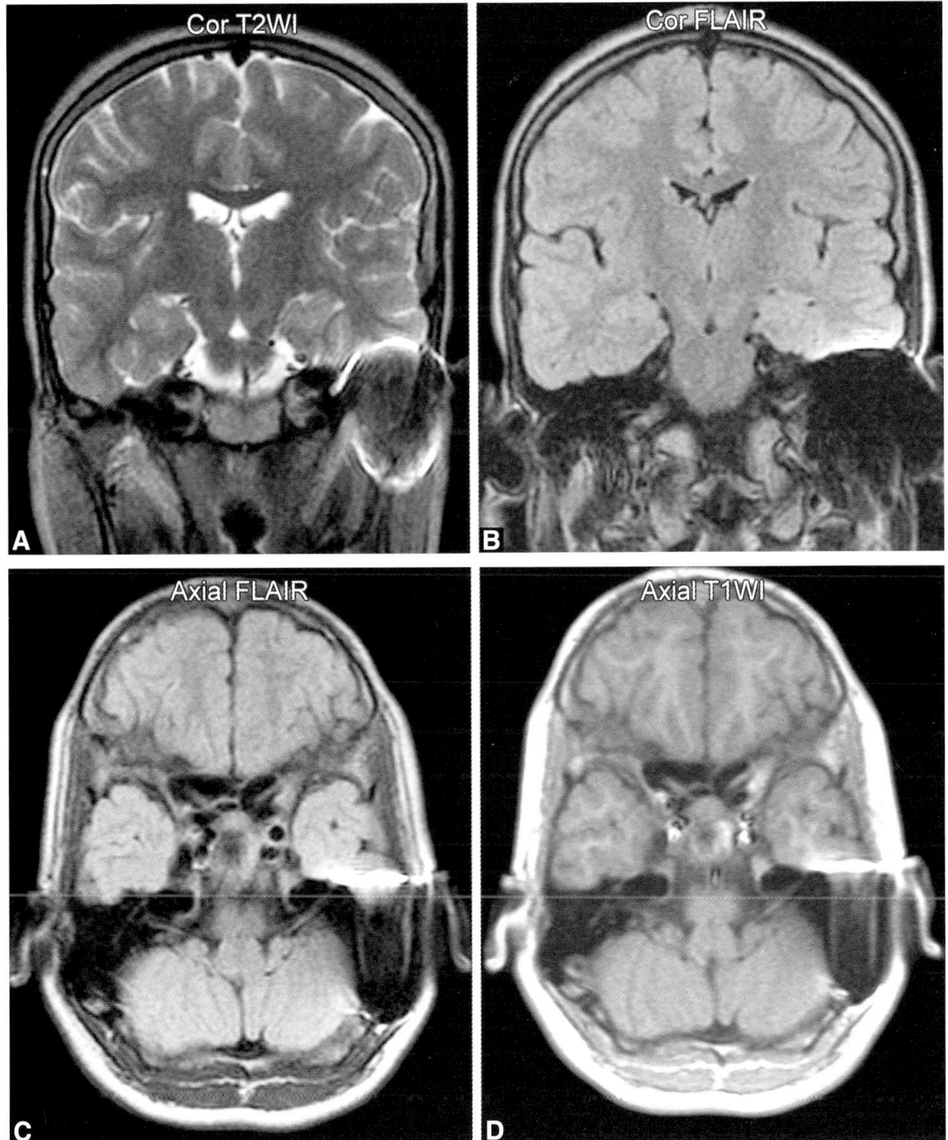

Figs 9A to D

Susceptibility artefact is seen in the petrous portion of the left temporal bone (Figs 9A to D).

Answer: Magnetic susceptibility artifact due to foreign body in left external auditory canal. Small pebble and plastic stud as foreign body was found and removed from the left external auditory canal.

Magnetic susceptibility is tendency of material to become magnetized when placed in magnetic field. Caused by material with large differences in susceptibility create local disturbance in magnetic field resulting in nonlinear changes of resonant frequency, which in turn creates image distortion and signal changes leading to signal void in image.

A 27-year-old male presented with abdominal distension and tremors since 2 years.

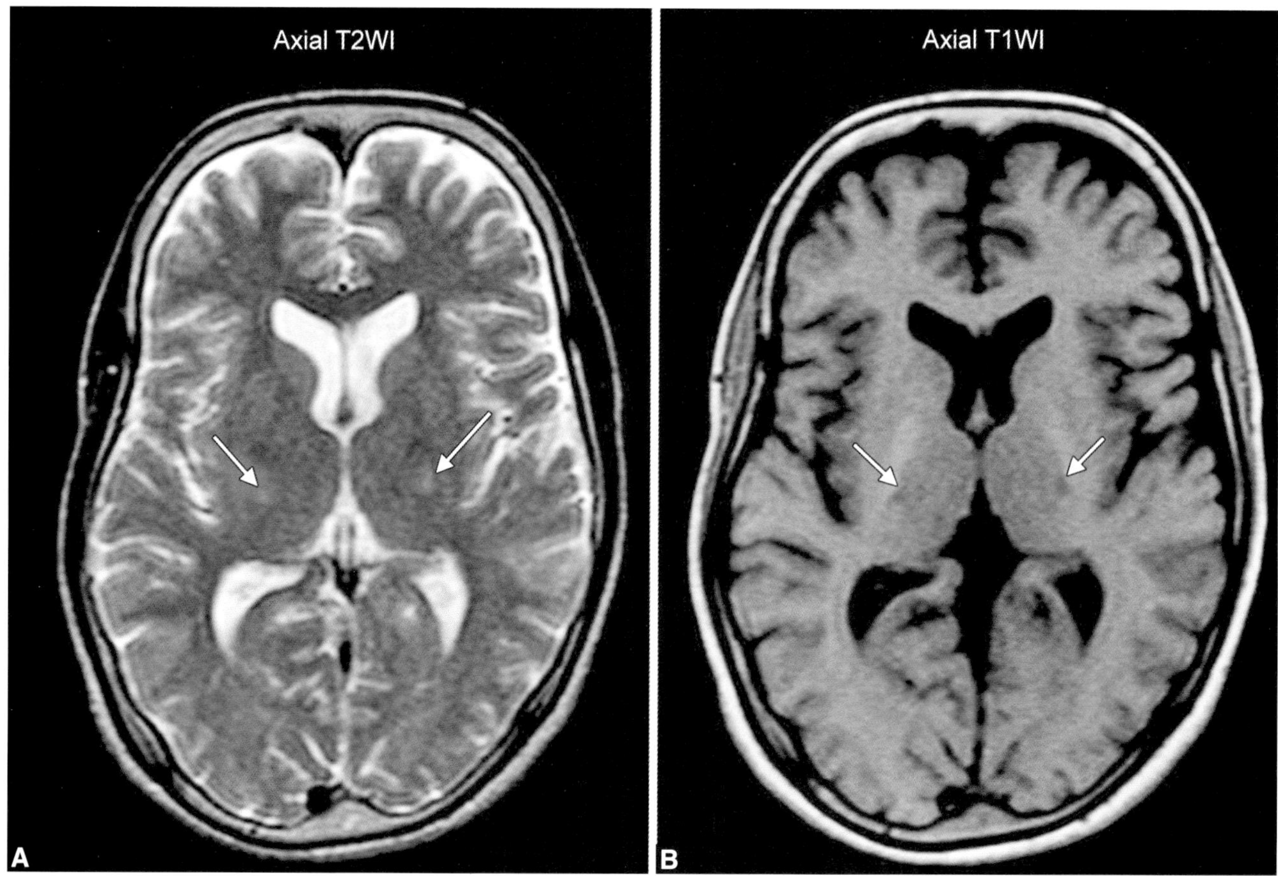

Figs 10A and B

Answer: Wilson's disease.

MR revealed symmetrical hyperintense signal in both lentiform nuclei (globus pallidi) on (Fig. 10A) T2W image (arrow) and hypointense on (Fig. 10B) T1W image (arrow) and represents hepatolenticular degeneration disease. Ophthalmic examination revealed bilateral Kayser Fleischer rings.

Wilson's disease is called as hepatolenticular degeneration, a disorder of copper metabolism with decreased biliary excretion of copper and accumulation of copper within organs. Copper gets accumulated in the CNS, liver, kidney and cornea. Biochemically, there is reduced or absent circulatory ceruloplasmin. The prevalence is about 1:30,000. Clinical symptomatology includes signs of hepatitis, liver cirrhosis and central nervous system disorders. Clinical manifestations are variable and may be acute with an acute psychotic onset or progressive lethargy, abdominal pain, malaise, tremors, dysarthria and disturbed motor function. On examination of the eye, there is the presence of Kayser-Fleischer (KF) rings around the cornea. KF rings are dark rings that appear to encircle the iris of the eye. They are due to copper deposition as a result of particular liver diseases. They are named after the German doctors Dr Bernhard Kayser and Dr Bruno Fleischer. KF rings do not cause any symptoms, they may be detected in early stages by slit-lamp examination before they become visible to the naked eye.

There may be renal dysfunction, jaundice and hepatomegaly. Radiological manifestations are nonspecific and include osteopenia, rickets and an enlarged liver. On MRI of the brain, there is bilateral decreased signal intensity on T1, with increased signal density on T2 weighted images in the lentiform nucleus, thalami, caudate and dentate nuclei, and occasionally in the brainstem.

A 27-year-old male presented with history of shoulder dislocation.

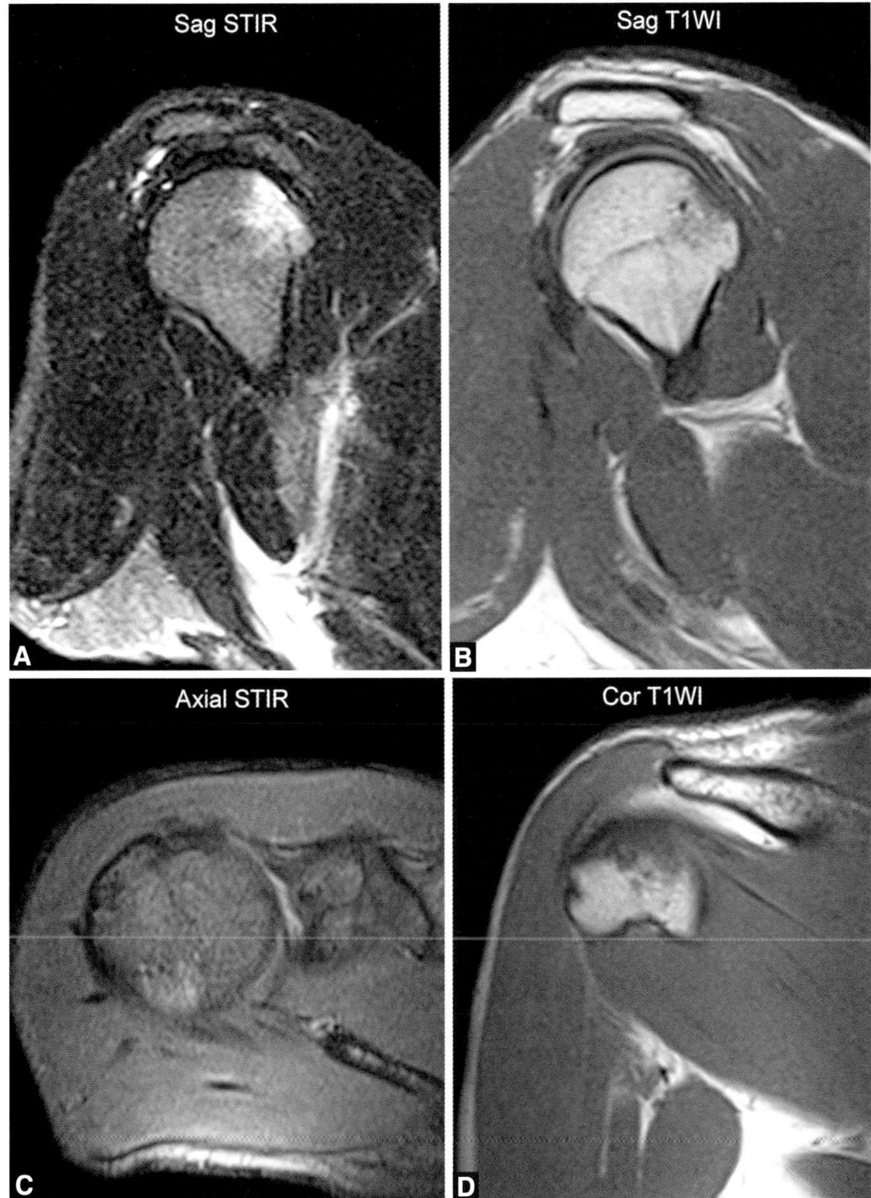

Figs 11A to D

Answer: Hill-Sachs lesion.

Hyperintense signal noted along the posterosuperior aspect of the humeral head on sagittal STIR and axial STIR images (Figs 11A and C) appearing hypointense on sagittal T1 W and coronal T1 WI images (Figs 11B and D), findings are suggestive of Hill-Sachs lesion.

Hill-Sachs lesions are associated exclusively with anterior shoulder dislocations. When the humerus is driven out from the glenohumeral cavity, head being relatively soft it impacts against the anterior edge of the glenoid. The result is a divot or flattening in the posteromedial aspect of the humeral head, typically referred to as a 3 to 6 o'clock lesion for the right humeral head if seen from the bottom. The mechanism which leads to shoulder dislocation is often traumatic but may occur with history of previous dislocations. Sports, fall, seizure, assault, throwing, pulling on the arm, or just turning over in bed can be a cause of anterior shoulder dislocation.

A 32-year-old male, athlete with history of ankle pain.

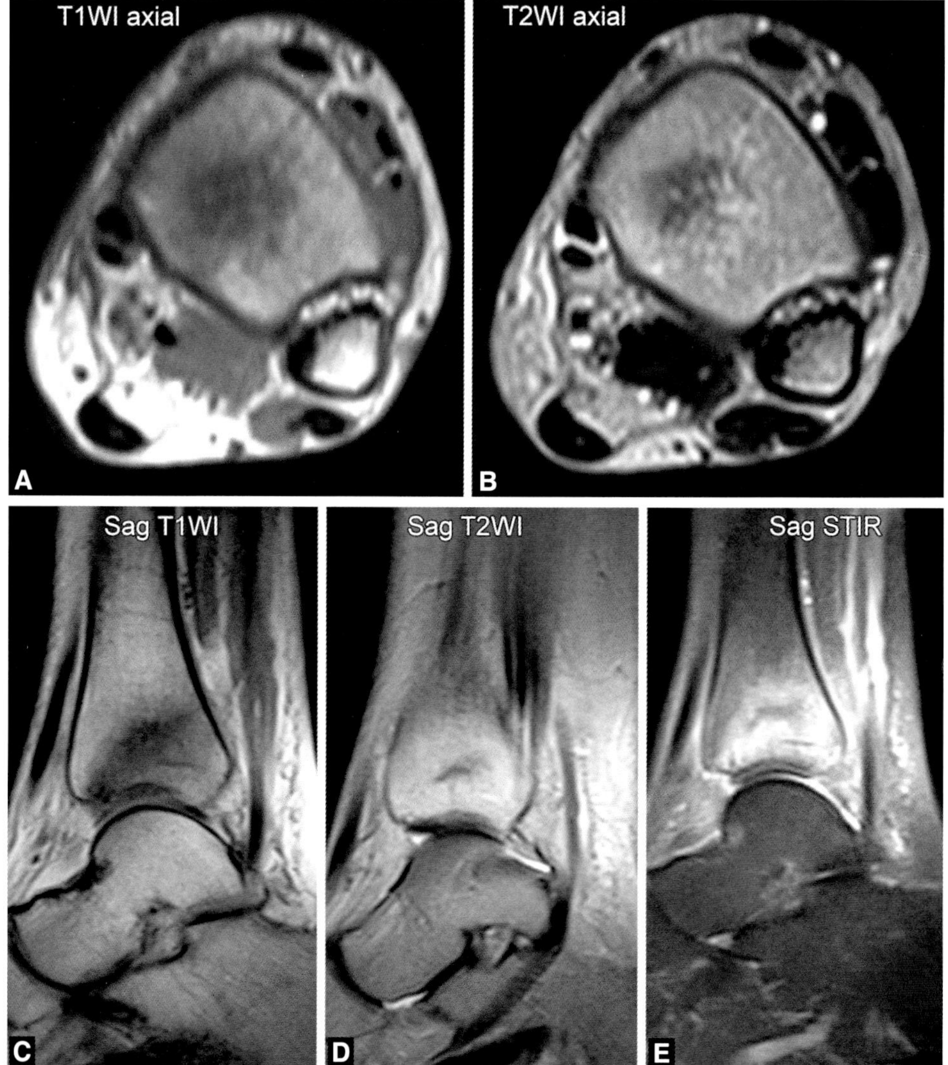

Figs 12A to E

Answer: Stress fracture at distal metaphysis of tibia.

A linear zone of low signal intensity which indicates fracture line with surrounding broader, poorly defined area of higher signal intensity suggestive of marrow edema on T2-weighted and STIR (Figs 12D and E) MR images and appearing hypointense on T1W image (Fig. 12C). Similar changes are seen on axial images (Figs 12A and B).

Stress fracture occurs due to injury to normal or abnormal bone that results from repeated cyclic loading. Two types of stress fracture are recognized: fatigue fracture, which occurs after application of abnormal stress to a bone with normal elastic resistance; and insufficiency fracture, which results when normal stress is placed on a bone with deficient elastic resistance. Typical examples of fatigue fractures are those occurring in the metatarsal bones of military recruits (march fracture), and in the lower extremities in athletes, joggers and dancers.

Routine radiography plays an essential role in the diagnosis of stress fractures; however, scintigraphy possesses greater diagnostic sensitivity. Stress fractures are associated with focal fusiform, sharply marginated areas of increased radionuclide activity. In addition, MR imaging has comparable sensitivity and superior specificity to bone scintigraphy in the assessment of stress fractures.

A 10-year-old female presented with pain and swelling in right lower leg.

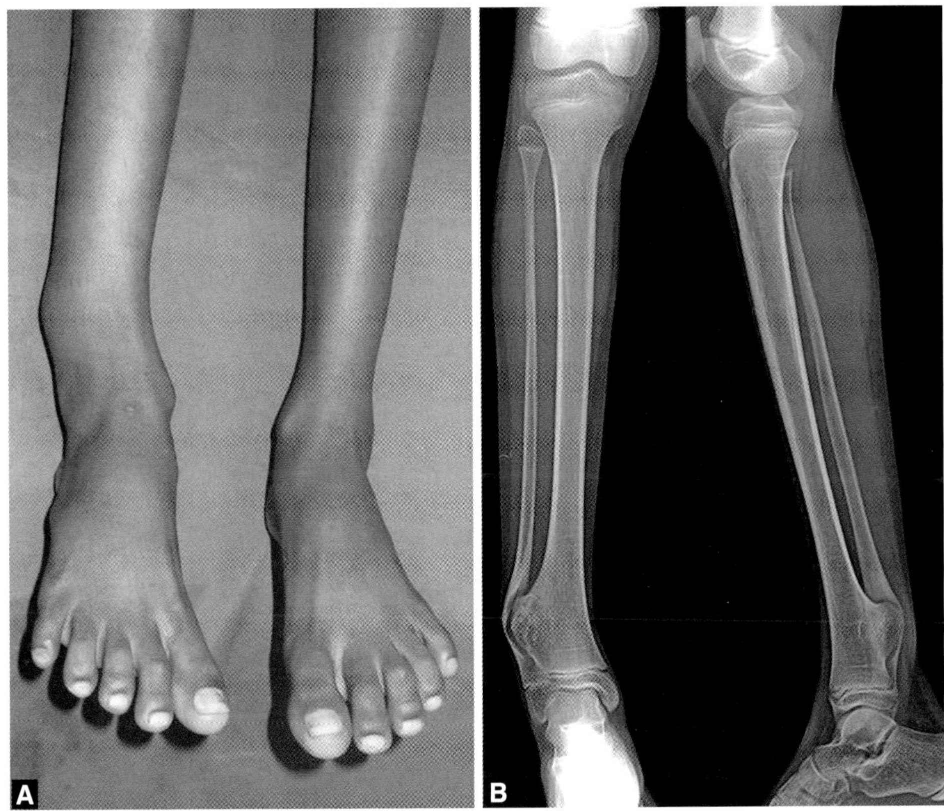

Figs 13A and B: (A) Photograph both legs and feet shows deformity at the distal part of right leg; (B) X-ray right leg and ankle, AP and lateral views reveal a sessile bony outgrowth from right lower tibia lateral aspect with continuity of cortex and medullary cavity with the parent bone, causing significant pressure erosion and thinning of the adjoining fibula

Osteochondroma is the most common benign tumor or tumorlike lesion of bone. An osteochondroma is a cartilage-covered bony excrescence (exostosis) that arises from the surface of a bone. The radiographic appearance of this tumor is often diagnostic and reflects its pathologic characteristics, that is, a lesion composed of cortical and medullary bone with an overlying hyaline cartilage cap. However, it is the continuity of this lesion with the underlying native bone cortex and medullary canal that is pathognomonic of osteochondroma (Figs 13A and B).

Osteochondromas may be solitary or multiple, and they may arise spontaneously or as a result of previous osseous trauma. An osteochondroma can affect any bone preformed in cartilage. Most solitary osteochondromas are discovered incidentally in children and adolescents. Hereditary multiple exostoses (HME), also known as osteochondromatosis, is an inherited, autosomal dominant disorder in which multiple osteochondromas are seen throughout the skeleton. Complications of osteochondromas include fractures, bony deformities, neurologic and vascular injuries, bursa formation, and malignant transformation.

Most osteochondromas, solitary or multiple, arise from tubular bones and are metaphyseal in location. The lesion is composed of cortical and medullary bone protruding from and continuous with the underlying bone. The areas of osseous continuity between parent bone and osteochondroma may be broad-sessile osteochondroma, or narrow, with a bulbous tip-pedunculated osteochondroma. Identifying the characteristic cortical and medullary continuity between lesion and parent bone on

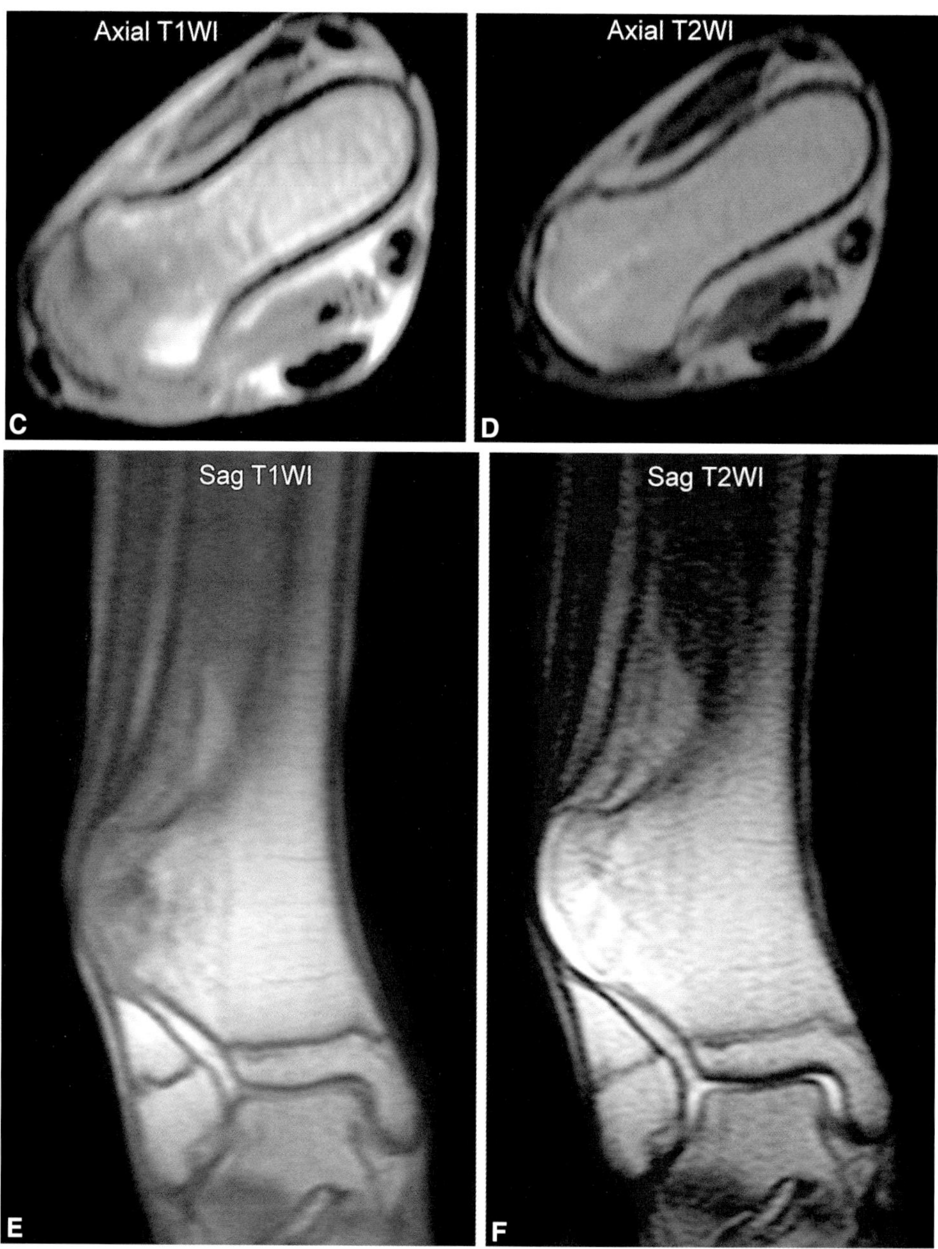

Figs 13C to F: Mineralized areas in the cartilage cap remain low signal intensity with all MR pulse sequences. The high water content in nonmineralized portions of the cartilage cap had intermediate to low signal intensity on T1-weighted images and very high signal intensity on T2-weighted MR images

radiographs is dependent on lesion type (sessile or pedunculated), location, and image projection. Pedunculated lesions usually point away from the nearest joint owing to the forces of the overlying tendons and ligaments.

MR imaging also demonstrates cortical and medullary continuity between the osteochondroma and parent bone, cortical bone remains low signal intensity with all pulse sequences, whereas the medullary component has an appearance of yellow marrow (Figs 13C to F). MR imaging is the best radiologic modality for visualizing the effect of the lesion on surrounding structures and evaluating the hyaline cartilage cap.

A 20-year-old male patient with history of wrist pain.

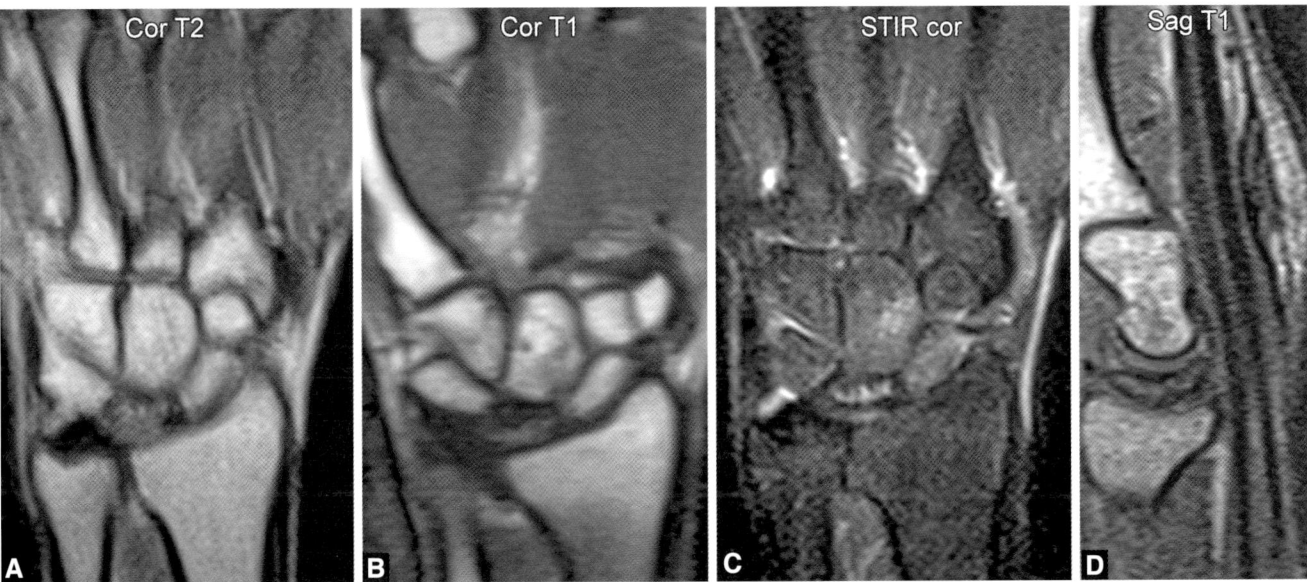

Figs 14A to D

Answer: Kienbock's disease.

Abnormal hyperintense signal with marrow edema noted on coronal T2WI (Fig. 14A) and STIR (Fig. 14C) images in lunate bone, appearing hypointense on coronal T1WI (Fig. 14B) and sagittal T1WI (Fig. 14D). Findings are suggestive of Kienbock's disease.

Kienbock's disease is osteonecrosis of the carpal lunate bone that often follows a history of trauma. It is more common in adults but is occasionally seen in children, typically athletic adolescents and particularly gymnasts. The patient may experience progressive pain, swelling and disability. On radiographs the lunate may have a normal architecture and density initially, although a linear or compression fracture may be present. Later the lunate bone becomes denser than the other carpal bones and eventually the entire lunate may collapse and fragment. Complications include scapholunate dissociation and secondary degenerative joint disease. The two features of the lunate that may predispose this bone to injury and subsequent osteonecrosis are its vulnerable blood supply and its fixed position in the wrist, which leads to stress.

MR imaging shows initial decreased signal on T1- and increased signal on T2-weighted or STIR sequences reflecting edema. Later there will be decreased signal or signal void on T1- and T2-weighted sequences reflecting bone death or sclerosis, this signal void may be limited to the body of the lunate. There may be an associated synovitis seen best on intravenous contrast-enhanced fat suppressed T1-weighted sequences.

A 15-year-old female patient presented with complaint of left leg pain since seven months.

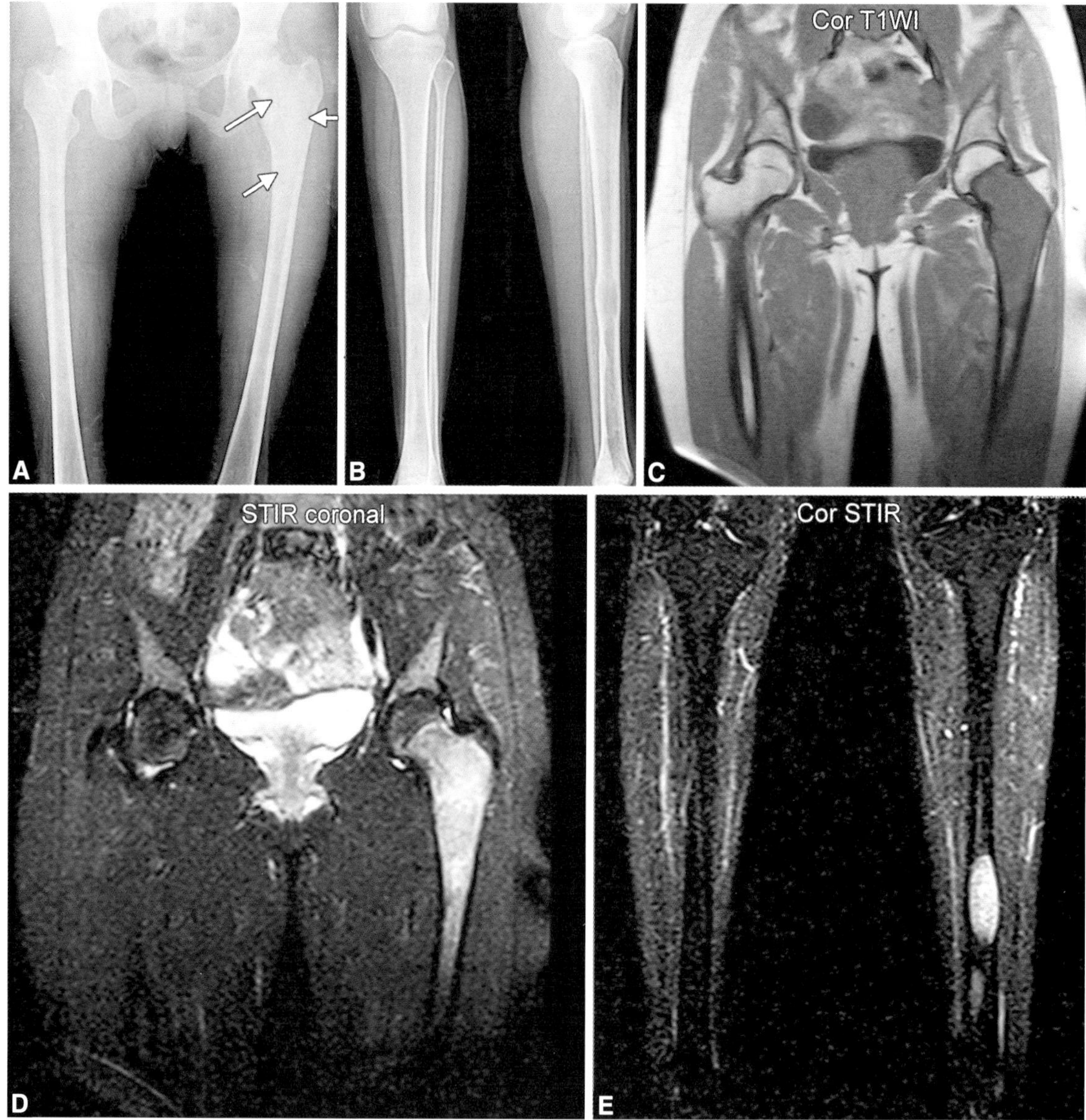

Figs 15A to E

Answer: Polyostotic fibrous dysplasia.

X-ray of both hips and thigh AP (Fig. 15A) view shows expansile trabeculated lytic lesion in left femoral meta-diaphysis causing expansion of medullary cavity with thinning of cortex. X-ray left leg including knee joint, AP and lateral view (Fig. 15B) shows expansile lytic lesion seen in distal third shaft of tibia causing expansion of medullary cavity and thinning of cortex. T1W coronal image shows iso to hypointense lesion in meta-diaphyseal region of left femur causing expansion of medullary cavity and thining of cortex (Fig. 15C). Coronal STIR image (Fig. 15D) shows the lesion as hyperintense. STIR coronal (Fig. 15E) image of left leg shows hyperintense lesion in distal third of left tibia causing expansion of medullary cavity and thinning of cortices. These findings suggest diagnosis of polyostotic fibrous dysplasia.

Fibrous dysplasia (FD) is a benign lesion, manifested as a defect in osteoblastic differentiation and maturation, with progressive replacement of normal bone with immature woven bone. Fibrous dysplasia can affect any bone. In 20 to 30 percent of cases multiple bones are involved (polyostotic FD). Polyostotic fibrous dysplasia typically present in early childhood (mean age of 8 years). Often unilateral and monomelic. Plain films demonstrate well circumscribed lesions with ground-glass opacities, may be completely lucent (cystic) or sclerotic. It may lead to premature fusion of growth plates leading to short stature, bowing deformities, Shepherd's crook deformity of femoral neck, discrepant limb length and looser zones. On MRI lesions show heterogeneous intermediate signal on T1W images and heterogeneously low signal on T2W images but may have regions of higher signal. Post-contrast T1W images show heterogeneous contrast enhancement (Figs 15A to E). Bone scans demonstrate increased tracer uptake on Tc^{99} bone scans.

A 45-year-old female with history of swelling along the medial aspect of right thigh.

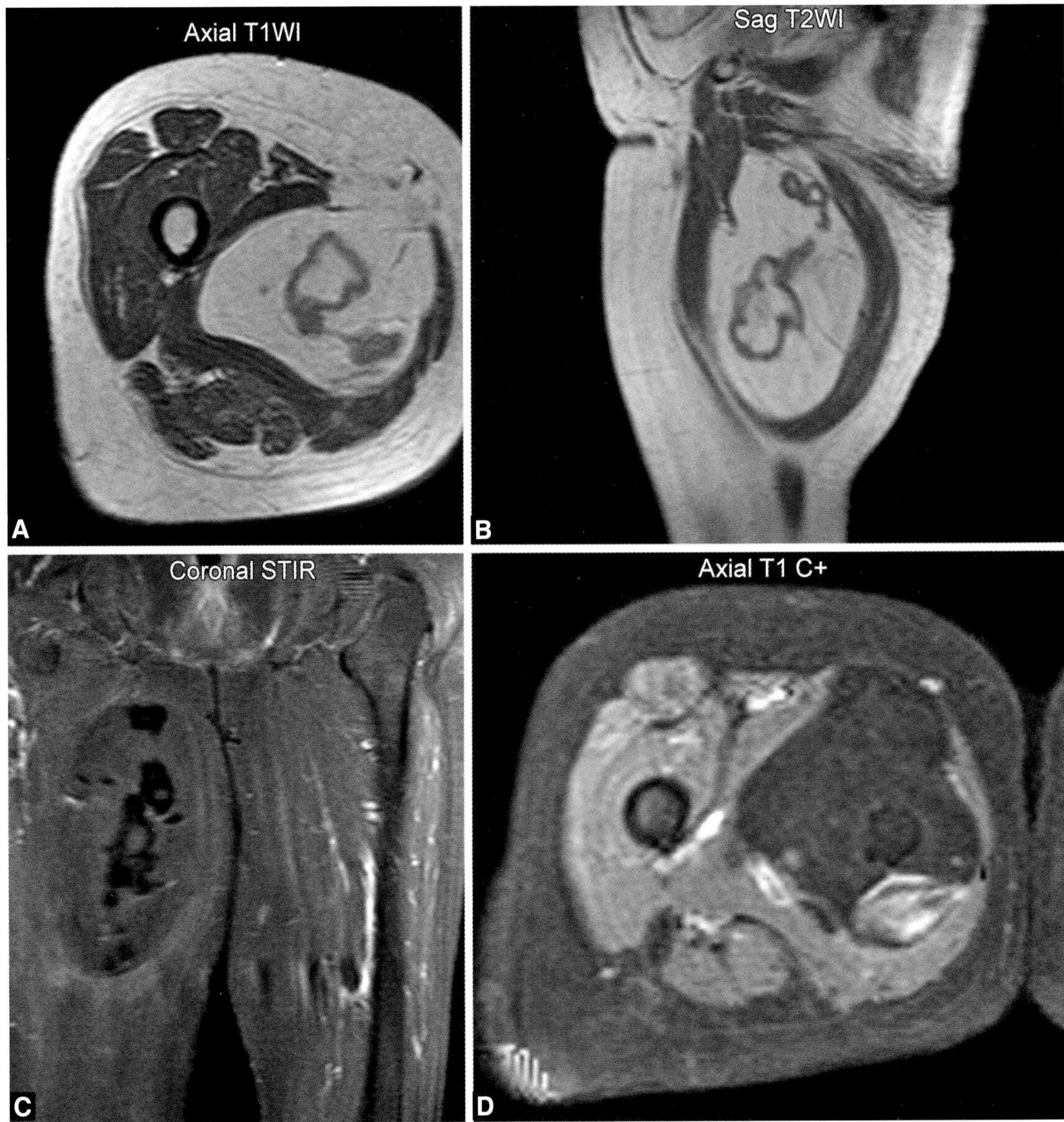

Figs 16A to D

Answer: Liposarcoma.

A large well-defined fat intensity lesion is seen in the medial aspect of thigh between the adductor and gracilis muscles on axial T1W1 (Fig. 16A) and sagittal T2W images (Fig. 16B). It is mildly heterogenous with few central septations. On coronal STIR image (Fig. 16C) there is homogeneous suppression of fat. Mild enhancement is seen on post-contrast image (Fig. 16D). No evidence of invasion or infiltration. Neurovascular bundle appears normal.

Liposarcoma is malignant tumor that arises in fat cells in deep soft tissue, such as that inside the thigh or in the retroperitoneum. Most frequent in middle-aged and older adults (above 40 years). Liposarcomas are the second most common of all soft-tissue sarcomas following malignant fibrous histiocytomas. Patients usually note a deep seated mass in their soft tissue. Only when the tumor is very large symptoms of pain or functional disturbances occur.

A 3-month-old baby with history of swelling over dorsolumbar region since birth.

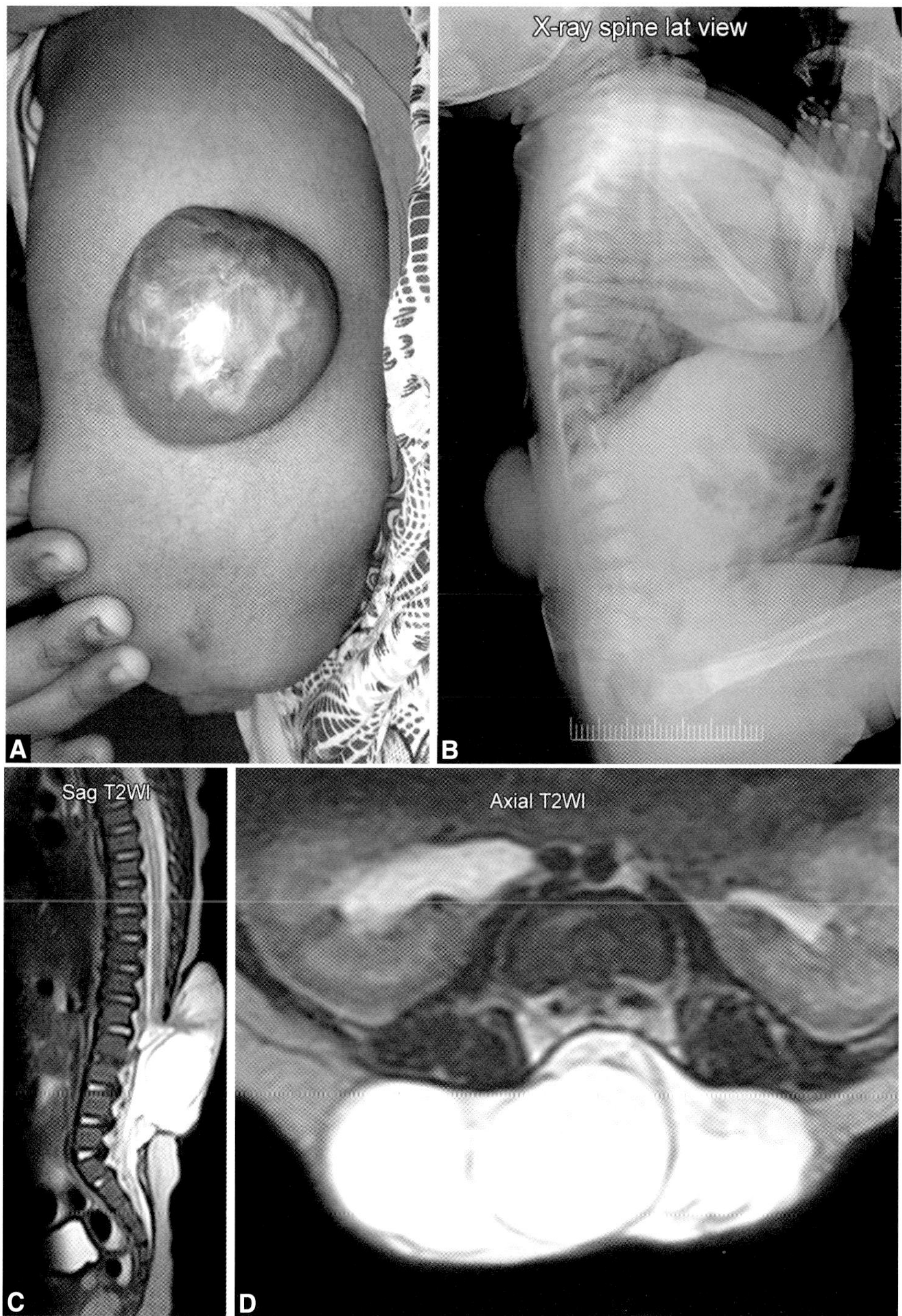

Figs 17A to D
(For color version of Figs A and B, see Plate 2)

Answer: Meningomyelocele.

X-ray spine reveals posterior soft tissue swelling in lower back overlying dorsolumbar spine (Figs 17A and B) with increased interpedicular distance (Figs 17C to F). On sagittal and axial T2W (Figs 17C and D) and T1W (Figs 17E and F) images reveals defect in the posterior elements of lumbar L2 to L5 vertebrae with herniation of meninges, lower end of cord and nerve roots in the CSF intensity pouch into the overlying subcutaneous region. Meningomyelocele is herniation of the spinal cord and meninges through a defect in the vertebral canal. The origin of meningomyelocele is not completely known. It is one of the commonest congenital CNS anomalies. There may be a slight female predilection. Patients present with a lower limb paralysis and sensory loss, bladder and bowel dysfunction as well as cognitive impairment. This defect is the most common cause of neuropathic osteoarthropathy in children, in whom the ankle and tarsal joints are the primary sites of involvement.

Myelomeningocele may be associated with vertebral hypoplasia, hemivertebra, laminar and pedicular fusion, diastematomyelia, kyphosis, scoliosis, pes cavus deformity and lipoma.

CT scanning, with or without the administration of contrast agents, or MR show the vertebral and neural abnormalities.

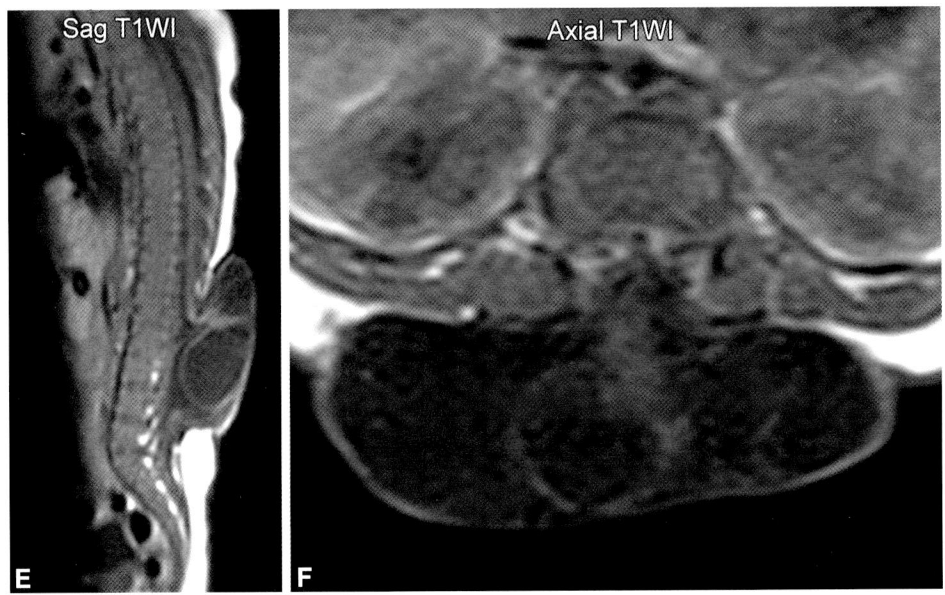

Figs 17E and F

An 8-month-old female infant presented with history of no neck holding, no rolling over, generalized tonic clonic convulsions and blindness.

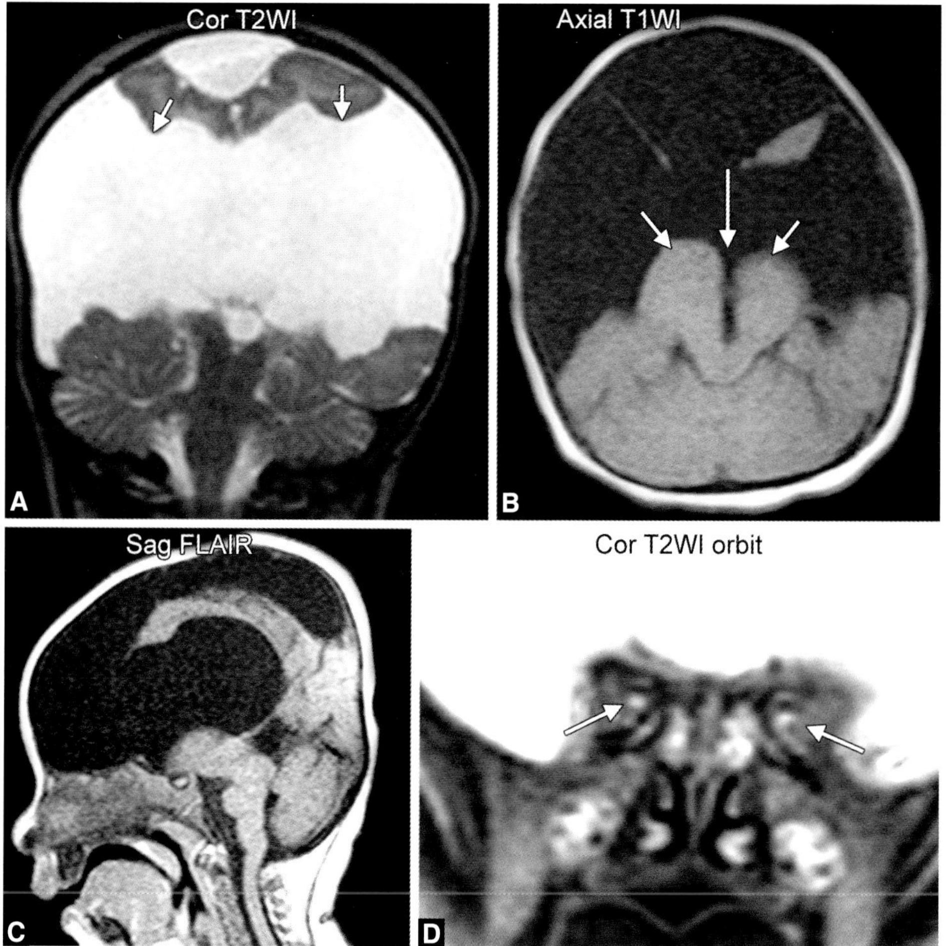

Figs 18A to D

Answer: Open lip schizencephaly with septo-optic dysplasia.

MRI revealed large, bilateral, fronto-parietal (arrows), wedge shaped CSF clefts (Fig. 18A). These clefts are lined with gray matter. The cerebral parenchyma in these regions is deficient. Both lateral ventricles are dilated. The thalami (small arrows) are separated by normal appearing third (long arrow) ventricle (Fig. 18B). Fourth ventricle, brainstem and cerebellum were normal. A small portion of frontal and temporal lobes was seen bilaterally. Corpus callosum and cavum septum pellucidum are absent (Fig. 18C). CSF spaces around the bilateral optic nerve were prominent (arrows) indicating optic atrophy (Fig. 18D).

Schizencephaly is an uncommon congenital disorder of cerebral cortical development, defined as a gray matter lined cleft extending from the pial surface to the ventricle.

It is known that schizencephaly and septo-optic dysplasia frequently coexist and that both are associated with absence of the septum pellucidum.

An 8-month-old child with developmental delay.

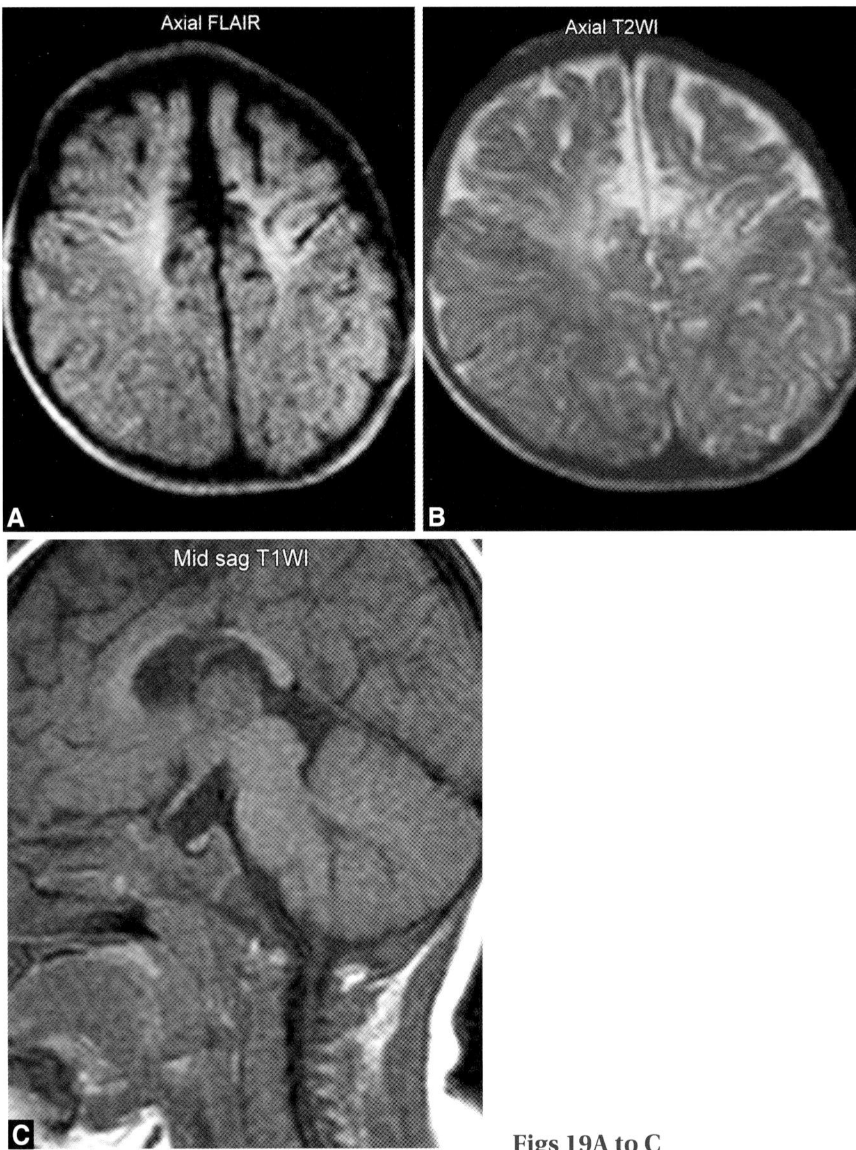

Figs 19A to C

Answer: Hypoxic ischemic encephalopathy.

MRI brain reveals on FLAIR and T2WI hyperintense signals (Figs 19A and B) in white matter of bilateral frontoparietal regions with crowding of gyri, deep sulci, and white matter volume loss and thinning of corpus callosum (Fig. 19C).

Areas of high signal intensity in the white matter dorsal and superior to the ventricular trigones occur in many children on long TR/TE images. These have been attributed to the known physiological delay in myelination of fiber tracts involving parietal and temporal association areas, and have been called "terminal zones."

Distinction between these periventricular areas of high signal and mild periventricular leukomalacia is difficult, but is facilitated by preservation of a layer of myelinated white matter between the ventricle and the areas of high signal in normal subjects. This layer is absent in periventricular leukomalacia.

An 11-year-old male child presented with history of convulsions.

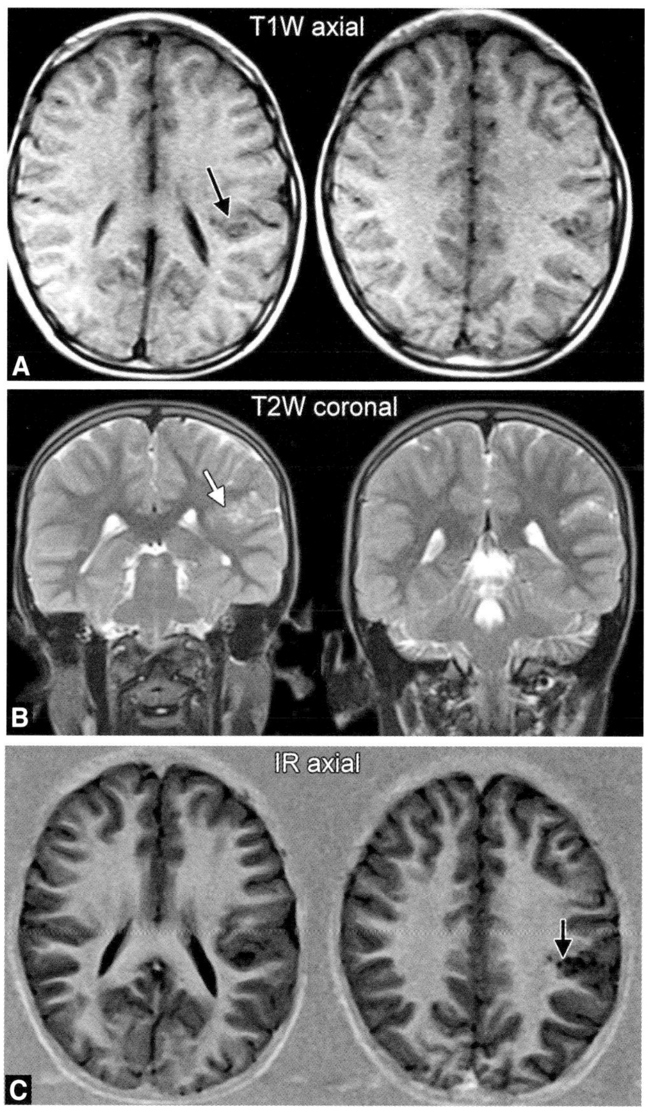

Figs 20A to C

Answer: Dysembryoplastic neuroepithelial tumor (DNET).

T1W axial images (Fig. 20A) of the brain show an area of thickened cortex (arrow) in left parietal region appearing heterogeneously hypointense. On T2W coronal images (Fig. 20B) the lesion appears heterogeneously hyperintense and shows cystic areas within it. There is no evidence of perilesional edema or mass effect or calcification. Inversion Recovery (IR) images (Fig. 20C) show thickened cortex and cystic hypointense areas (arrow) in left parietal region.

DNET is a benign (WHO Grade I) slow growing tumor arising in majority of cases from either cortical or deep gray matter. They are thought to arise from secondary germinal layer and are frequently (80% of cases) associated with coexistent cortical dysplasia, and are characteristically the cause of intractable partial seizures. On MRI, DNET is seen as a cortical lesion with hardly any surrounding vasogenic edema. The lesion appears hypointense on T1W sequence and hyperintense on T2W sequence.

A 68-year-old male with progressive pain and limp came to radiology department for MRI both hips.

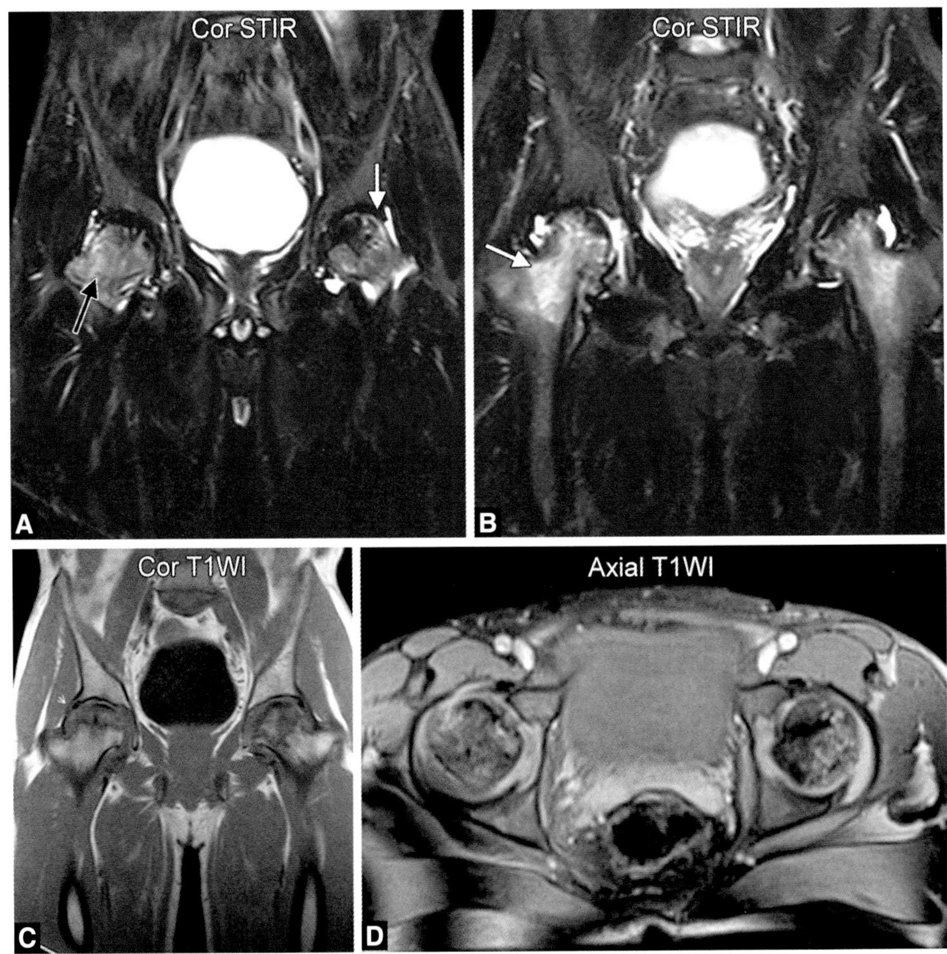

Figs 21A to D

Answer: Avascular necrosis both femoral heads.

Coronal STIR (Figs 21A and B) images show well defined crescents of altered marrow signal in the subchondral regions of bilateral femoral heads. Marrow within the crescent is hyperintense on T2W images and hypointense on coronal T1W images (Figs 21C and D). There is loss of normal contour of bilateral femoral heads with degenerative changes in the form of osteophytes (arrow). Marrow edema is seen in the bilateral femoral head, neck and acetabulum. Minimal joint effusion is noted on either side. Coronal T1W (Fig. 21C) and axial T1W (Fig. 21D) images. Well defined crescents of altered marrow signal are seen in the subchondral regions of bilateral femoral heads. Marrow within the crescent is hypointense on T1W images. Findings are consistent with Grade IV (AVN).

According to Ficat and Arlet classification for AVN of the femoral heads which uses a combination of clinical features, plain film and MRI, the features of Grade IV AVN are

- Clinical symptoms of pain and limp
- *X-ray:* The femoral head undergoes further collapse, leading to articular cartilage destruction and joint space narrowing with evidence of secondary degenerative change in hip joint
- *MRI:* Shows loss of normal contour and collapse of femoral head and secondary degenerative changes in hip joint.

A 25-year-old male patient with history of shoulder pain.

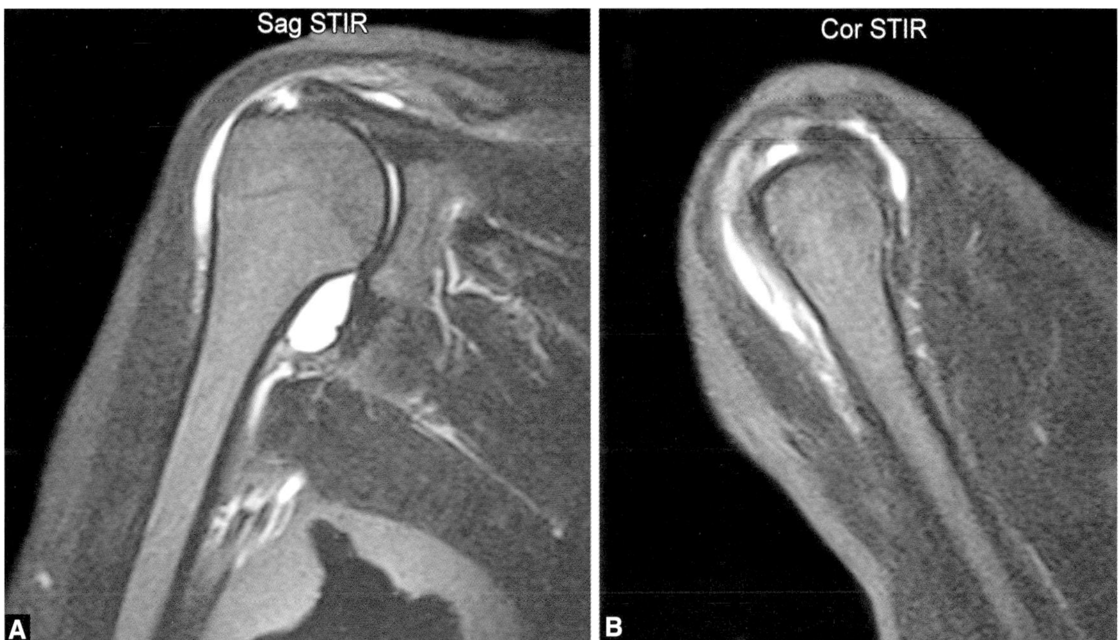

Figs 22A and B

Answer: Supraspinatus muscle tear.

Complete tear is seen in the supraspinatus tendon with mild joint effusion (Figs 22A and B). Tear of the rotator cuff may be complete (full thickness) or incomplete (partial thickness). Precipitating factors include trauma, attrition, ischemia, and impingement.

MR imaging is useful, where the high signal intensity of tendons on T2 weighted and STIR sequences, is indicative of tears. Full-thickness tears of the rotator cuff are characterized by presence of a tendinous defect that is filled with fluid or granulation tissue and retraction of the musculotendinous junction.

Partial-thickness tears often appear on MRI as only an intermediate signal, isointense to muscle, which disrupts the normal low-signal surface of the rotator cuff. Magnetic resonance arthrography can improve the differentiation of rotator cuff degeneration from partial or complete rotator cuff tears. In complete tears an abnormal communication between the glenohumeral joint and bursa allows contrast material to collect within the subacromial bursa.

MRI Artifacts 9

Manisha Hadgaonkar

Artifacts are imaging findings that are not actual part the original image or what the image should have been. It is important to recognize them, so that misdiagnosis can be avoided as they can sufficiently degrade images to cause a misdiagnosis; it can obscure pathology or create a false one. Sources of such artifacts can be broadly divided into:

- Motion related artifacts
- Nonmotional artifacts.

MOTION RELATED ARTIFACTS

Motion related artifacts can be again divided into:

- Gross body movement related artifacts
- Physiological motion related artifacts.

Gross Body Movement Related Artifacts

Magnetic resonance imaging (MRI) is motion sensitive as the images are based on timing sequences; these cause artifacts to appear in reconstructed images. Movement can occur during RF pulses, between RF pulses, during data sampling and between phase-encoding sequences. Gross body movement in the patient may occur in all three dimensions but the artifacts propagate in the two dimensional phase-encoding dimension. Random patient movement, gastrointestinal peristalsis or eyeball movements may cause such artifacts. When motion is periodic occurring in a cyclical pattern it results in complete or incomplete replication of the affected voxels, commonly referred to as "Ghosting".

Physiological Motion Related Artifacts

Artifact can be caused by respiratory motion, cardiac motion or fluid tissue pulsation (blood flow, CSF flow). The ghosting artifact can arise from respiration due to high signal intensity of tissue which moves with breathing. These artifacts can be minimized using techniques such as: breath hold technique, respiratory gating, respiratory ordered phase encoding (ROPE), navigator gating, fat suppression sequences such as STIR sequences. Abdominal movement during respiration can be suppressed by using a compression belt across the abdomen.

In cardiac MRI, continuous contraction and dilatation of the cardiac chambers constitute a physiological motion resulting in blurring of cardiac structures. To eliminate such artifacts cardiac gating technique is used, the imaging sequence is triggered by the R-wave and the data is collected during the same period of the cardiac cycle for each TR period. Fluid pulsation artifacts due to pulsatile CSF flow may show on MRI as areas of signal void and also as ghosting in phase-encoding direction. Gradient movement rephrasing (GMR) is a method of balancing the phase for both stationary and moving nuclear spins. This technique has been successful in eliminating CSF pulsatile flow artifacts in gradient echo images of head and spine.

Fluid pulsation artifacts due to blood flow may produce a range of artifacts:

- Pulsatile blood flow may produce ghost artifacts in the phase-encoding direction

- Flowing blood can cause an anomalously low or high signal intensity
- Flow signal can be mismapped on the image and appear outside the vessel in the frequency encoding direction.

Techniques such as cardiac (peripheral) gating, swapping phase frequency encoding axes, presaturation pulses are useful to eliminate artifacts due to blood flow. Presaturation bands are used in spin echo imaging of the head and whole body, since venous and arterial blood flow occur in opposite directions, "presaturation slabs" are applied on either side of the imaging volume to saturate flow in either direction, this principle is important in MR angiography .

NONMOTIONAL ARTIFACTS

These can be broadly divided into:

- Patient related artifacts
- MRI scanner related artifacts.

Patient Related Artifacts

- *Extrinsic type:* Ferromagnetic metal artifacts show up as characteristic geometric distortion with a region of near zero signal intensity adjacent to a bright region (Figs 1A and B). Removal of the metal object eliminates this type of artifact.
- *Intrinsic type (magnetic susceptibility):* Diamagnetic effects are apparent at anatomical interfaces like between adjacent tissues depending on their degree of polarization with respect to the magnetic field applied. Tissues such as cortical bone or air filled cavities have little polarisable hydrogen atoms whereas soft tissues have hydrogen atoms in greater number available to get polarized by the magnetic field. The patient may also disturb the magnetic field because of increase in concentration of hemoglobin that may occur following bleeding, as concentrated hemoglobin is ferromagnetic due to its high iron content. Spin echo sequences minimize these type of artifacts. Chemical shift artifacts arise from the frequency difference between the hydrogen nuclei in water and the hydrogen nuclei in fat and tissues when subjected to the magnetic field. This frequency difference is defined as chemical shift in MR spectroscopy. It is usually expressed as a fraction of the Larmor frequency. Thus two static artifacts can be generated by chemical shift-signal misrepresentation and phase cancellation.

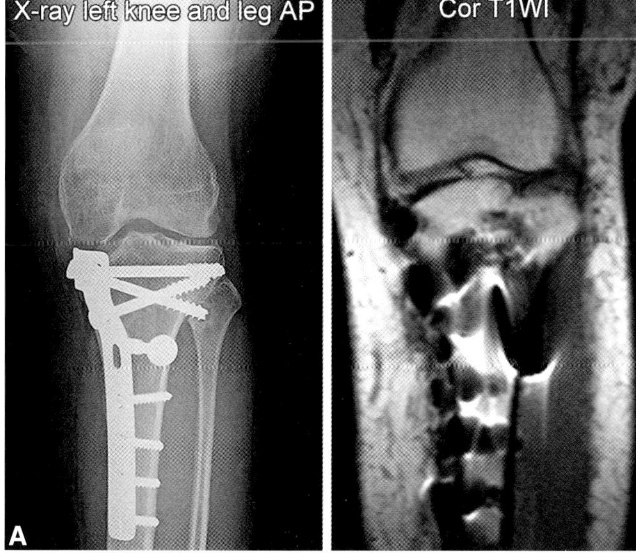

Fig. 1A: X-ray left leg AP view, tibia shows internal fixating metallic implant and coronal MR T1WI shows susceptibility artifact caused by the internal fixating metallic implant

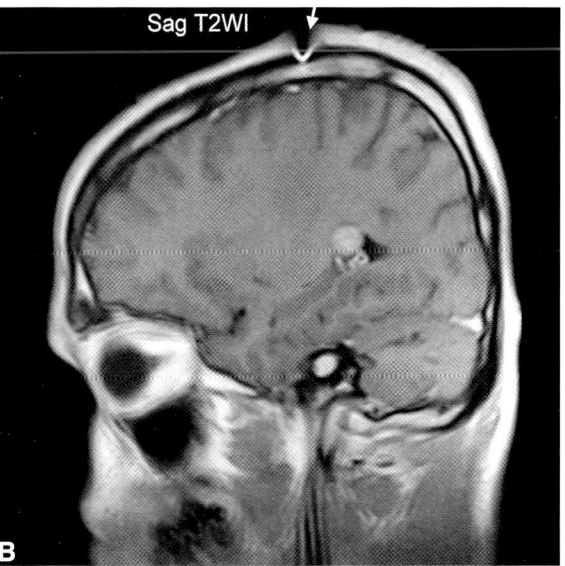

Fig. 1B: Sagittal T1WI shows susceptibility artifact over the scalp due to coupling gel used during EEG and patient was shifted for MRI

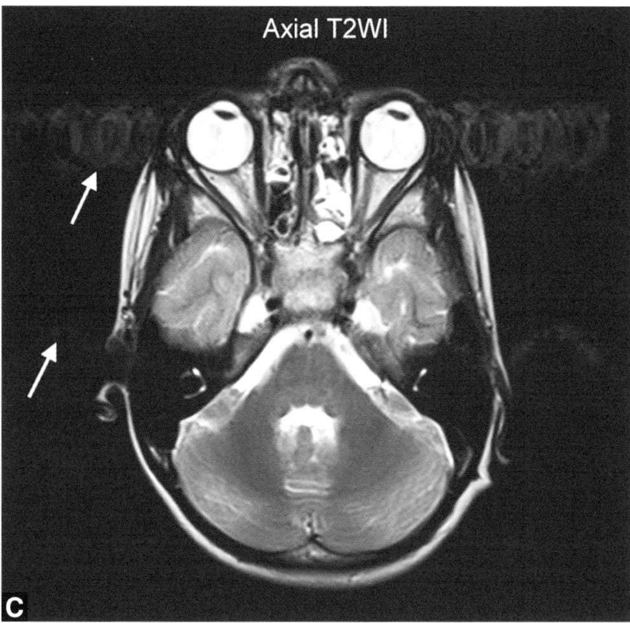

Fig. 1C: Multiple, regularly spaced parallel bands of alternating bright and dark signal seen parallel to the orbit and the petrous portion of the temporal bones. This is known as Gibbs artifact

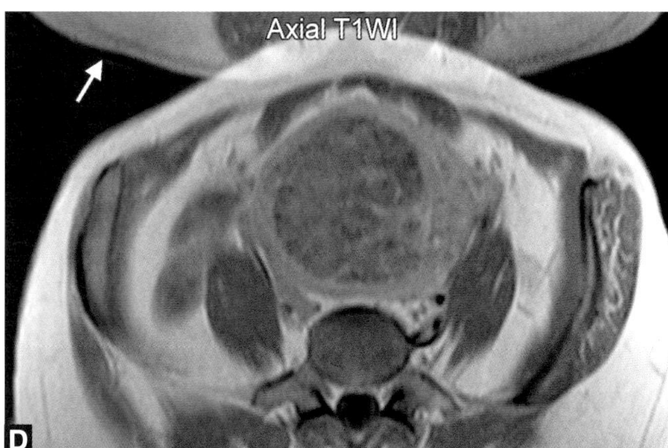

Fig. 1D: Axial T1WI shows overlapping wrap around of the posterior abdominal wall over the anterior known as wrap around artifact

Chemical shift artifacts can be minimized by performing imaging at low magnetic field strengths or by increasing the frequency bandwidth or by decreasing the field of view (FOV). This artifact can be used as advantage to confirm presence of fat in a lesion.

MRI Scanner Related Artifacts

- Gibbs phenomenon (ringing artifact) or truncation artifact. This is caused by the under-sampling of high spatial frequencies at sharp boundaries in the image. Lack of appropriate high-frequency components leads to an oscillation at a sharp transition known as a ringing artifact. The artifact occurs near the sharp boundaries, where high contrast transitions in the object occur. It appears as multiple, regularly spaced parallel ripples of alternating bright and dark signal parallel to tissue interface (Fig. 1C). This artifact can be eliminated by increasing the phase-encodings or reducing the FOV.
- Aliasing or wrap around artifact occurs when the FOV is smaller than the area to be scanned. The region to be scanned lies outside the FOV but within the slice volume. The region outside the FOV is seen wrapped around on the opposite side. It can be caused by under sampling of the frequencies contained within the return signal. This can be generally seen in the end slices of the 3D acquisition (Fig. 1D). It can be corrected by increasing the FOV, but it decreases resolution. It can be also reduced by oversampling the data in the frequency direction (standard) and increasing phase steps in the phase-encoded direction–phase compensation (time or SNR penalty). Surface coil can be used so no signal is detected outside of FOV.
- Zebra artifacts or bands occur due to instabilities of magnetic field gradients due to overheated or overloaded gradient coils, they can produce loss of spatial resolution or even image ghosting in the phase-encoding direction. Eddy current compensation and active shielding of gradient coils are needed to prevent such artifacts.
- Noise artifacts occur when radiofrequencies from sources like television, radio interfere with the MRI scanner RF signal. It can produce graininess to the MR images. In such situations RF distortion will be seen in images. To counter this problem a RF shielding cage (Faraday cage) is constructed around the MRI scan room. The shielding material often used is copper or aluminum grids.
- Zipper artifacts can occur due to RF surface coils placed close to the patient. Artifacts appear

as "image shading" or in worst cases as "linear serrated images" resembling a zipper. Adjusting the RF surface coil and selecting a smaller FOV helps to minimize this artifact.

- *Center line artifact:* In this the artifact appear in the center in frequency encoding direction or parallel to the phase encoding direction. It occurs due to RF interference as the RF transmitter and receiver are placed close together. This type of artifacts can be eliminated by alternating the phase of the RF pulse and by isolating the receiver amplifier chain.
- Shading artifacts are seen as foci of relatively reduced signal intensity involving some part of the MR image. Some causes for this type of artifact are magnetic field inhomogenity and partial volume averaging. Malfunction of the RF transmitter, amplifier or receiver and excessive absorption of power can all lead to shading artifacts. Reducing the slice thickness and scanning in two planes (transversely and sagittally) helps to eliminate shading artifacts.
- *Crosstalk:* Most MRI scans are acquired as multiple two dimensional slices. From one slice to the next only the RF is changed. So, if the slices are placed too closely, the tail of one RF slice excitation can partially excite the neighboring slice. This effect can be minimized by interleaving the slice acquisitions, so that within this time the magnetization of the adjacent slice will recover towards equilibrium value so that only the slice that is excited by the RF gives the signals back to the receiver.

Partial volume averaging: Although the MR image appears to be two-dimensional, all the information within the slice is averaged and contributes to the final image. For instance a tumor that is only partially contained within a slice will appear to be different from the one that spans the slice. This phenomenon is called partial volume averaging and it gives the radiologist an incomplete picture of the lesion. Thus to avoid missing the lesion due to this phenomenon it is necessary to image the region of interest in more than one orientation (sagittal, coronal and axial planes).

MRI Contrast 10

Subodh Laul

INTRAVENOUS CONTRAST AGENTS

In magnetic resonance imaging (MRI), the most commonly used intravenous contrast agents are gadolinium chelates. The paramagnetic property of gadolinium provides contrast. It has the ability to alter the magnetic characteristics of neighboring tissues. The effect of this is shortening of the T1 and T2 relaxation times. Shortening of T1 effects are exploited since shortening of T1 relaxation time leads to an increase in signal intensity.

Gadolinium containing contrast agents available are gadodiamide (Omniscan), gadobenic acid (Multihance), gadopentetic acid (Magnevist), gadoteridol (Prohance), gadofosveset (Ablavar), gadoversetamide (OptiMARK), gadoxetic acid (Eovist or Primovist).

Other MRI contrast agents gaining recognition are superparamagnetic agents, i.e. iron oxide and manganese.

Two types of iron oxide contrast agents exist: (1) Superparamagnetic iron oxide (SPIO) and (2) Ultrasmall superparamagnetic iron oxide (USPIO). These contrast agents consist of suspended colloids of iron oxide nanoparticles and are injectables, they reduce the T2 signals of absorbing tissues. SPIO and USPIO contrast agents have been used successfully in some liver tumor enhancement. Available iron oxide contrast agents are cliavist, combidex, resovist and sinerem.

Manganese chelates such as Mn-DPDP enhance the T1 signal and have been used for the detection of liver lesions. It is absorbed intracellularly and excreted in bile.

In MRI oral contrast can be used for enhancement of the gastrointestinal tract. Gadolinium, manganese chelates and iron salts are used for T1 signal enhancement.

SPIO, barium sulfate, air and clay have been used to lower T2 signal. Blueberry and green tea having high manganese concentration can also be used for T1 increasing contrast enhancement.

Perflubron, a type of perfluorocarbon, has been used as a gastrointestinal MRI contrast agent for pediatric imaging.

This contrast agent works by reducing the amount of protons in a body cavity. Gadolinium initially disperses through the vascular system and then diffuses into the extracellular space, before moving into the intracellular space. Whilst still circulating within the vessels, magnetic resonance angiography (MRA) can be performed.

Gadolinium does not cross the intact blood-brain barrier but helps identifying intracranial lesions with interruption of the barrier, like infection and tumors. It helps to discriminate tumors from edema, low-grade from high-grade tumors, scar tissue from a tumor tissue.

Oral gadolinium is used to highlight loops of bowel to distinguish from surrounding soft tissue.

Superparamagnetic agents are more specific hepatic agents and are specially taken up by the Kupffer cells in the liver and help make a distinction between normal liver and malignant tissue.

MAGNETIC RESONANCE ANGIOGRAPHY

All pulse sequences are sensitive to flow. There is a complex relationship between the type and rate of flow and the resultant signal intensity. As a general rule, fast or turbulent vascular flow results in a signal dropout, whilst slow vascular flow results in high signal. There are two principal flowsensitive sequences, time of flight and phase contrast. Magnetic resonance angiography (MRA) can also be performed with intravenous gadolinium whilst in the vascular phase of enhancement.

Glossary of MRI Terms 11

Algorithm: Computer program which modifies the raw data to alter the characteristics of the final image.

Aliasing: Aliasing, or wrap-around, can occur whenever any part of the object to be imaged extends outside the imaging field of view (FOV). Anatomy that exists outside the FOV is mapped inside the FOV, on the opposite side of the image. Anatomy outside the FOV still produces a signal if it is in close proximity to the receiver coil.

Angular frequency: Frequency of oscillation or rotation represented by the Greek symbol omega (ω).

Artifact: An artifact is a feature appearing in an image that is not present in the original object. Depending on their origin, artifacts are typically classified as patient-related, signal processing dependent and hardware (machine) related.

Averaging: A method for improving the signal-to-noise ratio (SNR). The data lines in k-space are acquired multiple times by repeat acquisitions of the same phase encoding steps. The same MR signal is added up and the sum divided by the number of signals. The number of averages is also referred to as the number of excitations (NEX) or the number of signal acquisitions (NSA).

B_0: The symbol used for the static main magnetic field in the MR system measured in Tesla. The orientation of this field is along the z axis.

B_1: The symbol used to denote the radiofrequency (RF) magnetic field in an MR system measured in Tesla.

Bandwidth: Bandwidth is a frequency range of the receiver. MR system is tuned to receive the signal (receiver bandwidth) or the range of frequencies within an RF pulse delivered by the transmitter (transmitter bandwidth). Alteration in the receiver bandwidth affects the SNR, with narrowing of the bandwidth increasing SNR and vice versa.

Coil: Single or multiple loops of wire used to produce a magnetic field from current flowing through the wire or measure (receive) an induced voltage in the loop arising from a changing magnetic field.

Contiguous: Sections which are nominally immediately adjacent to each other.

Diamagnetic: A substance with magnetic susceptibility less than zero that interact weakly with a magnetic field causing repulsion of magnetic field lines.

Diffusion: A movement of water molecules through a tissue by a process known as Brownian motion. MR is a sensitive technique for measuring diffusion effects, e.g. in strokes, differentiating cysts from solid tumor and in CSF dynamic studies.

Echo: An increase in the signal intensity due to RF or gradient pulses.

Echo time: The time between the RF excitation and the midpoint of signal sampling.

Echo train: The number of echoes acquired during a single TR of a fast spin echo pulse sequence.

Echo planar imaging: An ultrahigh-speed imaging technique.

Echo spacing: The time between successive echoes in a fast spin echo pulse sequence.

Echo rephasing: The re-establishment of MR signal coherence which is achieved with either a 180° RF pulse or by gradient switching.

Eddy currents: Small electrical currents induced by the changing magnetic fields within the gradients coils or the structure of the magnet.

Entry slice phenomenon: Flow related enhancement due to the entry of unsaturated spins into the slice at the edge of the imaged volume.

Even echo rephasing: Signal due to flow that results at the even echoes of a multiecho acquisition where all TEs are multiples of the first TE.

Excitation: Application of an RF pulse to generate magnetization.

Fat/water suppression: A method that suppresses the signal within the imaging volume from either fat or water protons by application of a frequency-selective saturation RF Pulse.

Ferromagnetic: A substance, such as iron, cobalt or nickel, with extremely high magnetic susceptibility that retain magnetization even after being removed from an externally applied magnetic field.

Field of view (FOV): The dimensions of the sample that are represented in the image, as long as receiver bandwidth is sufficient to accurately measure all frequencies in the sample.

Fast imaging employing steady state acquisition (FIESTA): Sequence provides images of fluid filled structures with very short acquisition times. This sequence uses the T2 steady state contrast mechanism to provide high SNR images with strong signal from fluid tissues while suppressing background tissue for contrast and anatomic detail of small structures.

Fluid attenuated inversion recovery (FLAIR): A MR sequence used to suppress fluid.

Flip angle: The angle through which the magnetization vector moves, relative to the longitudinal axis of the static magnetic field, as a result of the application of an RF pulse. This variation in flip angle is used in gradient echo imaging to obtain the various tissue-weighted.

Flow-related enhancement: High signal arising from moving spins that are less saturated than stationary spin within the imaging slice between successive RF pulses.

Fourier transform: A mathematical process by which the frequency components of a signal are separated from its amplitudes as a function of time, and vice versa.

Fractional anisotropy: A measure of the homogeneity of diffusion direction within a voxel.

Free induction decay (FID): A transient signal that occurs as the transverse magnetization decays towards zero following application of an RF pulse.

Frequency encoding: Spatial localization by applying gradient magnetic field during signal sampling.

Functional MRI: An MRI technique for detecting localized brain activation in response to a stimulus by measuring changes in blood flow, volume, or oxygenation.

Gating: Timing of MRI acquisition to begin at a specific time during, for example, the cardiac or respiratory cycle.

Gauss (G): An old unit used for measuring magnetic field strength. The internationally accepted unit is the Tesla (1 Tesla = 10,000 Gauss). The earth's magnetic field is approximately 0.5 Gauss.

Gradient coils: These are magnetic coils designed to alter the main magnetic field by a few percent. The magnetic field gradient generated by a coil is controlled by the electrical current passed through the coil.

Gradient echo (GE/GRE): A basic pulse sequence which only uses magnetic field gradient reversal to rephase the transverse magnetization and produce echoes of the MR signal. This allows shorter repetition times thus faster scanning, and flip angles less than 90°.

Gradient induced dephasing: Signal loss due to motion (e.g. flow) along the direction of a gradient magnetic field, leading to phase accumulation and dephasing.

Gyromagnetic ratio: A constant that describes the behavior of a specific nucleus when exposed to a magnetic field.

High velocity signal loss: Low signal seen in blood vessels on a spin echo images due to the fact that spins travel so fast that they are not refocused by the slice selective 180° refocusing pulse and thus have low signal relative to refocused stationary spins.

Image acquisition time: This is the scanning time to produce a set of images from a measurement sequence.

Inhomogeneity: The slight variation in uniformity of the static magnetic field expressed in parts per million (ppm) as a fractional deviation from the average value of the field.

Inversion recovery (IR): A basic pulse sequence which inverts the magnetization and measures the recovery rate as the nuclei return to equilibrium.

Inversion time (TI): The time from the center of the first exitation pulse (180°) to the beginning of the second (90°) excitation pulse in an IR sequence.

K-space: The time domain MRI data prior to application of the Fourier transform. By manipulating K-space faster sequences can be implemented as in fast or slow imaging.

Laminar flow: Flow through a straight cylinder such that higher-velocity flow is present in the center and lower velocity flow at the periphery adjacent to walls of the cylinder.

Larmor frequency: The frequency of precession at a given magnetic field strength.

Longitudinal magnetization: The component of magnetization whose vector is parallel to the vector describing B_0.

Magnetic susceptibility: The degree to which a substance becomes magnetized when exposed to a magnetic field, generating its own magnetic field and thereby causing variation in the strength of the applied magnetic field.

Magic angle artifact: In joint imaging if a tendon is orientated at a certain angle (55°) to the static main magnetic field, the tendon appears brighter on T1- and proton density weighted images but normal low signal on T2-weighted images. This artifactual increase in signal within the tendon is termed the magic angle effect.

Magnetic moment: A measure of the strength of nuclear paramagnetism of an object or particle that cause it to align with the static main field and create its own local magnetic field.

Maximum intensity projection MRI: A technique used to generate 3D images of the vasculature from MRA images.

MR angiography: An MR pulse sequence sensitive to motion that is used to generate images of blood vessels.

MR hydrography: Modification to a fast spin echo pulse sequence with filling of the periphery of k-space before the center to create images showing contrast between fluid and all other tissue but having poor soft tissue contrast. The technique is used for urogaphy, myelography, and so forth.

Multiecho imaging: Acquisition of two separate lines of data after a single RF excitation. Each signal is acquired after an 180° RF pulse and is written to a separate k-space to generate two images, each with a unique TE.

Multislice imaging: Excitation of multiple slices during the TR of the first slice to improve efficiency.

Multivoxel spectroscopy: Acquisition of spectra from a grid of multiple adjacent locations during a single acquisition.

Nuclear magnetic resonance: The basic phenomenon describing the behavior of nuclei in an applied magnetic field and their response to application of RF energy.

NEX: Number of signal excitations repeated in a given acquisition. This is a way of increasing SNR at the expense of time.

Parallel imaging: Accelerating imaging by simultaneously acquiring signal from more than one receiver coil and deriving spatial information from the location and sensitivity of the coil.

Paramagnetic: Substances with a magnetic susceptibility greater than zero that interact with a magnetic field causing attraction of magnetic field lines.

PD: Proton density weighted sequence. Signal intensity depends on the number of protons in the tissue.

Phase contrast MRA: An MRA technique that exploits the predictable phase shifts that will occur with movement along a gradient magnetic field at a given velocity.

RF: Radiofrequency pulse. A packet of energy delivered to tissue during acquisition of MR signal.

Single voxel spectroscopy: Acquisition of a spectrum from a single volume of tissue.

Signal to noise ratio (SNR) is used in MRI to describe the relative contributions to a detected signal of the true signal and random superimposed signals, i.e. background noise considered as a criterion for image quality.

Spectroscopy is MR technique designed to measure the signal strength of specific subpopulations of spins based on their unique precessional frequencies (chemical shift).

Spin: The smallest unit from which the NMR signal can be derived.

Spin echo: An increase in signal that occurs after an 180° RF pulse.

STIR: Short tau inversion recovery. A MRI sequence used to suppress fat.

Superconducting magnet: A type of electromagnet that requires no ongoing input of electric current because the material used to make the magnet coils, if kept at a temperature close to absolute zero, conducts electricity without resistance.

Surface coil: A single loop of conductive material placed adjacent to the sample and used to record the MR signal.

T1 shine through: High signal due to very short T1, but not due to flow, that appears in a TOF-MRA image.

T1 weighted image: T1 weighted image is the one in which the intensity contrast between any two tissues in an image is mainly due to the T1 relaxation properties of the tissues.

T2 shine through: High signal due to very short T2, but not due to low ADC, that appears in a diffusion-weighted image.

T2 weighted image: T2 weighted image is the one in which the intensity contrast between any two tissues in an image is mainly due to T2 relaxation properties of the tissues.

TE: Time to echo. Time period between application of RF pulse and generation of echo in tissue.

TR: Time of repetition of RF pulse in acquisition of MR signal.

12 MRI Acronyms

3D MP Rage	3D magnetization prepared rapid acquisition gradient echo
CE-FAST	Contrast enhanced Fourier acquired steady-state technique
CFAST	CSF flow artifact suppression technique
Chem Sat	Chemical saturation
C+	Post-contrast study
CHESS	CHEmical shift selective sequence
CISS	Constructive interference in steady state
CNR	Contrast to noise ratio
COR	Coronal
CSFSE	Contiguous slice fast spin echo
CSI	Chemical shift imaging
CYCLOPS	CYCLically ordered phase sequence
DESS	Double echo steady state
EPI	Echo planar imaging
FASE	Fast advanced SE
FAST	Fourier acquired steady-state technique
FAT SAT	FAT SATuration
FFE	Fast field echo (Gradient echo sequence)
FFT	Fast Fourier transform
FGR	Fast gradient recalled
FIESTA	Fast imaging employing steady state acquisition
FISP	Fast imaging with steady precession
FLAIR	Fluid attenuated inversion recovery
FLASH	Fast low angle SHot
FOI	Field of interest
FOV	Field of view
FSE	Fast spin echo
FSPGR	Fast spoiled gradient recalled
GE	Gradient echo
GFE	Gradient field echo
GRASE	Gradient and spin echo
GRASS	Gradient recalled acquisition in steady state
GRE	Gradient recalled echo
HASE	High angle spin echo
HASTE	Half Fourier single shot turbo spin echo
ILS	Image localized spectroscopy
IR	Inversion recovery
LASE	Low angle spin echo
MAST	Motion artifact suppression technique
MEDIC	Multi echo data image combination
MEMP	Multi echo multi planar
MIP	Maximum intensity projection
MOTSA	Multiple overlapping thin slab acquisition
MPGR	Multi planar gradient recalled
MPRAGE	Magnetization prepared rapid-acquisition gradient echo
MR	Magnetic resonance
MRA	MR angiography
MRI	MR imaging
MRM	MR mammography
MRS	MR spectroscopy
MRSI	MR spectroscopy imaging
MSE	Modified spin echo
MSMP	Multi slice multi phase
MSOFT	Multi slice off-resonance fat suppression technique
MTC	Magnetization transfer contrast
MTS	Magnetization transfer suppression
NMR	Nuclear magnetic resonance

PCA	Phase contrast angiography
PD	Proton density
PRESS	Point resolved spectroscopy
RACE	Real-time acquisition and evaluation
RAGE	Rapid acquisition gradient echo
RARE	Rapid acquisitions with relaxation enhancement
RASE	Rapid acquisition spin echo
RFOV	Rectangular field of view
RISE	Rapid inversion spin echo
SAG	Sagittal
SAT	Saturation
SE	Spin echo sequence
SSFP	Steady state free precession
SHORT	SHORT repetition techniques
SNR	Signal to noise ratio
SPGR	Spoiled gradient recalled
SPIR	Spectral presaturation with inversion recovery
SSFP	Steady state free precession
SSMP	Single slice multi phase
STAGE	Small tip angle gradient echo
STEAM	STimulated echo acquisition mode
STIR	Short T1/Tau inversion recovery
T1	Longitudinal relaxation time (spin-lattice)
T2	Transverse relaxation time (spin-spin)
TE	Echo time
TI	Inversion time
TFE	Turbo field echo
TOF	Time-of-flight
TR	Repetition time
True IR	True inversion recovery
TSE	Turbo spin echo
UFGRASS	Ultra fast gradient recalled acquisition in steady state
UFGRE	Ultra fast gradient recalled echo

Index

Page numbers followed by *f* refer to figure

S

T

U

V

W

X

Z